D0596871

OXFORD MEDICAL PUBLICATIONS

Urological
Surgery

Published and forthcoming Oxford Specialist Handbooks

General Oxford Specialist Handbooks
A Resuscitation Room Guide (Banerjee and Hargreaves)

Oxford Specialist Handbooks in End of Life Care
Cardiology: From advanced disease to bereavement
(Beattie, Connelly, and Watson eds.)
Nephrology: From advanced disease to bereavement
(Brown, Chambers, and Eggeling)

Oxford Specialist Handbooks in Anaesthesia
Cardiac Anaesthesia (Barnard and Martin eds.)
Neuroanaesthesia (Nathanson and Moppett eds.)
Obstetric Anaesthesia (Clyburn, Collis, Harries, and Davies eds.)
Paediatric Anaesthesia (Doyle ed.)

Oxford Specialist Handbooks in Cardiology
Cardiac Catheterization and Coronary Angiography
(Mitchell, West, Leeson, and Banning)
Echocardiography (Leeson, Mitchell, and Becher eds.)
Heart Failure (Gardner, McDonagh, and Walker)
Nuclear Cardiology (Sabharwal, Loong, and Kelion)
Pacemakers and ICDs (Timperley, Leeson, Mitchell, and Betts eds.)

Oxford Specialist Handbooks in Neurology
Epilepsy (Alarcon, Nashaf, Cross, and Nightingale)
Parkinson's Disease and Movement Disorders
(Edwards, Bhatia, Quinn, and Swinn)

Oxford Specialist Handbooks in Paediatrics
Paediatric Gastroenterology, Hepatology, and Nutrition
(Beattie, Dhawan, and Puntis eds.)
Paediatric Nephrology (Rees, Webb, and Brogan)
Paediatric Neurology (Forsyth and Newton eds.)
Paediatric Oncology and Haematology (Bailey and Skinner eds.)
Paediatric Radiology (Johnson, Williams, and Foster)

Oxford Specialist Handbooks in Surgery
Cardiothoracic Surgery (Chikwe, Beddow, and Glenville)
Hand Surgery (Warwick)
Neurosurgery (Samandouras)
Operative Surgery (McLatchie and Leaper eds.)
Otolaryngology and Head and Neck Surgery (Warner and Corbridge)
Plastic and Reconstructive Surgery (Giele and Cassell eds.)
Renal Transplantation (Talbot)
Urological Surgery
(Reynard, Sullivan, Turner, Feneley, Armenakas, and Mark eds.)
Vascular Surgery (Hands, Murphy, Sharp, and Ray-Chaudhuri eds.)

Oxford Specialist Handbooks in Surgery
Urological Surgery

John Reynard
Consultant Urological Surgeon,
Churchill Hospital, Oxford, UK

Stephen Mark
Consultant Urological Surgeon,
Christchurch Hospital, New Zealand

Kevin Turner
Consultant Urological Surgeon,
Royal Bournemouth Hospital, UK

Noel Armenakas
Clinical Associate Professor, Cornell University
Weill Medical College, New York, USA

Mark Feneley
Senior Lecturer in Urology,
University College London, UK

Mark Sullivan
Consultant Urological Surgeon
The Churchill Hospital, Oxford, UK

OXFORD
UNIVERSITY PRESS

OXFORD
UNIVERSITY PRESS

Great Clarendon Street, Oxford OX2 6DP

Oxford University Press is a department of the University of Oxford.
It furthers the University's objective of excellence in research, scholarship,
and education by publishing worldwide in

Oxford New York

Auckland Cape Town Dar es Salaam Hong Kong Karachi
Kuala Lumpur Madrid Melbourne Mexico City Nairobi
New Delhi Shanghai Taipei Toronto

With offices in

Argentina Austria Brazil Chile Czech Republic France Greece
Guatemala Hungary Italy Japan Poland Portugal Singapore
South Korea Switzerland Thailand Turkey Ukraine Vietnam

Oxford is a registered trade mark of Oxford University Press
in the UK and in certain other countries

Published in the United States
by Oxford University Press Inc., New York

© Oxford University Press, 2008

The moral rights of the authors have been asserted

Database right Oxford University Press (maker)

First published 2008

British Library Cataloguing in Publication Data

Data available

Library of Congress Cataloging in Publication Data

Data available

Typeset by Newgen Imaging Systems (P) Ltd., Chennai, India
Printed in Italy
on acid-free paper by LegoPrint.

ISBN   978-0-19-929942-3

10 9 8 7 6 5 4 3 2 1

Preface

One of my great frustrations as a trainee surgeon was the absence of an operative surgical textbook that gave a 'cook book' type approach to descriptions of how to perform a particular operation. In their descriptions of operative technique, many books assumed a level of knowledge in the various steps of a procedure that I did not always have, and this required time consuming reference to other texts in order to 'dissect' out each relevant step. I therefore often found myself writing my own descriptions of the minutiae of operations with notes on the precise placement of stay stitches, or of retractor blades, or the precise gauge of suture material or drainage tube that should (or could) be used.

This book is borne out of those notes. It is specifically designed for the trainee surgeon and it provides, we hope, the level of detail that trainees need to know in order to be able to perform any given operation both competently and safely. The individual trainee may use it as an aid memoir in the coffee room between cases, but we hope also that it is detailed enough that for many it will serve as their main operative text.

Just as there are many ways to skin a cat, so there are many ways to perform an operation. Inevitably in a book written by 6 surgeons from different parts of the globe, there will be differences in operative approach and style. The reader will decide for themselves, as they 'mature' from trainee surgeon to trained surgeon, which approaches they like and which they don't. We hope this little book will prove to be a valuable starting point in this process.

I have been fortunate to have been able to work alongside my five colleagues, Mark Sullivan from Oxford, Noel Armenakas from New York, Stephen Mark from New Zealand, Mark Feneley from London and Kevin Turner latterly from Melbourne and now settled back in the UK in Bournemouth. Each has described the operative approach to procedures relevant to their area of specialist interest, areas in which each has a reputation for excellence in their own countries. When one writes a book one acts as a teacher, but in 'teaching' I have often learnt more than I have taught. Certainly in reading their contributions I have learnt much of great value. I thank each one for the many, many hours of labour that they have committed to the task.

Special thanks go to Anna Winstanley and Anita Petrie at OUP for all the hard work that they have put into the project during the writing and production phases. Producing the finished product from the many disparate pieces is their (tremendous) achievement.

Finally, I must thank my long suffering wife, Jane, and my three children, Sonya, Josh and Billy for the many hours that I should have spent with them, but did not.

John Reynard, Oxford 2008

Contents

Contributors

Noel Armenakas
Clinical Associate Professor,
Department of Urology,
Cornell University Weill
Medical College, New York,
USA, and Attending Urologic
Surgeon, Lenox Hill Hospital and
New York Presbyterian Hospital,
New York, USA.

Mark Feneley
Senior Lecturer in Urology,
University College London,
London, UK.

Stephen Mark
Consultant Urologic Surgeon
and Head of Department,
Department of Adult and
Paediatric Urology,
Christchurch Hospital,
New Zealand.

John Reynard
Consultant Urologic Surgeon,
Nuffield Department of Surgery,
The Churchill Hospital, Oxford, UK,
and Honorary Consultant Urologist,
The National Spinal Injuries Centre,
Stoke Mandeville Hospital, UK.

Mark Sullivan
Consultant Urologic Surgeon,
Department of Urology,
The Churchill Hospital, Oxford, UK,
and Honorary Senior Lecturer,
Oxford University, Oxford, UK.

Kevin Turner
Formerly Specialist Registrar in
Urology, East of Scotland Training
Programme in Urology,
Currently Consultant Urological
Surgeon, Royal Bournemouth
Hospital, Bournemouth, UK.

Detailed contents

3   **Bladder outlet obstruction**   **89**

Symbols and abbreviations

📖	cross reference
≥	greater than or equal to
~	Approximately
<	less than
>	greater than
≤	less than or equal to
5-FU	5-fluorouracil
AAOS	American Academy of Orthopaedic Surgeons
ABC	airway, breathing, circulation
ACCP	American College of Chest Physicians
ACE	angiotensin-converting enzyme
ACE	antegrade colonic enema
ACh	acetylcholine
ADPKD	autosomal dominant polycystic kidney disease
AFP	alpha fetoprotein
AIS	androgen insensitivity syndrome
AK-TEDs	above-knee thromboembolic stockings
APTT	activated partial thromboplastin time
ASAP	atypical small acinar proliferation
ASO	anti-streptolysin-O
ATP	adenosine triphosphate
AUA	American Urological Association
BCG	bacille Calmette–Guérin
bds	twice daily
BNI	bladder neck incision
BOO	bladder outlet obstruction
BP	blood pressure
BPH	benign prostate hypertrophy
BSE	bovine spongiform encephalopathy
BWS	Beckwith–Wiedemann syndrome
BXO	balanitis xerotica obliterans
CAH	congenital adrenal hyperplasia
cAMP	cyclic adenosine-3',5'-monophosphate
CAUTI	catheter-associated urinary tract infection
CCD	charge-coupled device
CCU	camera control unit
CFU	colony-forming unit
cGMP	cyclic guanosine-3',5'-monophosphate
CI	confidence interval
CIC	clean intermittent catheterization
CIRF	clinically insignificant residual fragment

CIS	carcinoma in situ
CJD	Creutzfeldt–Jakob disease
CMV	cisplatin, methotrexate, and vinblastine
CPA	cyproterone acetate
CT	computed tomography
CTPA	CT pulmonary angiogram
CTU	CT urography
CXR	chest X-ray
DESD	detrusor–external sphincter dyssynergia
DH	detrusor hyper-reflexia
DHT	dihydrotestosterone
DICC	dynamic infusion cavernosometry and cavernosography
DMSA	dimercaptosuccinic acid
DRE	digital rectal examination
DSD	detrusor–external sphincter dyssynergia,
	disorders of sexual development
DVC	dorsal vein complex
DVT	deep vein thrombosis
EAU	European Association of Urology
ECG	electrocardiogram
EHL	electrohydraulic lithotripsy
EMG	electromyography
ENT	ear, nose, and throat
ESWL	extra-corporeal shock-wave lithotripsy
FBC	full blood count
FEV1	forced expiratory volume in 1 sec
FSH	follicle-stimulating hormone
FVC	forced vital capacity
GA	gastric analysis,
	general anaesthesia
GCT	germ cell tumour
GFR	glomerular filtration rate
GI	gastrointestinal
Gy	gray
HbS	sickle haemoglobin
hCG	human chorionic gonadotrophin
HDR	high-dose-rate brachytherapy
HDU	high-dependency unit
HGF	hepatocyte growth factor
Ho:YAG	holmium:yttrium aluminium garnet
HoLAP	holmium laser ablation of the prostate
HoLEP	holmium laser enucleation of the prostate
HoLRP	holmium laser resection of the prostate
HPV	Human papilloma virus
HRP	horseradish peroxidase
HU	Hounsfield units
ICSI	intra-cytoplasmic sperm injection

IF	infundibular
IFB	infundibulopelvic
IIEF	International Index of Erectile Function
IL	interleukin
IM	intramuscular
INR	international normalized ratio
IPCs	intermittent pneumatic calf compression boots
IPSS	International Prostate Symptom Score
IRS	Intergroup Rhabdomyosarcoma Study
ISC	intermittent self-catheterization
ITGCN	intra-tubular germ cell neoplasia
ITU	intensive therapy unit
IV	intravenous
IVC	inferior vena cava
IVF	in vitro fertilization
IVU	intravenous urography
JVP	jugular venous pressure
K	potassium
KUB	kidneys–ureter–bladder
LDH	Lactate dehydrogenase
LDR	low-dose-rate brachytherapy
LDUH	low-dose unfractionated heparin
LFT	liver function tests
LH	luteinizing hormone
LHRH	luteinizing hormone-releasing hormone
LMWH	low molecular weight heparin
LSA	lichen sclerosus et atrophicus
LUT	lower urinary tract
LUTS	lower urinary tract symptoms
MAG3	mercaptoacetyl triglycine
MAOI	monoamine oxidase inhibitor
MAST	military antishock trousers
MCDK	multicystic dysplastic kidney
MCU	micturating cysto-urethrography
MCUG	micturating cysto-urethrogram
MESA	microsurgical epididymal sperm aspiration
MI	myocardial infarction
MIS	Müllerian inhibitory substance
MMC	mitomycin C
MRSA	methicillin-resistant Staphylococcus aureus
MS	multiple sclerosis
MVAC	methotrexate, vinblastine, adriamycin, and cisplatin
Na	sodium
NA	not available
NHS	UK National Health Service
NIH	National Institutes of Health
NO	nitric oxide

NSAID	non-steroidal anti-inflammatory drug
NSGCT	non-seminomatous germ cell tumour
PAG	peri-aqueductal grey matter
PCNL	percutaneous nephrolithotomy
PCO_2	partial pressure of carbon dioxide
PD	Parkinson's disease
PE	pulmonary embolism
PESA	percutaneous epididymal sperm aspiration
PIFS	pedicled island foreskin
PIN	penile intra-epithelial neoplasia,
PIN	prostatic intra-epithelial neoplasia
PIPS	pedicled island penile skin
PLAP	placental alkaline phosphatase
PMC	pontine micturition centre
po	by mouth
PO_2	partial pressure of oxygen
PR	pulse rate
PrP	prion protein
PSA	prostate-specific antigen
PTN	posterior tibial nerve
PTNS	posterior tibial nerve stimulation
PUJ	pelvi-ureteric junction
PUJO	pelvi-ureteric junction obstruction
PUV	posterior urethral valve
RBC	red blood cell
RCC	renal cell carcinoma
RMS	rhabdomyosarcoma
RPLND	retroperitoneal lymph node dissection
RR	respiratory rate
RT	radiotherapy
SARS	sacral anterior root stimulator
SCI	spinal cord injury
SI	sacro-iliac
SNS	sacral nerve stimulation
SPC	suprapubic catheter
SSRI	selective serotinin-reuptake inhibitor
STD	sexually transmitted disease
STDS	sodium tetradecylsulfate
TB	tuberculosis
TCC	transitional cell carcinoma
tds	three times daily
TESA	testicular sperm aspiration
TIP	tubularized incised plate
TRUS	transrectal ultrasonography
TUIP	transurethral incision of the prostate
TURBT	transurethral resection of bladder tumour
TURP	transurethral resection of prostate

TVT	tension-free vaginal tape
U&E	urea and electrolytes
UDT	undescended testis
US	ultrasound
UTI	urinary tract infection
vCJD	variant Creutzfeldt–Jakob disease
VCUG	voiding cysto-urethrogram
VQ	ventilation–perfusion
VTE	venous thromboembolism
VUJ	vesico-ureteric junction
VUR	vesico-ureteric reflux
WBC	white blood cell
WHO	World Health Organization
YAG	yttrium aluminium garnet

Chapter 1

General principles of urological surgery

Preparation of the patient for urological surgery

The degree of preparation is related to the complexity of the procedure. Certain aspects of examination (pulse rate, blood pressure) and certain tests (haemoglobin, electrolytes, creatinine) are important not only to assess fitness for surgery, but also as a baseline against which changes in the post-operative period can be measured.

- Assess cardiac status (angina, arrhythmias, previous MI, blood pressure, ECG, CXR).
- Assess respiratory function by pulmonary function tests (FVC, FEV_1) for all major surgery and any surgery where the patient has symptoms of respiratory problems or a history of chronic airways disease (e.g. asthma. Arrange an anaesthetic review where there is for example, cardiac or respiratory comorbidity.
- Culture urine, treat active (symptomatic) infection with an appropriate antibiotic starting a week before surgery, and give prophylactic antibiotics at the induction of anaesthesia.
- Stop aspirin and non-steroidal anti-inflammatory drugs (NSAIDs) 10 days prior to surgery.
- Measure haemoglobin and serum creatinine.
- Investigate and correct anaemia, electrolyte disturbance, and abnormal renal function.
- If blood loss is anticipated, group and save a sample of serum or cross-match several units of blood, the precise number depending on the speed with which your blood bank can deliver blood if needed. In our unit the policy is:
  - TURBT: group and save.
  - TURP: group and save.
  - Open prostatectomy: cross-match 2 units.
  - Simple nephrectomy: cross-match 2 units.
  - Radical nephrectomy: cross-match 4 units.
  - Cystectomy: cross-match 4 units.
  - Radical prostatectomy: cross-match 2 units.
  - PCNL: group and save.

Patients may choose to store their own blood prior to the procedure.

Bowel preparation

Indicated if large bowel is to be used for bladder reconstruction, for example. We use a simple mechanical preparation (Citramag® or Picolax® (magnesium salts)), two doses starting the morning before surgery, with clear fluid diet only.

Antibiotic prophylaxis in urological surgery

The precise antibiotic prophylaxis policy used will depend on local microbiological flora. The local microbiology department will provide regular advice and updates on which antibiotics should be used, both for prophylaxis and for treatment. The policy shown below and in Table 1.1 is our own local policy.

Culture urine before any procedure, and use specific prophylaxis (based on sensitivities) if culture is positive. We avoid ciprofloxacin in inpatients because it is secreted onto the skin and causes MRSA colonization. For most purposes, nitrofurantoin provides equivalent cover without being secreted onto the skin. We use ciprofloxacin if there is known *Proteus* infection (all *Proteus* species are resistant to nitrofurantoin).

Patients with artificial heart valves

Patients with heart murmurs and with prosthetic heart valves: IV amoxicillin 1 g with gentamicin 120 mg should be given at induction of anaesthesia, with an additional dose of oral amoxicillin 500 mg 6 hr later (substituting vancomycin 1 g for those who are penicillin allergic).

Patients with joint replacements

The advice is conflicting.

Joint advice of the American Academy of Orthopaedic Surgeons (AAOS) and the American Urological Association (AUA): antibiotic prophylaxis is not indicated for urological patients with pins, plates, or screws, or for most patients with total joint replacements. It is recommended for all patients undergoing urological procedures, including TURP *within 2 years of a prosthetic joint replacement*, for those who are immunocompromised (e.g. rheumatoid patients, those with systemic lupus erythematosus, drug-induced immunosuppression including steroids), and for those with a history of previous joint infection, haemophilia, HIV infection, diabetes, and malignancy. Antibiotic regime: single dose of a quinolone (e.g. ciprofloxacin 500 mg) 1–2 hr pre-operatively + ampicillin 2 g IV + gentamicin 1.5 mg/kg 30–60 min pre-operatively (substituting vancomycin 1 g IV for penicillin-allergic patients).

In the UK a Working Party of the British Society for Antimicrobial Chemotherapy has stated that patients with prosthetic joint implants (including total hip replacements) do not require antibiotic prophylaxis and consider that it is unacceptable to expose patients to the adverse effects of antibiotics when there is no evidence that such prophylaxis is of any benefit. This advice is based on the rationale that joint infections are caused by skin organisms that get onto the prosthesis at the time of the operation and that the role of bacteraemia as a cause of seeding outside the immediate post-operative period, has never been established.

We use the same antibiotic prophylaxis as for patients without joint prostheses.

Table 1.1 Specific antibiotic prophylaxis protocol for urological surgery

Procedure	Antibiotic prophylaxis
Catheter removal	Nitrofurantoin, 100 mg po 30 min before removal
Change of male long-term catheter	Gentamicin 1.5 mg/kg IM or IV 20 min before change*
Flexible cystoscopy or GA cystoscopy	Nitrofurantoin, 100 mg po 30–60 min before procedure
Transrectal prostatic biopsy	Ciprofloxacin 500 mg po and metronidazole 400 mg 20 min pre-biopsy and for 48 hr post-biopsy (ciprofloxacin 500 mg bds, metronidazole 400 mg tds)
ESWL	500 mg oral ciprofloxacin 30 min before treatment (nitrofurantoin does not cover *Proteus*, as common 'stone' bacterium)
PCNL	Augmentin 1.2 g IV tds starting the day before operation and three doses post-operatively. Gentamicin at induction
Ureteroscopy	Gentamicin 1.5 mg/kg IV at induction
Urogynaecological procedures (e.g. colposuspension)	Augmentin 1.2 g IV and metronidazole 500 mg IV at induction of anaesthesia
TURPs and TURBTs for both non-catheterized patients (i.e. elective TURP for LUTS) and patients with catheters (undergoing TURP for retention)	Nitrofurantoin 100 mg + gentamicin 1.5 mg/kg IV at induction. Nitrofurantoin 100 mg po 30 min before catheter removal
Radical prostatectomy	Augmentin 1.2 g IV + gentamicin 240 mg IV + metronidazole 500 mg IV at induction. Gentamicin 240 mg for 24 hr post-operatively. Cefuroxime 750 mg IV tds for 48 hr. Ciprofloxacin po for 5 days
Cystectomy or other procedures involving use of the bowel (e.g. augmentation cystoplasty)	Augmentin 1.2 g IV + metronidazole 500 mg IV at induction. Further two doses of augmentin 1.2 g IV and metronidazole 500 mg are given post-operatively
Artificial urinary sphincter insertion	Vancomycin 1 g 1.5 hr before leaving the ward (infuse over 100 min).† Augmentin 1.2 g IV + gentamicin 3 mg/kg IV at induction. Continue IV augmentin, gentamicin, and vancomycin (1 g bds) for 48 hr

* Sepsis rate (necessitating admission to hospital) may be as high as 1% without antibiotic cover.
† OR teicoplanin if vancomycin allergic: 400 mg at induction and bds thereafter for a total of 48 hr. Meropenem may be substituted for vancomycin in 'vancomycin-free hospitals'.

Additional reading

1 Hargreave TB, Botto B, Rikken GHJM, *et al. Eur Urol* 1993; **23**:437–43.
2 *British National Formulary*. BMA and Royal Pharmaceutical Society, London (2003). ISBN 0-85369-56-3.
3 AAOS and AUA. Advisory statement. *J Urol* 2003; **169**:1796.

Complications of surgery in general: DVT and PE

Venous thromboembolism (VTE) is uncommon after urological surgery, but it is considered the most important non-surgical complication of major urological procedures. Following TURP, 0.1–0.2% of patients experience a pulmonary embolus[1] and 1–5% of patients undergoing major urologic surgery experience symptomatic VTE.[2] The mortality of PE is of the order of 1%.[3]

Risk factors for DVT and PE

Increased risk: open (versus endoscopic) procedures, malignancy, increasing age, duration of procedure.

Categorization of VTE risk

American College of Chest Physicians guidelines on prevention of venous thromboembolism[1] and British Thromboembolic Risk Factors (THRIFT) Consensus Group[2] categorize the risk of VTE.

- Low risk patients: those aged <40 years undergoing minor surgery (surgery lasting <30 min) and no additional risk factors. No specific measures to prevent DVT are required in such patients other than early mobilization.
- Increasing age and duration of surgery increases risk of VTE.
- High-risk patients include those undergoing non-major surgery (surgery lasting >30 min) aged >60 years.

Prevention of DVT and PE

See box opposite.

Diagnosis of DVT

Signs of DVT are non-specific, e.g. cellulitis and DVT share common signs (low-grade fever, calf swelling, and tenderness). If you suspect a DVT arrange a Doppler ultrasound. If the ultrasound probe can compress the popliteal and femoral veins, there is no DVT; if it cannot, there is a DVT.

Diagnosis of PE[8-10]

- Small PEs may be asymptomatic.
- Symptoms include breathlessness, pleuritic chest pain, haemoptysis.
- Signs: tachycardia, tachypnoea, raised JVP, hypotension, pleural rub, pleural effusion.

Options for prevention of VTE

- Early mobilization
- Above knee thromboembolic stockings (AK-TEDs) provide graduated static compression of the calves, thereby reducing venous stasis. More effective than below knee TEDS for DVT prevention.[5]
- Subcutaneous heparin (LDUH or LMWH). In unfractionated preparations heparin molecules are polymerized (molecular weight 5000–30 000 Da). LMWH is depolymerized (molecular weight 4000–5000 Da).
- Intermittent pneumatic calf compression boots (IPCs), which are placed around the calves, are intermittently inflated and deflated, thereby increasing the flow of blood in calf veins.[6]

For patients undergoing major urological surgery (radical prostatectomy, cystectomy, nephrectomy), AK-TEDS with IPC intra-operatively, followed by SC heparin (LDUH or LMWH) should be used. For TURP, many urologists use a combination of AK-TEDS and IPCs; relatively few use SC heparin.[7]

Tests
- CXR: may be normal or show linear atelectasis, dilated pulmonary artery, oligaemia of affected segment, small pleural effusion.
- ECG: may be normal or show tachycardia, right bundle branch block, inverted T waves in V1–V4 (evidence of right ventricular strain). The 'classic' S1, QIII, TIII pattern is rare.
- Arterial blood gases: low PO_2 and low PCO_2.
- Imaging: CT pulmonary angiogram (CTPA) has superior specificity and sensitivity compared with ventilation–perfusion (VQ) radio-isotope scan.
- Spiral computed tomography: a negative CTPA rules out a PE with similar accuracy to a normal isotope lung scan or a negative pulmonary angiogram.

Treatment of established DVT

- Below knee DVT: AK-TEDs; if no peripheral arterial disease (enquire about claudication and check pulses) unfractionated heparin 5000 units SC every 12 hr.
- Above knee DVT: start LMWH and warfarin; stop LMWH when INR is between 2 and 3. Continue treatment for 6 weeks for post-surgical patient, lifelong if underlying cause (e.g. malignancy).

Treatment of established PE

Fixed-dose subcutaneous LMWH seems to be as effective as adjusted-dose intravenous unfractionated heparin for the treatment of PE found in conjunction with a symptomatic DVT.[3] Rates of haemorrhage are similar with both forms of heparin treatment. Start warfarin at the same time and stop heparin when INR is 2–3. Continue warfarin for 3 months.

References

1 Donat R, Mancey-Jones B. Incidence of thromboembolism after transurethral resection of the prostate (TURP). *Scan J Urol Nephrol* 2002; **36**:119–23.

2 Geerts WH, Heit JA, Clagett PG et al. Prevention of venous thromboembolism (American College of Chest Physicians (ACCP) Guidelines on prevention of venous thromboembolism) *Chest* 2001; **119**:132S–75S.

3 Quinlan DJ, McQuillan A, Eikelboom JW. Low molecular weight heparin compared with intravenous unfractionated heparin for treatment of pulmonary embolism. *Ann Intern Med* 2004; **140**:175–83.

4 Lowe GDO, Greer IA, Cooke TG et al. Risk of and prophylaxis for venous thromboembolism in hospital patients. Thromboembolic Risk Factors (THRIFT) Consensus Group. *BMJ* 1992; **305**:567–74.

5 Howard A et al. Randomized clinical trial of low molecular weight heparin with thigh-length or knee-length antiembolism stockings for patients undergoing surgery. *Br J Surg* 2004; **91**:842–7.

6 Soderdahl DW, Henderson SR, Hansberry KL. A comparison of intermittent pneumatic compression of the calf and whole leg in preventing deep venous thrombosis in urological surgery. *J Urol* 1997; **157**:1774–6.

7 Golash A, Collins PW, Kynaston HG, Jenkins BJ. Venous thromboembolic prophylaxis for transurethral prostatectomy: practice among British urologists. *J R Soc Med* 2002; **95**:130–1.

8 British Thoracic Society Guidelines for management of suspected acute pulmonary embolism. *Thorax* 2003; **58**:1–14.

9 Kruip MJH, Slob MJ, Schijen JH et al. Use of a clinical decision rule in combination with D-dimer concentration in diagnostic workup of patients with suspected pulmonary embolism. *Arch Intern Med* 2002; **162**:1631–5.

10 Kelly J, Rudd A, Lewis RR, Hunt BJ. Plasma D-dimers in the diagnosis of venous thromboembolism. *Arch Intern Med* 2002; **162**:747–56.

Fluid balance and the management of shock in the surgical patient

Daily fluid requirement

Can be calculated according to patient weight:
- For the first 10 kg: 100 mL/kg/24 hr (= 1000 mL).
- For the next 10 kg (i.e. from 10 to 20 kg): 50 mL/kg/24 hr (= 500 mL).
- For every kilogram above 20 kg: 20 mL/kg/24 hr (= 1000 mL for a patient weighing 70 kg).

Thus, every 24 hr a 70 kg adult will require 1000 mL for their first 10 kg of weight plus 500 mL for their next 10 kg of weight plus 1000 mL for their last 50 kg of weight, giving a total 24 hr fluid requirement of 2500 mL.

The daily sodium and potassium requirements are ~100 mmol and ~70 mmol, respectively. Thus, a standard 24 hr fluid regimen is 2 L of 5% dextrose + 1 L of normal saline (equivalent to ~150 mmol Na), with 20 mmol K for every litre of infused fluid.

Fluid losses from drains or nasogastric aspirate are similar in composition to plasma and should be replaced principally with normal saline.

Shock due to blood loss

Inadequate organ perfusion and tissue oxygenation. The causes are hypovolaemic, cardiogenic, septic, anaphylactic, and neurogenic. The most common cause in the surgical patient is hypovolaemia due to loss of blood and other fluids. Haemorrhage is an acute loss of circulating blood volume.

Haemorrhagic shock can be classified as follows:
- Class I: up to 750 mL blood loss (15% of blood volume), normal pulse rate (PR), respiratory rate (RR), blood pressure, urine output, and mental status.
- Class II: 750–1500 mL blood loss (15–30% of blood volume), PR >100, decreased pulse pressure due to increased diastolic pressure, RR 20–30, urinary output 20–30 mL/hr.
- Class III: 1500–2000 mL blood loss (30–40% of blood volume), PR >120, decreased blood pressure and pulse pressure due to decreased systolic pressure, RR 30–40, urine output 5–15 mL/hr, confusion.
- Class IV: >2000 mL blood loss (>40% of blood volume), PR >140, decreased pulse pressure and blood pressure, RR >35, urine output <5 mL/hr, cold clammy skin.

Management
- Remember ABC; 100% oxygen to improve tissue oxygentation.
- ECG, cardiac monitor, pulse oximetry.
- Insert two short wide intravenous cannulae (e.g. 16G) in the antecubital fossa; a central venous line may be required.
- Infuse 1 L of warm Hartmann's solution, or if severe haemorrhage start a colloid instead (e.g. gelofusin). Aim for a urinary output of 0.5 mL/kg/hr and maintenance of blood pressure.
- Check FBC, coagulation screen, U&Es, and cardiac enzymes.
- Cross-match 6 units of blood.
- Arterial blood gases to assess oxygenation and pH.

Obvious and excessive blood loss may be seen from drains, but drains can block. Therefore assume that there is covert bleeding if there is tachycardia (and low blood pressure). If this regimen fails to stabilize pulse and blood pressure, return the patient to the operating room for exploration.

Reference
1 American College of Surgeons Committee on Trauma. *Advanced trauma life support for doctors—student course manual.* 6th edn., 1999.

Chapter 2

Basic urological surgical skills and equipment

Cystoscopy

Indications

Diagnostic

- Haematuria (specifically looking for macroscopic evidence of bladder cancer).
- Suspected carcinoma in patients with marked 'storage' lower urinary tract symptoms (frequency, urgency, suprapubic pain).

Therapeutic

- Cystodiathermy or laser ablation of small bladder tumours.
- Intravesical injection of therapeutic agents (e.g. botulinum toxin for bladder overactivity).
- Access to the upper tract for retrograde ureterography, ureteroscopy, JJ stent insertion, or ureteric catheter insertion prior to PCNL.

Rigid versus flexible cystoscopy

Flexible cystoscopy has a number of advantages. It can be done using only local anaesthesia (or just lubricating gel[1,2]) on a supine patient. The combination of rotation of the cystoscope and deflection of the tip allows inspection of parts of the bladder inaccessible to a rigid cystoscope, even when using a 70° rigid cystoscope. Rigid cystoscopy gives better views (superior optics and faster irrigant flow) and allows passage of more and larger accessory instruments (larger working channel). For these reasons, choose rigid cystoscopy when haematuria is heavy or when the bladder needs a washout: the views and irrigation channel of the flexible cystoscope are inadequate in this situation. Rigid cystoscopy is also indicated when you know that you need to do more than just look (e.g. take a biopsy, diathermy a small TCC, pass a ureteric catheter). If necessary and with practice cystodiathermy and laser ablation of tumours and ureteric catheterization can be done with a flexible cystoscope (see below), but they are technically easier with the rigid cystoscope.

References

1 Kobayashi T, Nishizawa K, Mitsumori K, Ogura K. Instillation of anesthetic gel is no longer necessary in the era of flexible cystoscopy: a crossover study. *J Endourol* 2004; **18**:483–6.
2 Chen YT, Hsiao PJ, Wong WY, Wang CC, Yang SS, Hsieh CH. Randomized double-blind comparison of lidocaine gel and plain lubricating gel in relieving pain during flexible cystoscopy. *J Endourol* 2005; **19**:163–6.

Cystoscopy (rigid)

Equipment

Rigid cystoscopes consist of an outer sheath (through which irrigant fluid flows), a 'telescope', a light source, and a camera which is mounted on the 'eyepiece' of the telescope allowing video monitoring (Fig. 2.1).

The sheath is made of steel and may have an insulated tip made of plastic or ceramic to allow safe use in electroresection. An insulated tip is only needed if an electrode may come into contact with the end of the sheath (e.g. in TURP/TURBT), and not when using an insulated wire electrode for cystodiathermy. Continuous flow sheaths allow simultaneous inflow and outflow of fluid. They are useful during TURP and TURBT to prevent over-distension of the bladder and to keep the view clear.

Light sources are fibre-optic and attach to the cystoscope by a flexible cable. They transmit light along fine glass fibres by total internal reflection (each glass fibre is coated with glass of a different refractive index so that light entering at one end is totally internally reflected and emerges at the other). Although they are flexible, the glass fibres can break (with consequent impairment of light transmission). Handle the cables carefully, avoid bending them acutely, and have spares to hand. The intensity of the light source can be varied. Maximum output is not always best; too high an output can cause glare from the surface of the urothelium, obscuring the view. Check with the manufacturer of your system as to how the camera and light source should best be set up.

All modern rigid telescopes use a rod lens system invented by Harold Hopkins. In this system the light is transmitted along glass rods with air gaps between them which function as lenses. This system allows much more efficient transmission of light than glass lenses and simplifies manufacture (small lenses are much more difficult to manufacture than rod lenses). The image obtained with a cystoscope depends upon the angle of view (varied by a prism behind the objective telescope) which ranges from 0° to 120°.

The telescope is passed through a 'bridge' which connects the telescope to the sheath. Biopsy forceps have their own integral bridge. The bridge allows simultaneous passage of other instruments (e.g. guidewires) via a catheterizing channel and may have a deflecting mechanism (an Albarran bridge) (Fig. 2.2b). Obturators are passed within the outer sheath to facilitate passage of the sheath in to the bladder. Most surgeons tend to use a visual rather than a blind obturator, to allow safer instrumentation of the urethra (Fig. 2.2c). Sheaths range in size from 8Fr to 27Fr. A 21Fr or 22Fr would be typical for diagnostic cystoscopy for an adult and 24–27Fr for transurethral resection.

A 0° cystoscope is used for urethroscopy. Most surgeons use a 30° cystoscope for examining the bladder and employ abdominal pressure on the anterior abdominal wall of the deflated bladder to demonstrate the anterior recesses of the bladder at the bladder neck.

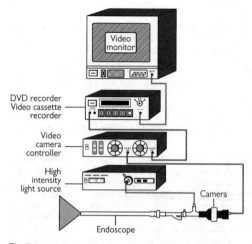

Fig. 2.1 A typical cystoscopic set-up.

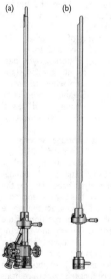

Fig. 2.2 (a) An Albarran bridge used, for example, for deflecting guidewires and ureteric catheters to allow easier access to the ureteric orifice. (b) A visual obturator. Reproduced with permission of Karl Storz Endoscope.

Preparation

Ensure that the urine is sterile or that appropriate antibiotics have been administered (we administer prophylaxis for all patients, even those with sterile urine). We use oral antibiotic prophylaxis (nitrofurantoin 100 mg) in patients undergoing simple (diagnostic) cystourethroscopy (we treat infection with antibiotics for a few days where we have evidence of infection pre-cystoscopy, using a culture-determined appropriate antibiotic). For high-risk patients, including those who are immunosuppressed, those who have prosthetic heart valves, or with a history of urosepsis, we add gentamicin 120 mg IV and amoxicillin 500 mg). Position the patient in a low lithotomy position with the perineum perpendicular to the operating table.

Technique

Assemble the cystoscope and turn on the camera and light source. The camera should be white balanced so that the colour of the image is true to life. Hold the tip of the telescope close to, but not right up against, a white surface (e.g. a gauze swab) and press the white balance button on the camera head or video system. Check and adjust the camera focus. As in all endoscopy, never use force, follow the lumen, and if you lose the lumen withdraw the instrument until you find it again. If your chosen instrument will not pass, choose a smaller one, dilate the urethra, or perform an Otis urethrotomy. Hold the penis vertically on a gentle stretch with your left hand. Inject 10 mL of anaesthetic gel along the urethra. Pick up the cystoscope with your right hand and hold it vertically. Turn on the irrigation. Pass the cystoscope along the urethra whilst viewing the monitor. Visualize the penile and bulbar urethra. The external sphincter is recognized as a narrowing of the lumen with mucosal folding. As you reach the sphincter, advance and lower the instrument simultaneously so that it is parallel to the floor as you pass through the sphincter and over the verumontanum into the prostate. Further depression of the cystoscope may be needed when advancing through the prostate and bladder neck. Observe (and subsequently record) the size of the lobes of the prostate and the patency and 'height' of the bladder neck (a 'high' bladder neck provides supplementary* evidence of possible bladder neck obstruction).

Once in the bladder, remove the telescope and bridge, leaving the sheath *in situ*. Empty the bladder, record the volume drained (NB this is not necessarily a true reflection of residual volume, which strictly speaking is the volume of urine left in the bladder post-micturition) and consider sending urine for bacteriological or cytological analysis depending on the clinical situation. Start by inspecting the mucosa of the trigone and note the positions and features of the ureteric orifices. Then inspect the whole bladder systematically. This is done by a combination of rotation of the cystoscope and moving it in and out of the bladder. The way in which the bladder is inspected is not important; completeness is. Imagine the bladder as a sphere divided into segments. Our preference is to inspect the central strip (from trigone to dome to bladder neck) and then to inspect the lateral walls. As the cystoscope is rotated, ensure that the camera remains vertical or orientation will be lost. Pressure with your left hand on the

* Supplementary to video-urodynamics

anterior abdominal wall will bring the anterior wall of the bladder in to view. A 30° telescope is adequate for many patients; for others you may need to switch to a 70° telescope to visualize the area around the bladder neck. Keep the irrigation fluid running until the bladder is sufficiently distended to visualize the entire mucosa. If the bladder is overfilled, some parts (especially the anterior wall) may be hard to reach. Record mucosal abnormalities (tumours, cystitis) and the presence of trabeculation, diverticulae, and stones.

Upon completion of the cystoscopy, leave the bladder full or partially full if you intend to pass a catheter at the end of the procedure (when you pass the catheter you will be sure that you are in the bladder when fluid drains); otherwise empty the bladder by removing the telescope and bridge and allowing the bladder to drain via the sheath. When withdrawing the sheath, reverse the angulation that was used on insertion (i.e. initially raise your hands to allow the sheath to run down the slope of the prostatic urethra). This minimizes trauma to the urethra.

Useful aside

The end of the light cable can become very hot. Do not set it down on the drapes for more than a few seconds before the light source is switched to standby. If the light appears poor, you can make a rough assessment of the integrity of the light cable by disconnecting it and holding the end ~15 cm from a dark drape. Broken fibres show up as dark patches in an otherwise bright circular field. If there are many broken fibres, change the cable. Never look directly at the light source (you can damage your eye) and take care not to shine the light at theatre staff when disconnecting the cable.

Flexible cystourethroscopy

Equipment

Flexible cystoscopes use fine glass fibres to transmit light. For transmission of the image the orientation of the fibres at each end of the cystoscope must be the same (coordinated). Like light leads, flexible cystoscopes can be damaged by rough handling. Flexible cystoscopes are typically 17Fr. A light source and irrigant fluid are connected to the handpiece. With most flexible cystoscopes the surgeon looks directly into the eyepiece since use of a camera system often complicates orientation. Some modern video flexible cystoscopes incorporate a camera in the handpiece and use video monitoring. The tip can be deflected up to 220° using a thumb lever. There is a working channel which allows passage of instruments (guidewires, biopsy forceps). Some flexible cystoscopes can be used with a diathermy electrode (or laser fibre) for fulguration of small bladder tumours. Check with the manufacturer of the cystoscope.

Technique

The patient lies supine (male) or in the frog-leg position (female). Prepare, drape, and instill lidocaine gel (or simple lubricant gel) as you would for a catheterization. Hold the penis vertically using the fourth and fifth fingers of the left hand (palm facing up) and guide the tip of the scope into the meatus using the thumb and index finger. Start irrigation. When you reach the sphincter ask the patient to try to void; this helps to open the sphincter and reduces discomfort. Make only a cursory examination of the urethra, prostate, and bladder neck on the way in; these areas are better viewed on withdrawal of the telescope. Inspect the bladder in systematic fashion. Many cystoscopes deflect more in one direction than the other. If this is the case, rotation through 180° helps to bring all areas in to view. To inspect the bladder neck, perform a 'J manoeuvre'. This is done by fully deflecting the scope and advancing it towards the dome of the bladder (Fig. 2.3). Gently withdraw the scope under vision.

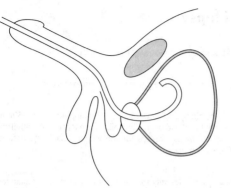

Fig. 2.3 The 'J manoeuvre' in flexible cystoscopy for inspecting the region of the bladder neck.

Bladder biopsy

Indication
For the diagnosis of mucosal abnormalities.

Preparation
As for cystoscopy. Ensure that the patient is not anticoagulated.

Equipment
Biopsy forceps passed along a rigid cystoscope allow biopsies of size ~5 mm. Most forceps are 'cold cup', although some allow connection of diathermy ('hot forceps'). Flexible biopsy forceps for use with a flexible cystoscope take biopsies of size 1–2 mm.

Technique
Perform a cystoscopy and identify the intended biopsy site. The bladder should be partially distended but not full (the wall of the full bladder is thinner than that of the partially full one, and is therefore more prone to perforation). Pass the biopsy forceps, open the jaws, and push gently against the mucosa. Close the jaws firmly, and partially withdraw the forceps smartly to take the biopsy. If using hot forceps, touch the biopsy site with the closed forceps and apply diathermy until haemostasis is secured. If using cold forceps, withdraw the forceps completely and pass a wire electrode along the bridge. Identify the biopsy site, bring the electrode into contact with the mucosa, and apply diathermy. Diathermy is not usually necessary when taking biopsies with the flexible cystoscope since the biopsies are small.

Useful aside
- Make a mental note of exactly where you have taken the biopsy from. If the site bleeds briskly, the view may be impaired by the time you pass the diathermy electrode and only your mental 'image' will guide you back to the biopsy site.
- If the biopsies are combined with another procedure (e.g. cystodistension), take the biopsies at the end. Avoid distending a bladder that has just been biopsied: The risk of perforation is increased.
- Take particular care when taking a biopsy from a scarred area of the bladder (previous biopsy or resection site): The bladder may have a very thin wall here.

Drains and catheters in urological surgery

Drains

Indications

Drains are placed to prevent the accumulation of fluid (blood, urine, serum, lymph) and thereby reduce the risk of such fluid acting as a focus for infection and abscess formation. Consider the indication for a drain carefully and weigh up the risks and benefits. Placing a drain theoretically increases the risk of bacterial colonization of the wound or surgical site. Traditional teaching holds that a drain should be placed whenever the urinary tract has been opened, since the closure will never be truly watertight and urine will tend to leak from the closure, causing the development of a urinoma. When placing a drain, try to avoid the tip of the drain coming into direct contact with an anastomosis or operation site. The presence of a drain may enhance drainage if the drain itself is irritating the surgical site. Use a tube drain (non-suction) (Fig. 2.4) rather than a suction drain (Fig. 2.5) adjacent to an anastomosis, as a suction drain will tend to promote leakage of fluid through the wound closure and prevent healing of the anastomosis.

There is little evidence regarding the optimal time for drain removal. In most situations an abdominal drain can be removed safely when it is draining less than 50 mL in 24 hr. If drainage is persistent, many surgeons feel that it is worthwhile 'shortening' the drain (i.e. pull out a few centimetres and re-secure it with a stitch or adhesive dressing) in order to reduce the drainage. If there is concern that the drain fluid is urine, then comparison of the creatinine concentration in that fluid with that in a serum and urine sample may be helpful (check that the units are the same). Non-suction drains rely on the pressure in the abdomen or wound to promote drainage. Such drains are appropriate for most urological operations. Suction drains are more useful in superficial operations such as inguinal lymphadenectomy or to prevent accumulation of lymph in the superficial tissues of a wound in an obese patient. Bring drains out through a separate stab incision to reduce the chance of contamination of the main wound.

Useful aside

If a drain tube needs to be cut shorter at the time of insertion, always cut the drain between rather than across drainage holes. When a drain is difficult to remove there can be concern that it has snapped and a fragment has been retained. Drains tend to break across drain holes (the weakest point). If a drain has been cut across drain holes it can be harder to differentiate a snapped drain from one which was deliberately shortened. If in doubt that a fragment of drain has been retained, request an X-ray; the drain has a radio-opaque marker strip which allows it to be identified radiographically.

(a)

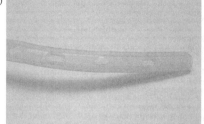

Fig. 2.4 A Robinson's tube drain. Detail of the tip of the drain showing the eye-holes. Reproduced with permission from Reynard et al., *Oxford Handbook of Urology*, 2006, Oxford University Press.

(a)   (b)

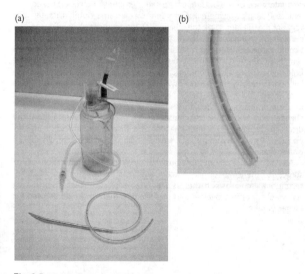

Fig. 2.5 (a) A Redivac suction drain showing the drain tubing attached to the needle used for insertion and the suction bottle. (b) The eye holes at the tip of the suction drain. Reproduced with permission from Reynard et al., *Oxford Handbook of Urology*, 2006, Oxford University Press.

Catheters

Indications

- Relief of urinary retention.
- Irrigation of the bladder when there is haematuria (e.g. after TURP/ TURBT) to prevent clot retention.
- Drainage of the bladder when it has been opened (traumatic or deliberate).
- To keep the bladder empty (peri-operatively during pelvic surgery, chronically in neurogenic detrusor overactivity).
- To allow precise measurement of urine output.
- For administration of intravesical therapy.
- For investigations (urodynamics, cystography).

Equipment

Catheters are sized on the Charriére French (Fr) scale which is the circumference of the outside of the catheter in millimetres (1Fr is equivalent to 0.33 mm diameter). Catheters of the same outer diameter may vary in the diameter of the channel(s) inside them depending on the number of channels and the material from which the catheter is made. Simple catheters (without a retaining mechanism) are used for intermittent self-catheterization (ISC), but most indwelling catheters are of the Foley type (named after Frederic Foley) and are retained by an inflatable balloon (5–50 mL) (Fig. 2.6). 'Two-way catheters' (a misnomer for there is only one drainage channel) have one channel for balloon inflation and one for drainage or instillation. 'Three-way catheters' have an inflation channel and two other channels allowing simultaneous instillation and drainage (Fig. 2.7). The inlet channel of a three-way catheter is usually positioned obliquely and is of a smaller calibre than the centrally placed outlet channel.

Always enquire about previous pathology of, instrumentation of, or surgery to the lower urinary tract. Consider the likely duration of catheterization. Simple latex catheters are suitable for short-term use (up to a few weeks) but hydrogel-coated or silicone catheters should be used for longer durations (up to 3 months before changing).

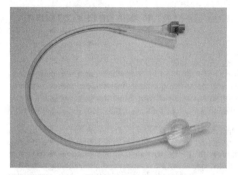

Fig. 2.6 A Foley self-retaining balloon catheter. Reproduced with permission from Reynard et al., *Oxford Handbook of Urology*, 2006, Oxford University Press.

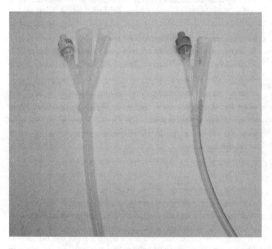

Fig. 2.7 Two- and three-way catheters. Reproduced with permission from Reynard et al., *Oxford Handbook of Urology*, 2006, Oxford University Press.

Technique of urethral catheterization

Male catheterization

Prepare the urethral meatus and cover the patient with a fenestrated drape. Inject 10 mL of lubricant (e.g. KY Jelly or lidocaine jelly) into the urethra (there is no absolute need for anaesthesia, as lubricant gels containing no anaesthetic provide equivalent analgesia to those containing anaesthetic[1,2]). Start with a 14Fr catheter. Hold the penis vertically with a gentle stretch and advance the catheter. Never use force. Continuous gentle pressure may be needed to overcome resistance from the sphincter or prostate. Insert the catheter to the hilt. Never inflate the balloon until you are sure that the catheter is in the bladder (urine drains). If drainage is not prompt, gentle suction on the catheter with a syringe may dislodge anaesthetic jelly from the lumen and allow drainage. Replace the foreskin to prevent paraphimosis. If catheterization is unsuccessful, try to decide at what level obstruction exists (e.g. penile urethra, bulb, prostate, bladder neck). A single attempt with a 12Fr catheter (e.g. if previous urethral stricture) may be successful. If unsuccessful after two attempts, STOP. Consider suprapubic catheterization or direct visualization with a flexible cystoscope.

Flexible cystoscopy assisted catheterization

Perform a flexible cystoscopy. Try to ascertain why the catheterization has been difficult (stricture, false passage, irregular prostatic fossa). Enter the bladder with the cystoscope. Pass a guidewire along the cystoscope until you see the wire in the bladder. Remove the cystoscope, advancing the wire as you do so. As the cystoscope emerges from the meatus, grasp the wire to prevent further displacement. Either attempt passage of a catheter alongside the wire (the wire will often direct it into the bladder) or cut a few millimetres off the end of the catheter (do not damage the balloon as you do so) and slide it over the wire into the bladder. Remove the wire and ensure urine drainage before inflating the balloon.

Using an introducer

Catheter introducers are metal instruments used to negotiate the natural angle of the male urethra (30° upward slope from veru montanum to bladder neck). There are two main types of introducers.

- Wire introducers pass down the lumen of the catheter and can be bent to the required shape (Fig. 2.8).
- Gutter type (e.g. Merryfield) introducers are more rigid; the catheter is mounted alongside the introducer lying within a gutter (Fig. 2.9).

Many urologists use introducers routinely on completion of a TURP where the posterior wall of the prostatic cavity may be thin or where there has been undermining of the bladder neck. An introducer guides the catheter tip anteriorly, thereby avoiding the potential hazard of running the catheter beneath the bladder neck. Introducers are also useful when passing a catheter in a man who has had previous bladder outlet surgery. Do not use an introducer unsupervised until you are confident. They can do a great deal of damage.

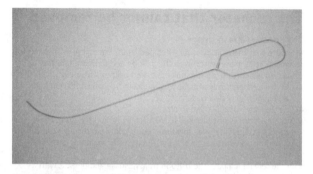

Fig. 2.8 A wire type catheter introducer.

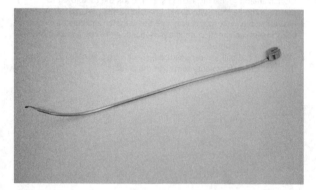

Fig. 2.9 A gutter type (Merryfield) catheter introducer.

Female catheterization

Part the labia and clean the introitus and meatus, drape, inject anaesthetic jelly, and pass a 12Fr or 14Fr catheter. Shorter catheters are available for females. In post-menopausal women the meatus may be difficult to locate. A lubricated finger or swab placed in the vagina with gentle downward pressure may bring the meatus into view. Sometimes you have to proceed more by feel than by vision.

References
1 Kobayashi T, Nishizawa K, Mitsumori K, Ogura K. Instillation of anesthetic gel is no longer necessary in the era of flexible cystoscopy: a crossover study. *J Endourol* 2004; **18**:483–6.
2 Chen YT, Hsiao PJ, Wong WY, Wang CC, Yang SS, Hsieh CH. Randomized double-blind comparison of lidocaine gel and plain lubricating gel in relieving pain during flexible cystoscopy. *J Endourol* 2005; **19**:163–6.

The catheter that cannot be removed

Try these steps in order

- Ensure that the balloon is fully deflated by aspirating the inflation valve.
- Inject a little more water in to the balloon and then aspirate the balloon again (this can unblock a blocked balloon channel).
- Leave a syringe firmly attached to the balloon channel for ~30 min. The balloon may slowly deflate.
- Cut the valve of the inflation channel.
- If the catheter is not blocked leave it for 24 hr and try again. Most balloons will deflate over this time (put a safety pin through the stump of the inflation channel to prevent the catheter migrating proximally while you wait).
- In the female, palpate the balloon transvaginally and burst it with a spinal needle placed alongside your examining finger. Gently advance it through the vaginal wall and into the bladder.
- Obtain an abdominal ultrasound scan and ask the radiologist to puncture the balloon with a spinal needle passed percutaneously.
- Pass a flexible cystoscope alongside the catheter and puncture the balloon with an injection needle passed along the instrument channel of the flexible scope.
- Whenever the balloon is punctured, check with a flexible cystoscope that no balloon fragments remain in the bladder.

Technique of suprapubic catheterization

Indications
- Failed urethral catheterization in urinary retention.
- Preferred site for long-term catheters.
- Bladder drainage in cases of pelvic fracture with urethral disruption. (NB Avoid percutaneous drainage in such cases; insert the catheter by open cystostomy to avoid inadvertent entry into a large pelvic haematoma and to assess the bladder for perforation and bone fragments from the pelvic fracture).

Long-term *urethral* catheters commonly lead to acquired hypospadias in males (ventral splitting of glans penis due to pressure erosion of the external meatus (see Fig. 2.10a)) and patulous urethra in females due to bladder neck and peri-urethral pressure atrophy (leading to frequent balloon expulsion and bypassing of urine around the catheter). Hence the suprapubic site is preferred to the urethral site for long-term catheters.

Contraindications
Suprapubic catheterization is best avoided in:
- Patients with clot retention, the cause of which may be an underlying bladder cancer (the cancer could be 'spread' along the catheter track to involve the skin).
- Patients with lower midline incisions (bowel may be 'stuck' to the deep aspect of the scar, leading to the potential for bowel perforation).
- Pelvic fractures, where the catheter may inadvertently enter the large pelvic haematoma which always accompanies severe pelvic fracture. This can lead to infection of the haematoma, and the resulting sepsis can be fatal! Failure to pass a urethral catheter in a patient with a pelvic fracture usually indicates a urethral rupture (confirmed by urethrography) and is an indication for formal open suprapubic cystotomy.

Technique
Prior to insertion of the trocar, be sure to confirm the diagnosis by:
- Abdominal examination (palpate and percuss the lower abdomen to confirm bladder is distended).
- Ultrasound (not usually available in practice).
- Aspiration of urine (using a green needle or a spinal needle in obese patients).

Patients with lower abdominal scars may have bowel interposed between the abdominal wall and bladder, and this can be perforated if the trocar is inserted near the scar and without prior aspiration of urine (Fig. 2.10b). In such cases, ultrasound-guided catheterization may be sensible. If this is not available, place the catheter some distance to one side of the scar.

Suprapubic catheter insertion is most easily and safely performed under anaesthetic (spinal or general) in an operating theatre, but it can be done safely on the ward (e.g. in patients with acute urinary retention), as long as you do not digress from the rules stated above. It is essential to fill the bladder (if not already distended by urinary retention) so that you have a 'target' of fluid to hit and adjacent structures (i.e bowel) are pushed upwards and out of harm's way. Fill the bladder as much as the patient will tolerate (≥500 mL), because discomfort for a few minutes is worth tolerating to avoid the potentially catastrophic consequences of bowel perforation. In the spinal cord injury patient, filling the bladder to such volumes can induce autonomic dysreflexia and cause a dangerous elevation of blood pressure. If the patient reports episodes of dysreflexia, give serious consideration to a general or spinal anaesthetic. This will make the whole procedure more pleasant and safer for the patient and less stressful for you.

If feasible, tilt the patient so that they are in the head-down position to encourage the bowel to move cephalad. In women with a patulous urethra, fill the bladder cystoscopically while compressing the urethra with the index and middle finger inserted into the vagina, so that the urethra can be compressed and occluded against the sheath of the cystoscope. Stay well away from lower abdominal scars.

Use a wide-bore trocar if you anticipate that the catheter will be in place for more than 24 hr (small-bore catheters will block within a few days). Aim to place the catheter about two to three finger-breadths above the pubis symphysis. Placement too close to the symphysis will result in the trocar hitting the symphysis. Instil a few millilitres of local anaesthetic into the skin of the intended puncture site and down to the rectus sheath. Confirm the location of the bladder by drawing back on the needle to aspirate urine from the bladder. This helps guide the angle of trocar insertion. Make a 1 cm incision with a sharp blade through the skin. Hold the trocar handle in your right hand, and steady the needle end with your left hand (this hand helps prevent insertion too deeply). Push the trocar in the same direction in which you previously aspirated urine. Aim the trocar towards the pelvis (i.e angled acutely) rather than passing it perpendicular to the skin. As soon as urine issues from the trocar, withdraw the latter, holding the attached sheath in place. Push the catheter in as far as it will go. Inflate the balloon. Peel away the side of the sheath and remove it.

Complications of suprapubic catheter insertion

- Bowel perforation is reported to occur in 2–3% of cases (Ahluwalia et al.,[1] 60% of cases were neuropaths; Sheriff et al.,[2] 100% of cases were neuropaths) (Fig. 2.10c).
- Perforation of the posterior wall of the bladder (and even perforation into the vagina in females or the rectum in males).
- Haematoma formation. Rare, but extensive bruising in the suprapubic area can occur, particularly in patients on anticoagulants or with clotting disorders.
- 30-day mortality rate 0.8–1.8%,[1,2] reflecting partly the infirm nature of patients undergoing suprapubic catheter insertion, but also the potentially fatal consequences of delayed recognition of bowel perforation and subsequent peritonitis.

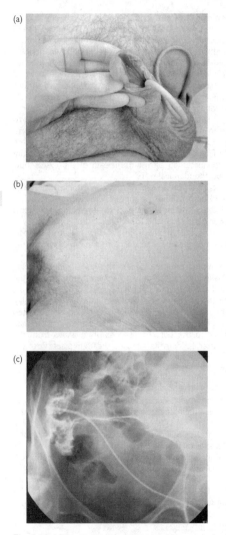

Fig. 2.10 (a) Acquired hypospadias in a patient managed with a long-term urethral catheter. The ventral aspect of the glans and penile shaft has eroded. (b) Beware the patient with lower abdominal scars. The bowel may be adherent to the deep surface of the scar. (c) The suprapubic catheter is sitting in the colon!

References

1 Ahluwalia RS, Johal N, Kouriefs C, et al. The surgical risk of suprapubic catheter insertion and long-term sequelae. Ann R Coll Surg Engl 2006; 88:210–3.
2 Sheriff MK, Foley S, McFarlane J, et al. Long-term suprapubic catheterization: clinical outcome and satisfaction survey. Spinal Cord 1998; 36:171–6.

Guidewires

Guidewires are a basic part of an urologist's armamentarium. They are used to guide other instruments (e.g. ureteroscopes, retrograde catheters, stents) along a path (usually up (or down) the ureter, but occasionally through a urethral stricture or along a conduit). There are a multitude of types. All are radio-opaque so they can be positioned using radiological guidance with an image intensifier. Wires are sized by their diameter in inches. Wires of diameter 0.035 inches (2.7Fr) or 0.038 inches (2.9Fr) are typically used, although wires as small as 0.018 inches (1.4Fr) are available. Most wires are about 150 cm long although extra-long wires (up to 260 cm) may be useful when you need a wire to span the whole urinary tract (e.g. in some complex stone procedures). Wires vary in thickness, length, stiffness, slipperiness, and configuration of the tip.

Stiffness

Most wires have a floppy (or at least less rigid) tip (the first few centimetres) and a semi-rigid body. Stiff wires (or even 'super-stiff' wires) are useful to straighten a difficult (tortuous) ureter for passage of instruments to the upper tract. A basic wire consists of a solid wire core with a tightly coiled wire wrapped around it like a spring. In most wires the core and spring are bonded to each other, but in some wires the core can be moved longitudinally within the spring. This enables the surgeon to vary the stiffness of the tip. Super-stiff wires use a thicker core and flattened wire as the spring (so that the overall diameter of the wire is not increased). Wires with a nitinol core are more resistant to kinking, which is useful for procedures where there are multiple exchanges of instruments over the wire.

Tips

Straight-tip wires are appropriate for most situations. An angled tip may be useful for accessing a difficult ureteric orifice. A J-tipped wire (also known as an angled wire) may be useful when trying to get past an impacted stone (the convexity pushes against the stone and the tip may then flip past the stone).

Slipperiness

Most standard wires are coated with PTFE to reduce friction when passing stents or instruments over the wire. Slippery wires are polymer coated so that they become very slippery when wet. Such wires are more awkward to handle but easier to negotiate past an obstruction such as an impacted ureteric calculus. In this situation the guidewire may initially coil back on itself, but may then suddenly 'flip' past the obstructing stone. They should not be used as safety wires as they have an irritating tendency to fall out of the ureter the moment you turn your back on them! Thus, if you have to use a slippery guidewire, once past the obstructing stone replace it with a 4Ch ureteric catheter and then exchange this for a more rigid wire which is less likely to fall out.

Irrigating fluids

Bladder irrigation is frequently used during and after urological endoscopy. Some absorption of irrigant fluid is inevitable when blood vessels (veins) have been opened. If this fluid is isotonic, then volume expansion results, but in reality this is rarely a problem. If the fluid is hypotonic then there is a risk of dilutional hyponatraemia. This complication (manifested in TUR syndrome) can be very serious (📖 p.120). The ideal irrigant fluid would be minimally conductive (so that during electrosurgery the current is not dissipated from the electrode and is maximized at its point of contact with the tissues) and harmless when absorbed in the intravascular space. Such a fluid does not exist.

The types of irrigant fluids in common use

- Saline (normal saline 0.9%, 154 mmol Na^+, 154 mmol Cl^-, osmolality 308 mosm/L) conducts electricity and therefore is not suitable for use with diathermy. It is the irrigant of choice for diagnostic procedures (including cystoscopy, ureteroscopy, and PCNL) and for bladder irrigation post-operatively. Suitable for use with laser resection/vaporization.
- Glycine (1.5%) is a poor electrical conductor and hence is used for conventional electrosurgery. Relatively hypotonic (200 mOsm/L) but not cytolytic. Risk of dilutional hyponatraemia. Glycine is an amino acid which inhibits neurotransmission in the retina, spinal cord, and mid-brain. It can cause visual disturbances such as flashing lights and temporary blindness which both the patient and the surgeon will find very alarming!
- Water is a poor conductor and can be used for small bladder tumour resections where bleeding is minimal. It is hypotonic compared with plasma and there is a risk of dilutional hyponatraemia if it is used for prolonged periods of time. In addition it is cytolytic. This has the disadvantge of causing haemolysis if absorbed during TURBT or TURP, but the advantage of lysing floating tumour cells after TURBT. If you use it, do so for just a few minutes. Therefore reserve its use for resection of small bladder tumours.

Useful aside

- Always check the type of irrigant fluid *yourself* before you start a procedure. Do not assume that the nurse will know which irrigant should be used for which situation.
- Switch immediately from glycine to saline upon completion of a procedure. Do not allow the remaining glycine to run through, especially if absorption is a concern.

Bladder washout

Bladder irrigation is used to prevent the formation of clots. If clots form post-operatively then the catheter may block resulting in urinary retention. The following procedure may be useful and applies equally to the patient presenting in clot retention.

• Check the vital signs and resuscitate if necessary.
• Consider checking FBC, renal function, and clotting, and ordering cross-matched blood.
• Give some analgesia. Your patient will be distressed.
• Set up a trolley with a sterile drape, one empty receiver, and one full of saline.
• Flush the catheter smartly down both the inlet and outlet channels using a catheter-tip 50–60 mL syringe filled with saline. It is often easiest to use two syringes, one on each channel.
• Aspirate firmly on the outlet channel. Occasionally a single clot will be aspirated and the catheter will then drain freely.
• If there is a lot of clot in the bladder, repeat the process of flushing and aspiration until no further clot can be aspirated and the aspirated fluid is only lightly blood-stained. Persistence is required to shift a lot of clot.
• If fluid flushes in easily but cannot be withdrawn, there may be clot adhering to the end of the catheter. Deflation of the balloon followed by further flushing/aspiration may dislodge this clot. Re-inflate the balloon.
• If either the inflow or outflow is blocked and cannot be cleared, the catheter will need to be changed. Reinsert a larger size if possible and re-commence washout. Consider a dose of intravenous antibiotics.
• If the replacement catheter also blocks with clot then you will need to take your patient to theatre for evacuation of clot.
• Once irrigation is re-established run it fast enough to prevent further clotting.
• Consider putting more fluid in the catheter balloon to tamponade the bleeding (a '30 mL' balloon will easily accommodate 50 mL).
• If profuse bleeding persists, put the catheter on traction for ~20 min. Do not do this by hanging the catheter bag over the end of the bed—it will fill up and become very heavy. Instead, wrap a crepe bandage around the leg just above the knee, loop an elastic band over the catheter and attach to the crepe bandage with a safety pin.
• If bleeding is profuse or the patient is unstable, return to theatre to stop the bleeding.

- In theatre, pass a resectoscope sheath and perform a cystoscopy.
- Evacuate the clot using a bulb evacuator. A glass evacuator allows generation of greater pressure than the more widely available plastic evacuators.
- If the clot is too tenacious or mature to be evacuated, proceed to resection of the clot using a loop electrode. It is often possible to use the loop to fragment the clot without actually applying current.
- When all the clot is cleared, try to identify and control the bleeding sites.
- When the clot is very large and has matured into a fibrinous mass or where the view is so poor that resection of the clot is hazardous, it is quicker and safer to perform an open cystotomy to remove it.

JJ stents and stent insertion

JJ stents are hollow tubes with a coil at each end which are positioned within the ureter with one end lying within the bladder and one within the renal pelvis. They are usually inserted in retrograde fashion via the bladder, by passing a guidewire through the VUJ, up the ureter, and thence into the renal pelvis. They are designed to bypass a ureteric obstruction (e.g. due to a stone) or drain the kidney (e.g. after renal surgery). They have a coil at each end, hence the alternative names of 'double-pigtail' stent (the coils have the configuration of a pig's tail), double 'g' stents (coiled like the letter 'g'), or the less accurate name of J stent. The coils prevent migration downwards (out of the ureter) or upwards (into the ureter). Therefore they are self-retaining.

They are made of polymers of variable strength and biodurability. Some stents have a hydrophilic coating which absorbs water and thus makes them more slippery and easier to insert. Stents are impregnated with barium- or bismuth-containing metallic salts to make them radio-opaque, so that they can be visualized radiographically to ensure correct positioning.

Types
- Classified by size and length.
- Common sizes are 6Ch or 7Ch (Fig. 2.11).
- Common lengths for adults are 22–28 cm.
- Multilength stents are of variable length, which allows them to accommodate to ureters of different lengths.

Stent materials
The material used to make stents must be strong enough to allow the stent to pass over a guidewire without kinking, but flexible enough for it to accommodate to the shape of the patient's ureter. Materials used for stents include polyurethane, silicone, C-flex, Silitek, Percuflex, and biode-gradable materials (experimental—obviates need for stent removal and eliminates possibility of the 'forgotten stent').

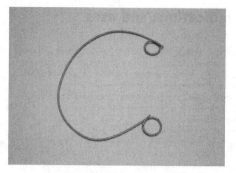

Fig. 2.11 A JJ stent. Reproduced with permission from Reynard et al., *Oxford Handbook of Urology*, 2006, Oxford University Press.

JJ stents: indications and uses

Therapeutic

- Relief of obstruction: ureteric stones; benign (i.e. ischaemic) ureteric strictures; malignant ureteric strictures (e.g. prostate or cervical cancer obstructing the lower ureter). The stent will relieve the pain caused by obstruction and reverse renal impairment if present.
- Following endopyelotomy (endopyelotomy stents have a tapered end from 14 to 7Ch, to keep the incised ureter 'open').
- Post renal transplantation.
- 'Passive' dilatation of ureter prior to ureteroscopy.
- To ensure antegrade flow of urine following surgery to ureter (e.g. pyeloplasty) or injury of ureter.
- Drainage of pus in the collecting system of the kidney, i.e. a pyonephrosis. Nephrostomy tube drainage is probably a more usual method of dealing with a pyonephrosis. However, a randomized trial of JJ stenting versus nephrostomy drainage for decompression of an obstructed or infected kidney due to a ureteric stone failed to demonstrate superiority of one method over the other in terms of adequacy of drainage or relief of symptoms.[1]

Prophylactic

- Prevention of obstruction: post ureteroscopy.

Stenting for malignant ureteric obstruction

Pelvic malignancies such as prostatic, bladder, cervical, uterine, ovarian, and colorectal can cause ureteric obstruction through a combination of direct compression of the lower ureter by the primary tumour mass or by compression from lymph nodes infiltrated with tumour. Standard JJ stents can relieve such obstruction. However, stents can themselves become compressed by the cancer. In this situation permanent nephrostomy drainage may be used. Alternatively, two JJ stents placed side by side can provide improved 'resistance' to external compression.[2] Rigid permanently sited metallic stents ('wallstents') are an alternative for such patients.[3]

References

1 Pearle MS, Pierce HL, Miller GL, *et al*. Optimal method of urgent decompression of the collecting system for obstruction and infection due to ureteral calculi. *J Urol* 1998; **160**:1260–4.

2 Liu JS, Hrebinko RL. The use of two ipsilateral ureteral stents for relief of ureteral obstruction from extrinsic compression. *J Urol* 1998; **159**:179–81.

3 Kulkarni R, Bellamy E. Nickel-titanium shape memory alloy Memokath 051 ureteral stent for managing long-term ureteral obstruction: 4-year experience. *J Urol* 2001; **166**:1750–4.

Symptoms and complications of stents

- Stent symptoms: common—as many as 80% of patients report bother-some LUTS and haematuria and >80% have pain affecting their daily life.[1,2] Suprapubic pain, LUTS (frequency, urgency (constant feeling of wanting to pass urine) stent irritating trigone), incontinence, haema-turia, inability to work. An excellent booklet is available online.[3]
- Urinary tract infection: development of bacteriuria after stenting is common. In a small proportion of patients sepsis can develop. In such cases consider placement of a urethral catheter to lower the pressure in the collecting system and prevent reflux of infected urine.
- Incorrect placement:
  - too high—distal end of stent in ureter; subsequent stent removal requires ureteroscopy which can be technically difficult; percutaneous removal may be required.
  - too low—proximal end not in renal pelvis; therefore stent may not relieve obstruction.
- Stent migration (up the ureter or down the ureter and into bladder).
- Stent blockage: catheters and stents become coated with a biofilm when in contact with urine (a protein matrix secreted by bacteria colonizing the stent). Calcium, magnesium, and phosphate salts are deposited. Biofilm build-up can lead to stent blockage or stone formation on the stent (Fig. 2.12).
- The 'forgotten stent': rare, but potentially very serious as biofilm may become encrusted with stone, making removal technically very difficult.

Management of the encrusted stent

Assess renal function with a MAG3 renogram or DMSA scan. It is possible that the kidney may no longer be functioning, in which case nephrectomy will be necessary. If the proximal end only is encrusted, try ESWL followed by a gentle attempt to remove the stent. If the stent will not come out with gentle traction, this means thit is well and truly stuck and further attempts to remove it risk either the stent breaking or, much worse, avulsion of the ureter from the renal pelvis at the PUJ. If ESWL fails to free the stent, PCNL will be required to remove the stone and the stent. If the entire stent is encrusted, open removal via several incisions in the ureter may be necessary.

It goes without saying that the problem is best avoided. Warn patients prior to stone surgery that stent insertion may be necessary. If you do insert one, tell the patient (when they have fully recovered from the anaesthetic or any sedative drugs) and explain why removal of the stent is so important. Advise them that failure to remove the stent can lead to stone formation, requiring further surgery and even ultimately leading to loss of the kidney. Make arrangements for the stent to be removed, and let the patient know this date prior to their discharge. Record all these details in the patient's notes.

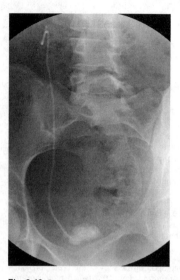

Fig. 2.12 Encrustation of a JJ stent. Reproduced with permission from Reynard et al., *Oxford Handbook of Urology*, 2006, Oxford University Press.

Further reading

1 Borboroglu PG, Kane CJ. Current management of severely encrusted ureteral stents with a large associated stone burden. *J Urol* 2000; **164**:648–50.
2 Mohan-Pillai K, Keeley Jr FX, Moussa SA *et al*. Endourological management of severely encrusted ureteral stents. *J Endourol* 1999; **13**:377–9.

References

1 Joshi HB, Okeke A, Newns N, Keeley FX Jr, Timoney AG. Characterization of urinary symptoms in patients with ureteral stents. *Urology* 2002; **59**:511–16.
2 Joshi HB, Stainthorpe A, MacDonagh RP, Keeley FX Jr, Timoney AG. Indwelling ureteral stents: evaluation of symptoms, quality of life and utility. *J Urol* 2003; **169**:1065–9.
3 *Ureteric stents: what to expect and how to manage.* Available online at http://www.blackwell publishing.com/products/journals/suppmat/BJU/BJU2356/hrishi.pdf

Commonly asked stent questions

Does urine pass though the centre of the stent?
No, it passes around the outside of the stent. Reflux of urine occurs through the centre.

Should I place a JJ stent after ureteroscopy?
A stent should be placed if:
- There has been ureteric injury (e.g. perforation, indicated by extravasation of contrast).
- There are residual stones that might obstruct the ureter.
- The patient has had a ureteric stricture that required dilatation.

Routine stenting after ureteroscopy for distal ureteric calculi is unnecessary[1] Many urologists will place a stent after ureteroscopy for proximal ureteric stones. Not placing a stent may lead to a higher complication rate.

Do stents cause obstruction?
In normal kidneys stents cause a significant and substantial increase in intra-renal pressure which persists for up to 3 weeks[2] (this can be prevented by placing a urethral catheter).

Do stents aid stone passage?
Ureteric peristalsis requires coaptation of the wall of the ureter proximal to the bolus of urine to be transmitted down the length of the ureter. JJ stents paralyse ureteric peristalsis and, at least in a canine model, actually impede stone passage. In dogs, the amplitude of each peristaltic wave (measured by an intraluminal ureteric balloon) falls (from 50 to 15 mmHg) and the frequency of ureteric peristalsis falls (from 11 to 3 waves/min). Peristalsis takes several weeks to recover. Ball bearings (3 mm) placed within a non-stented dog ureter take 7 days to pass, compared with 24 days in a stented ureter.[3] One study suggested that J stenting facilitates stone passage in humans, possibly by causing ureteric dilatation.[4]

Are stents able to relieve obstruction due to extrinsic compression of a ureter?
Stents are less effective at relieving obstruction due to extrinsic obstruction by, for example, a tumour or retroperitoneal obstruction.[5] They are much more effective for relieving obstruction by an intrinsic problem (e.g. a stone). Placement of two stents may provide more effective drainage (figure-of-eight configuration may produce more space around the stents for drainage).

For acute ureteric stone obstruction with a fever, should I place a JJ stent or a nephrostomy?

In theory, one might imagine that a nephrostomy is better than a JJ stent: it can be done under local anaesthetic (JJ stent insertion may require a GA); it lowers the pressure in the renal pelvis to zero or a negative value, whereas a JJ stent results in a persistently positive pressure; it is less likely to be blocked by thick pus; it allows easier subsequent imaging (contrast can be injected down the ureter (nephrostogram) to determine if the stone has passed). In practice, both seem to be effective for relief of acute stone obstruction and associated infection.[6]

References

1 Srivastava A et al. Routine stenting after ureteroscopy for distal ureteral calculi is unnecessary: results of a randomized controlled trial. *J Endourol* 2003; **17**:871–44.
2 Ramsay JW et al. The effects of double J stenting on obstructed ureters: an experimental and clinical study. *Br J Urol* 1985; **57**:630–4.
3 Lennon GM, Thornhill JA, Grainger R, et al. Double pigtail ureteric stent versus percutaneous nephrostomy: effects on stoen transit and ureteric motility. *Eur Urol* 1997; **31**:24–9.
4 Leventhal EK, Rozanski TA, Crain TW, Deshon Jr GE. Indwelling ureteral stents as definitive therapy for distal ureteric calculi. *J Urol* 1995; **153**:34–6.
5 Docimo SG. High failure rate of indwelling ureteral stents in patients with extrinsic obstruction: experience at two institutions. *J Urol* 1989; **142**:277–9.
6 Pearle MS, Pierce HL, Miller GL, et al. Optimal method of urgent decompression of the collecting system for obstruction and infection due to ureteral calculi. *J Urol* 1998; **160**:1260–4.

Additional Reading

1 Ryan PC et al. The effects of acute and chronic JJ stent placement on upper urinary tract motility and calculus transit. *Br J Urol* 1994; **74**:434–9.

Percutaneous nephrostomy: indications and complications (see 📖 p. 658)

Lasers in urological surgery

The term 'laser' is derived from light amplification by stimulated emission of radiation

Photons are emitted when an atom is stimulated by an external energy source and the excited electrons revert to their steady state. In a laser the light is coherent (all the photons are in phase with one another), collimated (the photons travel parallel to each other), and of the same wavelength (monochromatic). Thus the light energy is 'concentrated', allowing delivery of a high energy at a desired target.

The holmium: YAG (yttrium aluminium garnet) laser is currently the principal urological laser. It has a wavelength of 2140 nm and is highly absorbed by water, and therefore by tissues which are composed mainly of water. The majority of the holmium laser energy is absorbed superficially, resulting in a superficial cutting or ablation effect. The depth of the thermal effect is no greater than 1 mm. The holmium: YAG laser produces a cavitation bubble wh generates only a weak shock wave as it expands and collapses. Holmium laser lithotripsy occurs primarily through a photothermal mechanism wh causes stone vaporization.

Uses
- Laser lithotripsy (ureteric stones, small intra-renal stones, bladder stones).
- Resection of the prostate (holmium laser prostatectomy).
- Division of urethral strictures.
- Division of ureteric strictures including PUJO.
- Ablation of small bladder, ureteric and intra-renal TCCs.

Advantages
- Holmium laser energy is delivered via a laser fibre (Fig. 2.13) which is thin enough to allow it to be used down a flexible instrument without affecting the deflection of that instrument. Therefore it can be used to gain access to otherwise inaccessible parts of the kidney.
- The zone of thermal injury adjacent to the tip of the laser fibre is limited to no more than 1 mm. The laser can safely be fired at a distance of 1 mm from the wall of the ureter.
- Can be used for all stone types.
- There is minimal stone migration effect because of minimal shock wave generation.

Disadvantages

- High cost.
- Produces a dust cloud during stone fragmentation which temporarily obscures the view.
- Can irreparably damage endoscopes if inadvertently fired near or within the scope.
- Relatively slow stone fragmentation: the laser fibre must be 'painted' over the surface of the stone to vaporize it.

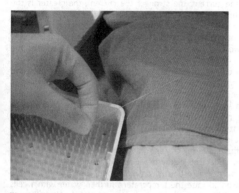

Fig. 2.13 A laser fibre used for delivery of holmium laser energy. Reproduced with permission from Reynard et al., *Oxford Handbook of Urology*, 2006, Oxford University Press.

Principles of diathermy

Diathermy is the coagulation or cutting of tissues by application of heat.

Monopolar diathermy

When an electric current passes between two contacts on the body there is an increase in temperature in the tissues through which the current flows. This increase in temperature depends on the volume of tissue through which the current passes, the resistance of the tissues, and the strength of the current: the stronger the current, the greater is the rise in temperature. If one contact is made large, the heat is dissipated over a wide area and the rise in temperature is insignificant. This is the earth or neutral electrode, and the rise in temperature under this is only 1 or 2°C. The working electrode or diathermy loop is thin, so that the current density is maximal and therefore so is the heating effect.

When a direct current is switched on or off, nerves are stimulated and muscles will twitch. If the switching on and off is sufficiently rapid, there is the sustained contraction familiar to the physiology class as the 'tetanic contraction.' If a high-frequency alternating current is used (300 kHz to 5 MHz), there is no time for the cell membranes of nerve or muscle to become depolarized, and nerves and muscles are not stimulated (they are stimulated at lower frequencies).

The effect of the diathermy current on the tissues depends on the heat that is generated under the diathermy loop. At relatively low temperatures coagulation and distortion of small blood vessels occurs. If the current is increased to raise the temperature further, water within cells vaporizes and the cells explode. This explosive vaporization literally cuts the tissues apart.

Bipolar diarthermy

Bipolar diathermy involves the passage of electric current between two electrodes on the same handpiece. It is inherently safer than monopolar diathermy, since the current does not pass through the patient and therefore diathermy burns cannot occur.

Potential problems with diathermy

The diathermy is not working

- Do not increase the current.
- Check that the irrigating fluid is glycine (sodium chloride conducts electricity, causing the diathermy to short-circuit).
- Check that the diathermy plate is making good contact with the patient's skin.
- Check that the lead is undamaged.
- Check that the resectoscope loop is securely fixed to the contact.

Modern diathermy machines have a warning circuit which sounds an alarm when there is imperfect contact between the earth plate and the patient.

Diathermy burns

If current returns to earth through a small contact rather than the broad area of the earth pad, the tissues through which the current passes will be heated just like those under the cutting loop. If the pad is making good contact, the current will find it easier to run to earth through the pad and no harm will occur even when there is accidental contact with some metal object. The real danger arises when the diathermy pad is not making good contact with the patient. It may not be plugged in or its wire may be broken. Under these circumstances the current must find its way to earth somehow, and any contact may then become the site of a dangerous rise in temperature.

Pacemakers and diathermy: problems and their prevention

- Pacemaker inhibition: the high frequency of the diathermy current may simulate the electrical activity of myocardial contraction and so pacemakers can be inhibited. If the patient is pacemaker dependent the heart may stop.
- Phantom reprogramming: the diathermy current may also simulate the radiofrequency impulse by which the pacemaker can be reprogrammed to different settings, so-called phantom reprogramming. The pacemaker may then start to function in an entirely different mode.
- The internal mechanism of the pacemaker may be damaged by the diathermy current if this is applied close to the pacemaker.
- Ventricular fibrillation: if the diathermy current is channelled along the pacemaker lead, ventricular fibrillation may be induced.
- Myocardial damage: another potential effect of channelling the diathermy current along the pacemaker lead is burning of the myocardium at the tip of the pacemaker lead. This can subsequently result in ineffective pacing.

It was formerly recommended that a magnet should be placed over the pacemaker to overcome pacemaker inhibition and make it function at a fixed rate. However, this can result in phantom reprogramming. For demand pacemakers, it is better to programme the pacemaker to a fixed rate (as opposed to demand pacing) for the duration of the operation. Consult the patient's cardiologist for advice.

Other precautions

- The patient plate should be sited so that the current path does not go right through the pacemaker. Ensure that the indifferent plate is correctly applied, as an improper connection can cause earthing of the diathermy current through the ECG monitoring leads, and this can affect pacemaker function. The indifferent plate should be placed as close as possible to the prostate (e.g. over the thigh or buttock).
- The diathermy machine should be placed well away from the pacemaker and should certainly not be used within 15 cm of the pacemaker.
- The heartbeat should be continually monitored, and a defibrillator and external pacemaker should be at hand.
- Try to use short bursts of diathermy at the lowest effective output.
- Give antibiotic prophylaxis (as for patients with artificial heart valves).
- Because the pacemaker-driven heart will not respond to fluid overload in the normal way, the resection should be as quick as possible and fluid overload should be avoided.

Sterilization of urological equipment

All surgical equipment should be dismantled and cleaned to reduce the degree of contamination. Sterilization is complete destruction of all micro-organisms including spores. Disinfection is reduction in the number of viable micro-organisms but not necessarily inactivation of viruses and spores.

- Most simple surgical instruments, rigid cystoscopes, rigid ureteroscopes, and light leads can be sterilized by steam (standard autoclave regimens: 134°C for 3–4 min or 121°C for 15 mins at 2 atm pressure). Steam sterilization is efficient and widely available.
- Steam sterilization is harmful to more complex instruments such as flexible cystoscopes (which cannot tolerate temperatures >65°C) and cameras. Flexible cystoscopes and cameras should be cleaned after use and detachable parts removed. They are then disinfected in automated processors which use chemical disinfectants and water rinses. A variety of disinfectants are available:
  - Chlorine dioxide (Tristel) is an oxidizing agent which causes cell wall lysis. It is effective against most pathogens and is minimally irritant. It requires regular replacement.
  - Chlorine dioxide solutions kills bacteria, viruses (including HIV and hepatitis B and C), spores, and mycobacteria.
- Peracetic acid (NuCidex) also works by oxidation. It has variable activity against spores and microbacteria. It may irritate skin/mucous membranes and may be harmful to cystoscopes.
- Superoxidized water electrolysis (Sterilox) is potent and non-irritant but is single use.

Sterilization and prion diseases

Variant Creutzfeldt–Jakob disease (vCJD) is a neurodegenerative disease caused by a prion protein (PrP). Other examples of neurodegenerative prion diseases include classic CJD, kuru, sheep scrapie, and bovine spongiform encephalopathy (BSE). vCJD and BSE are caused by the same prion strain, and represent a classic example of cross-species transmission of a prion disease.

There has been much recent concern about the potential for transmission of vCJD between patients via contaminated surgical instruments. Classic CJD may be transmitted by neurosurgical and other types of surgical instruments, because normal hospital sterilization procedures do not completely inactivate prions.[1] It is not possible at present to quantify the risks of transmission of prion diseases by surgical instruments. To date, iatrogenic CJD remains rare, with 267 cases having been reported worldwide up to 2000.[2]

The risk of transmission of CJD may be higher with procedures performed on organs containing lymphoreticular tissue, such as tonsillectomy and adenoidectomy, because vCJD targets these tissues and is found in high concentrations there. For this reason there was a move towards the use of disposable, once-only use instruments for procedures such as tonsillectomy. However, these instruments have been associated with a higher post-operative haemorrhage rate[3] and as a consequence

ENT departments in the UK are no longer obliged to use disposable instruments.

In the UK, the Advisory Committee on Dangerous Pathogens and Spongiform Encephalopathy provides advice on appropriate methods of cleaning and sterilization of surgical instruments.[4] Prions are particularly resistant to conventional chemical (ethylene oxide, formaldehyde, and chlorine dioxide) and standard autoclave regimens, and dried blood or tissue remaining on an instrument could harbour prions that will not then be killed by the sterilization process. Once proteinaceous material such as blood or tissue has dried on an instrument, it is very difficult subsequently to be sure that the instrument has been sterilized. Sterilization should include:

- *Pre-sterilization cleaning* Initial low temperature washing (<35°C) with detergents and an ultrasonic cleaning system removes and prevents coagulation of prion proteins. Ultrasonic cleaners essentially 'shake' attached material from the instrument.
- *Hot wash.*
- *Air drying.*
- *Thermal sterilization* Longer autoclave cycles at 134–137°C for at least 18 minutes (or six successive cycles with holding times of 3 min) or 1 hr at conventional autoclave temperatures may result in a substantial reduction in the level of contamination with prions.

The latest models of pre-sterilization cleaning devices (automated thermal washer disinfectors) are designed to perform all these cleaning tasks in one unit. Enzymatic proteolytic inactivation methods are under development.

References

1 Collinge J. Variant Creutzfeldt-Jakob disease. *Lancet* 1999; **354**:317–23.
2 Collins SJ, Lawson VA, Masters CL. Transmissible spongiform encephalopathies. *Lancet* 2004; **363**:51–61.
3 Nix P. Prions and disposable surgical instruments. *Int J Clin Pract* 2003; **57**:678–80.
4 Advisory Committee on Dangerous Pathogens and Spongiform Encephalopathy. *Transmissible spongiform encephalopathy agents: safe working and the prevention of infection.* London: Stationery Office, 1998.

Urological incisions: midline, trans-peritoneal

Indications

Access to peritoneal cavity and pelvis for radical nephrectomy, cystectomy, reconstructive procedures etc.

Technique

Divide skin, subcutaneous fat. Divide fascia in midline (Fig. 2.14). Finding the midline between the rectus muscles is not always as easy as it sounds. Traditionally one looks for the decussating fibres of the anterior rectus sheath, but this is not always a reliable anatomical indicator and not infrequently the surgeon finds that the incision is too lateral and therefore through the rectus muscle itself. Mobilize fat to adequately expose the rectus sheath. Then place your index finger in the apex of the incision and pull it in a cephalic direction. This will raise a ridge of rectus sheath that can be seen and palpated with your other hand (Fig. 2.15). This ridge represents the attachment of the median umbilical ligament (the urachal ligament) to the back of the rectus sheath as it passes upwards from the bladder to the umbilicus. The incision should be made along the ridge.[1] Dissect the muscles free from the underlying peritoneum. Place two clips on either side of the midline, pinch between the two to ensure no bowel has been trapped, elevate the clips, and divide between them with a knife. As air enters the peritoneal cavity the underlying bowel will fall away. Insert your index and middle fingers to push the bowel out of the way and extend the incision in the peritoneum by cutting between these two fingers.

Closure

Use a non-absorbable (e.g. nylon) or very slowly absorbable (e.g. PDS) suture, using Jenkins rule to reduce risk of dehiscence by taking 1 cm bites 1 cm apart (so that the suture length is four times the wound length). Be particularly careful not to inadvertently lacerate the underlying bowel with the needle.

Specific complications

Dehiscence (classically around day 10 post-operatvely and preceded by pink serous discharge, then sudden herniation of a bowel through incision).

Reference

1 Bariol SV, Lambrakis P, Cozzi PJ. Simple technique for identifying the linea alba in lower abdominal incisions. *Aust NZ J Surg* 2003; **73**:649.

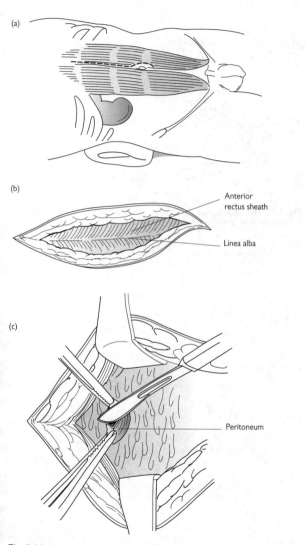

Fig. 2.14 Midline trans-peritoneal incision: (a) skin incision; (b) the anterior rectus sheath and linea alba are exposed; (c) once the rectus sheath has been divided in the midline, fat is cleared from the peritoneum, which is picked up between two clips and carefully divided with the belly of a scalpel blade.

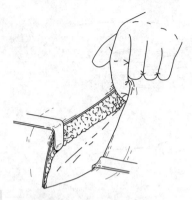

Fig. 2.15 The index finger is placed in the apex of the incision and pulled in a cephalic direction, thus raising a ridge of rectus sheath.

Transperitoneal anterior transverse incision (Chevron incision)

Indications

Access to peritoneal cavity and pelvis for radical nephrectomy, removal of large adrenal masses. Excellent exposure of the retroperitoneum can be achieved with this incision.

Technique

Start at the tip of the right 11th rib and divide the skin towards the midline, keeping just below the costal margin. At the midline continue onto the left side for a shorter distance (this may be extended if greater access is required). Divide the subcutaneous fat. Divide the rectus fascia on both sides. Insert a finger underneath each rectus muscle and divide it (beware the underlying superior epigastric artery which should be indentified, ligated, and divided). Divide the fascia over external oblique in the line of the incision, then the muscle itself, and then internal oblique. The fibres of transverses abdominis can be split. Divide the underlying transversalis fascia and then pick up the peritoneum between 2 clips (make sure there is no underlying bowel).

Closure

Use a non-absorbable (e.g. nylon) or very slowly absorbable (e.g. PDS) suture material to close each fascial layer to its divided neighbour.

Specific complications

Dehiscence (rare); denervaton of the uppermost part of the rectus muscles (due to division of the terminal branches of the intercostals nerves) and numbness of the overlying skin.

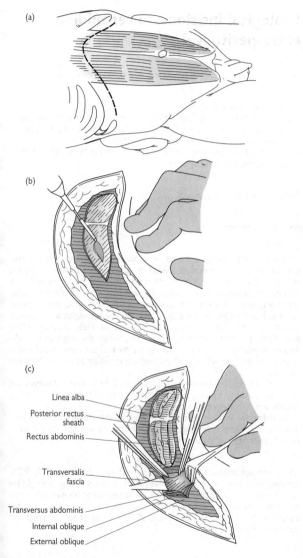

(a)

(b)

(c)

Linea alba

Posterior rectus
sheath

Rectus abdominis

Transversalis
fascia

Transversus abdominis

Internal oblique

External oblique

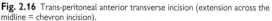

Fig. 2.16 Trans-peritoneal anterior transverse incision (extension across the midline = chevron incision).

Urological incisions: lower midline extra-peritoneal

Indications

Access to pelvis (e.g. radical prostatectomy, colposuspension).

Technique

- Divide skin, subcutaneous fat.
- Divide fascia in midline. Find the midline between the rectus muscles and dissect the muscles free from the underlying peritoneum. If you make a hole in it repair the defect with Vicryl.
- Divide the fascia posterior to the rectus muscles in the midline, thus exposing the extravesical space.

Closure

As for midline, trans-peritoneal.

Indications

Radical nephrectomy.

Technique

Divide skin and subcutaneous fat down to the fascia overlying external oblique and the rectus muscle. Divide the anterior rectus sheath and the rectus muscles. Ligate and divide the superior epigastric artery and vein. Elevate the posterior rectus sheath between clips and divide it to enter the peritoneum. Extend the incision laterally to divide the external oblique, internal oblique, and transverses abdominis muscles and transversalis fascia in the line of the incision. This is most easily done by cutting with diathermy (use coagulating current) between the index and middle fingers of your opposite hand. During this part of the incision the round ligament of the liver will be encountered and it should be divided between sutures.

During this incision the terminal branches of the intercostal nerves will be divided, leading to atrophy of the upper part of the rectus abdominis muscle and numbness of the overlying skin.

Extending the incision across the midline (a chevron incision) can provide improved access for large renal tumours, but will lead to a greater risk of denervation of these structures.

Closure

Use a non-absorbable (e.g. nylon) or very slowly absorbable (e.g. PDS) continuous suture. Approximate the round ligament of the liver. Close the incision on layers starting with the peritoneum and transversalis fascia and more medially the posterior rectus sheath. The anterior rectus sheath is then closed and more laterally the fascia of the external and internal oblique muscles.

Urological incisions: Pfannenstiel

Indications

Access to pelvis (e.g. colposuspension, open prostatectomy, open cysto-lithotomy).

Technique

- Divide the skin 2 cm above the pubis (Fig. 2.17a) and the tissues down to the rectus sheath which is cut in an arc (Fig. 2.17b), avoiding the inguinal canal (a higher incision leaves the lower flap to fall into the wound, interfering with exposure). This incision is carried laterally dividing the aponeuroses of the three abdominal wall muscles, thereby providing greater exposure than that afforded by separation of the rectus muscles alone (beware both the inferior epigastric vessels and the iliohypogastric nerve deep to internal oblique).
- Apply clips to top flap (and afterwards the bottom flap) (Fig. 2.17c) and use a combination of scissors and your fingers to separate the rectus muscle from the sheath (Fig. 2.17d). For maximum exposure you must elevate the anterior rectus sheath from the recti cranially to just below the umbilicus and caudally to the pubis (Fig. 2.17e). Take care to diathermy a perforating branch of the inferior epigastric artery on each side.
- Apply two Babock's forceps to the inferior belly of the rectus on either side of the midline (Fig. 2.17f). Elevate and cut the lower part of the fascia (transversalis fascia) in the midline between the recti (in the absence of a posterior rectus sheath the transversalis fascia is not adherent to the linea alba). Separate the recti in the midline (do not divide them unless exposure is not adequate—division of the rectus muscles from the
pubis is the Cherny incision).
- You are now confronted by pre-peritoneal fat. Use a combination of the sucker and diathermy to tease this away from the underlying organ you are trying to expose. If this is the bladder, it can be very helpful to inflate it (catheter attached to an elevated bag of water or glycine) so as to avoid inadvertently entering the peritoneal cavity. You will see the urachus (the median umbilical ligament) lying within this pre-peritoneal fat, anterior to the peritoneum and posterior to the transversalis fascia.

NB In the neuropathic patient (e.g. spinal cord injury) the rectus muscle may be very atrophied.

Closure

Tack the divided transversalis fascia together and then close the transversely divided rectus sheath with Vicryl.

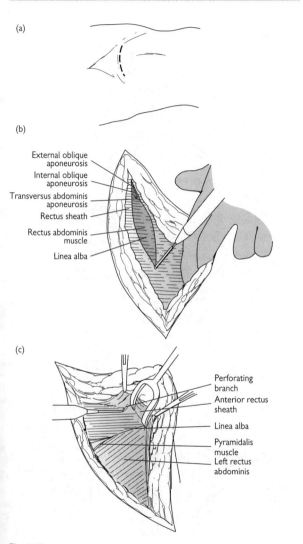

(a)

(b)

External oblique
aponeurosis

Internal oblique
aponeurosis

Transversus abdominis
aponeurosis

Rectus sheath

Rectus abdominis
muscle

Linea alba

(c)

Perforating
branch

Anterior rectus
sheath

Linea alba

Pyramidalis
muscle

Left rectus
abdominis

Fig. 2.17 A Pfannenstiel incision: (a) skin incision; (b) transverse incision across the rectus sheath; (c) the rectus fascia is elevated cranially off the underlying rectus muscle.

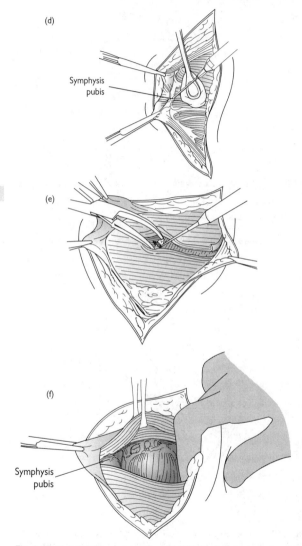

Fig. 2.17 (*Contd.*) A Pfannenstiel incision: (d) the rectus fascia is elevated caudally off the underlying rectus muscle down to the pubic symphysis; (e) the rectus muscles are separated in the midline; (f) the transversalis fascia is exposed.

Urological incisions: supra-12th rib incision

Indications

Access to kidneys, renal pelvis, upper ureter.

Technique

Make the incision over the tip of the 12th rib through skin and subcutaneous fascia (Fig. 2.18a). Palpate the tip of the 12th rib. Make a 3 cm cut with diathermy through the muscle (latissimus dorsi) overlying the tip of the 12th rib so that you come down onto the tip of the 12th rib. Then cut anterior to the tip of the 12th rib, down through external and internal oblique and transversus abdominis to Gerota's fascia and the peri-renal fat. Sweep anteriorly with a finger to push the peritoneum and intra-peritoneal organs out of harm's way. Cut the muscles overlying the rib, cutting centrally along the length of the rib, thus avoiding the pleura (Fig. 2.18b). Cut with scissors along the top edge of the rib to free the intercostal muscle from the rib—beware the pleura! (Fig. 2.18c,d). Insert a Gillies forceps between the pleura and the overlying intercostal muscle and divide the muscle fibres, thus protecting the pleura. Dissect fibres of the diaphragm away from the inner surface of the 12th rib. As you do so the pleura will rise upwards with the detached diaphragmatic fibres, out of harm's way. If you make a hole in the pleura do not repair it now (at the end of the operation, pass a Jacques catheter through the hole, close all the muscle layers, inflate the lung, and then remove the catheter before closing the skin).

At the posterior end of the incision feel for the sharp edge of the costovertebral ligament. Insert heavy scissors, with the blades just open, on the top of the rib (to avoid intercostal nerve XI) and divide the costovertebral ligament. You should now be on top of Gerota's fascia. Before incising this feel for the lower pole of the kidney to orientate yourself. Now pick up the fascia and cut it. Extend this incision lengthways. Expose the lower pole of the kidney (just so you can see it—there is no need to expose all of it, although it does not matter if you do).

Closure

Use an absorbable suture (e.g. Vicryl) to close the muscles and fascia in layers, being careful to avoid catching the intercostal nerve in the closure.

Specific complications

Damage to the pleura. If you make a hole in the pleura repair it at the end of the operation. Pass a small-bore catheter (e.g. Jacques catheter) through the hole, close all the muscle layers, inflate the lung, and then remove the catheter before closing the skin.

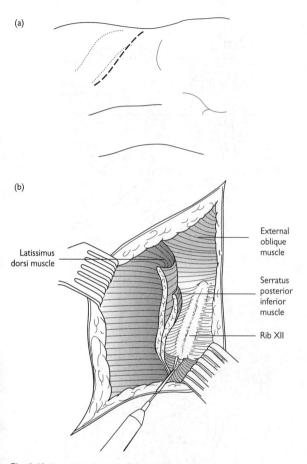

(a)

(b)

Latissimus
dorsi muscle

External
oblique
muscle

Serratus
posterior
inferior
muscle

Rib XII

Fig. 2.18 Supra-12th rib incision: (a) skin incision; (b) cut through the muscles overlying the 12th rib (latissimus dorsi and serratus posterior inferior);

(c)

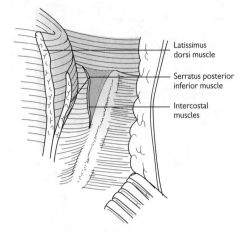

Latissimus dorsi muscle

Serratus posterior inferior muscle

Intercostal muscles

(d)

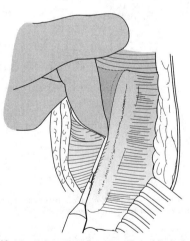

Fig. 2.18 (*Contd.*) Supra-12th rib incision: (c) carefully divide the intercostals muscles, keeping close to the upper border of the 12th rib; (d) as you progress posteriorly, insert a finger beneath the intercostal muscles to protect the underlying pleura. Cut down onto your finger. At the posterior aspect of the 12th rib, divide the costovertebral ligament to allow the rib to be swung downwards.

Complications common to all incisions

Hernia, wound infection, chronic wound pain

Neuropathies related to incisions and patient positioning

A number of peripheral nerves are in danger of injury during the process of making anterior incisions (midline, Pfannestiel) and during placement of retractors in these incisions. Placement of sutures can also damage nerves, most notably the femoral and genitofemoral nerves.

- The course of the femoral nerve: nerve roots (L2,3,4) join together to form the femoral nerve which emerges from the anterolateral aspect of psoas major, just below the level of the false pelvic brim. It descends in the groove between iliacus and psoas major, deep to the iliacus fascia, and it is here that pressure from the blade of a retractor can lead to a femoral nerve palsy[1] (Fig. 2.19a). After positioning a self-retaining retractor, insert your fingers beneath the retractor blades bilaterally to be sure that there is clearance between the ends of the retractor and the psoas muscle.[2]
- Remember that there are other structures that may be injured or compressed by the blades of your retractor. Much easier than damaging the femoral nerve with the blades of the self-retaining retractor is to compress the external iliac vein against the pelvic side wall. If you are lucky enough not to tear the vein, the patient may be unlucky enough to develop a DVT.
- The lateral (femoral) cutaneous nerve of the thigh, which supplies an area of skin over the upper outer aspect of the thigh is vulnerable to damage from the blades of retractors as it courses around the inner surface of the ilium on its way towards the inguinal ligament at the latter's origin from the anterior superior iliac spine (Fig. 2.19b).
  The genitofemoral nerve may be damaged during a psoas hitch procedure, since its lies on the belly of psoas major. If the nerve is caught within one of the hitch stitches the patient may either complain of loss of sensation in the skin overlying the hemi-scrotum or labia or develop chronic pain in this location. The femoral nerve may also be damaged by placement of hitch stitches deep into the psoas major (if the psoas minor tendon, the usual site for the stitches, is absent).
- Acute flexion of the thigh against the abdomen can lead to obturator nerve compression as it crosses the obturator crest of the superior pubic ramus. Paralysis of thigh abduction results. Acute flexion of the thigh can also compress the femoral nerve against the superior pubic ramus. Positioning a patient in an exaggerated lithotomy position carries these risks. Take care to avoid pressure on the saphenous nerve against leg supports and of the common peroneal nerve as its loops around the head of the fibula.
- Upper limb nerve palsies can also occur in relation to patient positioning, e.g. an ulnar nerve palsy can occur when the arm is abducted by as little as 90° for a lengthy procedure

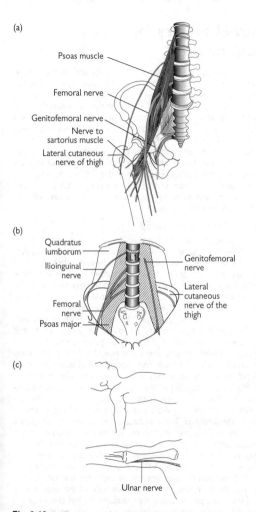

(a)

Psoas muscle

Femoral nerve

Genitofemoral nerve
Nerve to
sartorius muscle
Lateral cutaneous
nerve of thigh

(b)

Quadratus
lumborum
Ilioinguinal
nerve

Genitofemoral
nerve

Lateral
cutaneous
nerve of the
thigh

Femoral
nerve
Psoas major

(c)

Ulnar nerve

Fig. 2.19 (a) The course of the femoral nerve in the abdomen and pelvis; (b) Other abdominal wall nerves that can be injured; (c) A traction injury to the ulnar nerve is possible if the area is abducted for a prolonged time. Redrawn from Notley *et al.*, 2007, *Urology and the law*. Informa Healthcare, permission sought.

References

1 Hall, Koch, Smith (1995).
2 Burnett, Brendler (1995).

Small bowel surgery for urological surgery

Small bowel is frequently used in urinary diversions and reconstructive surgery. Avoid using bowel at a point of anastomosis from a previous bowel resection, bowel which has been irradiated, or bowel which is involved by coexistent bowel disease (e.g. inflammatory bowel disease). Be prepared to be flexible during the operation; the segment of bowel you intend to use may be unsuitable. For small bowel, 24–48 hr of clear fluids pre-operatively provides sufficient bowel preparation. Formal bowel preparation is not necessary. Where large bowel is used, some surgeons use formal mechanical bowel preparation, while others no longer formally prep the bowel. Ensure that the patient is seen by a stoma therapist pre-operatively and several potential stoma sites are marked, giving you the option of an alternative site if the bowel will not safely reach the preferred site without tension.

Small bowel anastomosis: sutured

There are many ways to join small bowel. The principles of all anastamoses are the same. An anastomosis should be tension free, well vascularized, and have mucosa-to-mucosa apposition. The best anastomosis is one that does not leak, bleed, or devascularize—it matters less how it is done. For a sutured anastomosis, our preference is a single-layer sero-muscular anastomosis. We avoid the use of bowel clamps (even soft ones) so as to minimize any trauma to the vascular supply of the bowel (efflux of bowel contents from the cut ends of the bowel can usually be removed with small swabs). Support the two ends to be joined on a large swab, and oppose the two ends. Place your first sutures on the mesenteric border, the so-called angle of grief, since it is here that bowel leaks are most likely to occur (because the fat at the mesenteric border can obscure the bowel wall, thereby preventing adequate bites of the serosa and submucosa from being taken). Place a 3/0 absorbable stitch through the serosa and submucosa (Fig. 2.20) on this mesenteric border, taking care not to damage mesenteric vessels. Cut one end short and leave one end long; secure an artery forceps to the long end. This stay suture can be used to manipulate the bowel, thereby avoiding the need to use forceps which can crush the bowel and impair its vascularity and subsequent healing. Do the same on the anti-mesenteric border Place the two opposing stay sutures on a gentle stretch. Place interrupted serosal/submucosal sutures between the stays roughly 3–4 mm apart. Take care not to catch the opposite side of the bowel as you do so. Having completed one side of the anastamosis, release one of the stays, pass it under the anastomosis, and grasp again in artery forceps. As you do this the anastomosis flips over to expose the open side. Place interrupted sutures as before to complete the anastomosis. Before cutting the stays, check the patency of the anastomosis by squeezing it gently between thumb and forefinger.

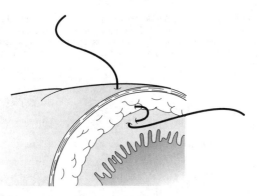

Fig. 2.20 Serosal and submucosal suture placement for small bowel anastomosis.

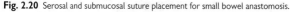

Small bowel anastomosis: stapled

Types of stapler

Two broad types of stapler are used in open urological surgery: those that simply lay down a row (usually a double row of offset staples), and those that lay down staples (usually two double rows of staples) and cut between the rows. Within each broad type of stapling device the staplers vary in the length of the staple line (typically 45–100 mm) and in the depth of the staples for different tissue thicknesses (e.g. 2.5–4.8 mm). Staples are either titanium or absorbable. Most staplers are 'single use' (i.e. they can only be used for a single case and cannot be re-sterilized), but they can be reloaded during the case and fired several times (check with the manufacturer) before the stapler has to be discarded.

It is our preference to to staple a small bowel anastomosis side to side (Fig. 2.21). A side-to-side anastomosis gives a larger lumen size than an end-to-end anastomosis, and it also overcomes the potential difficulty of performing an end-to-end anastomosis when there is a discrepancy in the size of the lumens of the bowel loops. When dividing the bowel (e.g. in the preparation of an ileal conduit), use a 60 mm long straight cutting stapler (e.g. GIA60, Autosuture). This leaves you with two ends of bowel sealed by a double row of offset staples. Lay the two ends of bowel to be joined next to each other with the anti-mesenteric borders together. Using heavy scissors, trim the corner off the staple line on the anti-mesenteric border of both limbs of the anastomosis. Insert one blade of the GIA60 stapler down each limb of the anastomosis; use the full length of the blades (Fig. 2.21). Before locking the blades, check that the mesentery will not be squeezed between the blades of the stapler. Lock the blades together and activate the stapler. Inspect the staple line on the inside and outside of the anastamosis. Check for haemostasis and use diathermy or place 3/0 absorbable sutures as required to stop any bleeding. Place 3/0 absorbable sutures through the serosal surface of the bowel at the apices of the anastamotic staple lines (one on each side) to take tension off the staples. Place two 3/0 stay sutures through the ends of the bowel towards the mesenteric borders and use these to hold the open anastamosis in a straight line. Place a linear stapler (e.g. TA55, Autosuture) across the open anastamosis and fire the stapler to close the anastamosis (Fig. 2.22). Alternatively close the end of the bowel with a hand-sewn anastamosis. Check again for haemostasis.

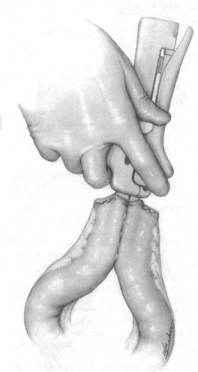

Fig. 2.21 A side-to-side small bowel anastomosis using a stapler. © 2006 United States Surgical, a division of Tyco Healthcare Group LP. Reprinted with permission.

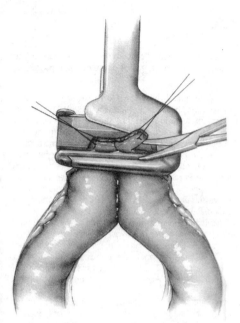

Fig. 2.22 Closure of a side-to-side small bowel anastomosis using a TA55 stapler. © 2006. United States Surgical, a division of Tyco Healthcare Group LP. Reprinted with permission.

Ileal conduit

Indications

Urinary diversion in the context of radical cystectomy, or for profound urinary incontinence where other techniques have failed or are not appropriate.

Technique

Midline trans-peritoneal incision. A minimum 15 cm segment of ileum is used, at least 15 cm from the ileocaecal junction (Fig. 2.23). When isolating a loop of ileum the distal mesenteric incision (i.e. the mesentery adjacent to the distal end of the loop) will be longer than the proximal mesenteric incision because the distal end needs to go all the way through the anterior abdominal wall, whereas the proximal end is going to sit on the retroperitoneum. Therefore there is no need to make a long proximal mesenteric incision, but the distal mesenteric incision needs to be longer. In fact, by making the proximal mesenteric incision as short as possible you minimize the number of blood vessels which need to be divided, thus maximizing the blood supply to the loop. Rejoin the bowel from which the segment of ileum has been isolated. The ileo-ileal anastomosis should be above the conduit (Fig. 2.24). Anastomose the small bowel using your preferred technique.

The divided ureters should be trimmed to the correct length. Insert stay sutures to avoid the need to handle the ureter with metal instruments. Spatulate the ureters for 2–3 cm using Pott's scissors. To join the ureters start at the heel. Use 4/0 Vicryl suture. Start on the left ureter. Pass from outside of the left ureter at the apex of the spatulation, and then from inside the right ureter to outside, again at the apex of the spatulation. Tie the knot on the outside and apply a clip to one end as a stay suture. This helps identify where the small bowel of the conduit

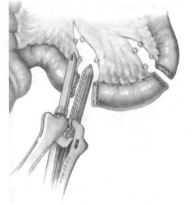

Fig. 2.23 Harvesting a segment of ileum for ileal conduit formation. © 2006. United States Surgical, a division of Tyco Healthcare Group LP. Reprinted with permission.

should be anastomosed to the ureters. Pass the needle underneath the conjoined ureters so that the suture lies between the two ureters. Now enter the right ureter from outside to inside, pass the suture across to the left ureter, and go from inside to outside on the left ureter. Continue in this fashion progressing distally, thereby creating a 'plate' of ureters onto which the isolated loop of small bowel will be anastomosed. Pass two 8Ch adult feeding tubes up the ureters, having first passed them through the conduit (we use 'Bardic' feeding tubes (BARD®)).

Make sure that the conduit lies below the anastomosed small bowel. To anastomose the isolated loop of small bowel to the ureteric plate, starting on the bowel pass a 3/0 Vicryl suture from outside the bowel to inside and then from inside the right ureter to outside the right ureter at the heel of the ureteric plate, previously marked by a long stay suture (Fig. 2.25). Thus the knot is on the outside. The anastomosis is completed on the outside of the bowel and ureter (i.e. not from the inside), going from outside to inside the bowel and then from inside to outside the ureter. Pass a second suture from outside to inside the bowel at the same point, roughly, as the first suture, and then from inside to outside the left ureter at the heel. Go up the right side of the bowel and the right ureter with the right-hand stitch, and then up the left side of the bowel and the left ureter with the left-hand stitch.

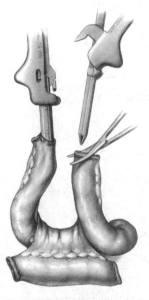

Fig. 2.24 Perform the small bowel anastomosis above the segment of small bowel that has been isolated for the conduit. © 2006. United States Surgical, a division of Tyco Healthcare Group LP. Reprinted with permission.

Check the integrity of your uretero-ileal anastomosis by filling a bladder syringe with 50 mL of saline and gently flush this into the conduit, looking for leaks. Place 'rescue' sutures of Vicryl as necessary.

Now retro-peritonealize the proximal end of the conduit (the uretero-ileal anastomosis) by fixing the cut edges of the peritoneum to the conduit. This contains post-operative urine leaks. It also protects the uretero-ileal anastomosis from damage if the abdomen is opened subsequently for another reason (e.g. general surgical operation).

(a)

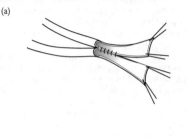

(b)

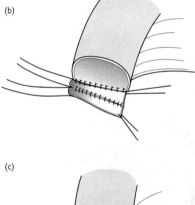

(c)

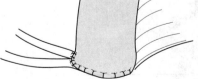

Fig. 2.25 Anastomosing the ureteric plate to the isolated segment of ileum.

Pick up the skin in an Allis forceps, tent it upwards, and then cut transversely with a scalpel. Cut out a disk of skin over the site which has been marked by the stoma therapist. Grab the underlying fat in an Allis forceps and use the coagulating diathermy finger switch to cut out a disk of fat until you reach the rectus sheath. Make a cruciate incision in the rectus sheath (Fig. 2.26). Place a 3/0 absorbable suture at each corner (four in total); keep the needles on the sutures and clip them. These will be used to secure the serosa of the bowel to the rectus fascia to prevent parastomal hernia formation. Insert a Babcock's forceps through the hole thus created and clip it onto the feeding tubes. It is often easier to deliver these through the skin hole before pulling the conduit through. Pass the Babcock's forceps back through the hole and gently grab the end of the ileal conduit. Ease it through the hole, pulling with the forceps and coaxing the conduit through with your fingers. Leave enough bowel sitting proud of the skin such that you will be able to produce a conduit that protrudes well above the skin surface (so that urine does not drip directly onto the skin). Then pass the previously placed sutures at each corner of the cruciate incision in the rectus fascia through the serosa of the bowel and tie them. Now pass a series of interrupted absorbable sutures through the skin, picking up the ileum about 1–2 cm from its distal end, and then, with the same suture, pick up the cut distal end of the ileum (Fig. 2.27). Tie the suture. This will have the effect of everting the edges of the conduit so that it sits proud of the skin surface rather than being flush with it.

Close the 'lateral space' (i.e. the space between the lateral abdominal side wall and the ileal conduit) with a few absorbable sutures. This will help prevent a loop of small bowel herniating through this space— a potential cause of post-operative bowel obstruction.

Place a tube drain down to the uretero-ileal anastomosis, making sure that this is adjacent to, but not touching, the anastomosis.

In very obese patients or where there is limited mobility of the bowel, a Turnbull loop stoma may be helpful. Here the distal end of the bowel is closed in two layers. A knuckle of the terminal loop is delivered through the stomal defect and the bowel is incised with the cutting diathermy on its anti-mesenteric border. The serosa is sutured to the anterior rectus fascia. The cut edges of the bowel are sutured to the skin edge. The blind end of the stoma should be cephalad (to allow adequate drainage).

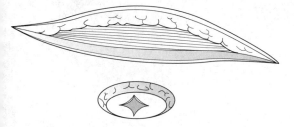

Fig. 2.26 Make a cruciate incision in the rectus sheath.

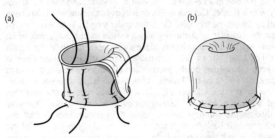

Fig. 2.27 (a) Pass a series of interrupted absorbable sutures through the skin, picking up the ileum about 1–2 cm from its distal end, and then, with the same suture, pick up the cut distal end of the ileum. (b) The bowel is turned back on itself once the sutures are tied, so securing the cut end of ileum to the skin.

Ileal conduit: post-operative care and complications and their management

Wound infection

Treat with antibiotics and wound care. Open the superficial layers of the wound to release pus.

Wound dehiscence

Rare. Requires resuturing in theatre under general anaesthetic.

Ileus

Common. Usually resolves spontaneously within a few days.

Small bowel obstruction

From herniation of small bowel through the mesenteric defect created at the junction between the two bowel ends. Continue nasogastric aspiration. The obstruction will usually resolve spontaneously. Reoperation is occasionally required where the obstruction persists or where there are signs of bowel ischaemia.

Leakage from the intestinal anastomosis

Leads to:
- Peritonitis: requires reoperation and repair, or refashioning of the anastomosis.
- Entero-cutaneous fistula: bowel contents leak from the intestine and through a fistulous track onto the skin. If low-volume leak (<500 mL/ 24 hr) it will usually heal spontaneously. Normal (enteral) nutrition can be maintained until the fistula closes (usually within a matter of days or a few weeks. If high-volume lek, spontaneous closure is less likely, and reoperation to close the fistula may be required.

Leakage from the uretero-ileal junction

May be suspected because of a persistently high output of fluid from the drain. Test this for urea and creatinine. Urine will have a higher urea and creatinine concentration than serum. If the fluid is lymph, the urea and creatinine concentration will be the same as that of serum. Arrange a loopgram (conduitogram). This will confirm the leak. Place a soft small catheter (12Ch) into the conduit to encourage antegrade flow of urine and assist healing of the uretero-ileal anastomosis. If the leakage continues, arrange bilateral nephrostomies to divert the flow of urine away from the area, and encourage wound healing.

Occasionally a uretero-ileal leak will present as a urinoma (this causes a persistent ileus). Radiologically assisted drain insertion can result in a dramatic resolution of the ileus, with subsequent healing of the uretero-ileal leak.

Hyperchloraemic acidosis

May be associated with obstruction of the stoma at its distal end or with infrequent emptying of the stoma bag (leading to back pressure on the conduit). Catheterize the stoma; this relieves the obstruction. In the long term, the conduit may have to be surgically shortened.

Acute pyelonephritis

Caused by the presence of reflux combined with bacteriuria.

Stomal stenosis

The distal (cutaneous) end of the stoma may become narrowed, usually as a result of ischaemia to the distal part of the conduit. Revision surgery is required if this stenosis causes obstruction leading to recurrent UTIs or back pressure on the kidneys.

Parastomal hernia formation

Around the site through which the conduit passes through the fascia of the anterior abdominal wall. Many hernias can be left alone. The indications for repairing a hernia are:
• Bowel obstruction.
• Pain.
• Difficulty with applying the stoma bag (distortion of the skin around the stoma by the hernia can lead to frequent bag detachment).

Repair the hernia defect by placing mesh over the hernia site via an incision sited as far as possible from the stoma itself so as to reduce the risk of wound infection.

Use of omentum in urological surgery

The excellent vascularity and lymphatic supply of the omentum provides it with excellent healing properties which can be used to assist healing of anastomoses (e.g. uretero-ileal, bowel) and fistula repairs by providing vascular support and assisting drainage of infected material.

Anatomy

The blood supply of the omentum is derived form the gastro-epipolic artery. The right gastro-epipolic artery is usually larger and in a more caudal position than the left gastroepipolic artery (Fig. 2.28). As a consequence it needs less mobilization to reach into the pelvis where the omentum is often used (in approximately a third of individuals the omentum can reach into the pelvis without the need for mobilization).

Technique of omental mobilization

The omentum is draped over the transverse colon and attached to it by adhesions. Start mobilization of the omentum by lifting it off the colon and, using a combination of blunt and sharp dissection, divide the adhesions which attach it to the transverse colon. Once the adhesions have been freed, lift the omentum upwards. In so doing the posterior wall of the stomach will be lifted upwards and exposed, and the gastro-epiploic artery will be seen along its free edge. If the omentum will not reach into the pelvis without tension, divide the left gastro-epiploic artery (a branch of the splenic artery) and sequentially divide the short gastric arteries as they pass between the gastroepipolic artery and the stomach. This is most easily done using a Ligasure cautery device. Alternatively, ligate each artery and divide it with scissors. Be sure that these ties are secure, because if they slip off the subsequent haemorrhage can be severe and difficult to control as the vessels retract within the fat of the omentum (Fig. 2.29). It is important to ligate each artery individually, partly to help prevent the ties from slipping off, but also to avoid 'bunching up' the omentum and so shortening it.

Anticipate an ileus lasting a few days after extensive omental mobilization.

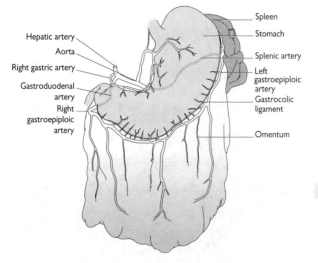

Fig. 2.28 The blood supply to the greater omentum.

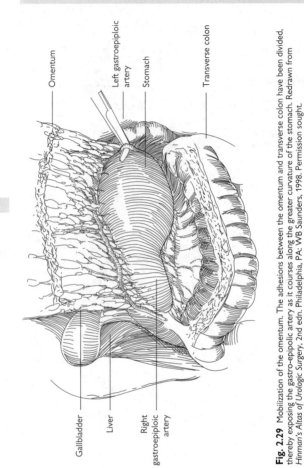

Fig. 2.29 Mobilization of the omentum. The adhesions between the omentum and transverse colon have been divided, thereby exposing the gastro-epipolic artery as it courses along the greater curvature of the stomach. Redrawn from *Hinman's Atlas of Urologic Surgery*, 2nd edn. Philadelphia, PA: WB Saunders, 1998. Permission sought.

Chapter 3

Bladder outlet obstruction

'LUTS' versus 'prostatism'

The terminology used to describe the symptom complex that was traditionally associated with obstruction due to BPH changed in the 1990s as
a consequence of finding that:

- Age-matched men and women have equivalent American Urological
  Association (AUA) symptom scores.[1,2]
- The 'classic' prostatic symptoms of hesitancy, poor flow, frequency,
  urgency, nocturia, and terminal dribbling have little relationship to
  prostate size, flow rate, residual urine volume, or urodynamic evidence
  of bladder outlet obstruction.[3]

The term 'lower urinary tract symptoms' (LUTS) is now used to describe
symptoms previously known as prostatism.[4] More recently, 'LUTS/BPH'
has been used to describe the symptoms of BPH. Precisely how you refer
to these symptoms does not matter very much. What is important is that
you remember the non-prostatic causes of urinary symptoms so that you
avoid operating on the prostate when the problem lies elsewhere.

References

1 Barry MJ, Fowler FJ Jr, O'Leary MP et al. The American Urological Association symptom index for benign prostatic hyperplasia. *J Urol* 1992; **148**:1549–57.

2 Lepor H, Machi G. Comparison of AUA symptom index in unselected males and females between fifty-five and seventy-nine years of age. *Urology* 1993; **42**:36–41.

3 Reynard JM, Yang Q, Donovan JL et al. The ICS-'BPH' study: uroflowmetry, lower urinary tract symptoms and bladder outlet obstruction. *Br J Urol* 1998; **82**:619–23.

4 Abrams P. New words for old: lower urinary tract symptoms for 'prostatism'. *BMJ* 1994; **308**:929–30.

Indications for treatment for LUTS/BPH

The indications are relative, since a catheter (urethral or suprapubic) can be used to bypass the obstructing prostate in cases of urinary retention:

- Troublesome lower urinary tract symptoms which fail to respond to changes in lifestyle or medical therapy.
- Recurrent acute urinary retention.
- Renal impairment due to bladder outlet obstruction (high-pressure *chronic* urinary retention).
- Recurrent haematuria due to benign prostatic enlargement.
- Bladder stones due to prostatic obstruction.

Clinical practice guidelines for LUTS/BPH

A number of clinical practice guidelines have been developed to help diagnosis and treatment decisions in men presenting with urinary symptoms.[1] There is considerable variation between guidelines in terms of the diagnostic tests that they recommend. Some recommend that a flow rate and residual urine volume should be measured, while in other guidelines these tests are optional. Guideline 'quality' has been assessed according to a set standard. Those that have been deemed high quality (they rank the evidence upon which they are based according to whether it is derived from randomized controlled trials or based on descriptive evidence such as case series or case reports) keep the diagnostic approach to the man presenting with LUTS simple, recommending measurement of symptom scores, urinalysis, completion of a voiding diary, and no other tests. Since there is such variability between the various guidelines, it is not possible to recommend one over the other. What guidelines you use will depend on what part of the world you practise in.

Reference

1 Irani J, Brown CT, van der Meulen J, Emberton M. A review of guidelines on benign prostatic hyperplasia and lower urinary tract symptoms: are all guidelines the same? *Br J Urol* 2003; **92**:937–42.

Assessment of men with LUTS thought to be due to BPH

Take a history, do a basic examination, and arrange simple investigations to determine whether the cause of the patient's symptoms is likely to lie in the prostate, in the urethra or bladder, or elsewhere.

'Red flag' symptoms and signs

- Macroscopic haematuria or dipstick or microscopic haematuria: arrange flexible cystoscopy and upper tract imaging to exclude the presence of bladder or renal cancer.
- Marked frequency and urgency, particularly when also combined with bladder pain, can occasionally be due to carcinoma *in situ* of the bladder. Have a low threshold for obtaining urine for cytology and for performing flexible cystoscopy.
- Bedwetting in an elderly man is very suggestive of high-pressure chronic retention.
- Rare causes of LUTS (e.g. neurological disease causing spinal cord or cauda equina compression, or pelvic or sacral tumours) suggested by:
  - Back pain.
  - Sciatica.
  - Ejaculatory disturbance.
  - Sensory disturbance in the legs, feet, and perineum.
  - Examine for loss of pericoccygeal or perineal sensation (sacral nerve roots 2–4); indicates an interruption to the sensory innervation of the bladder.
  - Arrange a sacral/lumbar/cauda equina MRI scan.

Examination

Look for:
- Gross distension of the abdomen (chronic retention).
- Digital rectal examination to detect prostate cancer.
- Adequate abduction and flexion of patient's hip joints if considering TURP, so you can be sure that you can gain access to perform a TURP.

Prostate size

Prostate size does not correlate with severity of symptoms and is not in itself an indication for treatment, but it is useful to have an idea of prostate size prior to embarking upon surgical treatment. DRE gives a *rough* estimate of prostate size, and if you suspect that the prostate is markedly enlarged, a transrectal ultrasound scan can be performed to provide a more accurate assessment of its volume. A large prostate could be an indication for an open prostatectomy.

Tests

PSA

Most current 'BPH' guidelines recommend a discussion with the patient about the pros and cons of PSA testing.

Urine culture

- In some cases infection may be the cause of the symptoms.
- Where you plan to do a TURP, a short course of antibiotics for a few days beforehand reduces the likelihood of post-operative septicaemia.

Frequency—volume chart

In patients with nocturia an estimatation of night-time voided volume will establish the presence or absence of nocturnal polyuria.

Serum creatinine

Measure serum creatinine to detect renal failure secondary to high-pressure urinary retention.

Post-void residual urine volume

Optional in some guidelines; recommended by others. Its day-to-day and even hour-to-hour variability limits the usefulness of residual urine estimation as a diagnostic test,[1] as does its inability to predict symptomatic outcome from TURP.[2]

Flow rate measurement

Optional in some guidelines and '*obligatory* prior to undertaking surgical treatment' in other guidelines. As with residual urine, flow rate measurements vary substantially on a given day.[3] Uroflowmetry cannot distinguish between low flow due to bladder outlet obstruction and low flow due to a poorly contractile bladder. While some studies suggest that men with poor outcomes are more likely to have had higher flows pre-operatively compared with those with good outcomes, others report equivalent symptomatic improvement whether pre-operative flow rate is high or low. In a trial of TURP versus watchful waiting, flow rate could not predict the likelihood of a good symptomatic outcome after TURP.[2]

Pressure—flow studies

Pressure–flow studies are probably better than residual urine volume and flow rate at predicting symptomatic outcome after TURP. However, most patients without obstruction have a good outcome and the time and cost of performing pressure—flow studies routinely is perceived by most urologists as not worth the effort.

Renal ultrasound

Useful if serum creatinine is elevated above the normal range. The percentage of patients with upper tract dilatation on ultrasound according to their serum creatinine level was: creatinine <115 μmol/L, 0.8%; creatinine 115–130 μmol/L, 9%; creatinine >130 μmol/L, 33%.[4]

References

1 Dunsmuir WD, Feneley M, Corry DA et al. The day-to-day variation (test–retest reliability) of residual urine measurement. Br J Urol 1996; 77:192–3.

2 Bruskewitz RC, Reda DJ, Wasson JH et al. Testing to predict outcome after transurethral resection of the prostate. J Urol 1997; 157:1304–8.

3 Reynard JM, Peters TJ, Lim C, Abrams P. The value of multiple free-flow studies in men with lower urinary tract symptoms. Br J Urol 1996; 77:813–18.

4 Koch WF, Ezz el Din KE, De Wildt MJ et al. The outcome of renal ultrasound in the assessment of 556 consecutive patients with benign prostatic hyperplasia. J Urol 1996; 155:186–9.

Transurethral resection of prostate (TURP)

Transurethral resection of prostate (TURP) remains the gold standard treatment for LUTS/BPH, recurrent urinary retention, and high-pressure chronic retention. While some alternative and less invasive treatments have approached TURP in terms of symptomatic outcome and improvement in voiding parameters (flow rates, residual urine volume and pressure—flow relationships), none has surpassed it. No other treatment has yet surpassed TURP in terms of durability of symptomatic improvement. Better patient selection, improved technology, and a greater awareness and earlier recognition of complications have resulted in a substantial reduction in morbidity and mortality from TURP.

Preparation for TURP in the weeks before surgery
Stopping anti-platelet drugs and NSAIDs
The risk of post-operative bleeding in patients taking these drugs should be balanced against the risks of stopping antiplatelet therapy. There are no hard and fast rules. The majority of studies support stopping these agents several days prior to elective surgery (10 days before for aspirin and 7 days before for the newer agents such as clopidogrel). It is our current practice to stop antiplatelet drugs, including NSAIDs, 10 days prior to surgery.

Typing and saving serum
Group and save serum (UK National Prostatectomy Audit found that approximately 8% of patients undergoing TURP for retention and 3% of those undergoing TURP for symptoms required >2 units of blood).

Immediate pre-operative preparation for TURP
Antibiotics
Positive blood cultures and the risk of septicaemia are reduced by routine antibiotic prophylaxis.[1,2] The optimum antibiotic prophylaxis prior to TURP has not been established. Seek the advice of your local microbiology department with regard to the local bacterial flora and patterns of antibiotic resistance. We give antibiotic prophylaxis for all patients undergoing TURP. Our choice of antibiotic is based on urine culture results done some weeks before surgery (a midstream specimen in those not in retention and a catheter specimen in those who present with urinary retention). If an organism is grown which is sensitive to a specific antibiotic, start treatment with this antibiotic 48 hr before operation and continue for a total of 10 days. If the urine is sterile, we use oral nitrofurantoin 100 mg taken 1 hr before the patient is called to the operating theatre, with a dose of IV gentamicin (1.5 mg/kg weight) at induction of anaesthesia. When the catheter is removed a few days after surgery, we again administer a prophylactic dose of oral nitrofurantoin 100 mg 1 hr before catheter removal.

Antibiotics for patients with heart murmurs and artificial heart valves

For patients with heart murmurs or with prosthetic heart valves give IV amoxicillin 1 g plus gentamicin 120 mg at induction of anaesthesia, with an additional dose of oral amoxicillin 500 mg 6 hr later. Substitute vancomycin 1 g for those who are penicillin allergic.[3]

Antibiotic prophylaxis for patients with joint replacements

Bacteraemia can cause haematogenous seeding of total joint replacements, both soon after joint replacement and for many years post-joint replacement. Advice (conflicting!) about antibiotic prophylaxis in such patients is available from two sources.

AAOS and AUA joint guidelines[4]

Urological procedures can be stratified according to risk of bacteraemia.
- Higher risk for bacteraemia—prophylaxis should be considered:
  - Stone manipulation including ESWL.
  - Any procedure involving transmural incision into the urinary tract.
  - Any endoscopic procedure of upper tract (ureter, kidney).
  - Any procedure involving the use of bowel segments.
  - Transrectal prostate biopsy.
  - Any procedure or condition that involves entry into the urinary tract (ISC, urinary retention, indwelling catheter, history of recurrent UTIs, urinary diversion).
- Lower risk for bacteraemia—prophylaxis not indicated on the basis of the orthopaedic implant alone (but may be indicated because of the urological procedure itself):
  - Endoscopic procedures in urethra or bladder not involving stone manipulation or incision (e.g. fulguration of bladder lesions, biopsy of bladder).
  - Open or laparoscopic procedures without stone manipulation or incision into the urinary tract.
  - Catheterization for drainage (both transurethral or percutaneous).
- Antibiotic prophylaxis is *not* indicated for:
  - Urological patients who have pins, plates or screws, or most patients with total joint replacements.
- Antibiotics should be given to:
  - All patients undergoing urological procedures, including TURP, within 2 years of a prosthetic joint replacement.
  - Those who are immunocompromised (e.g. rheumatoid patients, those with systemic lupus erythematosus, those with drug-induced immunosuppression including steroids).
  - Those with comorbidities including a history of previous joint infection, haemophilia, HIV infection, diabetes, and malignancy.

Recommended prophylaxis A single dose of a quinolone, e.g. ciprofloxacin 500 mg 1–2 hr pre-operatively plus ampicillin 2 g IV and gentamicin 1.5 mg/kg 30–60 min pre-operatively (substitute vancomycin 1 g IV for penicillin-allergic patients). It is obviously sensible to culture the patient's urine pre-operatively and use alternative drugs if a specific organism is grown.

Working Party of the British Society for Antimicrobial Chemotherapy[3]
States that 'patients with prosthetic joint implants (including total hip replacements) do not require antibiotic prophylaxis ... The Working Party considers that it is unacceptable to expose patients to the adverse effects of antibiotics when there is no evidence that such prophylaxis is of any benefit.'

This advice is based on the rationale that joint infections are caused by skin organisms that get onto the prosthesis at the time of the operation and that the role of bacteraemia as a cause of seeding, outside the immediate post-operative period, has never been established.

Prophylaxis against deep venous thrombosis and pulmonary embolism

Patients undergoing TURP are in a hypercoagulable state.[5] In contemporary studies of complications following TURP, 0.1–0.2% of patients experience a pulmonary embolus.[6]

Use above knee TED stockings (thromboembolism stockings) until the patient is discharged and intermittent pneumatic compression boots during the operation and until the patient starts to mobilize after the operation. Encourage early post-operative mobilization. We avoid low-dose heparin unless there is a history of DVT or PE.

Management of patients on warfarin therapy (the same protocol can be used for <u>all</u> major surgery)[7]

A patient on warfarin for atrial fibrillation has a risk of stroke of up to 0.3% during the 4–6 days for which their INR is subtherapeutic.[8] For a patient on warfarin because of venous thromboembolism, the risk of a recurrent DVT while off warfarin is approximately 40% within a month of the first DVT and approximately 10% at 3 months. For such patients it is best to postpone surgery for 3 months. For patients on warfarin because of a prosthetic heart valve, the risk of a stroke when warfarin is stopped is up to ~0.4% per day during which INR is subtherapeutic.[8]

One study suggests that transurethral resection may be performed safely despite warfarin treatment.[9] For those who are not happy to perform TURP on a fully warfarinized patient (and this includes the author), the ACCP Consensus Conference on Antithrombotic Therapy gives advice on management of oral anticoagulation around the time of surgical procedures.[10]

For patients with a **low risk of thromboembolism** (e.g. DVT >3 months ago or atrial fibrillation with no prior history of stroke), warfarin should be stopped approximately 4 days prior to surgery to allow the INR to return to a near-normal level, and prophylaxis such as subcutaneous unfractionated heparin (e.g. 5000 units every 8–12 hr) or LMWH should be administered only at the time of surgery (the last dose of heparin should be given 12 hr before surgery). It takes approximately 4 days for the INR to return to ≤1.5 in most patients, at which level surgery is safe.[11] For patients with an intermediate risk of thromboembolism (e.g. DVT 1–3 months previously, those with artificial aortic valves) warfarin should be stopped approximately 4 days prior to surgery to allow the INR to return to a near-normal level, and low-dose subcutaneous unfractionated heparin (5000 units every 8–12 hr) or LMWH should be started 2 days before surgery.

For patients with a **high risk of thromboembolism** (e.g. DVT within the last month, those with mechanical mitral heart valves or old model (ball and cage) aortic valves, atrial fibrillation with a history of stroke), stop warfarin approximately 4 days prior to surgery, allow INR to return to a near-normal level and start unfractionated heparin as an IV infusion in hospital or SC LMWH. The activated partial thromboplastin time (APTT) should be kept at ~2.5. Intravenous heparin is stopped 3–4 hours before surgery so that the anticoagulant effect has worn off at the time of surgery and is restarted as soon as possible after surgery. The precise timing depends on the colour of the urine in the irrigant fluid. A controversial group is those with non-caged prosthetic aortic valves and no other risk factor. It is acceptable not to use 'bridging' therapy with a treatment dose of heparin, particularly if the bleeding risk is high.

Anaesthesia for TURP

Spinal anaesthesia is routinely used by many anaesthetists. There are certain advantages to the patient being awake during the procedure. Alhough TUR syndrome is uncommon, one of the earliest indications that this is occurring can come from the awake patient reporting visual distur-bance such as flashing lights. This early warning can allow the surgeon to end the procedure rapidly.

Position on the table

Tables adapted for endoscopic surgery have the advantage that they can be raised or lowered by the surgeon. Many different types of leg support are available. Ensure that the legs are kept in the correct position with the thighs making an angle of no more than 45° with the plane of the table. The lithotomy position produces an awkward angulation of the prostate as well as sometimes causing backache afterwards.

Operative technique
Urethrotomy
Use a 24 or 26Ch resectoscope sheath. If the urethra is at all tight, gently dilate the meatus with Clutton's sounds (Fig. 3.1) or pass an Otis urethrotome and incise the urethra at 12 o'clock along its last 4 or 5 cm. The urethrotome is passed with its blades closed, right into the bladder (Fig. 3.2a). Withdraw it past the external sphincter, open the blades to 30Ch in the mid-bulb (Figs 3.2b and 3.2c), advance the knife and withdraw the instrument.

The basic skills of transurethral resection
Cutting off the chip
Cut the chip either against the edge of the resectoscope sheath or by bringing the loop out completely before entering the sheath. Cut canoe-shaped chips (Fig. 3.3). Avoid bringing the loop too far inside the sheath, since sparks may 'jump' between the loop and the metal of the sheath and can damage the lens of the telescope (Fig. 3.4).

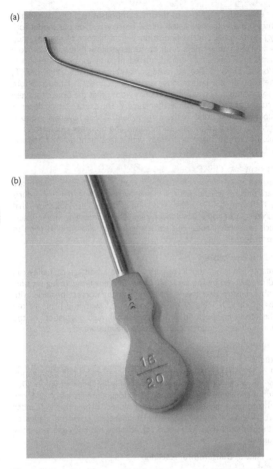

Fig. 3.1 (a) A Clutton's sound. (b) The Cluttons sound is 16Ch at the tip and 20Ch at the proximal end.

(a)

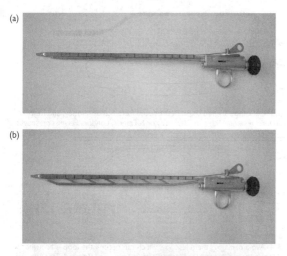

(b)

(c)

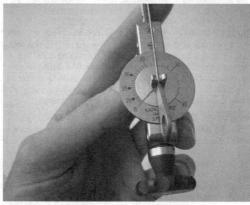

Fig. 3.2 (a) The Otis urethrotome is passed with its blades closed. (b) The blades of the urethrotome have been opened. (c) The dial of the urethrotome is used to calibrate the instrument to the appropriate dimensions.

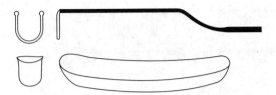

Fig. 3.3 Cut canoe-shaped chips. Reproduced from Blandy, Notley, and Reynard, *Transurethral resection*, 5th edn. 2005, Taylor & Francis, London. Permission sought.

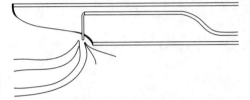

Fig. 3.4 Avoid damaging the telescope, which can occur if the loop is brought too far inside the sheath. Reproduced from Blandy, Notley, and Reynard, *Transurethral resection*, 5th edn. 2005, Taylor & Francis, London. Permission sought.

Develop a rhythm when resecting. Lift up the handpiece and sink the loop into the prostate at the start of the stroke (Fig. 3.5). Once you have safely established the landmarks, save time by making sure that every stroke removes the maximum amount of tissue (the depth of the chip should be at least that of the loop and its length as long as that of the lateral lobe, even if this means moving the sheath outwards, always making sure that you know the exact situation of the verumontanum).

Haemostasis
Most of the light bleeding during TURP is from small veins which are cut as you resect the adenoma. This type of bleeding is minimized by using a continuous flow irrigating system, but it should be stopped as you go along in order to keep a clear view. Any arterial bleeder should be controlled as soon as you see it by touching it with the loop and applying the coagulating current briefly. Once you have dealt with the bleeding arteries, slow down the irrigant flow to check for venous bleeding. Veins are more difficult to detect than arteries because of their lower pressure—venous bleeding may be tamponaded by high-pressure irrigation.

Maintain a clear view
You must able to see what you are doing. The view may be obscured by:
• Bubbles on the lens caused by hydrolysis of the water by the electric sparks cannot be avoided. However, larger bubbles can be caused by faulty connections of the tubing and bag of irrigating fluid. Continuous flow resectoscopes minimize both types of bubble, but do not entirely avoid them. When bubbles form, stop the flow of irrigant briefly and allow water to run out. If the bubbles persist, tap the telescope smartly a few times.

- Check the eyepiece of the scope and also that the camera is clean. Avoid getting them wet or covered in lubricating gel.
- The most common cause of sudden loss of vision is loss of irrigant flow, usually because an inattentive nurse has let the bag run out. This happens on a boringly regular basis, so keep an eye on the bag from time to time and warn the nurse that you need more fluid well in advance. Sometimes the inflow becomes kinked or twisted. In continuous flow systems there may be imbalance between the negative pressure in the suction and the rate of inflow of the irrigating fluid. For this reason inflow and outflow taps must be under the control of the surgeon.
- Whatever system of irrigation is used the inflow will stop when the bladder is so full that it can take no more. Since this means that the pressure inside the bladder has risen, this is a state of affairs which should never be allowed to occur. This can occur with continuous irrigation, although it is much less likely to do so. If it does, the balance between inflow and outflow is wrong and must be adjusted. Most surgeons develop a sixth sense as to when the bladder is nearly full and when it is time to empty it out, and most resectoscopes begin to leak before this critical moment has been reached.
- Sometimes a chip of prostate or bladder tumour will be stuck to the lens or jammed between loop and sheath. In either case it is necessary to remove the handpiece. The lens should be cleaned using the jet of irrigating fluid or a piece of sterile lint. Blood that has been allowed to coagulate on the lens is a different matter. Use a broken wooden orange stick such as used for microbiological cultures; the wood does not scratch the optical glass.

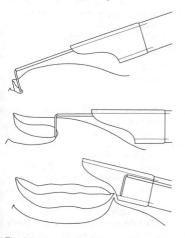

Fig. 3.5 Lift up the handpiece and sink the loop into the prostate at the start of the stroke; depress the sheath to cut the chip off. Reproduced from Blandy, Notley, and Reynard, *Transurethral resection*, 5th edn. 2005, Taylor & Francis, London. Permission sought.

Evacuation of the chips

Use an Ellik evacuator to evacuate resected chips. The bulb allows the irrigating fluid to pass in and out of the bladder, while allowing the chips and clot to float out of the bladder and fall down into the chamber. Used it gently—vigorous 'Elliking' can rupture the bladder (particularly in the context of TURBT in old ladies with thin bladders and who have undergone bladder tumour resection). The irrigation inflow valve can be left open as a 'safety valve' to take some of the pressure off the bladder each time the Ellik is squeezed. Disposable single-use sterile Elliks are now used in many hospitals, partly because of concern about adequacy of sterilization of the components of the old multi-use Elliks and also as a specimen pot to send the chips to the pathologist (Fig. 3.6). Disposable Elliks have the added advantage of a flap valve which stops evacuated tissue from flying back into the bladder. Also, they do not break when you drop them on the floor!

Technique of prostate resection for benign prostatic enlargement

Several different techniques of transurethral resection have been described. All aim to remove all the adenomatous tissue from the inner zone, leaving the compressed outer zone intact—the so-called 'surgical capsule.' The idea is to mimic enucleation of the prostate at open prostatectomy. Many resectionists resect far less tissue than what would be removed at open surgery. Radical TURP (resection right down to the prostatic capsule) compared with 'minimal' TURP gives equivalent reduction in symptom score and residual urine volume and equivalent improvement in flow rate at 10 years, although treatment failure is somewhat higher in the minimal resection group than in the radical resection group.[12] This somewhat higher failure rate in the minimal TURP group must be balanced against the higher stricture rate in the radical TURP group (3% versus 14%).

The key to prostatic resection is to:
- Establish the landmarks.
- Remove the main bulk of tissue.
- Tidy up.

Landmarks

The distal limit of resection is the verumontanum, which lies just proximal to the membranous urethra (the external sphincter). The proximal limit of resection is the bladder neck. Having identified the verumontanum and the external sphincter, the next step is to find the ring of muscle at the bladder neck in the posterior middle line. Define this proximal limit so as to prevent inadvertent resection of the trigone or the ureteric orifices. In some patients there is virtually no adenoma in the region of the middle lobe, and the first cut in the midline may reveal muscle fibres immediately under the urothelium. In others it is necessary to resect a considerable volume of adenoma (middle lobe) before the bladder neck is exposed (Fig. 3.7). Once the middle lobe has been resected, coagulate Badenoch's arteries at 5 and 7 o'clock if these have not been completely controlled already (Fig. 3.8).

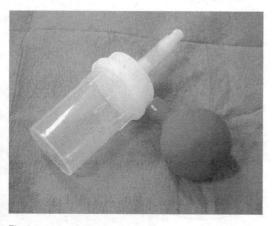

Fig. 3.6 Disposable Ellik evacuator.

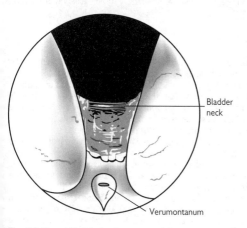

Bladder neck

Verumontanum

Fig. 3.7 The middle lobe has been resected. Reproduced from Blandy, Notley, and Reynard, *Transurethral resection*, 5th edn. 2005, Taylor & Francis, London. Permission sought.

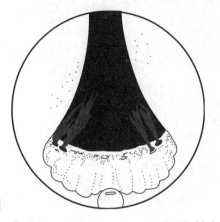

Fig. 3.8 Coagulate Badenoch's arteries at 5 and 7 o'clock. Reproduced from Blandy, Notley, and Reynard, *Transurethral resection*, 5th edn. 2005, Taylor & Francis, London. Permission sought.

Removing the adenoma
Method 1
Rotate the resectoscope to the 12 o'clock position. Your goal is to remove one of the lateral lobes from the capsule. Start by taking one or two careful chips at 1 o'clock until the bladder neck fibres and the capsule are disclosed, remembering that the prostate is very thin anteriorly (Fig. 3.9). Deepen the trench that you have started until the lateral lobe falls backwards into the space left by removal of the middle lobe. You may now see the arteries of Flocks at 2 o'clock. Coagulate these.

Now remove the lump of lateral lobe which has fallen inwards and away from the capsule. This part of the resection is usually relatively bloodless since the main arteries have already been controlled at 2 and 5 o'clock. Trim the top of the lateral lobe away in a series of even cuts, keeping the surface flat rather than hollowing out the lateral lobe (Fig. 3.10).

Check the position of the veru montanum and bladder neck, and then turn your attention to the other side, again making a trench to detach the other lateral lobe and resecting it once it has fallen into the midline (Fig. 3.11).

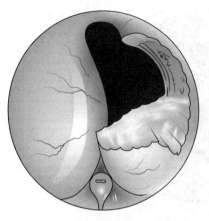

Fig. 3.9 Cut a lateral trench starting at 1 o'clock and working downwards, thus deepening the trench. Reproduced from Blandy, Notley, and Reynard, *Transurethral resection*, 5th edn. 2005, Taylor & Francis, London. Permission sought.

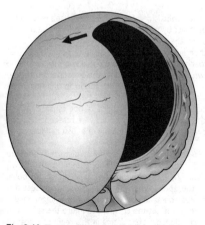

Fig. 3.10 The lateral lobe has been removed. Reproduced from Blandy, Notley, and Reynard, *Transurethral resection*, 5th edn. 2005, Taylor & Francis, London. Permission sought.

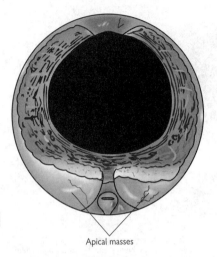

Apical masses

Fig. 3.11 Both lateral lobes have been removed. Reproduced from Blandy, Notley, and Reynard, *Transurethral resection*, 5th edn. 2005, Taylor & Francis, London. Permission sought.

Method 2
Here the bulk of the lateral lobes is removed in a circular sequence after removing the middle lobe. Start by taking one lateral lobe from the bottom upwards (Fig. 3.12), across the commissure between the lateral lobes, and then down the other lateral lobe to the starting point (Fig. 3.13) As your resection approaches the anterior commissure, a mass of tissue will be seen hanging down. Remember again that the prostate is very thin here. Do not hollow it out, but trim it away with the loop pointing laterally rather than upwards. The resection can then be carried across the midline at 12 o'clock, bearing in mind that there is not much depth of adenoma in this part of the gland. Continue the clockwise resection until the rest of the lateral lobe is removed, sparing only the tissue adjacent to the veru montanum.

When the adenoma is very large the anatomy is distorted, and the lumps of adenoma in the apex of each lateral lobe extend well down below the verumontanum. The external sphincter is in danger of being damaged when resecting the apex. When the time comes to resect this apical tissue, great care must be taken to lift it up with a finger in the rectum so that the loop does not cut the corner and injure the sphincter. It is equally important to refrain from coagulating in this region for fear of injuring the sphincter.

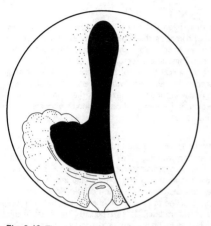

Fig. 3.12 The right lateral lobe is resected, starting at the 7 o'clock position. Reproduced from Blandy, Notley, and Reynard, *Transurethral resection*, 5th edn. 2005, Taylor & Francis, London. Permission sought.

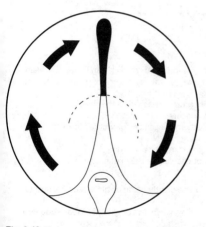

Fig. 3.13 The resection is continued in a clockwise direction. Reproduced from Blandy, Notley, and Reynard, *Transurethral resection*, 5th edn. 2005, Taylor & Francis, London. Permission sought.

Tidying up

The apical tissue which has been left behind is removed very carefully, taking great care to avoid damaging the sphincter. Repeatedly check the position of the veru montanum and sphincter. Take only very short chips. It often helps to insert one finger in the rectum to lift up the veru montanum, effectively offering the apical tissue to the loop rather than digging into the tissue. The finger in the rectum provides a very precise sensation of the amount of tissue remaining and the nearness of the loop. Bleeding is seldom severe in the region of the apex, and one should be very sparing in the use of the coagulating current.

Perforations

At the end of a resection it is usual to see little patches of fat which are essentially small capsular perforations. Small perforations are not dangerous, and there is no need to drain the retropubic space even though there is always some extravasation of the irrigating fluid into it. Perforations under the trigone can occur during resection of the middle lobe and it is possible for the resectoscope to pass under the trigone, between the bladder muscle and Denonvilliers fascia. It is particularly important in this situation to pass a catheter on an introducer so that the catheter rides up over the trigone, rather than under it.

Once all the chips have been evacuated, pass a 22Ch catheter, inflate the balloon with 30–40 mL of water and irrigate the bladder continuously with saline. Do not hesitate to remove the catheter and reinsert the resectoscope if haemostasis is not perfect. A few minutes of extra care at this stage may save hours of misery later on.

Trouble-shooting

The loop won't cut

Check that:

- The loop is sitting firmly in its holder. A 'click' can be felt and heard as the loop fits into the holder on the hand-piece of the resectoscope.
- The loop is not broken.
- The diathermy plate is securely attached to the thigh.
- The diathermy lead is attached to the machine.
- The wire within the diathermy lead has not worked loose at either end.
- The irrigating fluid is glycine, rather than saline.
- If the loop still does not cut, change the diathermy machine.

I can't stop the bleeding

- Compress the tissue to one or other side of the bleeding artery to compress the artery.
- Check for 'bounce' bleeding, when a strong jet of blood rebounds off the opposite wall of the prostatic fossa to that where you think the bleeding is coming from.
- Is the bleeding artery shooting straight out at you? Advance the resectoscope beyond the bleeder, angulate it to compress the vessel, and then slowly withdraw the sheath until the opening of the artery is seen by the emergence of a puff of blood.

- Look just inside the bladder neck, particularly at the 12 o'clock position where a small bleeding artery can be easily missed.
- Tamponade venous bleeding by passing a catheter into the bladder and inflate the balloon with 40–50 mL of water. Then pull it firmly down to compress the bladder neck where many of the bleeding veins are located. Maintain traction for 10 min. Make sure that the scrub nurse does not to clear the equipment away, so you can re-insert the resectoscope to achieve better haemostasis. It is far easier and faster to sort the bleeding out while the patient is on the operating table anaesthetized and the equipment is still available, than to bring them back from recovery and start all over again.
- Once you are happy that there are no more bleeding vessels to control, reinsert the catheter and maintain traction by means of a Salvaris swab: two gauze swabs are tied moderately tightly around the catheter and pushed up against the glans penis. These swabs should be removed after 20–30 min, otherwise a pressure sore may develop on the glans.

Additional reading

1 Mak S, Amoroso P. Stop those antiplatelet drugs before surgery. *Br J Urol* 2003; **91**:593–4.
2 Meyer JP, Gillatt DA, Lush R, Persad R. Managing the warfarinized uological patient. *BJU Int* 2003; **92**:351–4.

References

1 Hall JC, Christiansen KJ, England P et al. Antibiotic prophylaxis for patients undergoing transurethral resection of the prostate. *Urology* 1996; **47**:852.
2 Hargreave TB, Botto B, Rikken GHJM et al. European Collaborative Study of Antibiotic Prophylaxis for Transurethral Resection of the Prostate. *Eur Urol* 1993; **23**:437–43.
3 *British National Formulary*. London:BMA and Royal Pharmaceutical Society, 2003.
4 American Academy of Orthopaedic Surgeons (AAOS) and the American Urological Association (AUA). Advisory statement. *J Urol* 2003; **169**:1796.
5 Bell CR, Murdock PJ, Pasi KJ, Morgan RJ. Thrombotic risk factors associated with transurethral prostatectomy. *BJU Int* H1999; **83**:984–9.
6 Donat R, Mancey-Jones B. Incidence of thromboembolism after transurethral resection of the prostate (TURP). *Scand J Urol Nephrol* 2002; **36**:119–23.
7 Dunn AS, Turpie AG. Perioperative management of patients receiving oral anticoagulants: a systematic review. *Arch Int Med* 2003; **163**:901–8.
8 Spandorfer JM. The management of anticoagulation before and after procedures. *Med Clin North Am* 2001; **85**:1109–16.
9 Parr NJ, Lohn CS, Desmond AD. Transurethral resection of the prostate without withdrawal of warfarin therapy. *Br J Urol* 1989; **64**:623–5.
10 Ansell J, Hirsh J, Dalen J et al. Managing oral anticoagulant therapy. Sixth ACCP Consensus Conference on Antithombotic Therapy. *Chest* 2001; **119**:22S–38S.
11 Kearon C, Hirsh J. Management of anticoagulation before and after elective surgery. *New Engl J Med* 1997; **336**:1506–11.
12 Aagaard J, Jonler M, Fuglsig S et al. Total transurethral resection versus minimal transurethral resection of the prostate: a 10 year follow-up study of urinary symptoms, uroflowmetry and residual urine volume. *Br J Urol* 1994; **74**:333–6.

Transurethral resection of bladder tumours (TURBT)

Indications
- To provide accurate information with regard to bladder tumour grade and local stage.
- To treat superficial bladder tumours. TURBT is the mainstay of treatment for the majority of such tumours (supplemented by intravesical chemotherapy and immunotherapy).
- To palliate symptoms, such as bleeding, in invasive cancers where cystectomy or radiotherapy are not appropriate.
- To debulk large tumours prior to radiotherapy.

A small percentage of patients may be cured of their muscle invasive tumours by TURBT alone, but this is usually only apparent once they have undergone cystectomy and there is no tumour, as suggested by the absence of any residual tumour when the bladder is inspected by the pathologist.

Preparations for TURBT
As for TURP. Since TURBT is usually a shorter procedure than TURP above-knee TEDS may be all that is necessary for DVT prophylaxis (as long it is anticipated that the procedure will not last too long). If there are additional risk factors for venous thromboembolism, additional prophylaxis such as intermittent pneumatic calf compression may be necessary. Culture the urine beforehand and using a similar antibiotic regime to that used for TURP.

Some surgeons prefer to stop antiplatelet drugs. Heavy bleeding after TURBT is uncommon, but checking the patient's blood group and saving some serum prior to TURBT is a sensible precaution.

Formal resection versus fulguration of bladder tumours
Before deciding whether to resect a bladder tumour or to 'coagulate' it with a 'roly-ball', decide if your goal is removal of the tumour for accurate staging and grading in order to determine the need for adjuvant treatment such as cystectomy or radiotherapy. If this is the goal, a formal resection is required. However, if adjuvant treatment in the form of chemotherapy, radiotherapy, or cystectomy is not appropriate (e.g. the patient is very elderly and frail or has significant medical problems), simple coagulation of the tumour may be more appropriate. There is little point in resecting a tumour aggressively, thereby exposing the patient to the risk of uncontrollable bleeding or bladder perforation, if accurate staging information is not required and the tumour can be confidently removed by coagulation alone. The bladders of little old ladies can be particularly thin and not infrequently discretion (in the form of roly-ball diathermy coagulation) is the better part of valour. Rather than coagulating the tumour, it is easier to use the roly-ball with the cutting current, as the tissue treated in this way is vaporized rather than coagulated. Coagulated tissue tends to stick to the electrode, which has to be frequently cleaned as a consequence.

Small tumours

When the tumour is very small, remove it together with its base and some underlying bladder muscle with the sharp 'cold' cup forceps. Diathermy the base to stop any bleeding. When there are multiple superficial tumours, remove a few of them in this way for histological examination and coagulate the remainder with the roly-ball.

Moderate sized pedunculated tumours

The majority of superficial tumours are 1–3 cm in diameter and have a well-defined stalk. One or two large vessels can be seen entering the stalk from the adjacent mucosa.

Coagulate these with the roly-ball prior to formal resection. These tumours are too large to be removed with the cup biopsy forceps. Cut off the tumour, together with some underlying muscle, by a single cut of the diathermy loop. Coagulate the base. If you have not obtained a sample of the base of the tumour and the adjacent bladder wall, use the cold-cup forceps or the loop of the resectoscope to take an additional biopsy from the base of the stalk. This specimen can be sent in a separately labelled pot to indicate that it represents the part of the tumour that was immediately adjacent to the bladder wall. The cold-cup forceps may allow better preservation of the tumour architecture, which makes subsequent histological examination of the tumour easier.

Larger papillary tumours 4–6 cm in diameter

Use a continuous flow resectoscope to prevent the tumour moving away from you as the bladder fills up. Coagulate large blood vessels in the stalk of the tumour. Start resecting at the stalk, removing the fronds of tumour which hide the stalk from view. As soon as you see the edge of the stalk, apply the roly-ball electrode to the stalk to coagulate it so that the remainder of the resection is less vascular. Continue to resect more and more of the overlying tumour until it has all been removed. Haemostasis must be complete for, unlike the prostate, there is no way of effecting tamponade in the bladder.

Once resection is complete, empty the bladder and perform a careful bimanual examination; induration in the wall of the bladder remaining after resection suggests invasion of muscle. Once haemostasis is complete, set up continuous irrigation as for a routine prostatectomy.

Second-look TURBT

In some circumstances a second TURBT is carried out some weeks after the first resection. This is done where the preliminary pathology report suggests a high-grade non-invasive tumour. The rationale for second-look TURBT is to establish whether there really is no muscle invasion. In such cases, be particularly careful when taking further biopsies from the original tumour site, as the bladder wall here may be very thin and therefore prone to perforation. A cold-cup biopsy may be safer than a formal loop resection where the bladder appears especially thin.

Very large papillary tumours

Very rarely one encounters a large tumour or tumours which bleed heavily as soon as you start to resect. You have two options. Resect as many of the tumours that you can see, as long as you are able to maintain a clear field of view, and then come back to finish the job another day, rather than risk perforating the bladder. Alternatively, consider using prolonged high-pressure cystodistension (Helmstein's technique). This is very rarely used nowadays, and the majority of younger urologists will probably never have seen it, let alone used it. The technique is described here for the rare situations where it may still be required.[1,2] The technique requires a very long period of continuous epidural anaesthesia because it relies on compression of the tumour by the balloon to produce ischaemic necrosis.

Under continuous epidural anaesthesia, which will produce a measure of hypotension, a large balloon tied to a catheter is placed in the bladder. Specially made and tested balloons are available for this purpose, but initially Helmstein and others used ordinary toy balloons. The pressure inside the balloon is monitored continuously, as it is distended with glycine and the pressure is kept up for 6 hr. After the balloon is let down the ischaemic tissue of the tumour sloughs and an irrigating catheter may be necessary for the next few days until all the necrotic debris has come away. The bladder is re-examined after 3 weeks, by which time only the stumps of the previous tumours will be found. These are resected for staging in the usual way.

Invasive solid tumours

The purpose of TURBT for solid tumours, where the patient is a candidate for aggressive adjuvant treatment such as radiotherapy or cystectomy, is to provide accurate grading and local staging information. It is not necessary to resect all the tumour, particularly if cystectomy is planned, since the purpose of the cystectomy (obviously) is to remove all residual cancer. For patients where radiotherapy is contemplated many surgeons feel that TURBT controls bleeding and provides symptomatic relief from frequency and strangury, and many radiotherapists prefer that the bulk of the intravesical tumour should be removed, leaving less to be destroyed by irradiation. A good deep biopsy that reaches well into bladder muscle is required to obtain evidence of tumour grade and stage.

Resecting tumours in inaccessible places

Tumours on the anterior wall and in the dome can sometimes be very difficult to reach. In this situation, decompress the bladder slightly. This, combined with your free hand applying suprapubic pressure, may bring the tumour within reach of the loop of the resectoscope. It is sometimes easier to use the roly-ball to treat such tumours as this can be controlled more safely than the loop of the resectoscope. Sometimes inclining the table so that the patient is in the head-down position may make the resection a little easier, particularly where there is a large 'overhang' of lower abdomen. If these tricks fail, ask for the long resectoscope.

Tumours in diverticula can present a problem. The bladder wall in the depths of a diverticulum is thin, and it is safer to use cold-cup biopsy forceps to remove tumours here, with roly-ball diathermy for coagulation.

Resecting tumours in the region of a ureteric orifice

Resection of tumours located right over the ureteric orifice only rarely leads to subsequent scarring of the ureter. The usual outcome is a gaping ureteric orifice ('golf-hole' ureteric orifice). Management of this theoretical problem is based on anecdote. The use of pure cutting current will reduce the likelihood of scarring occurring, but clearly coagulating current may be required to stop bleeding. You can simply resect the tumour, leave the resected ureteric orifice alone, and hope for the best. Alternatively, an insulated guidewire can be positioned in the ureter before the resection is done, so that you can subsequently place a JJ stent easily. This can be left in place for a couple of weeks and then removed. Follow-up IVU will establish whether there is any significant hold-up in the flow of contrast through the ureter.

Occasionally the tumour completely obscures the ureteric orifice and in this situation one has no choice other than to resect it and then try to find the lumen of the ureter to allow placement of a JJ stent. Sometimes the lumen instantly becomes apparent; at other times it cannot be found. Again, follow-up IVU will determine whether the ureteric orifice is obstructed, in which case a nephrostomy with antegrade balloon dilatation and stenting can be used to deal with the stricture. It is our cumulative experience that ureteric obstruction is very rare and therefore such precautions are probably unnecessary.

References

1 Helmstein K. Treatment of bladder carcinoma by a hydrostatic pressure technique. *Br J Urol* 1972; **44**:434.

2 England HR, Rigby C, Shepheard BGF, Tresidder GC, Blandy JP. Evaluation of Helmstein's distension method for carcinoma of the bladder. *Br J Urol* 1973; **45**:593.

Immediate complications of TURP and TURBT

Extraperitoneal perforation during TURP

This occurs in 0.25% of cases.[1] In itself the perforation is not a problem, but the absorption of a large volume of irrigant fluid can be. Where it is obvious that you have created an exptraperitoneal perforation, achieve haemostasis as quickly as possible, abandon the resection if there is still much tissue to remove, and place a catheter. Come back another day for further resection if necessary.

Extraperitoneal and intraperitoneal perforation during resection of a bladder tumour

Small perforations into the perivesical tissues are not uncommon when resecting small tumours of the bladder. As long as you have secured good haemostasis and all the irrigating fluid is being recovered, no additional steps are required except that perhaps the catheter should be left in for about 5 days rather than 2 days.

Is the perforation extraperitoneal or intraperitoneal?

Sometimes this is difficult to determine, because both can cause marked distension of the lower abdomen—an intraperitoneal perforation by allowing escape of irrigating solution directly into the abdominal cavity, and an extraperitoneal perforation by expanding the retroperitoneal space, with fluid then diffusing directly into the peritoneal cavity. The fact that a suspected intraperitoneal perforation is actually extraperitoneal becomes apparent only at laparotomy when no hole can be found in the bladder.

When there is no abdominal distension, the volume of extravasated fluid is likely to be low and, if the perforation is small, it is reasonable to manage the case conservatively. Achieve haemostasis, pass a catheter, and send the patient to the recovery room. Make frequent visits to see the patient. If the patient remains well, you may continue conservative management. If things are not right—worsening abdominal pain and distension—proceed to laparotomy. In most cases everything will settle down and the hole in the bladder will heal spontaneously if a catheter is left *in situ* for 10 days. The patient can go home in a few days and will have been spared the morbidity and longer hospital stay that is required after laparotomy.

Where there is marked abdominal distension, whether the perforation is extraperitoneal or intraperitoneal is academic. Explore the abdomen to drain the large amount of fluid, which can compromise respiration in an elderly patient by splinting the diaphragm, and to check that loops of bowel adjacent to the site of perforation have not been injured at the same time.

Failing to make the diagnosis of an intraperitoneal perforation, particularly if bowel has been injured, is a worse situation than performing a laparotomy for a suspected intraperitoneal perforation, but then finding that the perforation was 'only' extraperitoneal.

The diagnosis of an intraperitoneal perforation is obvious if you can see loops of bowel. The tell-tale sign of the Ellik evacuator not sucking back can occur with both intraperitoneal and extraperitoneal perforation and therefore this tells you that something is wrong, rather than what is wrong.

When there is marked abdominal distension, or where it is obvious that the perforation has been made right through into the peritoneum or, as is often the case, the perforation is obscured and accompanied by haemorrhage, then it is necessary to explore the abdomen.

Approach the bladder through a Pfannenstiel incision or a lower abdominal incision, open it between stay sutures, evacuate the clot, control the bleeding, and sew up the hole. Open the peritoneum to see if there is any blood-stained fluid inside. Pull out adjacent loops of small and large bowel and look for diathermy damage. Close a hole in the small bowel transversely. Give serious consideration to 'covering' repair of a hole in the colon with a temporary loop-colostomy.

Peritoneal seeding of tumour has been reported following perforation at the time of TURBT.[2]

Perforation into the rectum

Rare: 0.25% of 4226 TURPs in the UK National Prostatectomy Audit.[1] Management is decided on a case-by-case basis. Involve a colorectal surgeon in subsequent management decisions. If the perforation is large, seriously consider a defunctioning colostomy with a catheter left *in situ* for about 3 weeks. If the perforation is small, an indwelling catheter for a few weeks may be all that is necessary. However, bear in mind that the injury will have been caused by the diathermy, rather than by a sharp knife, and as a consequence the edges of the perforated bowel will have been devitalized and may not heal. If in doubt, err on the side of performing a colostomy. If a defunctioning colostomy and a suprapubic cystostomy are used, most fistulae will heal within about 6 weeks.

Explosions in the bladder

Very rare.[3] The hydrogen and oxygen formed by hydrolysis of water by diathermy sparks, along with air introduced in the irrigating fluid, collects in a bubble at the vault of the bladder. This is sometimes an explosive mixture, so if you are resecting tumour from the vault, push down on the suprapubic region to indent the vault and displace the bubble away from the loop.

Obturator jump

If a bladder tumour is located on the lateral wall of the bladder or near the ureteric orifice, application of a low-frequency current may cause sudden contraction of the adductors as a consequence of stimulation of the obturator nerve. Perforation of the wall of the bladder with the cutting loop may occur. It is particularly easy to stimulate the obturator nerve just above and lateral to the ureteric orifice. If you see a tumour in this location, and it is small and the purpose of treating the tumour is for local control only, use the roly-ball to coagulate it rather than trying to resect it formally. If the patient is not a candidate for radical treatment of a muscle invasive bladder tumour, there is little point in exposing them to the potential risk of bladder perforation from an aggressive resection which causes an obturator kick.

If it is important to determine the precise stage of the tumour because you need to decide whether radical treatment such as cystectomy or radiotherapy will be required, and then you will have to perform formal resection of the tumour. Even if you do not need precise staging information, the tumour may simply be too large for adequate local control by roly-ball vaporization.

In these situations minimize obturator nerve stimulation and its effects:

- Turn down the current until it is barely cutting.
- Get two assistants to stand one on either side of the patient, and to grasp the patient's thighs and lower abdomen firmly, underneath the sterile drapes. This stabilizes the pelvis, preventing it from rocking to one side or the other if the obturator nerve is stimulated.
- Ask the anaesthetist to intubate the patient and paralyse their muscles. Curare-related agents work by blocking depolarization of the neuro-muscular end plates, but this blockade can be overcome by supra-maximal nerve stimulation.
- Just as you are about to start resecting, be prepared to withdraw the resectoscope quickly into the prostatic urethra so that if an obturator kick does occur, the end of the resectoscope will not go shooting through the bladder.

Erection occurring during resection

In the UK National Prostatectomy Audit[1] an erection caused the operation to be stopped in 0.2% of cases. The first sign that anything is amiss may be that the resectoscope seems to be unduly tight in the urethra, or that the view has become obscured by new bleeding. Feel the penis; early engorgement is quite obvious. Stop now, before it is too late.

The erection can be reversed by injecting phenylephrine 200 mcg diluted in normal saline directly into the corpus cavernosum.[4] This can be repeated. If the erection fails to subside immediately then you should seriously consider terminating the operation. It is better to come back another day rather than to lose one's way and risk damaging the sphincter.

Failure to recognize that an erection is taking place and failure to reverse it may result in the resectoscope being forced out of the urethra, with the result that the operator may easily mistake the external sphincter for the prostate, and resect it.

References

1 Neal DE. The National Prostatectomy Audit. *Br J Urol* 1997; **79**(suppl 2):69–75.
2 Myldo JH, Weinstein R, Shah S *et al.* Long term consequences from bladder perforation and/or violation in the presence of transitional cell carcinoma: results of a small series and a review of the literature. *J Urol* 1999; **161**:1128–32.
3 Hansen RE, Iversen P. Bladder explosions during uninterrupted transurethral resection of the prostate. *Scand J Urol Nephrol* 1979; **13**:211.
4 Montague DK, Jarow J, Broderick GA *et al.* American Urological Association guideline on the management of priapism. *J Urol* 2003; **170**:1318–240.

Length of resection and the TUR syndrome

How long can you safely resect for—the 1 hour rule

It has been handed down from generation to generation that resection must be completed within 60 min because of the risk of TUR syndrome. The origin of this rule seems to lie in the early days of transurethral resection when surgeons often gave their own spinal anaesthetic, and patients began to recover sensation after about an hour. Clearly, the longer the operation goes on, the more time there is for blood to be lost and irrigating fluid to enter the veins, and if the resection takes more than 1 hr, it usually means that the gland is very large.

TUR syndrome

Occurred in 0.5% of cases in the National Prostatectomy Audit.[1]

Symptoms and signs

Confusion, nausea, vomiting, hypertension, bradycardia, and visual disturbances.

Pathophysiology

Although 1.5% glycine avoids the risk of haemolysis, absorption of large quantities of irrigant fluid dilutes serum electrolytes. The TUR syndrome is characterized by biochemical, haemodynamic and neurological disturbances. Dilutional hyponatraemia is the most important and serious factor leading to the symptoms and signs. The serum sodium usually has to fall to below 125 mmol/L before the patient becomes unwell. The hypertension is due to fluid overload. Visual disturbances may be due to the fact that glycine is a neurotransmitter in the retina.

Predicting and preventing development of the TUR syndrome and definitive treatment

Try to avoid the development of the TUR syndrome by limiting resection time, avoiding aggressive resection near the capsule, and reducing the height of the irrigant solution. Increasing the height of the irrigation fluid from 60 to 70 cm above the patient increases fluid absorption by a factor of 2.[2]

For long and bloody resections assume that the patient is going to develop the TUR syndrome and take corrective measures before symptoms occur. Send a sample of blood for sodium measurement, and give IV frusemide 20–40 mg to start off-loading the excess fluid that has been absorbed.

It is possible to measure the quantity of fluid escaping into the patient if a special weighing machine is added to the ordinary operating table.[3] It is also possible to monitor the concentration of sodium in the blood with a sodium-sensing electrode[4] or, more easily, by adding a little alcohol to the irrigating fluid and constantly monitoring the expired air with a breathalyser.[5] This allows the volume of excess fluid that has been absorbed to be estimated.

Many techniques have been used to avoid the TUR syndrome. A continuous irrigating resectoscope is helpful.[6] In practice the TUR syndrome is rarely seen in most modern departments, partly because of these precautions, and perhaps because of sparing use of intravenous fluids and careful measurement of the volumes of fluid that are irrigated in and out of the bladder.

References

1 Neal DE. The National Prostatectomy Audit. *Br J Urol* 1997; **79**(suppl 2):69–75.
2 Madsen PO, Naber KG. The importance of the pressure in the prostatic fossa and absorption of irrigating fluid during transurethral resection of the prostate. *J Urol* 1973; **109**:446–52.
3 Coppinger SW, Lewis CA, Milroy EJG. A method of measuring fluid balance during transurethral resection of the prostate. *Br J Urol* 1995; **76**:66.
4 Watkins-Pitchford JM, Payne SR, Rennie CD, Riddle PR. Hyponatraemia during transurethral resection: its practical prevention. *Br J Urol* 1984; **56**:676.
5 Hahn RG. Ethanol monitoring of extravascular absorption of irrigating fluid. *Br J Urol* 1993; **72**:766.
6 Iglesias JJ, Stams UK. How to prevent the TUR syndrome. *Urologe* 1975; **14**:287.

TURP: mortality

Roos et al.[1] reported that the death rate within 90 days of TURP was significantly higher than after open prostatectomy. The 90 day mortality after TURP amongst the 37 000 Danish men in this study who formed the most recent group of patients operated on (between 1977 and 1985) was 2.5%. Ninety day mortality after open prostatectomy was 2.7% in the Danish patients, but was lower at the other centres when compared with TURP. For the entire group of patients in the Roos study, the relative risk of death 90 days after TURP compared with open prostatectomy was 1.45. Roos and colleagues admitted that it was not possible to 'rule out potential confounding effects of unmeasured characteristics of patients' and it is likely that the higher mortality after TURP was due to a greater degree of comorbidity in those patients undergoing TURP when compared with those undergoing open prostatectomy. This view is supported by data from Western Australia.[2] In this large population based cohort study of mortality after TURP and open prostatectomy, the relative mortality of TURP over open prostatectomy, after adjusting for comorbidity, was 1.2 (CI 0.99–1.23). In a study of almost 66 000 TURPs performed in Scotland between 1968 and 1989, Hargreave et al.[3] found that the relative risk of death after TURP compared with open prostatectomy was 1.1. There had been suggestions that the changes in fluid balance occurring as a consequence of using irrigation fluid during the process of TURP could in some way lead to an increased 'strain' on the heart of frail patients, but interestingly no difference in the risk of dying from ischaemic heart disease (including myocardial infarction) was found between the TURP and open prostatectomy groups in the Australian study.

In contemporary series of TURPs, the National Prostatectomy Audit[4] reported a hospital mortality rate (death before discharge) of 0.8% for patients undergoing TURP for urinary retention and 0.2% for those with symptoms alone. Overall mortality in the UK Northern Region Audit[5] was 0.9% at 30 days: 0.5% for elective admissions and 2.4% for emergency admissions. In the series reported by Mebust et al.,[6] 0.23% of patients died within 30 days of surgery.

Further reading

1 Hahn RG, Farahmand BY, Hallin A et al. Incidence of acute myocardial infarction and cause-specific mortality after transurethral treatments of prostatic hypertrophy. *Urology* 2000; **55**:236–40.
2 Shalev M, Richter S, Kessler O et al. Long term incidence of acute myocardial infarction after open and transurethral resection of the prostate for benigh prostatic hyperplasia. *J Urol* 1999; **161**:491–3.

References

1 Roos NP, Wennberg J, Malenka DJ et al. Mortality and reoperation after open and transurethral resection of the prostate for benign prostatic hyperplasia. *New Engl J Med* 1989; **320**:1120–4.
2 Holman CD, Wisniewski ZS, Semmens JB et al. Mortality and prostate cancer risk in 19,598 men after surgery for benign prostatic hyperplasia. *BJU Int* 1999; **84**:37–42.
3 Hargreave TB, Heynes CF, Kendrick SW et al. Mortality after transurethral and open prostatectomy in Scotland. *Br J Urol* 1996; **77**:547–53.
4 Pickard R, Emberton M, Neal DE. The management of men with acute urinary retention. *Br J Urol* 1998; **81**:712–20.
5 Thorpe AC, Cleary R, Coles J et al. Deaths and complications following prostatectomy in 1400 men in the Northern Region of England. *Br J Urol* 1994; **74**:559–65.
6 Mebust WK, Holtgrewe HL, Cockett ATK et al. Transurethral prostatectomy: immediate and postoperative complications. A cooperative study of 13 participating institutions evaluating 3885 patients. *J Urol* 1989; **141**:243–7.

Immediate or early post-operative complications of TURP

Deep venous thrombosis and pulmonary embolism

- DVT: 0.2%.[1]
- PE: 0.1–0.5%.[2]

Bacteraemia

Highly variable reported rates: 1.6–58%. More common when the urine is infected before operation.[3–5] As many as 55% of men were found to have positive blood cultures even though their preoperative urine had been sterile,[6] while if bacterial endotoxins were measured the proportion rose even higher.[7] Only a small proportion of men in whom bacteria or endotoxins are found go on to develop septicaemic shock.

Septicaemia

- National Prostatectomy Audit: TURP for retention, 2%; TURP for LUTS, 1.3%.[1]
- Northern Region Audit: 8% (varying from 0% to 17% depending on the hospital).[8]
- European Collaborative Study of Antibiotic Prophylaxis for TURP: 1.5% of patients with sterile urine prior to surgery, where no antibiotic prophylaxis had been given at the time of surgery.[9]

Avoid by culturing the urine prior to TURP and treating any bacterial growth with antibiotics several days in advance of surgery. If the urine is sterile, give prophylactic antibiotics according to your local hospital policy (we use oral nitrofurantoin and IV gentamicin).

Bleeding

- Bleeding severe enough to require the operation to be stopped occurs in 0.7% of prostatectomies.
- Bleeding severe enough to require packing of the prostate to stop the bleeding occurs in 0.4% of prostatectomies.
- Return to the operating theatre to control major bleeding reported in 0.6% of cases.[10]

Urinary infection

Highly variable rates: from 6% to 100%. In the National Prostatectomy Audit[1] proven UTI occurred either before or after discharge in 13% of patients undergoing prostatectomy for retention and 4.6% of those undergoing prostatectomy for symptoms alone. Routine antibiotic prophylaxis in patients with sterile urine prior to TURP substantially reduces the chance of post-operative symptomatic UTI.[9]

References

1 Neal DE. The National Prostatectomy Audit. *Br J Urol* 1997; **79**(suppl 2):69–75.

2 Donat R, Mancey-Jones B. Incidence of thromboembolism after transurethral resection of the prostate (TURP). *Scand J Urol Nephrol* 2002; **36**:119–23.

3 Kiely EA, McCormack T, Cafferkey MT, Faliner FR, Butler MR. Study of appropriate antibiotic therapy in transurethral prostatectomy. *Br J Urol* 1989; **64**:61.

4 Ibrahim AIA, Bilal NE, Shetty SD, Patil KP, Gomaa H. The source of organisms in the post-prostatectomy bacteremia of patients with pre-operative sterile urine. *Br J Urol* 1993; **72**:770.

5 Hall JC, Christiansen KJ, England P et al. Antibiotic prophylaxis for patients undergoing tran-surethral resection of the prostate. *Urology* 1996; **47**:852.

6 Robinson MRG, Arudpragasam ST, Sahgal SM et al. Bacteraemia resulting from prostatic surgery: the source of bacteria. *Br J Urol* 1982; **37**:551.

7 Sohn MH, Vogt C, Heinen G et al. Fluid absorption and circulating endotoxins during tran-surethral resection of the prostate. *Br J Urol* 1993; **72**:605.

8 Thorpe AC, Cleary R, Coles J et al. Deaths and complications following prostatectomy in 1400 men in the Northern Region of England. *Br J Urol* 1994; **74**:559–65.

9 Hargreave TB, Botto B, Rikken GHJM et al. European Collaborative Study of Antibiotic Prophylaxis for Transurethral Resection of the Prostate. *Eur Urol* 1993; **23**:437–43.

10 Emberton M, Neal DE, Black N et al. The National Prostatectomy Audit: the clinical management of patients during hospital admission. *Br J Urol* 1995; **75**:301–16.

Other early post-operative complications of TURP

Failure to void

Failure to remove enough obstructing tissue is rarely the cause, and the majority of patients will void successfully after a second 'trial of catheter removal' a few weeks later. In the National Prostatectomy Audit[1] 9% of those with acute retention and 2.3% in those who had a TURP for symptoms alone failed to void on catheter removal after the operation. A permanent catheter was required in 1% and 0.1% of men, respectively.

Failure to void is surprisingly frequent after TURP done for retention.[2] It can be predicted from the retention volume, i.e. the volume of urine drained at the initial presentation. One per cent of patients ultimately failed to void at repeat catheter removal 6 weeks later (thus requiring a long-term catheter), all having presented with chronic retention.

It is presumably due to a degree of swelling of the residual prostatic tissue, possibly combined with post-operative urethral pain which inhibits normal voiding and in some cases with the added problem of a poorly contractile bladder. Given a few additional weeks of catheterization after TURP, the oedema has settled down, the resection margin has shrunk a little, and the patient has recovered from the effects of surgery. Successful voiding is the norm. There is some evidence that detrusor pressure increases over the course of several months in patients who initially fail to void after TURP, but ultimately regain the ability to void spontaneously.[3]

Incontinence

The incidence of incontinence after TURP falls with time. This is probably due to spontaneous resolution of bladder over-activity (detrusor instability) in a substantial proportion of patients. Long-term incontinence occurs in approximately 1–2% of men after TURP. Technical error at the time of operation can also cause incontinence. In such a patient endoscopy may show a defect in the external sphincter, usually at 10 or 2 o'clock. The investigation of post-TUR incontinence requires uro-dynamic investigations to determine the state of the detrusor, and endoscopy to reveal the sphincter. Management options include pads, a long-term catheter, injection of bulking agents in the region of the sphincter, or insertion of an artificial sphincter.[4]

Urethral stricture or bladder neck contracture

Occurs in 3–4% of men after TURP, usually just inside the external meatus, and is often easily treated by regular dilatation using a short straight sound. The patient can be taught to pass a Lofric® catheter of appropriate calibre on himself. Other sites for post-operative stricture are at the penoscrotal junction, the bulb, and the external sphincter. Prophylactic internal urethrotomy may reduce the incidence of urethral strictures.[5]

Table 3.1 Risk of failure to void is surprisingly frequent after TURP

Type of retention	Type of retention	Failure to void (% of men)
Acute retention	Painful inability to void with a catheter volume of <800 mL urine	10
Chronic retention	Maintenance of voiding with a residual urine volume of >500 mL	38
Acute on chronic retention	Painful inability to void with a catheter volume of >800 mL of urine	44

Sexual dysfunction

- Common.
- National Prostatectomy Audit found that 40% of men were unhappy with their post-operative sexual function.[6]
- Retrograde ejaculation occurs in approximately 80% of men (caused by removal of the bladder neck which normally closes during ejaculation, and is necessarily removed along with the obstructing adenoma).
- Erectile dysfunction: averages 6.5% after TURP.[7] However, in the trial of watchful waiting versus TURP by Wasson et al.,[8] erectile dysfunction rates were equivalent in both arms, and 20% of men in the UK National Prostatectomy Audit[6] reported an *improvement* in erectile function after TURP.
- 52% of men describe absent or altered sensation of orgasm.[9]

References

1 Emberton M, Neal DE, Black N et al. The National Prostatectomy Audit: the clinical management of patients during hospital admission. Br J Urol 1995; 75:301–16.

2 Reynard JM, Shearer RJ. Failure to void after transurethral resection of the prostate and mode of presentation. Urology 1999; 53:336–9.

3 Djavan R, Madersbacher S, Klingler C et al. Urodynamic assessment of patients with acute urinary retention: is treatment failure after prostatectomy predictable? J Urol 1997; 158:1829–33.

4 Gundian JC, Barrett DM, Parulkar BG. Mayo Clinic experience with the AS800 artificial urinary sphincter for urinary incontinence after transurethral resection of prostate or open prostatectomy. Urology 1993; 41:318.

5 Edwards LI, Lock R, Powell C, Jones P. Post-catheterization urethral strictures: a clinical and experimental study. Br J Urol 1983; 55:53.

6 Dunsmuir WD, Emberton M. Surgery, drugs and the male orgasm. BMJ 1997; 314:319.

7 Madersbacher S, Marberger M. Is transurethral resection of the prostate still justified? Br J Urol 1999; 83:227–37.

8 Wasson JH, Reda DJ, Bruskewitz RC et al. A comparison of transurethral surgery with watchful waiting for moderate symptoms of benign prostatic hyperplasia. The Veterans Affairs Cooperative Study Group on Transurethral Resection of the Prostate. New Engl J Med 1995; 332:75–9.

9 Dunsmuir WD, Emberton M. There is significant sexual dysfunction following TURP. Br J Urol 1996; 77:39 (abstract).

Additional reading

Hanbury DC, Sethia KK. Erectile function following transurethral prostatectomy. Br J Urol 1995; 75:12.

Symptomatic and other outcomes of TURP

Symptomatic improvement

70% of men are pleased with the symptomatic outcome following TURP:
- Improvement in flow rate: averages ~10 mL/s (~100% improvement).
- Reduction in residual urine volume: ~60% reduction.

Need for to redo TURP

This is required in ~1–2% of men per year.

Predicting poor outcome after TURP

Poor outcome after TURP (failure of symptom resolution and/or development of complication such as incontinence or impotence) is more likely in:
- Patients with frequency, urgency, and nocturia: these LUTS seems to be particularly resistant to treatment.
- Parkinson's disease (PD): risk of incontinence as high as 20%.[1] This may be due in part to a higher prevalence of bladder overactivity in PD combined with an inability to recruit sufficient perineal and/or sphincteric muscular activity to inhibit unstable bladder contractions and to prevent leakage when such contractions occur. It is difficult to know whether a patient with PD and frequency/urgency/nocturia has these LUTS because of BOO-related bladder overactivity, PD-related bladder overactivity, or a combination of both.
- Patients with a history of pelvic fracture leading to disruption of the membranous urethra: such patients may be totally reliant on their bladder neck for maintenance of continence. Division of the bladder neck during TURP may render then incontinent.

Reference

1 Staskin DS, Vardi Y, Siroky MB. Post-prostatectomy continence in the Parkinsonian patient: the significance of poor voluntary sphincter control. *J Urol* 1988; **140**:117–8.

Minimally invasive surgery management of BPH

In the late 1980s a number of factors combined as catalysts prompting the search for less invasive treatments for LUTS/BPH:
- The report by Roos et al.[1] of a seemingly higher mortality and reoperation rate after TURP when compared with open prostatectomy.
- Studies suggesting poor symptomatic outcome after TURP in a substantial proportion of patients.
- Reports of substantial morbidity in a proportion of patients undergoing TURP.

The two broad categories of alternative surgical techniques are minimally invasive and invasive. All are essentially heat treatments, delivered at variable temperature and power, and producing variable degrees of coagulative necrosis of the prostate or vaporization of prostatic tissue.

Transurethral radiofrequency needle ablation of the prostate (TUNA)

Low-level radiofrequency is transmitted to the prostate via a transurethral needle delivery system which is deployed within the prostate once the instrument has been advanced into the prostatic urethra. It is done under local anaesthetic, with or without intravenous sedation. The resultant heat causes localized necrosis of the prostate.

Improvements in symptom score and flow rate when compared with TURP are modest.[2] Side-effects include bleeding in one-third of patients and urinary retention in 10–40% of patients, but this is short lived with 95% of patients being catheter free at 1 week post-treatment.[3] UTI occurs in 10% and urethral stricture in 2%. Irritative urinary symptoms can last for a month or more. No adverse effects on sexual function have been reported.[4] The UK National Institute for Clinical Excellence[5] has endorsed TUNA as a minimally invasive treatment option for symptoms associated with prostatic enlargement. Concerns remain with regard to long-term effectiveness.

Transurethral microwave thermotherapy (TUMT)

Microwave energy can be delivered to the prostate via an intraurethral catheter which incorporates a microwave generator (antenna), a temperature measurement system, and a cooling system to prevent damage to the adjacent urethra. The microwave energy produces prostatic heating and coagulative necrosis. Subsequent shrinkage of the prostate and thermal damage to adrenergic neurons (i.e. heat-induced adrenergic nerve block) relieves obstruction and symptoms. Cavities can be demonstrated 3 months post-treatment by TRUS. Low-energy, high-energy, and high-intensity protocols are available.

Low-energy protocol (e.g. Prostatron® version 2.0)

In this system there is a stepwise increase in temperature together with urethral temperature sensing. Clinical efficacy (symptom improvement, flow rate improvement of 3–4 mL/s) has been confirmed in several studies comparing 'sham' treatment (where the microwave catheter is inserted, but no microwave energy is given) with active treatment.[6,7] The treatment effect seems to be durable over 5 years.[8] The improvement in symptoms, flow rates, residual urine volumes, and pressure–flow studies with low-energy TUMT is almost equivalent to that after TURP.

High-energy protocol (e.g. Prostatron® version 2.5)

Improvements in symptom scores, and flow rates after TUMT compare favourably with those after TURP.[9]

High-intensity protocol

The stepwise increase in temperature and urethral temperature sensing is not used with this software. Energy delivery is determined by measurement of rectal temperature and the treatment session lasts just 30 min (as opposed to 1 hr with the lower-energy systems). At 12 months post-treatment substantial reductions in symptom scores from a mean of 18 to 5 on the IPSS have been reported, with flow rates improving from 9 to 18 mL/s.[10, 11]

Post-treatment problems

Perineal discomfort is common after TUMT, as is urgency, but these symptoms usually resolve in a few days. Sexual side-effects after TUMT (e.g. impotence, retrograde ejaculation) are less frequent that after TURP, but a catheter may be required for about a week because of urinary retention in up to 25% of patients with lower-energy protocols.[7,9,12] In higher-energy protocols retention is common, and a catheter is required for about 2 weeks in a substantial proportion of patients.

High intensity focused ultrasound (HIFU)

A focused ultrasound beam can be used to induce a rise in temperature in the prostate, or indeed in any other tissue to which it is applied. A transrectal probe is used for HIFU treatment of the prostate A general anaesthetic or heavy IV sedation is required during the treatment. There are no randomized trials comparing its effectiveness against other treatment modalities. It is regarded as an investigational therapy.

References

1 Roos NP, Wennberg J, Malenka DJ et al. Mortality and reoperation after open and transurethral resection of the prostate for benign prostatic hyperplasia. New Engl J Med 1989; 320:1120–4.

2 Zlotta AR, Giannakopoulos X, Maehlum O et al. Long-term evaluation of transurethral needle ablation of the prostate (TUNA) for treatment of symptomatic benign prostatic hyperplasia: clinical outcome up to five years from three centres. Eur Urol 2003; 44:89–93.

3 Chapple CR, Issa MM, Woo H. Transurethral needle ablation (TUNA): a critical review of radiofrequency thermal therapy in the management of benign prostatic hyperplasia. Eur Urol 1999; 35:119–28.

4 Fitzpatrick JM, Mebust WK. Minimally invasive and endoscopic management of benign prostatic hyperplasia. In Campbell's Urology 8th edn, ed Walsh PC, Retik AB, Vaughan ED, Wein AJ. Philadelphia PA: WB Saunders, 2002.

5 National Institute for Clinical Excellence Transurethral radiofrequency needle ablation of the prostate. Interventional Procedure Guidance, October 2003.

6 Blute ML, Patterson DE, Segura JW et al. Transurethral microwave thermotherapy vs. SHAM: a prospective double-blind randomized study. J Endourol 1996; 10:565–73.

7 De la Rosette JJM, de Wildt MJ, Alivizatos G et al. Transurethral microwave thermotherapy (TUMT) in benign prostatic hyperplasia: placebo versus TUMT. Urology 1994; 44:58–63.

8 Keijzers GB, Francisca EA, d'Ancona FCH et al. Long-term results of lower energy transurethral microwave thermotherapy. J Urol 1998; 159:1966–72.

9 D'Ancona FC, Francisca EA, Witjes WP et al. High energy thermotherapy versus transurethral resection in the treatment of benign prostatic hyperplasia (BPH): results of a prospective randomized study with 1-year follow-up. J Urol 1997; 158:120–5.

10 Pace G, Selvaggio O, Palumbo F, Selvaggi FP. Initial experience with a new transurethral microwave thermotherapy treatment protocol '30-minute TUMT'. Eur Urol 2001; 39:405–11.

11 D'Ancona FCH, Francisca EAE, Witjes WPJ et al. Transurethral resection of the prostate vs high-energy thermotherapy of the prostate in patients with benign prostatic hyperplasia: long-term results. Br J Urol 1998; 81:259–64.

12 Dahlstrand C, Walden C, Deirsson G et al. Transurethral microwave thermotherapy versus transurethral resection for symptomatic benign prostatic obstruction: a prospective randomized study with a 2 year follow-up. Br J Urol 1995; 76:614–18.

Invasive surgical alternatives to TURP

TUIP (bladder neck incision (BNI))

Advantages over TURP
- Simpler to learn, teach, and perform.
- Quicker to perform.
- Blood loss is less.
- Shorter in-hospital stay.

Indications
- Bladder neck obstruction (including bladder neck dyssynergia in patients with neurological voiding dysfunction, such as spinal cord injury, or idiopathic bladder neck obstruction where there is no underlying neurological disease but the patient reports a poor flow rate and the bladder neck fails to open adequately during video-urodynamics).
- Bladder neck stenosis (i.e. bladder neck stricture, usually a consequence of prior TURP).
- BOO where the prostate is small.

Technique
Make a unilateral incision in the 7 o'clock position from just distal to the right ureter through the bladder neck and down to a point just proximal to the veru monatanum, using a Collings knife electrode. Alternatively, make a bilateral incision at both 5 o'clock and 7 o'clock. When you see fat in the depths of the incision, you have cut deeply enough. Achieve haemostasis either using the Collings knife with the coagulation current or with a roly-ball.

Outcomes of BNI compared with TURP
- Lower incidence of complications, particularly bleeding and need for blood transfusion.
- Lower rate of symptomatic improvement for larger prostates (>30 mL) and a higher need for re-treatment.

Several randomized trials have compared the symptomatic outcomes of TUIP and TURP. Where the prostate is small (<30 mL) and there is no middle lobe, outcomes are similar.[1] The risk of bladder neck contracture (0.5%) and urethral stricture (1.5%) is less after TUIP than after TURP. Retrograde ejaculation occurs in about 40% of men.

Transurethral electrovaporization of the prostate (TUVP)

This technique vaporizes and dessicates the prostate. TUVP seems to be as effective as TURP for symptom control and relief of bladder outlet obstruction, though there are few available data on the durability of these results.[2,3] Operating time and in-patient hospital stay are equivalent.[5,6] Requirement for blood transfusion may be slightly less after TUVP than after TURP. Retrograde ejaculation occurs 70–100% of patients and impotence in 0–15%. Irritative symptoms seem to be more troublesome than after TURP and can last for 4–6 weeks. TUVP does not provide tissue for histological examination, and so prostate cancers cannot be detected.

Laser prostatectomy

Holmium laser prostatectomy

The wavelength of the holmium:YAG laser is such that it is strongly absorbed by water within prostatic tissue. It produces vaporization at the tip of the laser fibre. Its depth of penetration is <0.5 mm and so it can be used to produce precise incisions in tissue. When the beam is 'de-focused,' it provides excellent haemostasis. It can be used with normal saline, thus avoiding the possibility of TUR syndrome. Three techniques of holmium laser prostatectomy have been developed in progression.

Vaporization

Holmium-only laser ablation of the prostate (HoLAP): time consuming, suitable only for small prostates.

Resection

Holmium laser resection of the prostate (HoLRP): similar symptomatic outcome to TURP.

Enucleation

Holmium laser enucleation of the prostate (HoLEP): lobes of the prostate are dissected off the capsule of the prostate and then pushed back into the bladder. A transurethral tissue morcellator is introduced into the bladder and used to slice the freed lobes into pieces which can then be removed. Improvements in symptom scores and flow rates are equivalent to TURP. Although the operation time with HoLEP is longer, catheter times and in-hospital stays are shorter (Gilling 2003). HoLEP is technically more demanding than other forms of laser prostatectomy, and this may have limited its widespread use. However, it can be done on large prostates (as large as 100 mL in volume) and on patients in urinary retention.

Greenlight PVP (Photoselective Vaporization of the Prostate)

The latest evolution of laser prostatectomy is photoselective vaporization of the prostate using an 80 Watt KTP (potassium titanyl phosphate) laser. The laser is green (hence the name 'greenlight' laser) and is absorbed by haemoglobin, generating a heating effect which causes vaporization of targeted tissue.

The procedure is done under general or spinal anaesthetic is using saline for irrigation (therefore no TUR syndrome).

Improvement in symptom scores and flow rates seem to be sustained over time.[7] There is only one published randomized study comparing PVP with TURP.[8] Outcomes from a recently introduced high power greenlight laser (120 Watt) remain to be determined.

References

1 Yang Q, Peters TJ, Donovan JL et al. Transurethral incision compared with transurethral resection of the prostate for bladder outlet obstruction: a systematic review and meta-analysis of randomised controlled trails. J Urol 2001; 165:1526–32.

2 Shokeir AA, Al-Sisi H, Farage YM et al. Transurethral prostatectomy: a prospective randomized study of conventional resection and electrovaporization in benign prostatic hyperplasia. Br J Urol 1997; 80:570–4.

3 Kaplan SA, Laor E, Fatal M, Te AE Transurethral resection of the prostate versus transurethral electrovaporization of the prostate: a blinded, prospective comparative study with 1-year follow-up. J Urol 1998; 159:454–8.

4 Gilling PJ, Kennett KM, Westenberg AM et al. Holmium laser enucleation of the prostate (HoLEP) is superior to TURP for the relief of bladder outflow obstruction (BOO): a randomised trial with 2 year follow-up. J Urol 2003; 169:1465.

5 McAllister WJ, Karim O, Plail RO et al. Transurethral electrovaporization of the prostate: is it any better than conventional transurethral resection of the prostate? BJU Int 2003; 91:211–14.

6 Hammadeh MY, Madaan S, Hines J, Philp T. Transurethral electrovaporization of the prostate after 5 years: is it effective and durable. BJU Int 2000; 86:648–51.

7 Malek R, Kuntzman R, Barrett D. Photoselective potassium-titanyl-phosphate laser vaporization of the benign obstructive prostate: observations on long term outcomes. J Urol 2005; 174: 1344–8.

8 Bouchier D, Anderson P, van Appledorn S et al. KTP laser versus transurethral resection: early results of a randomized trial. J Endourol 2006; 20:580–5.

Open prostatectomy for benign prostatic obstruction

Indications

- Large prostate (estimated weight >100 g. However, the precise weight at which an open rather than a transurethral prostatectomy should be done is determined by the skill of the operator in resecting large prostates).
- TURP not technically possible (e.g. limited hip abduction due to hip disease).
- Failed TURP (e.g. because of bleeding).

Contraindications

- Small fibrous prostate.
- Prior prostatectomy in which most of the gland has been resected or removed (this obliterates the tissue planes, making enucleation of the prostate impossible).
- Carcinoma of the prostate (this obliterates the tissue planes).

Diagnostic work-up

The decision to perform open prostatectomy will usually have been made pre-operatively based on a suspicion of marked prostatic enlargement on DRE, confirmed with either transrectal or transabdominal ultrasonography or cystoscopy.

Techniques

- Suprapubic (transvesical) where mainly the middle lobe of the prostate is enlarged.
- Simple retropubic where the lateral lobes are enlarged.

Suprapubic (transvesical) prostatectomy

The preferred operation if enlargement of the prostate involves mainly the middle lobe. First recorded at St Bartholomew's Hospital in 1884,[1] it was independently developed by Goodfellow[2] in Tombstone, Arizona, in 1885, McGill[3] in Leeds in 1887, Mansell-Moullin[4] at the London Hospital in 1892, Fuller[5] in New York in 1895, and Freyer[6] at St Peter's Hospital, London in 1901. Freyer reported 1600 cases with a mortality of just 5%!

Pre-operative preparation

Give antibiotic prophylaxis (see 📖 p. 4) and anti-thromboembolic prophylaxis (see 📖 p. 6), which will usually be AK-TEDs with subcutaneous heparin or intermittent pneumatic compression boots.

Technique

First perform a cystoscopic examination of the patient to assess size and check that there is no bladder pathology (incidental bladder tumours, stones). Pass a large catheter (22 Ch, 30 mL to the balloon). Instil 250 mL of saline into the bladder.

Make a low midline incision from the pubis to the umbilicus (stay extraperitoneal) or a Pfannenstiel incision. Separate the rectus muscles in the midline and insert a self-retaining retractor (e.g. Bookwalter). Divide the transversalis fascia. You are now in the prevesical/retropubic space. Bluntly push the peritoneum upwards away from the bladder. Clear the fat overlying the bladder (use a combination of the sucker to clear it out of the way, with diathermy to perivesical vessels which can cause irritating haemorrhage). Place two stay sutures (e.g. Vicryl) on either side of the midline of the bladder. The midline incision in the bladder is continued down to within 1 cm of the bladder neck. Readjust the retractor blades so that they are positioned within the bladder, thus allowing exposure of the inside of the bladder. Place a superior blade positioned over a swab inserted in the dome of the bladder.

The large adenoma of prostatic tissue will be seen protruding into the bladder. Incise the mucosa around the base of the adenoma taking care not to damage the ureteric orifices (Fig. 3.14). Develop the plane between the adenoma and prostatic capsule with curved scissors starting at 6 o'clock. Insert a finger into this plane and start to enucleate the prostate. This requires sweeping your finger from side to side around the bulk of the adenoma. A helpful manoeuvre is to force a finger into the prostatic urethra and then to exert anterior pressure to split the anterior commissure (Fig. 3.15). Move to another area if one area is stuck, leaving the adherent area until last. When the adenoma is nearly free, grasp it with a sponge forceps and use scissors to free the urethra where it is firmly attached at the apex, keeping close to the adenoma to avoid damaging the sphincter (Fig. 3.16).

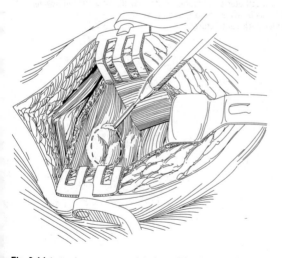

Fig. 3.14 Incise the mucosa around the base of the adenoma taking care not to damage the ureteric orifices. Reproduced from Hinman, *Hinman's Atlas of Urologic Surgery*, 2nd edn. 1998, WB Saunders, Philadelphia. Permission sought.

There will be brisk bleeding. Do not panic. Pack the prostatic fossa with a warm pack and apply pressure for ~5 min. The prostatic capsule will tend to contract and this, combined with pressure on the swab, can help stop some vessels from bleeding. Under-run bleeding vessels at 5 and 7 o'clock near the bladder neck. It is worthwhile doing this even if there is no active bleeding (vessels may go into spasm, only to haemorrhage later). Tack the mucosa of the bladder down over the proximal edge of the prostatic urethra with absorbable sutures.

Leave a 22Ch urethral catheter. Some surgeons leave a suprapubic catheter as well, brought out through a separate stab wound in the bladder (not through the bladder closure, because this is less likely to heal when the catheter is removed). Close the bladder in two layers with an absorbable suture (e.g. Vicryl). Place a retropubic drain (e.g. 20 Ch Robinson).

Remove the urethral catheter at 3 days and clamp the suprapubic catheter at 6 days, removing it 24 hr later. The drain can be removed 24 hr after this.

Complications of suprapubic (transvesical) prostatectomy for benign prostatic obstruction

- Post-operative bleeding: if traction on the over-inflated catheter balloon (50 mL) fails to tamponade the bleeding, endoscopic diathermy of bleeding vessels should be attempted.
- Wound infection.
- Epididymo-orchitis.
- Prolonged drainage of urine from the retropubic drain site: pass a urethral catheter to encourage distal drainage of urine and healing of the fistula between the bladder and skin.
- Bladder neck contracture.

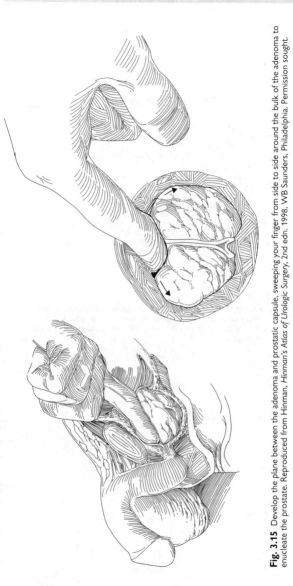

Fig. 3.15 Develop the plane between the adenoma and prostatic capsule, sweeping your finger from side to side around the bulk of the adenoma to enucleate the prostate. Reproduced from Hinman, *Hinman's Atlas of Urologic Surgery*, 2nd edn. 1998, WB Saunders, Philadelphia. Permission sought.

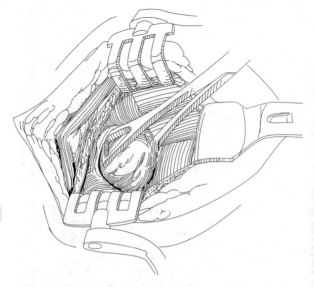

Fig. 3.16 Grasp the prostatic adenoma with a sponge forceps and use scissors to free the urethra where it is firmly attached at the apex. Reproduced from Hinman, *Hinman's Atlas of Urologic Surgery*, 2nd edn. 1998, WB Saunders, Philadelphia. Permission sought.

References

1 St Bartholomew's Hospital Reports. Statistical Tables 1885; **21**:79.
2 Goodfellow G. Prostatectomy in general especially by the perineal route. *JAMA* 1904; **Nov 12**:1448.
3 McGill AF. Suprapubic prostatectomy. *BMJ* 1887; **ii**:1104.
4 Mansell-Moullin CW. Enlargement of the prostate: its treatment and cure. London: Lewis, 1894.
5 Fuller E. Six successful and successive cases of prostatectomy. *J Cutan Genitourin Dis* 1895; **13**:229.
6 Freyer PJ. A clinical lecture on total extirpation of the prostate for radical cure of enlargement of that organ. *BMJ* 1901; **ii**:125.

Simple retropubic prostatectomy

First described by Millin[1] in 1947. Compared with the suprapubic (transvesical) approach it allows more precise anatomical exposure of the prostate, thus giving better visualization of the prostatic cavity. Better visualization allows:

- More accurate removal of the adenoma.
- Better control of bleeding points.
- More accurate division of the urethra, thus reducing the risk of incontinence.

Contraindications

As for suprapubic prostatectomy, but in addition simple retropubic prostatectomy is contraindicated where the middle lobe of the prostate is very large, because it is difficult to get behind the middle lobe through a transprostatic incision and so safely incise the mucosa distal to the ureters.

Pre-operative preparation

Give antibiotic prophylaxis (see 📖 p. 4) and anti-thromboembolic prophylaxis (see 📖 p. 6) which will usually be AK-TEDs with subcutaneous heparin or intermittent pneumatic compression boots. The patient is supine.

Technique

Perform a cystoscopic examination of the patient, specifically looking for incidental bladder tumours or stones. Catheterize the patient with a 22Ch catheter, 30 mL to balloon. Do not distend the bladder, as the enlarged bladder interferes with access to the retropubic space and prostate.

Pfannenstiel or lower midline incision. Separate the rectus muscles in the midline. Divide the transversalis fascia. You are now in the prevesical/retropubic space. Sweep the fat away from the anterior surface of the bladder and prostate. Use a combination of the sucker and long DeBakey's forceps to gently tease the more adherent fat away from the anterior surface of the prostate and bladder neck (as for a radical prostatectomy), using diathermy when necessary to coagulate larger veins. These vessels can be large and are easily torn.

Put in a Balfour or Millin retractor with a malleable middle blade which is used to push the bladder superiorly. Alternatively, use a Bookwalter retractor. Put a small swab on either side of the prostate to stop pooled blood from welling up in the wound and obscuring the view. Achieve haemostasis before enucleating the prostate by ligating the dorsal vein complex.[2] To do this place a large horizontal stay suture (0 or 1 gauge) deeply through the prostate, one inferiorly and one superiorly (Fig. 3.17). These sutures are principally haemostatic, but will also be used later to guide you in the closure of the capsule (by identifying where the capsule is).

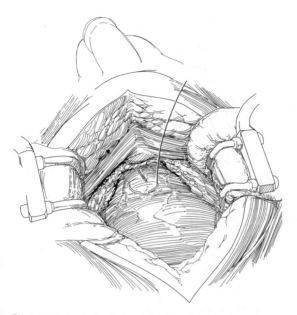

Fig. 3.17 Ligating the dorsal vein complex. Reproduced from Hinman, *Hinman's Atlas of Urologic Surgery*, 2nd edn. 1998, WB Saunders, Philadelphia. Permission sought.

About 1.5–2 cm distal to the bladder neck incise the prostatic capsule *transversely* with coagulating diathermy and continue down through the adenoma (Fig. 3.18). Do not use a longitudinal incision as it can extend through the prostate–urethral junction and cause incontinence. Continue this incision until you hit the catheter. Introduce a finger into the bladder and then down the urethra).

Define the plane between the capsule and the adenoma with McIndoe's scissors (Fig. 3.19). Develop this plane around the margins of your incision for about 1 cm. This will allow you to insinuate your finger between the capsule and the adenoma and thereby enuclate the prostate. Enucleate the adenoma by finger dissection. Initially place your finger in the urethra and lift it anteriorly to feel the left lateral lobe. Find the plane between the capsule and adenoma and sweep your finger laterally and anteriorly around both sides, so separating the adenoma from the capsule (Fig. 3.20). Gradually extend your finger posteriorly. Enucleation of the adenoma may be more easily done by turning your back to the operating table and manipulating your hand behind your back, particularly if you are right-handed and standing on the right side of the table. Be careful not to poke your finger through the rectum posteriorly. Work the prostatic adenoma free around the top and bottom. You should aim to free

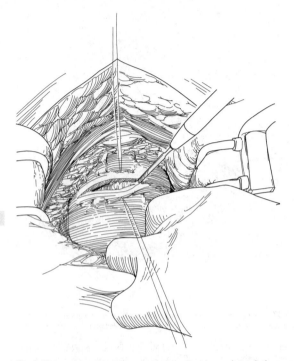

Fig. 3.18 Incise the prostatic capsule transversely with coagulating diathermy.
Reproduced from Hinman, *Hinman's Atlas of Urologic Surgery*, 2nd edn. 1998,
WB Saunders, Philadelphia. Permission sought.

the prostatic adenoma everywhere except distally, where it is attached to
the sphincter mechanism. Cut the last few strands distally (just proximal
to the veru montanum) rather than tearing the adenoma out at this point
(this could damage the sphincter). If enucleation is very difficult, place a
suprapubic tube close the capsular defect and proceed with TURP.

Once you have enucleated the adenoma, haemorrhage is likely to be
heavy. Place a large swab into the prostatic cavity and apply pressure while
you get your breath back. Some of the bleeding will stop by this manoeuvre alone. Achieve haemostasis of larger vessels with large absorbable
sutures (e.g. 0 or 1 gauge Vicryl). Take deep bites first down the right side
and then down the left side of the initial transverse incision which has
been opened longitudinally. You are trying to suture ligature arteries as
they penetrate the capsule; the main ones enter at 2 and 10 o'clock and at
5 and 7 o'clock. Start from outside the prostatic capsule and pass the
suture through the capsule to the inside. Then pass from inside to outside.
Start proximally and work distally.

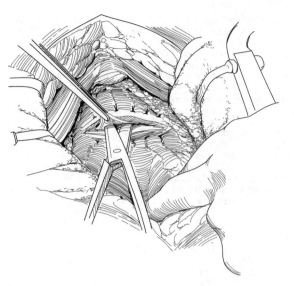

Fig. 3.19 Define the plane between the capsule and adenoma with McIndoe's scissors. Reproduced from Hinman, *Hinman's Atlas of Urologic Surgery*, 2nd edn. 1998, WB Saunders, Philadelphia. Permission sought.

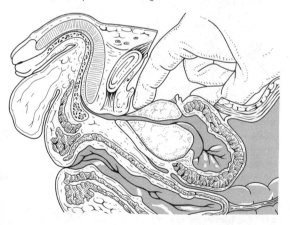

Fig. 3.20 Find the plane between the capsule and adenoma and sweep your finger laterally and anteriorly around both sides, thus separating the adenoma from the capsule. Reproduced from Whitfield, *Rob and Smith's Operative Surgery*, 1993, Elsevier. Permission sought.

Once good haemostasis is achieved, remove the swabs you positioned earlier and then resect a wedge of bladder neck. Do this using a Vullcellum forceps to hold the bladder neck and cut with the diathermy needle (Fig. 3.21). Beware the ureters! Infant feeding tubes help to protect them, as does staying near the midline and keeping your incision as distal as possible. Use a 1 gauge Vicryl for haemostasis, picking up the mucosa of the bladder neck with three or four sutures (some surgeons find it easier to use a smaller suture such as a 2/0 Vicryl). These sutures should also aim to advance the trigone, so that if the catheter has to be replaced later the new catheter will not under-run it (Fig. 3.22). Now put in a catheter—inflate the balloon to just 5 mL so that you do not burst it during closure. Use a 1 gauge Vicryl to close the transverse capsular incision, using your top and bottom haemostatic stay sutures to identify the capsule (Fig. 3.23). Fully inflate the catheter to 30 mL. Irrigate the bladder to check that your closure is watertight. Place a 30Ch Robinson's drain. Close the rectus sheath. Leave the drain for 24–48 hr. Take the catheter out in 5 days.

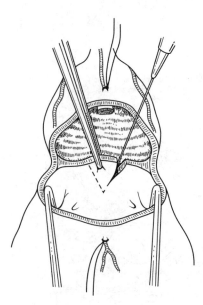

Fig. 3.21 Use forceps to hold the bladder neck and cut with a diathermy needle. Reproduced from Whitfield, *Rob and Smith's Operative Surgery*, 1993, Elsevier. Permission sought.

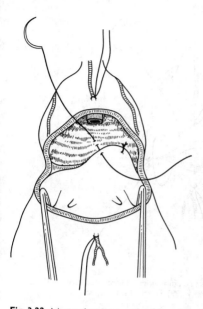

Fig. 3.22 Advance the trigone, so that if the catheter has to be replaced later the new catheter will not under-run the trigone. Reproduced from Whitfield, *Rob and Smith's Operative Surgery*, 1993, Elsevier. Permission sought.

Complications of retropubic prostatectomy for benign prostatic obstruction

- Rectal injury: if a tear is made in the rectum during enucleation, close the defect in two layers, apply a flap of omentum, place a cystostomy tube, and consider making a transverse colostomy or a four-finger anal stretch.
- Incontinence.
- Bladder neck stenosis (stricture).
- Haemorrhage.
- Ureteric obstruction as a consequence of placing a suture too high in the bladder neck region.
- Suprapubic fistula.
- Impotence (rare).
- Retrograde ejaculation.

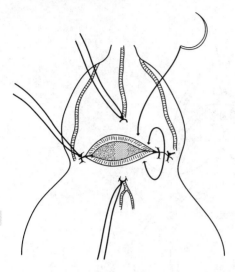
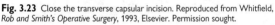

Fig. 3.23 Close the transverse capsular incision. Reproduced from Whitfield, *Rob and Smith's Operative Surgery*, 1993, Elsevier. Permission sought.

References

1 Millin T Retropubic urinary surgery Ireland, 1947.
2 Walsh PC, Oesterling JE Improved haemostasis during retropubic prostatectomy. *J Urol* 1990; **143**:1203.

Urethral stricture disease

A urethral stricture is an area of narrowing of the urethra due to formation of scar tissue in the tissues surrounding the urethra. Some surgeons restrict the term urethral stricture to a narrowing in the anterior urethra, excluding obliteration of the lumen of the posterior urethra arising from a pelvic fracture disruption injury from this definition.

Anterior urethra (penile and bulbar urethra)

The process of scar formation occurs in the spongy erectile tissue (corpus spongiosum) of the penis which surrounds the urethra and is known as spongiofibrosis. Most cases are idiopathic. Well-recognized aetiological factors are:

- Inflammation:
  - Balanitis xerotica obliterans (BXO).
  - Gonococcal infection leading to gonococcal urethritis (less common nowadays because of prompt treatment of gonorrhea).
- Trauma
  - Straddle injuries—blow to bulbar urethra, e.g. cross-bar injury (forgotten straddle injuries during childhood may account for many 'idiopathic' cases).
  - Iatrogenic—trauma to the anterior urethra during instrumentation, e.g. during catheterization, cystoscopy, TURP, bladder neck incision.

Iatrogenic 'trauma' (the process of catheterization, infection leading to spongiofibrosis around indwelling catheters, prostatectomy) may be the most common cause nowadays. The role of non-specific urethritis (e.g. *Chlamydia*) in the development of anterior urethral strictures has not been established.

Posterior urethra (membranous and prostatic urethra)

Fibrosis of the tissues in the space previously occupied by the posterior urethra results from pelvic fracture or surgical trauma (radical prostatectomy, TURP, urethral instrumentation). Where pelvic fracture is the cause, the mechanism is a *distraction* injury, as the posterior urethra is pulled apart. Strictly speaking, this is not a stricture since the urethra is not narrowed, but is completely disrupted. The space where the lumen was heals by the process of scar formation, and so there is no continuity between the prostatic urethra and the bulbar urethra.

Symptoms and signs of urethral stricture

- Voiding symptoms (there may be no symptoms): hesitancy, poor flow, post-micturition dribbling.
- Urethral bleeding.
- Urinary retention: acute or high-pressure acute-on-chronic.
- Urinary tract infection: prostatitis, epididymitis.
- Renal failure (rare).
- Urethrocutaneous fistula.
- Peri-urethral abscess.

Investigation of a suspected stricture

- Retrograde urethrography (plus an antegrade urethrogram via a previously placed suprapubic catheter).
- Ultrasound is advocated by some to establish the extent (length of urethra involved) and depth of spongiofibrosis.
- Where the calibre of the stricture is large enough to allow instrumentation with a cystoscope, urethroscopy can be used to assess its length.
- Visualization of the area of the sphincter to allow assessment of sphincter function in cases of posterior urethral disruption secondary to pelvic fracture can be done using a flexible cystoscope passed via the suprapubic track. However, whether this 'assessment' can predict the likelihood of continence after posterior urethroplasty has not been systematically studied.
- Some advocate the use of MRI in pelvic fracture urethral disruption injuries to allow assessment of anatomy, but this method is not in routine use.[1]

Management of urethral strictures: general principles

The reconstructive ladder versus modern management

In previous years there was a tendency to manage urethral strictures according to the principle of the reconstructive ladder, starting with the simplest procedure first, often repeating this when the stricture recurred and then moving on to more complex procedures when simple options had been exhausted. By extending the length and depth of spongiofibrosis it is possible that such 'treatment' may make subsequent open surgery technically more difficult and less likely to succeed.

Modern treatment is based on a decision made with the patient about whether the goal of treatment is cure or management. Strictures may be managed by repeat urethral dilatations or optical urethrotomies (the latter may sometimes cure a stricture), or cured (usually) by reconstructive surgery in the form of a urethroplasty. A stepwise progression up this 'reconstructive ladder' is appropriate for some patients, but not for all. In general terms curative treatment, which may involve complex reconstructive surgery, is more appropriate for the younger patient. The older less fit patient will often be most appropriately managed by repeat dilatations or optical urethrotomies, or in the case of a bulbar or penile stricture might be willing to undergo a perineal urethrostomy and accept the need to void sitting down.

Treatment in the context of mode of presentation

Where the patient presents with urinary retention, the diagnosis is usually made following a failed attempt at urethral catheterization. In such cases, avoid the temptation to 'blindly' dilate the urethra. Dilatation may be the wrong treatment option for this type of stricture: it may convert a short stricture, which could have been cured by urethrotomy or urethroplasty, into a longer and denser stricture, thus committing the patient to more complex surgery and a higher risk of recurrent stricturing. Instead, place a suprapubic catheter and image the urethra with retrograde and antegrade urethrography to establish the precise position and length of the stricture.

Similarly, avoid the temptation to inappropriately dilate a urethral stricture diagnosed at flexible cystoscopy (urethroscopy). Arrange retrograde urethrography so that appropriate treatment can be planned.

Options in general

Treatment options depend on location, cause, length, associated comorbidity, and patient preference.

- Urethral dilatation.
- Optical urethrotomy (visual internal urethrotomy).
- Excision with primary anastomotic urethroplasty.
- Incision and onlay urethroplasty. The stricture is not excised. An onlay graft of buccal mucosa or skin is applied ventrally (San Francisco technique of McAninch) or dorsally (Barbagli) on the stricture which has been longitudinally divided (the incision is extended into normal urethra on either side of the stricture). When the onlay graft is applied dorsally this is known as a 'dorsal patch substitution urethroplasty' or Barbagli procedure.
- Excision and onlay urethroplasty ('excisional augmented anastomotic urethroplasty'): the stricture is excised and the two urethral ends are mobilized to allow a tension-free anastomosis. They are opened longitudinally on their dorsal surface (spatulation) and are re-anastomosed over a dorsally applied onlay graft of buccal mucosa.
- Flap-based repair (penile skin flap).
- Staged repair, e.g. Johanson urethroplasty (staged linear urethroplasty).
- Perineal urethrostomy.
- Urolume stent: contraindicated in the posterior urethra, and its role in the anterior urethra is limited (Jordan).

Tube grafts have a high incidence of stricturing and are no longer employed.

Options depending on location

- Penile urethra: the technique of repair depends on the *aetiology* of the stricture. In general, a one-stage repair is suitable if the stricture is secondary to trauma, e.g. following urethral instrumentation. A multi-stage approach is usually required for strictures due to BXO or those occurring in the context of failed hypospadias repair.
- Bulbar urethra treatment depends on the *length* of the stricture.

Pendulous urethra

Recurrent stricturing is likely when urethral dilatation or optical urethrotomy is used in the pendulous urethra because the urethra has very little 'supporting' vascular spongiosal tissue (as opposed to the bulbar urethra where there is a large quantity of surrounding spongy tissue).

Pendulous urethra: no BXO present

Stricture excision and simple end-to-end anastomotic urethroplasty is not an option, unless the stricture is short (<1 cm in length), because the relatively immobile penile urethra prevents adequate mobilization for a tension-free anastomosis. Usually strictures of the pendulous urethra require repair by use of an island flap of skin used as a flap or tube.

- Onlay pedicled flap repair using foreskin if uncircumcised or penile shaft skin if circumcised. The stricture is incised longitudinally, leaving the stricture *in situ* and avoiding further vascular compromise of the tissues by stricture mobilization of excision. A longitudinal island flap based on a fasciocutaneous pedicle is raised and anastomosed to the incised urethral edges (Orandi flap) (Fig. 3.24), or a fasciocutaneous flap of preputial or penile skin (McAninch flap) can be used.
- Johanson urethroplasty. This is used when there is inadequate penile skin for a fasciocutaneous urethroplasty, the stricture is too long for a buccal graft, or the patient has had multiple operations or has fistulae. Typically used for penile urethral strictures (±BXO), with a buccal graft placed in the first stage. The first stage involves exteriorization of the urethra by incision of the urethra through the stricture, extending into normal urethra on either side of the stricture (Fig. 3.25). The edges of the urethra are then stitched to the skin. The second stage creates a 3 cm wide urethral plate which is rolled inwards to form a new urethra. The second stage need not be done in the elderly, those with comorbidity, or those unwilling to undergo further surgery, and the patient can void through a perineal urethrostomy.
- Perineal urethrostomy.

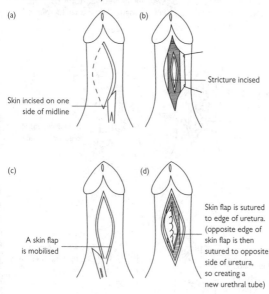

(a)

Skin incised on one side of midline

(b)

Stricture incised

(c)

A skin flap is mobilised

(d)

Skin flap is sutured to edge of uretura. (opposite edge of skin flap is then sutured to opposite side of uretura, so creating a new urethral tube)

Fig. 3.24 Orandi longitudinal island flap for penile urethral stricture repair. (a) skin incised on one side of midline. (b) stricture incised. (c) a skin flap is mobilized. (d) skin flap is sutured to edge of uretura (the opposite edge of skin flap is then sutured to opposite side of uretura, so creating a new urethral tube).

Pendulous urethra: BXO present

Balanitis xerotica obliterans (also known as genital lichen sclerosus et atrophicus) is the most common cause of stenosis of the meatus. Hyperkeratosis is seen histologically. It appears as a white plaque on the foreskin, glans of the penis, or within the urethral meatus. The foreskin becomes thickened and adheres to the glans, leading to phimosis (a thickened non-retractile foreskin). Patients with long-standing BXO and meatal stenosis often have more proximal urethral strictures, extending as far as the mid-bulbar urethra. Management options are:

- Topical steroids, e.g. 0.05% clobetasol two to four times weekly.
- Simple meatotomy for distal strictures.
- Perineal urethrostomy.
- Complex staged repair (Johanson urethroplasty).

Bulbar urethra

- Urethral dilatation: designed to stretch the stricture without causing more scarring. Bleeding post-dilatation indicates tearing of the stricture, i.e. further injury has been caused, and restricturing is likely.
- Optical urethrotomy (visual internal urethrotomy).
- Stricture <2 cm long: excision with primary anastomosis.
- Stricture 2–4 cm long: excision with augmented anastomosis (augmented with buccal mucosa) is in vogue ('excisional augmented anastomotic urethroplasty').

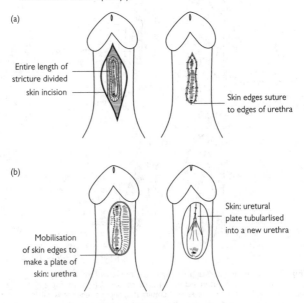

(a)

Entire length of stricture divided skin incision

Skin edges suture to edges of urethra

(b)

Mobilisation of skin edges to make a plate of skin: urethra

Skin: uretural plate tubularlised into a new urethra

Fig. 3.25 Johanson urethroplasty. (a) first stage. (b) second stage.

- Where excision is not feasible because the stricture is long, simple incision and augmentation with an onlay graft of buccal mucosa or skin is appropriate.
- Urolume stent: introduced in 1988 for the treatment of bulbar urethral strictures. Webster 'rarely uses it'.[2] When used for bulbar strictures, it can cause post-micturition dribbling, perineal pain, and erectile pain, and recurrent strictures can occur.

Techniques for treatment of urethral strictures

Optical urethrotomy (visual internal urethrotomy)

This is stricture incision. It is best suited for short (<1.5cm) bulbar urethral strictures with minimal spongiofibrosis.[3] Recurrent stricturing is less likely than when optical urethrotomy is used in the pendulous urethra, where the corpus spongiosum is thinner than in the bulbar urethra and therefore the vascularity of the urethra is more easily compromised (for this reason avoid optical urethrotomy in the pendulous urethra). Some surgeons incise at the 12 o'clock position, others at 3 o'clock, and others at 6 or 9 o'clock (the choice depends on surgeon). In the bulbar urethra bear in mind that the cavernosal nerves lie in the 1 and 11 o'clock positions, so incision here runs the risk of erectile dysfunction. A cold knife or Ho:YAG laser can be used. Leave a catheter for 3–5 days (longer catheterization does not reduce long-term restricturing). Consider ISC for 3–6 months, starting several times daily and reducing to once or twice a week towards the end of this period.

Outcomes between urethral dilatation and optical urethrotomy for short bulbar strictures are equivalent (randomized trial):[3,4] short bulbar stricture, 40–50% success rate; 10% with second urethrotomy. When optical urethrotomy is used for *penile* urethral strictures, the recurrence rate is 80–90%; hence optical urethrotomy is frowned upon as a treatment for penile urethral strictures.[3]

Some surgeons (Mundy, Roehrborn) argue that a previous optical urethrotomy compromises the outcome of anastomotic repair (though not of dorsal patch substitution urethroplasty).[5,6] Others (Webster, Barbagli) suggest that previous optical urethrotomy does not compromise the outcome of urethroplasty.[2,7] Mundy's feeling is that patients who have undergone previous optical urethrotomy should undergo dorsal patch substitution in preference to simple anastomotic urethroplasty (in patients who had had a previous optical urethrotomy, 40% of those who underwent bulbar anastomotic urethroplasty subsequently restrictured but only 6% of those who underwent dorsal patch substitution urethroplasty subsequently restrictured).

Excision and anastomotic urethroplasty

Of the various forms of urethroplasty this provides the best long-term stricture-free rates when used for bulbar strictures. A successful outcome depends on adequate mobilization of the urethra, and therefore it is only suitable for short strictures in the bulbar urethra which can be mobilized (the penile urethra cannot).

A perineal incision is made which may be a midline, inverted U, or Mercedes Benz shape. Divide the bulbospongiosus muscle to expose the urethra. Mobilize the urethra on either side of the stricture, the site of which is identified by a catheter passed down the urethra. Cut across the urethra at the stricture and incise each end of the urethra longitudinally until normal urethra is identified. Excise the abnormal areas. Spatulate the urethral ends on the ventral surface of the proximal urethra and the dorsal surface of the distal urethra (the anastomosis will shrink by 20%, hence the need for spatulation) (Fig. 3.26) Perform a tension-free anastomosis using fine absorbable interrupted sutures. Close the perineal wound. Leave a catheter for 2–3 weeks.

Incision and augmentation with onlay graft of buccal mucosa or skin

The patient position and incision site are determined by whether the stricture is penile or bulba in location. Position the patient in a simple rather than an exaggerated lithotomy position for bulbar strictures. Use a simple supine position for penile strictures. Pass a 16Ch Foley catheter to identify the distal end of the stricture.

A midline perineal incision is made for a bulbar stricture. Detach the urethra form the corpora cavernosa. The urethra is rotated 180°. The stricture is incised longitudinally on its dorsal surface to open it completely, extending the incision into healthy urethra both proximally and distally. The spongy tissue of the corpus spongiosum of the bulbar urethra is thicker and more vascularized ventrally, wit the lumen of the bulbar urethra lying in an offset dorsal location within the corpus spongiosum. A dorsal incision is thought to preserve the blood supply to the corpus spongiosum better than a ventral incision (the dorsal incision avoids dividing the well-vascularized ventral tissue), although good results have been reported by enthusiasts of both ventrally[8,9] and dorsally[10] placed buccal grafts. In the bulbar urethra long-term stricture-free rates of 80–90% have been reported ('success' can be defined on the basis of absent symptoms, improvement of Q_{max} and absence of stricturing on retrograde urethrography).

For a penile stricture use a circumcoronal degloving incision. Expose the penile urethra. Open the stricture using a ventral midline incision. A dorsal midline incision is then made in the urethra down to the albuginea of the corpora. The two halves of the urethra are mobilized on either side of the midline, thus creating a wide bed for the buccal graft which is sutured in a dorsal location with 6/0 absorbable sutures (e.g. polyglactin). Quilting sutures are used to further immobilize the graft. The urethra is closed over a 12Ch Foley catheter and this remains in place for 2 weeks.

(a)

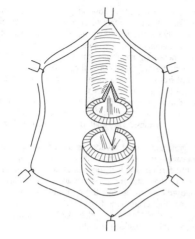

(b)

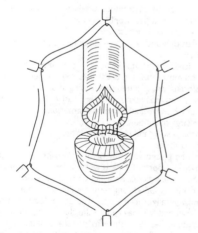

Fig. 3.26 (a). Anastomotic urethroplasty: spatulation. (b) Anastomotic urethroplasty: the anastomosis.

Ideally a second surgeon harvests the buccal graft while the other exposes the stricture. The patient is intubated through the nose to allow the mouth to be completely empty. The lower lip or inner surface of the cheek is infiltrated with saline containing adrenaline 1:100 000. A free graft of buccal mucosa measuring roughly 4 cm × 2–3 cm is harvested (use a marker pen to mark the site) in an ovoid shape (longer if necessary, and taking a second graft from the contralateral inner cheek if necessary) (Fig. 3.27). Avoid damage to Stensen's duct at the level of the 2nd upper molar tooth. Close the donor site with 4/0 polyglactin sutures. The graft is fixed to a cork board. All fibrovascular tissue and fat is removed from the graft, thereby reducing its thickness. The graft is fenestrated with a few small incisions.

For a dorsal onlay graft the buccal mucosa is placed on the ventral surface of the corpora cavernosa, which has been covered with fibrin glue to help stabilize the graft further, and is sutured in place. The two apices of the graft are sutured to the distal and proximal apices of the urethrotomy. The urethra is closed over the graft with interrupted 4/0 polyglactin sutures applied between the urethra and graft. The bulbocavernosus muscles are closed over the urethra followed by Colles' fascia and the skin. Remove the catheter after 2 weeks (Fig. 3.28).

Buccal mucosa
Used in excisional augmented anastomotic urethroplasty and in stricture incision combined with dorsal patch onlay urethroplasty (Barbagli procedure). The advantages of buccal mucosa are:
- A panlaminar plexus of blood vessels which optimize perfusion and hence graft survival.
- Thick epithelium rich in elastin, making it easy to handle and durable.
- Waterproof: buccal mucosa lives in the hostile environment of the mouth and therefore is ideally suited to surviving in the urethra.
- Thin lamina propria (oxygen and nutrients can easily diffuse from the underlying surface) which facilitates neovascularization.
- Easy to harvest in large quantities.
- The donor site heals quickly and relatively painlessly.
- Minimal tendency to shrink.

The buccal graft can be placed ventrally or dorsally with respect to the urethra. Barbagli favours a dorsal location which is believed to provide a well vascularized and non-elastic base on the corpora cavernosa (to prevent diverticula formation.[11] Good long-term results have been reported with both dorsal and ventrally placed grafts.[9] The dorsal location provides a fixed base for the graft and this may reduce the chance of graft shrinkage and diverticula formation. Results with onlay grafts are better than with tube grafts: 2–5 year results, 97% stricture free with patch graft versus 55% with tube graft.[12]

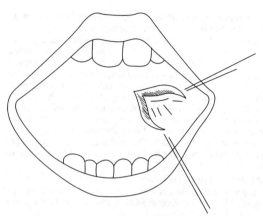

Fig. 3.27 Harvesting a buccal mucosal graft.

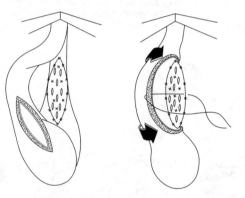

Fig. 3.28 The dorsally incised distal urethra is anastomosed to the buccal graft. Reproduced from Schreiter and Jordan, *Urethral Reconstructive Surgery*, 2006, Springer. Permission sought.

Excision with augmented anastomosis (augmented with buccal mucosa): 'excisional augmented anastomotic urethroplasty'

Here a segment of the most strictured part of the urethra is excised (up to 2 cm in length, but no more). The proximal and distal urethral segments are spatulated by a midline incision on their dorsal aspects. An onlay graft of buccal mucosa is sutured onto the exposed and underlying corpora cavernosa. Fibrin glue may be applied to the albuginea of the corpora cavernosa to immobilize the graft further. The dorsally spatulated distal urethra is pulled down and the proximal urethra is pulled up over a 16Ch catheter and they are anastomosed to the buccal graft. The distal and proximal urethral ends are sutured together in the midline, thereby closing the repair. The bulbocavernosus muscles are closed over the urethra, followed by Colles' fascia and the skin. Remove the catheter after 2 weeks (Fig. 3.29).

Penile flaps for reconstruction of bulbar urethral strictures

A flap is a segment of tissue with its own blood supply. A graft is a segment of tissue whose blood supply is obtained from another area (the adjacent tissue must have its own blood supply).

Ideally, flaps should be hairless, viable (good arterial blood supply and good venous drainage), and adaptable in terms of length and location. Extragenital dermal and tunica vaginalis grafts do not do well in the urethra, apart from those harvested from the posterior auricular area. Completely tubularized grafts do not do as well as onlay grafts.

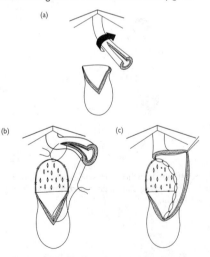

Fig. 3.29 (a) The proximal and distal urethral segments are spatulated. (b) An onlay graft of buccal mucosa is sutured onto the exposed and underlying corpora cavernosa. (c) The dorsally spatulated distal urethra is anastomosed to the buccal graft as is the proximal urethra. Reproduced from Schreiter and Jordan, *Urethral Reconstructive Surgery*, 2006, Springer. Permission sought.

Types of flap

- Penile skin flaps satisfy all of the criteria given above. They are created from pedicled island penile skin (PIPS) or, in uncircumcised men, from pedicled island foreskin (PIFS):
  - Preputial fasciocutaneous flap.[13]
  - Quartey longitudinal-transverse preputial island flap (this is a combination of the Orandi and McAninch flaps) (Fig. 3.30).
- Scrotal skin flaps (very hairy so are not generally used):
  - Distal penile fasciocutaneous circular flap (McAninch)[13] (Fig. 3.31).

Mark two parallel incisions 2 cm apart around the shaft of distal penis. Incise the distal skin mark, and continue the incision through Dartos fascia and the superficial layer of Buck's fascia. Buck's fascia has superficial and deep lamellae. The deep dorsal neurovascular bundle (dorsal artery, dorsal nerve, and deep dorsal vein) lie just deep to the *superficial* layer of Buck's fascia. Only the superficial lamella of Buck's fascia is raised with the fasciocutaneous flap, avoiding the underlying neurovascular bundle. Mobilize the skin of the penis back to its base so that the flap, once formed, can be tunnelled through to the bulbar urethra. Pull the skin back over the shaft of the penis and now incise the proximal skin mark and Dartos fascia deep to this, but do not incise Buck's fascia (to preserve a pedicle based on Buck's fascia). Split the ring of skin ventrally and rotate the flap dorsally. A subcutaneous tunnel is created into the perineal wound and sutured as an onlay graft onto the incised bulbar urethra.

Posterior urethra (membranous urethra) due to pelvic fracture urethral trauma

- Membranoprostatic (80%): sphincter stays with prostate (goes 'north').
- Bulbomembranous (20%): sphincter stays with bulbar urethra (stays 'south').
- Complex: recto-urethral fistula or combined with a bladder neck injury.

Retrograde urethrography and urethroscopy from above (via the suprapubic catheter track) and from below will help to distinguish where the stricture is. At retrograde urethrography if contrast flows beyond the bulbar urethra, this implies the membranous urethra is attached to the bulbar urethra (bulbomembranous).

Acute situation

If urethral injury is suspected (blood at meatus, known pelvic fracture) carry out retrograde urethrography. If there is free flow to the bladder and no leak of contrast pass a urethral catheter. If there is no free flow or extravasation, gently pass a urethral catheter. If it fails to pass, place a suprapubic catheter. Perivesical haematoma may make percutaneous placement technically very difficult; it may not be possible to pass the trocar through the haematoma and into the bladder. Furthermore, pelvic fracture associated bladder perforation may be missed with percutaneous placement. Open cystotomy not only allows safe placement of a suprapubic catheter, but also affords an opportunity to diagnose and repair bladder injuries.

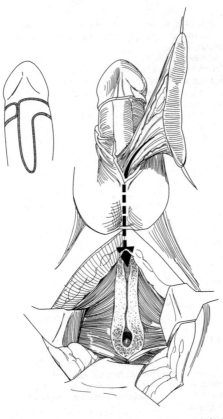

Fig. 3.30 The Quartey longitudinal-transverse preputial island flap. Reproduced from Hinman, *Hinman's Atlas of Urologic Surgery*, 2nd edn. 1998, WB Saunders, Philadelphia. Permission sought.

Leave the SPC for 3–6 months to allow perineal haematoma to resolve. As this occurs, the urethral defect will shorten making subsequent repair easier.

Realignment

This has the potential advantage (not always realized) of shortening the length of strictured urethra, thus reducing the depth of scar tissue that must be excised during subsequent posterior urethroplasty. In reality, sufficient expertise in these techniques is often unavailable in the initial treating hospital, and the majority of posterior urethral distraction injuries will be managed by suprapubic cystostomy, followed by delayed (3–6 months) repair.

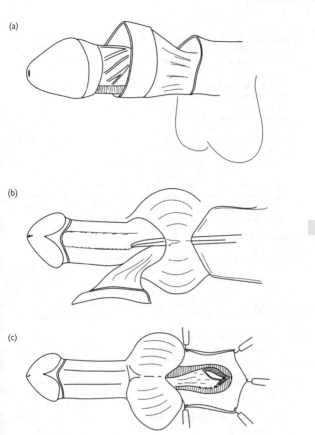

Fig. 3.31 The McAninch distal penile fasciocutaneous circular flap. (a) Harvesting the graft from the penile shaft skin. (b) Transferring the graft to the perineum. (c) Anastomosing the graft to the incised bulbar stricture.

Techniques
- Immediate (primary) realignment is used by some surgeons (using magnetic guides or interlocking sounds to pull the two distracted urethral ends together, or attempting to pull the ends together by an open perineal approach). Haemorrhage can be severe. Stricturing of the urethra is very common, and hence further endoscopic or open surgery is very often required.
- Delayed (primary) endoscopic realignment. In selected cases, and assuming the patient is fit enough to undergo surgery 5–10 days post-injury, endoscopic realignment can be attempted. A flexible cystoscope is passed, via the suprapubic track, down into the prostatic urethra and into the haematoma. A second surgeon passes a large-bore rigid cystoscope or resectoscope retrogradely along the penile and into the bulbar urethra. A guidewire can then be passed across the defect, and a urethral catheter can be passed over this. This is left *in situ* for several weeks. When removed a retrograde urethrogram is performed to confirm healing (absence of extravasation) and to determine the length of strictured urethra (stricturing is very common).

Delayed repair
Formal repair: with complete urethral distraction there is no urethral lumen. The lumen is completely obliterated by fibrosis.

Repair is carried out by a posterior urethroplasty. This is done via a perineal approach and can usually be completed in one procedure. There are four stages to the repair: the so-called 'progressive' perineal repair. Each stage is completed until a tension-free anastomosis has been achieved (this may be achieved with the first stage, but all four stages may be needed).
- Mobilization of the urethra, division of the distal urethra at the point where it is obliterated, identification of the proximal end of the urethra by passing a sound through the suprapubic track and into the proximal urethra, and excision of scar tissue around the proximal end of the urethra until healthy tissue is present (cut gently through the scar tissue and onto the end of the sound and then carefully excise scar tissue from the proximal end of the urethra until healthy circumferential mucosa is seen, or alternatively remove the scar tissue piecemeal using a scalpel).
- If a tension-free anastomosis cannot be achieved, develop the intercrural space (i.e. separate the two crura) to reduce the length of the defect.
- If a tension-free anastomosis still cannot be achieved, excise a wedge of inferior pubic ramus to reduce the length of the defect.
- If a tension-free anastomosis cannot be achieved, re-route the urethra around one corpora cavernosa.

Leave a 16Ch urethral catheter for 2–3 weeks and perform a micturating cystogram via the SPC. If there is no extravasation of contrast at the site of repair, clamp the SPC and, once the patient has voided satisfactorily for 2–3 weeks, remove it.

Post-radical prostatectomy vesico-urethral stenosis or obliteration

- Most vesico-urethral strictures respond to dilatation or optical urethrotomy.
- Stents.
- 'Cutting for the light'. A flexible cystoscope is passed via the suprapubic track and is positioned in the bladder neck. An optical urethrotome is passed retrogradely up the urethra to the stricture. The theatre lights and the light of the urethrotome are turned off, so that the light of the flexible cystoscope can be seen. The blade of the urethrotome is deployed to cut through the stricture.

Both stents and cutting to the light are associated with poor long-term outcomes.

References

1 Dixon CM, Hricak H, McAninch JW. Magnetic resonance imaging of traumatic posteror urethral defects and pelvic crush injuries. *J Urol* 1992; **148**:1162–5.
2 Peterson AC, Webster GD. Management of urethral stricture disease: developing options for surgical intervention. *BJU Int* 2004; **94**:971–76.
3 Pansadoro V, Emiliozzi P. Internal urethrotomy in the management of anterior urethral strictures: long term follow-up. *J Urol* 1996; **156**:73–75.
4 Steenkamp JW, Heyns CF, de Kock ML. Internal urethrotomy versus dilation as treatment for male urethral strictures: a prospective, randomized comparison. *J Urol* 1997; **157**:98–101.
5 Andrich DE, O'Malley K, Greenwell TJ, Mundy AR. Does urethrotomy jeopardize the outcome of urethroplasty? *BJU Int* 2003; **91**(Suppl):89.
6 Roehrborn CG, McConnell JD. Analysis of factors contributing to success or failure of 1-stage urethroplasty for urethral stricture disease. *J Urol* 1994; **151**:869–74.
7 Barbagli G, Palminteri E, Lazzeri M et al. Long-term outcome of urethroplasty after failed urethrotomy versus primary repair. *J Urol* 2001; **151**:869–74.
8 Kane CJ, Tarman GJ, Summerton DJ et al. Multi-institutional experience with buccal mucosa onlay urethroplasty for bulbar urethral reconstruction. *J Urol* 2002; **167**:1314–7.
9 Elliott SP, Metro MJ, McAninch JW. Long-term follow-up of ventrally placed buccal mucosa onlay graft in bulbar urethral anastomosis. *J Urol* 2003; **169**:1754–7.
10 Iselin CE., Webster GD. Dorsal onlay graft urethroplasty for repair of bulbar urethral stricture. *J Urol* 1999; **161**:815–18.
11 Barbagli G, Selli C, Tosto A, Palminteri E. Dorsal free graft urethroplasty. *J Urol* 1996; **155**:123–6.
12 Venn SN, Mundy AR. The use of buccal mucosa for substitution urethroplasty. *Eur Urol* (Suppl) 1998; **33**:154.
13 McAninch JW. Reconstruction of extensive urethral strictures: circular fasciocutaneous penile flap. *J Urol* 1993; **149**:488.

Perineal urethrostomy

Indications
- Management of urethral stricture disease where reconstruction is deemed inappropriate.
- Where access to the prostate for TURP is difficult, e.g. because of distal meatal narrowing or the presence of a penile prosthesis.

Technique
Place a Clutton's sound (i.e. a curved sound) with its tip resting in the prostatic urethra. The curved end is levered towards the perineal skin. While holding the sound between the thumb and finger, make a longitudinal midline incision, cutting through the skin and then through the urethra down onto the sound (Fig. 3.32a). Mobilize the urethra over a few centimetres so that you can bring it to the perineum (not the perineum to the urethra), thereby avoiding the creation of a perineal cleft which potentially can remain wet with urine after voiding, leading to maceration of the skin.

Grasp the cut edges of the urethra either with Allis forceps, one on each side of the incision in the urethra, or with stay sutures (Fig. 3.32b). Pull the sound gently out of the urethra and replace it with a Foley catheter which is passed into the bladder and the balloon inflated (Fig. 3.32c). For a permanent urethrostomy, close the divided urethra and skin around the catheter with absorbable sutures (Fig. 3.32d).

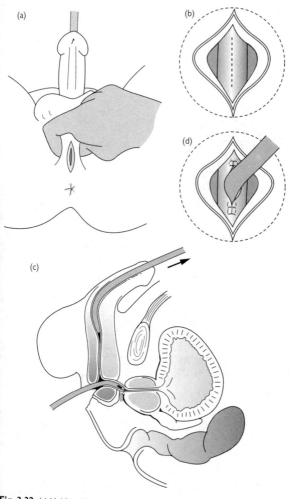

Fig. 3.32 (a) Holding the sound between the thumb and finger, make a longitudinal, midline incision through the skin. (b) Mobilize the bulbar urethra so it can come up towards the skin incision and then incise it in the midline, cutting onto the sound which remains positioned in the urethra; grasp the cut edges of the urethra with Allis forceps. (c) Replace the sound with a Foley catheter. (d) For a permanent urethrostomy, close the divided urethra and skin around the catheter with absorbable sutures.

Chapter 4

Surgery for urological cancer

Renal cell cancer: pathology and staging

Classification of renal cell cancer (WHO classification)[1]

- Clear cell (conventional) (65%):
  - Frequent 3p losses, including *VHL* gene (3p25-p26).
- Papillary, chromophil, (tubulo-papillary) (15%):
  - Trisomy common, particularly chromosomes 7 and 17.
- Chromophobe (8%):
  - Characterized by near-haploid genome, monosomy, and frequent loss of chromosomes (particularly 1, 2, 6, 10, 13, 17, 21, including 10q23.3 involving *PTEN/MMAC1*).
- Collecting duct (Bellini's duct).
- Medullary carcinoma.
- Other/unclassified.
- Oncocytoma (10%):
  - Typically benign, may be familial. Sometimes with losses of chromosomes 1 and Y; sometimes diploid chromosomes. Oncocytoma cannot be reliably distinguished from renal cell carcinoma by clinical and radiological criteria.

Benign tumours

Benign tumours of the kidney include cysts, angiomyolipoma, oncocyloma and adenoma (<0.5cc). Oncocytoma are sometimes multiple and familial. Angiomyolipoma also may be multiple, and are sometimes associated with tuberose sclerosis.

Distinguishing cell types

Oncocytoma, chromophobe carcinoma and the granular variant of clear cell carcinoma may have similar appearances on haematoxyin and eosin staining, and are distinguished by electron microscopy features and immunohistochemical markers. Oncocytoma is characterized on electron microscopy by cells packed with mitochondria, and thereby distinguished from chromophobe carcinoma whose cells contain microvesicles.

Classification of renal cysts[2-6]

Renal cysts can be evaluated with ultrasound, and for those that do not clearly fulfil the criteria for a simple or minimally complicated cyst, CT scanning and sometimes MRI are indicated for further evaluation. Infected and haemorrhagic cysts may have features that make underlying malignancy difficult to exclude by radiological criteria. The Bosniak classification was first described with CT, and has since been adapted with ultrasound criteria. In general, surgical intervention must be considered for Bosniak III and IV.

Bosniak classification

- Type I Simple benign cyst:
  - US: absence of internal echoes; sharply defined, thin, smooth, distinct wall and margin; good ultrasound transmission with acoustic enhancement behind the cyst; spherical shape.

- CT: sharp, thin, distinct, smooth walls and margins; spherical shape; homogenous; no contrast enhancement; density similar to that of water (−10 to +20 HU)
- Type II Minimally complicated (benign):
  - Septated or minimally calcified or infected or high density (20–90 HU) cysts.
  - Follow-up may be required.
- Type III Moderately complicated (require surgery):
  - Benign—haemorhagic, complex septated, multiloculated, irregularly, extensively or densely calcified cysts.
  - Malignant—irregular cyst wall; irregular, extensive, or dense calcification.
  - Includes multiloculated cystic nephroma and malignant cystic tumours which may be difficult to distinguish from Bosniak type III benign lesions (including post-infective changes) by radiological criteria.
- Type IV Malignant:
  - Tumours in wall of cyst, solid vascular elements, necrotic cystic neoplasms, and cystic carcinoma.

Familial types of renal cell carcinoma

- Clear cell carcinoma associated with von Hippel–Lindau disease:
  - Inherited tumour suppressor gene defect in von Hippel–Lindau disease (3p25).
- Familial non-VHL, non-papillary renal clear cell.
  - 3p chromosome abnormalities, commonly terminal deletion from 3p13.
- Hereditary papillary renal cell carcinoma.
  - Chromosomal changes include gains of chromosome 7 (trisomy), gains of chromosome 17p (trisomy).
  - Usually associated with mutation of c-*MET* gene (7q31) (MET codes for cellular receptor for hepatocyte growth factor (HGF); the mutant HGF receptor is unable to turn off when activated).
  - Non-MET hereditary papillary renal cancer may be more aggressive (particularly when there is loss of Xp).

Conditions associated with renal cell cancer having hereditary components

- Von Hippel–Lindau disease.
- Birt–Hogg-Dube syndrome.
- Tuberous sclerosis.
- Medullary (renal) carcinoma.
- Hereditary leiomyomatosis.
- Hyperparathyroidism–jaw tumour syndrome.
- Cowden's disease (multiple hamartoma syndrome).

Non-hereditary factors in renal cell cancer

Renal cell carcinoma is twice as common in men as women. The risk is substantially increased in chronic renal failure (×10 risk) and dialysis (acquired renal cystic disease, ×50 risk). Other non-heriditary risk factors include smoking (×2.5 risk), diet (high fat diet increases the risk, and inverse risk with fruit and vegetable consumption), obesity (particularly in female), oestrogen therapy (in animal model), hypertension (or its treatment), radiation exposure and occupation (exposure to carcinogens including asbestos, cadmium, petroleum, solvbents, tanning products, particularly in painters and fire-fighters).

2002 TNM (tumour, node, metastasis) classification for renal cell carcinoma[7]

The T, N, and M categories are each based on clinical examination and imaging.

Primary tumour

- TX   Primary tumour cannot be assessed
- T0   No evidence of primary tumour
- T1   <7.0 cm: limited to the kidney
- T2   >7.0 cm: limited to the kidney
- T3   Into major veins: adrenal or peri-nephric invasion
  - T3a Tumour invades adrenal gland or peri-nephric tissues
  - T3b Tumour extends grossly into renal vein(s) or vena cava below the diaphragm
  - T3c Tumour extends into the vena cava above the diaphragm
- T4   Tumour invades beyond Gerota's fascia

Regional lymph nodes

Hilar, para-aortic, and paracaval lymph nodes
- NX   Regional lymph nodes cannot be assessed
- N0   No regional lymph node metastases
- N1   Single regional node
- N2   More than one regional node

Metastases

- MX   Distant metastases cannot be assessed
- M0   No distant metastases
- M1   Distant metastases

Grading of renal cell carcinoma

Renal cell carcinoma is graded between 1 (well differentiated) and 4 (poorly differentiated) by Fuhrman grading.[8]

References

1 World Health Organization *Classification of Tumours. Pathology and Genetics of Tumours of the Urinary System and Male Genital Organs.* Lyon: IACR Press, 2004.

2 Aronson S, Frazier HA, Baluch JD, Hartman DS, Christenson PJ. Cystic renal masses: usefulness of the Bosniak classification. *Urol Radiol* 1991; **13**:83–90.

3 Curry NS, Cochran ST, Bissada NK. Cystic renal masses: accurate Bosniak classification requires adequate renal CT. *Am J Roentgenol* 2000; **175**:339–42.

4 Koga S, Nishikido M, Inuzuka S, Sakamoto I, Hayashi T, Hayashi K *et al.* An evaluation of Bosniak's radiological classification of cystic renal masses. *BJU Int* 2000; **86**:607–9.

5 Leder RA. Radiological approach to renal cysts and the Bosniak classification system. *Curr Opin Urol* 1999; **9**:129–33.

6 Bosniak MA. The use of the Bosniak classification system for renal cysts and cystic tumors. *J Urol* 1997; **157**:1852–3.

7 *TNM classification of malignant tumours*, 6th edn. New York: Wiley–Liss, 2002.

8 Fuhrman SA, Lasky LC, Limas C. Prognostic significance of morphologic parameters in renal cell carcinoma. *Am J Surg Pathol* 1982; **6**:655–63.

Radical nephrectomy

Radical nephrectomy includes removal the kidney within Gerota's fascia, including peri-renal fat and the adrenal gland.[1] It also includes removal of tumour thrombus that may extend for variable length from the renal vein to the right atrium, within the vena cava and adjacent major veins.[2] Lymphadenectomy is not routinely performed, but may have a limited place in selected cases.[3]

Diagnosis

Treatment of renal tumours is based on the clinical and radiological assessment of the patient and the location, extent, and stage of disease. Biopsy is not indicated unless lymphoma or metastatic disease to the kidney is suspected because of the risks of bleeding and difficulty in accurate histological assessment of primary renal tumours in needle biopsy material. Radiologically, a solid parenchymal mass of heterogenous density that enhances with intravenous contrast distinguishes renal cell carcinoma from normal renal parenchyma (including a Bertin's column), and renal cysts. The presence of a Bertin's column can otherwise be confirmed by DMSA nuclear scan. Complex renal cysts may require excision where there are suspicious features, based on the Bosniak classification, or there is diagnostic uncertainty concerning malignancy. 10–20% of renal masses prove to be benign on histological examination after their excision, depending on their size, but these cannot be distinguished reliably by pre-operative investigation or pre-operative biopsy.

Indications

Radical nephrectomy is indicated for treatment of a renal tumour with normal contralateral kidney and no evident metastases particularly when nephron-sparing surgery is not feasible or appropriate. The presence of a solitary metastasis may not be a contraindication, particularly where the metastasis is also amenable to resection. In the presence of more wide-spread metastatic disease, radical nephrectomy may be performed to reduce tumour burden where this may enhance the response to systemic therapies. It may also be carried out for symptomatic palliation, particularly intractable pain or recurrent bleeding.

Tumour assessment and staging

Treatment planning requires that the tumour is adequately assessed and staged with a contrast CT scan. This includes the assessment of tumour position, size, and extent, the presence of venous invasion and tumour thrombus, lymphadenopathy, and more distant metastases (particularly adrenal, liver and lung). The anatomic position of the kidney can be determined from the control film of an IVU or from CT scan by observing the relationship of the lateral border of the kidney to overlying ribs. Tumour multifocality and any other abnormality of the contralateral kidney must be assessed. Imaging also defines anomalous vasculature, and duplex ureter. MRI or ultrasound can be useful for assessing venous extension and for staging in patients allergic to intravenous contrast or with renal insufficiency. Bone scan may be carried out in patients with skeletal symptoms, abnormal serum alkaline phosphatase, or elevated calcium. The contralateral kidney must be further evaluated if there is a radiological abnormality, raised serum creatinine, or history of renal disease. This may include EDTA clearance (for GFR) and nuclear renography to estimate divided renal function. Assessment of cardiovascular and pulmonary function may also influence the surgical approach.

Patient preparation

The skin should be shaved according to the surgical approach and prepped with suitable antiseptic solution. Anti-thrombotic stockings, intermittent calf compression boots, low molecular weight heparin, and antibiotic prophylaxis should be used in accordance with local practice and guidelines. Blood should be cross-matched.

Surgical approach to the kidney

Incisions for nephrectomy are described in 📖 Chapter 2.

With flank extra-peritoneal approaches to the kidney, the retroperitoneal space is entered behind the peritoneum and below the diaphragm. The tip of the 12th rib is a safe and reliable landmark for entering this space, when this point can be incorporated into the incision. Damage to the intercostal neurovascular structures is avoided since these emerge from behind the tip of the inferior border of the 12th rib, deep to the thoracolumbar fascia. Using Mayo scissors, the muscular and tendinous attachments to the tip of the tip of the rib are cut, creating a small space through which the surgeon's finger can be insinuated to develop the underlying retroperitoneal space.

For higher intercostal approaches to the retroperitoneum, the layers of intercostal muscles are sequentially divided. Division of the internal intercostal muscle begins anteriorly and progresses posteriorly towards the pleural reflection; this is best done with dissecting scissors. Thus the retroperitoneal space will be approached under direct vision and exposed deep to the costal margin. As the incision proceeds in the posterior direction, the pleural reflection is identified. The pleura lies immediately deep to the internal (and innermost) intercostal muscles and the extrathoracic fascia; its costophrenic reflection will be encountered posterior to diaphragmatic attachments to the deep aspect of the rib. If it is not necessary to open the pleura, the diaphragmatic attachments to the rib should be divided carefully, so as to separate them without tearing the pleural attachments to the rib at the posterior limit of the incision. The pleura can be released by incompletely dividing the internal intercostal muscle where it overlies the pleura, and insinuating a finger over the superior aspect of the rib. Attachments of extra-thoracic fascia and pleura can then be pushed away and separated from the deep surface of the rib. If the pleural cavity is to be opened, the intercostal incision is extended posteriorly beyond the pleural reflection, and the diaphragm incised peripherally to maximize the retroperitoneal exposure.

Once the retroperitoneal space is entered, it is then relatively straightforward to extend the abdominal component of the incision. The peritoneum must be swept anteriorly, releasing it and the transversalis fascia from the abdominal wall musculature. This must be done gently with a finger or swab to avoid tearing the peritoneum. The intercostal neurovascular bundle passing from the inferior costal groove then between the transversalis and internal oblique layers can be felt digitally, directing the line of diathermy incision through the anterior abdominal wall musculature. In most situations, it is not necessary to extend the incision beyond the lateral border of the rectus muscle, but when the muscle is divided the epigastric vessels should first be formally ligated. The incision is extended for sufficient surgical access and exposure, and a retractor (e.g. a ring retractor with circumferential blades) positioned.

The transversalis fascia is opened where it overlies the kidney, *behind* the peritoneal reflection. This reveals the paranephric fat outside Gerota's fascia and represents the correct plane of dissection for radical nephrectomy. This surgical plane is extended by blunt dissection, and any fibrous or vascular attachments to Gerota's fascia are divided or diathermied. As the plane opens behind the right colon and its mesentery, the duodenum will be seen: its loose lateral fascial attachments should be cut (described by Kocher in 1902), allowing the plane of dissection to reach the inferior vena cava. On the left, the plane of dissection opens behind the spleen and tail of pancreas. In cases where the retroperitoneal plane between the kidney and colon does not open readily, because of peri-renal fibrosis or very bulky tumour, it may be necessary to open the peritoneum laterally to avoid unintentional or unrecognized bowel or vascular injury. Medially, Gerota's fascia merges with the adventitial layer of the great vessels. It is this attachment that prevents contralateral spread of a haematoma within the intact Gerota's fascia.

When an intraperitoneal approach to the kidney is made, through either an anterior laparotomy incision or a thoraco-abdominal exposure, the paranephric fat is approached by dividing the peritoneal reflection just medial to the line of Tolt, along the lateral margin of the colon and the hepatic/splenic flexure. The colon is then reflected medially. To enter the correct plane behind the colon and in front of Gerota's fascia, a thin fascial layer reflected from the back of the colon around the back of the kidney must be opened.

Gerota's fascia surrounds the kidney and proximal ureter. It also contains the peri-nephric fat, renal lymphatics, and ipsilateral adrenal gland. In radical nephrectomy, the kidney and adrenal gland should be removed with Gerota's fascia intact. Therefore the mobilization proceeds outside Gerota's fascia towards the great vessels and the kidney substance is not seen in the course of the dissection. This plane of dissection distinguishes the operation from 'simple nephrectomy' (for benign disease) and partial nephrectomy where the kidney or tumour is removed from within Gerota's fascia, having separated the kidney with its capsule from the peri-nephric fat. (In subcapsular nephrectomy, the kidney substance is removed from within the renal capsule.) In the region of the renal hilum, the plane of dissection and its proximity to the renal sinus determines the level of vascular branching that will be encountered.

Gerota's fascia is usually easily separated from the posterior thoracolumbar fascia and muscular posterior abdominal wall. Nevertheless, care should be taken to anticipate bleeding, particularly from collateral perforating veins. Dissect under vision with judicious use of diathermy.

When the kidney is mobilized, it can be rotated anteriorly, and thereby the renal artery(ies) are identified. The renal artery emerges from behind the vena cava on the right, or directly from the aorta on the left, and is directed towards the renal hilum. Once identified, the vessels can be slooped and controlled (Fig. 4.1 a, b). Further renal mobilization and anterior extra-hilar dissection are usually necessary for full anatomical display of the main renal vessels. Maintaining vascular control is imperative, and various possible combinations of multiple, aberrant, or normal displaced vessels

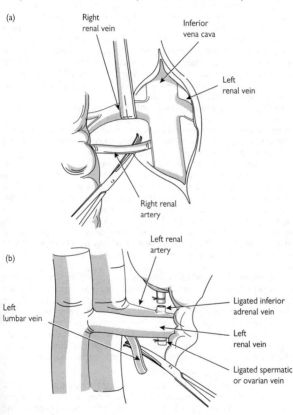

Fig. 4.1 (a) Right and (b) left renal hila at radical nephrectomy.

must always kept in mind. A large renal tumour may occasionally displace, rotate, or insinuate around normal structures, resulting in unexpected anatomical relationships to the great vessels (particularly vena cava) and their branches (e.g. the superior mesenteric artery), with potentially life-threatening consequences if midline or even contralateral vascular trunks are misidentified.

Early mobilization of the renal lower pole improves surgical access and enables the ureter to be identified. On the left, the gonadal vein will be encountered and should be ligated. The gonadal vessels (particularly veins) are easily torn in dissection or retraction which therefore requires due care. The plane between the great vessels and renal hilum is then dissected, and the small vessels therein controlled with diathermy. Dissection proceeds in a cranial direction alongside the lateral wall of the great vessels, until the main renal vessels are identified. This is facilitated by dissecting *within* the peri vascular adventitial layer. On the left the renal vein usually crosses anterior to the aorta, and on the right the renal artery emerges from behind the cava.

The right kidney and its hilum is situated lower than the left, because of its infra-hepatic position. At the renal hilum, the renal arteries usually lie behind their respective renal veins. The renal pelvis is located posteriorly and therefore the ureter can be a useful landmark when approaching the hilum from below. In front of the aorta, the left renal vein is crossed by the superior mesenteric artery. Each main renal artery divides outside the renal hilum into anterior and posterior branches from which the segmental arteries are derived. Segmental branches are variable in their origin but correspond to more constant renal vascular segments: superior, anterior superior, anterior inferior, inferior and posterior. The main segmental branches are end-arteries and (unlike the venous tributaries) have no collateral circulation. The renal artery also gives a named inferior adrenal branch. Supernumerary renal arteries may be present in ~30% of people, most commonly to the lower pole of the kidney and proximal ureter.

The left renal vein generally receives the gonadal vein, adrenal vein, tributaries of the phrenic vein, and a lumbar vein before coursing anterior to the aorta. The right renal vein has a shorter course to the inferior vena cava. It is generally considered that in the event of renal vein ligation, the collateral drainage of the left kidney may preserve some function, whereas on the right, renal function would be lost. Within the kidney, the segmental veins intercommunicate, providing collateral venous drainage. Therefore segmental veins can be ligated and divided as necessary.

Division of the renal vascular pedicle

The main renal arterial and venous trunks must be individually identified, and dissected clear of fibrous and lymphatic tissue. Having exposed the main vessels, tributaries should be identified, and sufficient length cleared for control and safe ligation (see below). Posterior tributaries, particularly a lumbar vein on the left, should be identified by careful dissection, as otherwise they may give rise to troublesome bleeding; there is no place for blind dissection with clamps. Vessel sloops enable the surgeon both to control vessels and to manipulate them for dissection and surgical exposure. Dissecting the renal artery and vein alongside the lateral margin of the great vessels allows control to be gained proximal to their divisions; dissecting too close to the renal hilum incurs the risk of both antegrade and retrograde bleeding, from retracting venous branches. Tributaries of the left venal vein are ligated and divided prior to ligation of the main renal vein (Fig. 4.16).

Usually, the renal artery is ligated before the renal vein to avoid renal congestion, swelling, and tendency to venous back-bleeding. Surgical exposure and vascular control thereby can be maintained. Due attention must also be given to venous invasion by tumour, avoidance of unnecessary venous manipulation, and early control of venous tributaries. Single or multiple renal arteries may be identified and ligated from their posterior aspect, with anterior rotation of the kidney. Alternatively, using an anterior approach, a vessel sloop placed around the main renal vein permits gentle retraction while the artery is identified behind it (Fig. 4.2). A ligature can then be passed around the artery and tied. With one secure ligature on the artery, still in continuity, attention can be turned to the venous dissection. Alternatively, two further ligatures are placed and the artery divided (see below), keeping in mind the possibility of supernumary vessels.

The main renal vein(s) should be ligated in continuity (i.e. before their division), with two ligatures proximal to the point of division and one distal (e.g. 0 Vicryl). Importantly, there must be sufficient distance between the two proximal ligatures, and between the more distal of these and the point of transection, to ensure security of the ties. Some surgeons use a vascular transfixion suture (4–0 polypropylene) as the distal of the two ligatures, although care is necessary to ensure that the vessel is not torn during this manoeuvre. The vessel can be precisely divided with a scalpel on a long handle, against the slightly opened jaws of a right-angled clamp

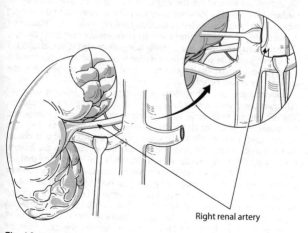

Right renal artery

Fig. 4.2 Ligation of the right renal artery.

positioned immediately behind the line of transection. Where renal vein involvement extends to the junction with the vena cava but not beyond, the cava can be side-clamped with a Satinsky clamp. The renal vein should then be divided with a scalpel a short distance from the clamp to provide sufficient cuff of caval wall for suturing. A running 4–0 polypropylene stitch can be used in one or two rows. In difficult situations, vessel loops around the cava and renal veins can be a wise precaution. Once the renal vein is divided, the renal artery can be dissected, ligated in continuity (with two proximal and one distal ligatures), and divided.

Where hilar dissection proceeds with difficulty and bleeding ensues, further dissection without adequate vascular control and blind clamping are dangerous. Hilar bleeding in these circumstances can sometimes be controlled by digital compression, permitting formal vascular ligation. Care must be taken to protect the great vessels (particularly the vena cava) from injury during bleeding, and sometimes proximal and distal control may be necessary. In some situations where the main renal vessels cannot be isolated, it may be feasible to pass a ligature around the entire vascular hilum, encircling all renal arteries and veins immediately lateral to the great vessels. Sometimes such a ligature can be manipulated under the vein to include only the renal artery for its selective ligation. However, it may be appropriate to control the artery and vein in the same ligature; separate ligation may be feasible at a later stage of the operation. Ligating the renal artery and vein together theoretically risks arteriovenous fistula, itself a very rare complication. Otherwise, where access is limited, the pedicle can be divided between two Satinsky clamps, allowing the kidney to be removed with subsequent completion of the vascular dissection.

Mobilization of the upper pole is often the most difficult aspect of the operation on account of restricted access and venous bleeding. Difficulties can arise where the surgical exposure is too low, and may be further confounded by inadequate retraction. Prior attention to the correct incision that can be extended as necessary will be rewarded. Mobilization is most safely carried out after the main renal vessels have been divided. Dissection may then proceed cranially alongside the great vessels around the upper pole. The surgeon must decide whether or not the adrenal is to be removed in continuity with the kidney; in radical nephrectomy, the adrenal is routinely resected.

Understanding the adrenal venous anatomy and its relation to larger retroperitoneal venous structures is key to maintaining vascular control. The left adrenal tends to lie above the upper pole of the left kidney, and the dissection proceeds above the adrenal towards the aorta. The right adrenal tends to lie medial to the upper pole of the kidney and its dissection proceeds across the upper pole of the kidney towards the inferior vena cava. Relatively fragile veins (particularly on the right, draining directly to the cava) are easily damaged by dissection or inappropriate traction. Ligaclips can be particularly useful for controlling small veins deep in the retroperitoneum. Bleeding from the adrenal bed if not controlled by diathermy can usually be managed with a transfixion suture. Bleeding from tributaries of the vena cava may be alarming; clamps may tear small veins or the cava itself, and blind clamping close to the cava must be avoided. Manouerves to control such bleeding are described on 📖 p. 288.

With the kidney fully mobilized and the renal vessels divided, remaining attachments of the kidney can be divided, allowing removal of the kidney. The ureter is ligated distal to the site of proposed division with an absorbable suture. Unless there is a history of urothelial malignancy, a normal ureter may be divided as low as convenient within the surgical field. On the proximal side, the ureter is ligated or clipped before division to prevent extraluminal spillage.

Inferior vena cava tumour extension

Intracaval tumour thrombus requires adequate exposure and access to the inferior vena cava, as well as the kidney. For right-sided tumours this usually necessitates a right flank thoraco-abdominal incision or right chevron (subcostal) at least, and for left-sided tumours a bilateral chevron or midline incision. The cava should be controlled and partially occluded with a vessel loop proximal to tumour thrombus prior to renal mobilization, particularly in cases of previous or pending embolism. This can be accomplished at the infra-hepatic or infra-diaphragmatic level unless there is more proximal tumour extension. The renal artery and ureter may then be ligated and divided before proceeding to full caval dissection. When tumour thrombus extends beyond the hepatic cava, cardiopulmonary bypass and circulatory arrest with heparinization are required. In these situations, the proximal thrombus in the renal vein may secured by double-clamping the vein, proximal suture ligation, and dividing the vein between the clamps; nephrectomy can then be completed prior to the caval dissection.

Tumour thrombus protruding just beyond the renal vein into the cava may be removed en bloc with the renal vein, using one (or two) Satinsky side-clamp(s) for partial caval isolation. The caval wall is opened around the renal vein with Pott's scissors, leaving a sufficient cuff within the clamp for caval closure (with a 4–0 polypropylene continuous suture). More extensive tumour extending into the cava, with a clear infra-hepatic margin, requires complete caval isolation. Rummel snuggers or vascular clamps are used to control the cava proximal to the level of intracaval tumour, and distal to the ipsilateral renal vein and its contained tumour, as well as the contralateral uninvolved renal vein (Fig. 4.3). Lumbar veins should be tied, and divided as necessary for adequate caval mobilization. The renal vein resection is continued into a longitudinal caval incision sufficient to allow dissection and extraction of the caval thrombus. Thrombus is everted through the cavotomy (in continuity with the renal vein stump), using a vascular dissector and suction.

Tumour extending to the infra-diaphragmatic cava requires hepatic mobilization and selective vascular clamping for adequate exposure and venous control. This includes the infra-diaphragmatic vena cava and small tributaries of the retrohepatic cava; hepatic inflow is controlled by isolation of the portal vein and use of the Pringle manoeuvre until the tumour thrombus is extracted. Where prolonged clamping is anticipated, veno-venous bypass may be used, or hypothermic systemic circulatory arrest and cardiopulmonary bypass.[4] Cardiopulmonary bypass is necessary for extensive and supra-diaphragmatic thrombus extension, or for extensive

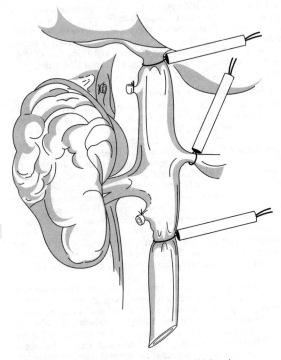

Fig. 4.3 Control of vena cava for extraction of level I thrombus.

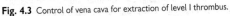

hepatic vein or retrohepatic caval wall infiltration. Occasionally, mural invasion necessitates local resection and vascular grafting. Surgery for caval tumour must be carefully planned and carried out by appropriately experienced surgical teams.

Lymph node dissection

Enlarged lymph nodes may be removed for histological assessment. This provides prognostic information, but to date has not influenced subsequent therapeutic options. In the absence of enlarged lymph nodes, lymphadenectomy is typically not performed. However, some surgeons advocate limited unilateral lymphadenectomy.[3,5–7] The extent of lymphadenectomy necessary to achieve any therapeutic or prognostic benefit is unknown. Future studies investigating adjuvant therapy for patients with nodal metastasis or other indicators of high-risk disease may be anticipated.[8]

Drains

A drain to the renal bed is not required after radical nephrectomy, unless pre-operatively there is underlying sepsis or collection. Where the chest has been opened, a chest drain is necessary. Small pleural tears at the posterior limit of a flank incision may sometimes be repaired after re-expanding the lung. A chest X-ray should be obtained immediately after surgery whenever the pleural cavity has been opened to ensure that the lung is re-expanded.

Closure

For closing a flank incision, preparatory placement of interrupted sutures prior to levelling the operating table facilitates secure mass closure of all muscular layers (O-PDS or nylon). The flexion should be taken out of the operating table before the sutures are tied. The overlying latissimus dorsi fascia and external oblique fascia are then closed in a second continuous suture.

Selective renal arterial embolization

Renal arterial embolization may sometimes be considered prior to nephrectomy for large or extensive renal tumour.[9] An embolization balloon is inflated within the main renal artery 24 hr prior to surgery and removed at surgery, with the kidney. Disadvantages include persistent tumour circulation from collateral vessels, longer hospital admission, and pain. Potential peroperative complications include tumour rupture and life-threatening haemorrhage.[10,11]

References

1 Robson CJ. Radical nephrectomy for renal cell carcinoma. *J Urol* 1963; **89**:37–42.
2 Blute ML, Leibovich BC, Lohse CM, Cheville JC, Zincke H. The Mayo Clinic experience with surgical management, complications and outcome for patients with renal cell carcinoma and venous tumour thrombus. *BJU Int* 2004; **94**:33–41.
3 Giberti C, Oneto F, Martorana G, Rovida S, Carmignani G. Radical nephrectomy for renal cell carcinoma: long-term results and prognostic factors on a series of 328 cases. *Eur Urol* 1997; **31**:40–8.
4 Ciancio G, Soloway MS. Renal cell carcinoma with tumor thrombus extending above diaphragm: avoiding cardiopulmonary bypass. *Urology* 2005; **66**:266–70.
5 Mickisch G, Carballido J, Hellsten S, Schulze H, Mensink H. Guidelines on renal cell cancer. *Eur Urol* 2001; **40**:252–5.
6 Minervini A, Lilas L, Morelli G et al. Regional lymph node dissection in the treatment of renal cell carcinoma: is it useful in patients with no suspected adenopathy before or during surgery? *BJU Int* 2001; **88**:169–72.
7 Terrone C, Guercio S, De Luca S et al. The number of lymph nodes examined and staging accuracy in renal cell carcinoma. *BJU Int* 2003; **91**:37–40.
8 Pantuck AJ, Zisman A, Dorey F et al. Renal cell carcinoma with retroperitoneal lymph nodes: role of lymph node dissection. *J Urol* 2003; **169**:2076–83.
9 Schwartz MJ, Smith EB, Trost DW, Vaughan ED, Jr. Renal artery embolization: clinical indications and experience from over 100 cases. *BJU Int* 2007; **99**:881–6.
10 Munro NP, Woodhams S, Nawrocki JD, Fletcher MS, Thomas PJ. The role of transarterial embolization in the treatment of renal cell carcinoma. *BJU Int* 2003; **92**:240–4.
11 Lin PH, Terramani TT, Bush RL, Keane TE, Moore RG, Lumsden AB. Concomitant intra-operative renal artery embolization and resection of complex renal carcinoma. *J Vasc Surg* 2003; **38**:446–50.

Partial nephrectomy

Partial nephrectomy may be recommended where it is possible to preserve ipsilateral normal renal tissue without compromising adequate pathology excision.[1-4] It may be imperative when removal of the entire kidney would either result in or lead to renal insufficiency, requiring renal dialysis or (later) renal transplantation. Twenty per cent of total normal renal function is necessary to avoid the need for dialysis. In patients electing for partial nephrectomy for management of malignant tumours, traditional concerns related to local recurrence and pathological multifocality.[5] However, the risk arising from ipsilateral multifocality appears similar to that from contralateral metachonous tumours,[6] and in well-selected cases local recurrence is rare. Partial nephrectomy can be carried out for a malignant or benign renal tumour, subject to its size and position. Although partial nephrectomy can be considered for larger masses, concerns are fewer and experience greater with tumours of ≤4 cm.[7-9] Radical nephrectomy should be performed where there is extensive local invasion, renal vein or inferior vena cava tumour thrombus, or regional lymphadenopathy.

The indication for partial nephrectomy is imperative with tumour in a solitary functioning kidney (e.g. renal agenesis, previous nephrectomy), with bilateral tumours, with a poorly functioning contralateral kidney, and with established underlying renal disease of the contralateral kidney that will progressively affect its function. Similar considerations include primary nephrological disease (e.g. chronic pyelonephritis), renovascular disease (e.g. renal artery stenosis), concurrent or previous significant calculus disease, or renal impairment secondary to systemic disease (such as diabetic or hypertensive nephropathy). Elective indications for partial nephrectomy include suitable tumours in patients with bilateral or multiple renal masses or an underlying genetic predisposition. It has gained its place in the management of small renal tumours, not least following the increasing presentation of low-stage or benign disease through incidental investigations.

In patients with bilateral renal tumours, the side with the tumour most amenable to partial nephrectomy may be undertaken as the first of two procedures to allow recovery of ipsilateral function, avoid temporary dialysis, and plan surgery for the major tumour. Pre-operative angiography may be undertaken for surgical planning with central or large tumours, particularly in a solitary kidney. Where the need for dialysis is anticipated, vascular access should be established prior to renal surgery.

Surgical approach

The surgical approach must provide good access for exposure of the tumour and, as necessary, hilar exposure, renal mobilization, and selective vascular control. Exposure is ensured by the most appropriate incision, adequate retraction, and lighting. Flank incisions generally provide better exposure than anterior approaches.

In contrast to radical nephrectomy, Gerota's fascia is opened, and the kidney mobilized within this fascial layer. Peri-renal fat overlying the tumour may be left *in situ*. Digital compression or an appropriately positioned soft bowel clamp may be sufficient for vascular control when enucleating small peripheral tumours. More secure vascular control is achieved using vascular bulldog clamps on individual segmental arteries. If necessary, segmental arteries should be dissected within the renal hilum (using Gil Vernet pyeloplasty retractors). Sloops may aid dissection and control of individual arteries. Branches of the main renal artery may be temporarily occluded to demonstrate their respective renal segment prior to renal incision. Methylene blue injected into a segmental artery (particularly polar) is an alternative method of defining the corresponding renal segment.

For polar tumours and small tumours within a single renal segment, where only a short period of ischaemia is required, excision may be possible while temporarily clamping a segmental parenchyma. Otherwise, segmental arteries supplying tumour and adjacent parenchyma can be selectively ligated and divided. Care should be taken to avoid ischaemia to the proximal ureter, or its vascular supply derived from the lower polar vessel and its branches. For small peripheral renal tumours, the renal vein need not be occluded routinely, to reduce intra-renal ischaemia. In an otherwise healthy kidney, warm ischaemia for maximum of 40–50 min can be tolerated.[10] Intravenous mannitol may be given prior to renal occlusion to maintain diuresis and renal function. Hypovolaemia, haemorrhage, and nephrotoxic medication should be avoided.

Larger tumours and mid-pole tumours may involve more than one renal segment; in this situation, or where more complex excision and reconstruction is anticipated, tumour excision should be carried out under cold ischaemia. Cooling is achieved using slushed iced saline around the kidney, separated from the surgical field by plastic sheet, bowel bag, or large cotton swabs. Up to 3 hr renal ischaemia may be tolerated at a renal core temperature of 20°C; this degree of core cooling is achieved after 15–20 min, with surface cooling having temporarily occluded the renal artery. Cold perfusion is not used because of the risk of intravascular tumour dissemination.

Partial nephrectomy must not compromise the principle of complete local tumour excision. Techniques include tumour enucleation (benign tumours), excision (with normal tissue margin), wedge resection, polar excision, and hemi-nephrectomy (Figs. 4.4, 4.5, 4.6). Consideration must be given to vascular control, warm or cold ischaemia, duration of ischaemia, renal incision, adequate excision margin, and renal reconstruction. Simple enucleation is appropriate for benign tumours, but when carried out for malignant disease, it incurs an unnecessary risk of a positive surgical margin and local recurrence.

Renal tissue may be incised with a knife, scissors, diathermy, harmonic scalpel, or argon laser. Preserving a strip of capsule at the resection margin aids later closure of the renal defect, particularly for benign disease, but may not be possible or appropriate in malignant disease. A combination of sharp and blunt dissection is used, with a sucker and adequate lighting. Larger vessels are transfixed as they are encountered with a fine prolene suture. A 1 cm macroscopic clearance margin is traditionally recommended, but there is not strong evidence to support this,

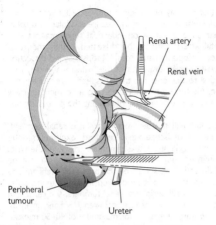

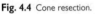

Fig. 4.4 Cone resection.

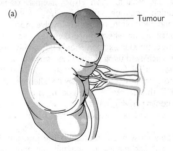

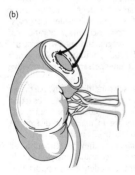

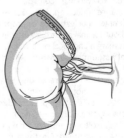

Fig. 4.5 Polar nephrectomy.

(a)

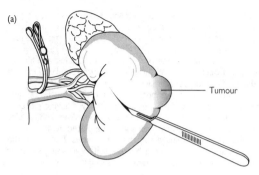

Tumour

(b)

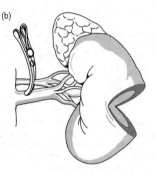

(c)

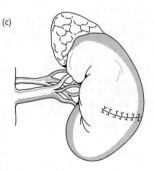

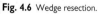

Fig. 4.6 Wedge resection.

particularly where patients are appropriately selected.[11] However, a biopsy from the margin of excision should be sent for frozen section histological examination to avoid an inadvertent positive surgical limit. Intra-operative ultrasound may help distinguish and characterize individual renal masses when multiple, for correlation with other imaging modalities, and also to guide intra-renal dissection. Bench surgery, and autotransplantation are options in the hands of surgeons familiar with these techniques.

When the collecting system has been opened, it is reconstructed and closed with an absorbable suture (e.g. 3–0 monocryl), having placed a ureteric stent to ensure urinary drainage to the bladder. Where an ongoing leak is anticipated, a nephrostomy tube should be placed at the time of surgery and kept on free drainage for at least 10 days. Defects in the collecting system and their repair can be assessed by injecting saline or methylene blue into the collecting system via a syringe and needle.

Haemostasis and closure of the renal defect

Individual bleeding vessels are ligated with a fine prolene cross-stitch. A bolster created from haemostatic gauze (e.g. Surgicel™) is placed across the raw surface of the renal defect. The edges of the renal parenchyma are re-approximated around the bolster with an absorbable suture through the capsule and parenchyma, securing the bolster in position. Alternatively adjacent vascularized fat, fascia, or a free peritoneal patch can be used to create a bolster (Fig. 4.7). Haemostatic paste (e.g. FloSeal™) can also be applied to the raw parenchymal surface and to the bolster. A retroperitoneal drain should be placed adjacent to the kidney.

Post-operative care

Post-operative care is similar to that for nephrectomy. However, there is a greater risk of post-operative haemorrhage than after nephrectomy, and potential for urinary fistula. Such complications must be recognized early for optimal management. The drain should be removed at 24–48 hr provided that there is no evidence of urinary leak. The absence of blood in the drain does not exclude the possibility of bleeding.

Radiofrequency ablation and cryotherapy

Technologies for ablation of renal masses include radiofrequency and cryotherapy.[12,13] Many of the technical difficulties associated with partial nephrectomy can be avoided, but oncological equivalence is not yet established. Patient choice is often a significant factor in selecting these treatments. Indications are similar to those for nephron-sparing surgery, with additional considerations of access, tumour location, and size. Tumour should not impinge on the renal pelvis or ureter during treatment, and its diameter should not generally exceed 4 cm. Indications also include small renal metastases. Bleeding coagulopathy is an absolute contraindication. CT or MRI is essential for case selection and treatment planning.

(a)

(b)

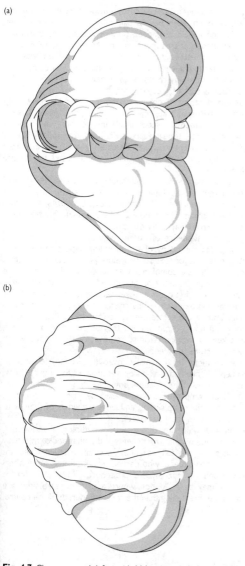

Fig. 4.7 Closure at renal defect with (a) haemostatic bolster and (b) omental patch.

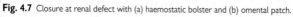

Access can be percutaneous, laparoscopic transperitoneal, laparoscopic retroperitoneal, or open. Each has its particular merits, disadvantages, and suitability for the individual patient, tumour access, and anatomical manipulation. Percutaneous treatment can be carried out with sedo-analgesia or general anaesthesia, in a prone or flank position, with CT guidance. The percutaneous technique is less suitable for anterior tumours, for tumours in close proximity to bowel, or where other viscera would interfere with probe access (e.g. colon, liver, spleen, lung). In some such situations, immediately adjacent organs can be displaced by injection of saline; in others, a laparoscopic approach may be feasible. With a laparo-scopic approach, the patient is placed in a flank position, and either a retroperitoneal or transperitoneal approach is used. The kidney is then mobilized and closely adjacent structures dissected to a safe distance from the therapeutic zone. Endoluminal ultrasound can be used for precise tumour localization.

Radiofrequency ablation delivers a monopolar alternating electric field directly to the target tissue. Ionic movement generates tissue heat (rather than its conduction from the probe itself), producing a predict-able zone of tissue necrosis. The tumour can be biopsied after treatment (rather than before, which may cause bleeding).

Cryotherapy uses a sequence of freeze–thaw cycles to induce tissue necrosis, achieving destruction by effects including hyperosmosis, dehy-dration, membrane destruction, cellular explosion, vascular stasis, ischaemia, and cell destruction. This is accomplished with needle probes placed in the target tissue. Multiple probes may be placed through an extracorporeal template. Reliable destruction ocurs at tissue temperatures below $-40°C$, creating both intra- and extracellular ice crystals; its extent is monitored with ultrasound. Usually three freeze–thaw cycles to $-180°C$ are used, including a margin of up to 5 mm around the tumour. After treatment, care must be taken to avoid premature removal of the probes which could cause tissue fracture and bleeding.

Potential complications of minimally invasive technologies include bleeding, peri-nephric haematoma, major vascular injury, urinary leak, urinoma, urinary fistula, ureteric stricture, bowel injury, and tumour recur-rence.[14] The risk of complications is increased by prior renal surgery, multiple treatments at the same setting, and close proximity of tumour to the renal hilum or other adjacent structures.

Case selection and availability of subsequent radiological monitoring during follow-up are important. The benefits and limitations of minimally invasive techniques are not fully defined. Percutanous techniques are currently most suited to patients who decline or are unsuitable for alter-native standard open or laparoscopic procedures. Minimally invasive ablative treatment may be an option where age or comorbidities are more immediately life-threatening than the renal tumour, but local control is nevertheless desirable.

The advantage of minimally invasive techniques is the minimization of surgical trauma, and ablation appears to be effective for control of renal tumours in the medium term. As long-term outcomes have not been defined in relation to alternative therapies, issues relate to completeness of tumour kill, reliability of needle biopsy for histological assessment, lack of complete histological examination, local recurrence, and consequences of multifocality. Where tumour excision is performed after minimally invasive ablation, viable residual disease has occasionally been demonstrated. High-intensity focused ultrasound, interstitial laser, radiosurgery with CT guidance, and respiratory tracking (Cyberknife) are among a number of other minimally invasive modalities under investigation.

References

1 Nieder AM, Taneja SS. The role of partial nephrectomy for renal cell carcinoma in contemporary practice. *Urol Clin North Am* 2003; **30**:529–42.

2 Shuch B, Lam JS, Belldegrun AS. Open partial nephrectomy for the treatment of renal cell carcinoma. *Curr Urol Rep* 2006; **7**:31–8.

3 Gill IS, Desai MM, Kaouk JH et al. Laparoscopic partial nephrectomy for renal tumor: duplicating open surgical techniques. *J Urol* 2002; **167**:469–7.

4 Uzzo RG, Novick AC. Nephron sparing surgery for renal tumors: indications, techniques and outcomes. *J Urol* 2001; **166**:6–18.

5 Polascik TJ. Pound CR, Meng MV, Partin AW, Marshall FF. Partial nephrectomy: technique, complications and pathological findings. *J Urol* 1995; **154**:1312–18.

6 Wunderlich H, Schlichter A, Zermann D, Reichelt O, Kosmehl H, Schubert J. Multifocality in renal cell carcinoma: A bilateral event? *Urol Int* 1999; **63**:160–3.

7 Lee CT, Katz J, Shi W, Thaler HT, Reuter VE, Russo P. Surgical management of renal tumors 4 cm. or less in a contemporary cohort. *J Urol* 2000; **163**:730–6.

8 Lerner SE, Hawkins CA, Blute ML et al. Disease outcome in patients with low stage renal cell carcinoma treated with nephron sparing or radical surgery. *J Urol* 1996; **155**:1868–73.

9 Leibovich BC, Blute ML, Cheville JC, Lohse CM, Weaver AL, Zincke H. Nephron sparing surgery for appropriately selected renal cell carcinoma between 4 and 7 cm results in outcome similar to radical nephrectomy. *J Urol* 2004; **171**:1066–70.

10 Kane CJ, Mitchell JA, Meng MV, Anast J, Carroll PR, Stoller ML. Laparoscopic partial nephrectomy with temporary arterial occlusion: description of technique and renal functional outcomes. *Urology* 2004; **63**:241–6.

11 Sutherland SE, Resnick MI, MacLennan GT, Goldman HB. Does the size of the surgical margin in partial nephrectomy for renal cell cancer really matter? *J Urol* 2002; **167**:61–4.

12 Janzen N, Zisman A, Pantuck AJ, Perry K, Schulam P, Belldegrun AS. Minimally invasive ablative approaches in the treatment of renal cell carcinoma. *Curr Urol Rep* 2002; **3**:13–20.

13 Aron M, Gill IS. Renal tumor ablation. *Curr Opin Urol* 2005; **15**:298–305.

14 Johnson DB, Solomon SB, Su LM et al. Defining the complications of cryoablation and radio frequency ablation of small renal tumors: a multi-institutional review. *J Urol* 2004; **172**:874–7.

Transitional cell carcinoma of the renal pelvis and ureter

Pathology

- In the upper urinary tract transitional cell carcinoma (TCC) accounts for 90% of urothelial tumours, the remainder being benign inverted papilloma, fibro-epithelial polyp, squamous cell carcinoma (associated with long-standing staghorn calculus disease), adenocarcimona (rare), and rare non-urothelial tumours including sarcoma.
- Renal pelvic TCC is uncommon, accounting for 10% of renal tumours, 4% of all TCC and 80% upper tract TCC. Ureteric TCC accounts for only 1% of all newly presenting TCC. 75% are located distally and only 3% involve the proximal ureter. Half are multifocal.
- Risk factors are similar to those of TCC in the bladder:
  - Males are affected three times as commonly as females.
  - Incidence increases with age.
  - Smoking confers a two-fold risk. There are various occupational risk factors, now mostly historical. Phenacetin use is associated with transitional cell carcinoma of the upper urinary tract and bladder, and analgesic nephropathy. Cyclophosphamide may cause cystitis, and urothelial malignancy.
  - TCC does not have a genetic hereditary form, although there is a high incidence of upper tract TCC in families from some villages in Balkan countries ('Balkan nephropathy') which remains unexplained.

Pathology and staging

The tumour usually has a papillary structure, but is occasionally solid. It is bilateral in 2–4%. It arises within the renal pelvis, and less frequently in one of the calyces or ureter. Histological features are most commonly TCC. Staging is by the TNM classification. Spread is by direct extension, lymphatic spread to para-aortic, and para-caval nodes and blood-borne spread most commonly to liver, lung, and bone.

2002 TNM (tumour, node, metastasis) classification for transitional cell carcinoma of the renal pelvis and ureter[1]

Primary tumour

- TX Primary tumour cannot be assessed
- T0 No evidence of primary tumour
- Ta Non-invasive papillary carcinoma
- Tis Carcinoma *in situ*
- T1 Invasion of subepithelial connective tissue
- T2 Invasion of muscularis
- T3 Renal pelvis
     Invasion beyond muscularis into peri-pelvic fat or renal parenchyma
     Ureter
     Invasion beyond muscularis into periureteric fat or renal parenchyma
- T4 Invasion of adjacent organs or through kidney into peri-nephric fat

Regional lymph nodes

Hilar, abdominal para-aortic, and para-caval lymph nodes for tumour of renal pelvis, and additionally intra-pelvic for ureteric tumour.

- Nx Regional lymph nodes cannot be assessed
- N0 No regional lymph node metastasis
- N1 Metastasis in a single lymph node ≤2 cm in greatest dimension
- N2 Metastasis in a single lymph node, >2 cm but ≤5 cm in greatest dimension, or multiple lymph nodes, none >5 cm in greatest dimension
- N3 Metastasis in a lymph node, >5 cm in greatest dimension

Metastases

- MX Distant metastases cannot be assessed
- M0 No distant metastases
- M1 Distant metastases

Reference

1 *TNM Classification of Malignant Tumours*, 6th edn. New York: Wiley–Liss, 2002.

Nephro-ureterectomy

Indications

Nephro-ureterectomy is most often carried out for transitional cell carcinoma in the upper urinary tract, where it involves the renal calyces, renal pelvis or ureter.[1] Upper tract urothelial malignancy is often associated with local invasion, multifocality, and carcinoma *in situ*, which together with its propensity for distal seeding in the urinary tract makes nephro-ureterectomy the most definitive management. Less radical treatment leaving the ureteral stump is associated with recurrence in a third to half of all patients.[2] The indication for nephro-ureterectomy can be based on the combination of uretero-renoscopy, imaging, selective cytology, and tumour biopsy.

Uretero-renoscopic or percutaneous surgery for upper urinary tract tumour ablation is sometimes employed in the treatment of small, solitary, well-differentiated, non-invasive, and therefore low risk tumours; it can also be considered in patients with a solitary functioning kidney.[3,4] However, careful surveillance follow-up is required, with the possibility of further surgery for disease recurrence or progression.[5] Tumour seeding in a percutaneous tract is a concern, even where prophylactic radiation is advised, as is the theoretical risk of systemic dissemination through pyelovenous reflux.[6,7] The presence of high-grade tumour and a normal contralateral upper tract makes minimally invasive treatment undesirable, other than for palliation, owing to its aggressive natural history.

Nephro-ureterectomy is performed with curative intent where there is no clinical evidence of metastatic spread, or to relieve local symptoms, bleeding, or other complications of upper tract tumour. Regional lymphadenopathy may be inflammatory rather than metastatic and is not necessarily a contraindication to surgery. In the absence of distant metastases, lymphadenectomy may be performed with nephro-ureterectomy for pathological staging and planning subsequent treatment.[8] The surgical approach and technique are modified according to the site and stage of the tumour, and the patient's habitus and comorbidities.

Preparation

Diagnostic and staging investigations must be completed, and the contralateral upper renal tract carefully evaluated. Associated bladder tumour must also be adequately assessed and treated, and at the time of nephro-ureterectomy, cystoscopy is carried out to ensure that the bladder is free of tumour. A urethral catheter should be placed, and water or other tumorcidal solution instilled into the bladder.

The skin should be shaved according to the surgical approach(es) to be made and prepped with suitable antiseptic solution. Anti-thrombotic stockings, intermittent calf compression boots, low molecular weight heparin, and antibiotic prophylaxis should be used in accordance with local practice and guidelines. Blood should be cross-matched.

Incision

There are a variety of surgical approaches to open nephro-ureterectomy. Their suitability depends on the site and size of the tumour, prior surgery, patient fitness and habitus. The patient is positioned according to the selected approach, with consideration to necessary intra-operative re-positioning.

A long midline abdominal incision, from xiphisternum to pubic symphysis, provides transperitoneal access for mobilization of the kidney the entire length of ureter and adjacent bladder cuff; it also provides access to the great vessels for lymphadenectomy, and to other intra-abdominal organs. Alternatively, an extra peritoneal dissection can be performed through a paramedian incision. However access to a high kidney or bulky renal tumour may be limited. An oblique flank incision provides optimal access to the kidney, upper ureter, and infra-diaphragmatic retroperitoneum but, unless endoscopic release of the lower ureter from the bladder is acceptable, a second incision will be required for the pelvic dissection. Lower ureteric mobilization with excision of the intramural ureter and the adjacent bladder cuff in continuity can be completed under direct vision through a Pfannelsteil or 'suprapubic V' incision.

Ligate the ureter below the tumour before renal and ureteric mobilization to minimize any risk of distal tumour spillage and seeding. Nephrectomy is carried out as described in 📖 p. 176. Mobilise the retroperitoneal ureter in continuity with the kidney to the common iliac artery. The pelvic ureter passes across the iliac bifurcation, and is itself crossed by the superior vesical artery. In the open pelvic dissection, the superior vertical artery must be ligated and divided. In the male, the ureter is also crossed by the vas deferens which is also routinely ligated and divided. Retract the bladder medially under a swab held in the left hand and dissect the ureter from its extravesical tunnel. This requires division of the loose fascia above the ureter that crosses anteriorly to it towards the pelvic sidewall, using diathermy forceps for haemostasis.

In the male, divide the thick band of lateral pelvic fascia above the prostate and lateral to the ureter to release the ureter from its extravesical tunnel. This manoeuvre opens the space under the ureter which becomes continuous with the retrovesical space behind the trigone and in front of Denonvillier's fascia. The dissection is facilitated by gentle anteromedial traction of bladder with the left hand, then passing a finger behind and medial to the ureter and thence behind the trigone, while releasing the previously mentioned lateral fascia.

In the female, open the fibrous tunnel ensheathing the ureter, within the lateral cervical ligament and adjacent to the vagina; the incision should be made on the ureter's lateral aspect guided with right-angled forceps. The medial aspect of the female ureter (and trigone) is very closely related to the vagina until the ureter is released by the lateral dissection.

In the operation of radical cystectomy, dissection of the very distal extravesical ureteric segment, as described above, is not necessary. The lateral fascial layer, encasing the ureter, remains on the bladder forming part of the surgical margin in front of the posterior pedicle and restraining the ureter as it angles anteromedially towards the trigone.

The bladder is opened by making a cystotomy between stay sutures (this technique is described elsewhere 📖 p. 215 and Fig. 4.8). The direction of the bladder incision should be angled obliquely so that it can be extended backwards towards the ipsilateral intramural ureter. After opening the bladder, the urethral catheter is removed and the ureteric orifices identified. The contralateral ureteric orifice should be located to avoid its inadvertent manipulation or injury. Good exposure, illumination, and suction are essential. A ureteric catheter can be used to guide the dissection of the intramural ureter and/or to protect the contralateral ureter.

The intramural ureter can be excised as an extension of the cystotomy incision, maintaining its continuity with the extravesical ureter, directed by a guiding finger lifting the trigone (Fig. 4.9). The bladder defect and cystotomy are closed in two layers, as described elsewhere (📖 p. 215 under ureteric re-implantation).

Alternatively, a purse-string suture (3–0 Vicryl) is placed around the ureteric orifice and through the intramural ureter, tied, and held in a small artery clip. Mark the urothelium adjacent to the ureteric orifice with a diathermy point. Dissect the orifice and intramural ureter with gentle traction on the purse string to bring this dissection within the bladder. Use sharp-pointed scissors and diathermy on vascular connections to release the intramural ureter from within the bladder. If the dissecting proceeds backwards beyond the posterior bladder wall defect, awkward bleeding may be encountered from retraction of bleeding vessels.

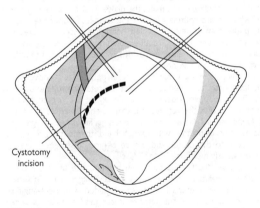

Cystotomy incision

Fig. 4.8 Cystotomy incision for excision of the intramural ureter is made with stay sutures in place.

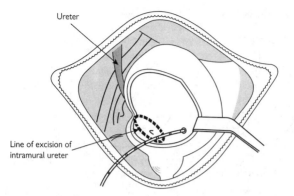

Fig. 4.9 Dissection of the pelvic ureter, incorporating the intramural ureter into the cystotomy incision.

To avoid open dissection of the pelvic ureter bladder, and a second incision, the lower ureter can be released endoscopically from the bladder.[9] This is accomplished by resecting the ureter itself, in the line of its intramural segment (with a resectoscope loop) (Fig. 4.10), or by circumcision of the ureteric orifice and intramural ureter (with a Collings knife). The pelvic ureter must be mobilized from above by blind digital dissection (i.e. with the retroperitoneal dissection), releasing it from its extravesical fascial attachments as far as the uretero-vesical junction. This technique is not suitable for tumours or multifocal disease involving the lower ureter or uretero-vesical junction because of the likelihood of tumour seeding, risk of local recurrence, and positive surgical margin.[10–12] Some surgeons address this concern by *beginning* with the renal and ureteric dissection, with early ligation of the lower ureter (without division). The lower ureter is fully mobilized to the bladder and the kidney then brought out through the flank wound which is then closed before endoscopic release of the ureter. After its distal release the ureter is then brought through the closed flank wound. Alternatively, the lower ureter is released endoscopically prior to the renal dissection, the ureter is fully mobilized and removed with the kidney.

Another technique for excising the intramural ureter is to place endoscopically a Braasch bulb-tipped ureteric catheter (Fig. 4.11) to the level of the mid-ureter, at the time of initial cystoscopy.[13,14] The kidney is then approached through a suitable incision and the ureter fully mobilized down to the bladder. Place a ligature above the ureteric catheter and two ligatures below the bulb of the catheter to ensure that it is well secured. Divide the ureter above the catheter. After removal of the kidney, perurethral traction on the ureteric catheter inverts the lower ureter into the bladder and urethra. Pass the resectoscope alongside the inverted ureter and resect the ureteric orifice and intramural ureter as previously described. This ensures complete removal of the intramural ureter, but is not suitable for tumours involving the middle or lower ureter.

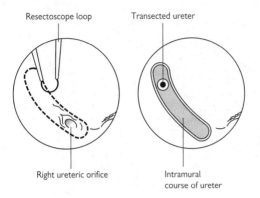

Resectoscope loop

Transected ureter

Right ureteric orifice

Intramural course of ureter

Fig. 4.10 Resection of the ureteric orifice.

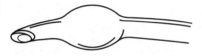

Fig. 4.11 Braasch-type ureteric catheter.

Place a drain in the lateral retropubic space in case of post-operative urinary leak from the bladder. Where an anterior lower abdominal incision has not been made, the tip of a retroperitoneal drain can be positioned adjacent to the bladder from above. A large (20F) urethral catheter should drain the bladder so that blood clots can be washed out as necessary.

Post-operative management

In addition to routine post-operative care, bladder drainage must be ensured until the cystotomy is shown to be healed by cystogram at 7–10 days. Bladder washouts should be done regularly to ensure that blood clots do not accumulate within the bladder. Irrigation of the bladder is then not usually necessary and preferably should be avoided as it risks extravesical leak, irrigation fluid absorption, and consequent complications.

Outcomes

The oncological benefit of radical nephro-ureterectomy relates to tumour clearance, negative surgical margins, and prevention of tumour implantation. Outcomes are adversely affected by higher tumour stage, with a strong correlation between tumour invasion and high grade. Any potential therapeutic advantage from lymphadenectomy can only be inferred from its role in the surgical treatment of bladder cancer. Nevertheless, lymphadenectomy may be worthwhile for pathological staging and guiding subsequent treatment, particularly when adjuvant chemotherapy can be offered.

Five-year survival

• Organ-confined	T1,2	60–100%
• Locally-advanced	T3,4	20–50%
• Node-positive	N+	15%
• Pulmonary, bone metastases	M+	<5%

References

1 McCarron JP, Mills C, Vaughn ED, Jr. Tumors of the renal pelvis and ureter: current concepts and management. *Semin Urol* 1983; **1**:75–81.

2 Cummings KB. Nephro-ureterectomy: rationale in the management of transitional cell carcinoma of the upper urinary tract. *Urol Clin North Am* 1980; **7**:569–578.

3 Roupret M, Hupertan V, Traxer O *et al.* Comparison of open nephro-ureterectomy and ureteroscopic and percutaneous management of upper urinary tract transitional cell carcinoma. *Urology* 2006; **67**:1181–7.

4 Jabbour ME, Smith AD. Primary percutaneous approach to upper urinary tract transitional cell carcinoma. *Urol Clin North Am* 2000; **27**:739–50.

5 Hrouda D, Ogden C, Morris SB, Wanendeya N, Fisher C, Woodhouse CR. Multiple frequent recurrences in superficial transitional cell carcinoma of the bladder: is survival compromised by a conservative management strategy? *Br J Urol* 1997; **79**:726–30.

6 Oefelein MG, MacLennan G. Transitional cell carcinoma recurrence in the nephrostomy tract after percutaneous resection. *J Urol* 2003; **170**:521.

7 Patel A, Soonawalla P, Shepherd SF, Dearnaley DP, Kellett MJ, Woodhouse CR. Long-term outcome after percutaneous treatment of transitional cell carcinoma of the renal pelvis. *J Urol* 1996; **155**:868–74.

8 Kwak C, Lee SE, Jeong IG, Ku JH. Adjuvant systemic chemotherapy in the treatment of patients with invasive transitional cell carcinoma of the upper urinary tract. *Urology* 2006; **68**:53–7.

9 Abercrombie GF, Eardley I, Payne SR, Walmsley BH, Vinnicombe J. Modified nephro-ureterectomy: long-term follow-up with particular reference to subsequent bladder tumours. *Br J Urol* 1988; **61**:198–200.

10 Arango O, Bielsa O, Carles J, Gelabert-Mas A. Massive tumor implantation in the endoscopic resected area in modified nephro-ureterectomy. *J Urol* 1997; **157**:1839.

11 Jones DR, Moisey CU. A cautionary tale of the modified 'pluck' nephro-ureterectomy. *Br J Urol* 1993; **71**:486.

12 Hetherington JW, Ewing R, Philp NH. Modified nephro-ureterectomy: a risk of tumour implantation. *Br J Urol* 1986; **58**:368–70.

13 Roth S, van Ahlen H, Semjonow A, Hertle L. Modified ureteral stripping as an alternative to open surgical ureterectomy. *J Urol* 1996; **155**:1568–71.

14 McDonald DF. Intussusception ureterectomy: a method of removal of the ureteral stump at time of nephrectomy without an additional incision. *Surg Gynecol Obstet* 1953; **97**:565–8.

Bladder cancer: pathology and staging

- Most primary bladder cancers are malignant and urothelial in origin:
  - \>90% are transitional cell carcinoma (TCC).
  - 1–7% are squamous cell carcinoma (SCC).
  - In areas where schistosomiasis is endemic 75% are SCC.
  - 2% are adenocarcinoma.
  - Rarities include phaeochromocytoma, melanoma, lymphoma and sarcoma.
  - Secondary bladder cancers are mostly metastatic adenocarcinoma from gut, prostate, kidney, or ovary.
  - Benign tumours of the bladder, including inverted papilloma and nephrogenic adenoma, are uncommon.
- Tumour spread:
  - Direct tumour invasion of the detrusor, ureters, prostate, urethra, uterus, vagina, perivesical fat, bowel, or pelvic side-walls;
  - Direct implantation into wounds/percutaneous catheter tracts.
  - Lymphatic infiltration and spread to the iliac and para-aortic nodes.
  - Haematogenous, most commonly to liver (38%), lung (36%), adrenal gland (21%), and bone (27%).
- Histological grading:
  - Well-differentiated (G1).
  - Moderately differentiated (G2).
  - Poorly-differentiated (G3).

WHO histological grading of non-invasive urothelial neoplasms[1,2]

- Urothelial carcinoma *in situ*.
- Non-invasive papillary urothelial carcinoma, high grade.
- Non-invasive papillary urothelial carcinoma, low grade.
- Non-invasive papillary urothelial neoplasm of low malignant potential.
- Urothelial papilloma.
- Inverted urothelial papilloma.

Transitional cell carcinoma

TCC may be single or multifocal. Because 5% of patients will have a synchronous upper tract TCC and metachronous recurrences may develop after several years, the urothelial 'field-change' theory of poly-clonality has been favoured over the theory of tumour monoclonality with transcoelomic implantation (seeding).

Primary TCC is considered clinically as muscle invasive or non-invasive:

- 70% of tumours are papillary, usually G1 or G2, exhibiting at least seven transitional cell layers covering a fibro-vascular core (normal transitional epithelium has approximately five cell layers). Papillary TCC is usually non-invasive and confined to the bladder mucosa (Ta) or lamina propria (T1). 10–15% of patients subsequently develop muscle-invasive or metastatic disease.
- 10% of TCC have mixed papillary and solid morphology and 10% are solid. These are usually G3, half of which are muscle invasive at presentation.

- 10% of TCC is flat carcinoma *in situ* (CIS). This is poorly differentiated carcinoma, often multifocal, confined by an intact basement membrane. 50% of CIS lesions occur in isolation; the remainder occur adjacent to tumour. CIS usually appears as a flat red velvety patch on the bladder mucosa; 15–40% of such lesions are CIS; the remainder are focal cystitis of varying aetiology. The cells are poorly cohesive; up to 100% of patients with CIS exhibit positive urine cytology, in contrast with much lower yields (17–72%) with G1/2 papillary TCC. 40–83% of untreated CIS lesions will progress to muscle-invasive TCC, making CIS the most aggressive form of non-invasive TCC.
- 5% of patients with G1/2 TCC and at least 20% with G3 TCC (including CIS) have vascular or lymphatic spread. Metastatic node disease is found in 15% Tis, 6% Ta, 10% T1, 18% T2 and T3a, 25–33% T3b and T4 TCC.

Squamous cell carcinoma

SCC is usually solid or ulcerative and muscle invasive at presentation. It accounts for only 1% of UK bladder cancers. SCC in the bladder is associated with chronic inflammation and urothelial squamous metaplasia, rather than CIS. In Egypt, 80% of SCC is induced by the ova of *Schistosoma haematobium*. 5% of paraplegics with long-term catheters develop SCC. Smoking is also a risk factor for SCC. The prognosis is better for bilharzial SCC than for non-bilharzial disease, probably because it tends to be lower grade and metastases are less common in these patients.

Adenocarcinoma

Adenocarcinoma is rare. It is usually solid/ulcerative, G3, and carries a poor prognosis. A third originate in the urachus, the remnant of the allantois, located deep to the bladder mucosa in the dome of the bladder. Adenocarcinoma is a long-term (10–20+ years) complication of bladder exstrophy and bowel implantation into the urinary tract, particularly bladder substitutions and urinary conduits after cystectomy. There is association with cystitis glandularis, rather than CIS. Secondary adenocarcinoma of the bladder may arise as discussed above.

2002 TNM (tumour, node, metastasis) classification for transitional cell carcinoma of the bladder[3]

For TCC of the bladder, the primary stage is based upon clinical examination, imaging, and endoscopy as well as appropriate tissue sampling and histological assessment. The N and M categories are based on physical examination, imaging and biopsy when indicated.

Primary tumour

- TX   Primary tumour cannot be assessed
- T0   No evidence of primary tumour
- Tis   Carcinoma *in situ*, 'flat tumour'
- Ta   Papillary non-invasive
- T1   Invasion of subepithelial connective tissue
- T2
  - T2a Invasion of superficial muscle (inner half)
  - T2b Invasion of deep muscle (outer half)

- T3   Invasion of perivesical tissue
  - T3a Microscopic extravesical invasion
  - T3b Extravesical mass
- T4
  - T4a Invasion of prostate or uterus or vagina
  - T4b Invasion of pelvic wall or abdominal wall

Although not in the TNM classification, T1 tumours are commonly subclassified.[2]

- T1a   Subepithelial invasion of a papillary process
- T1b   Invasion of lamina propria
- T1c   Invasion of muscularis mucosae

Regional lymph nodes
Pelvic lymph nodes below bifurcation of common iliac arteries

- NX   Regional lymph nodes cannot be assessed
- N0   No regional lymph node metastasis
- N1   Metastasis in a single lymph node ≤2 cm in greatest dimension
- N2   Metastasis in a single lymph node, >2 cm but ≤5 cm in greatest dimension, or multiple lymph nodes, none >5 cm in greatest dimension
- N3   Metastasis in a lymph node, more than 5 cm in greatest dimension

Metastases
- MX   Distant metastases cannot be assessed
- M0   No distant metastases
- M1   Distant metastases

2002 TNM (tumour, node, metastasis) classification for transitional cell carcinoma of the prostate and urethra[4]

The TNM stages of transitional cell carcinoma of the prostate and prostatic urethra are classified with urethral tumours. The primary stage is based upon clinical examination, imaging, and endoscopy. The N and M categories are based on physical examination and imaging.

Primary tumour
- TX   Primary tumour cannot be assessed
- T0   No evidence of primary tumour

Prostate and Prostatic Urethra (Male)
- Tis pu *In situ*, involving prostatic urethra
- Tis pd *In situ*, involving prostatic ducts
- T1   Invasion of subepithelial connective tissue
- T2   Invasion of prostatic stroma or peri-urethral muscle or corpus spongiosum
- T3   Invasion beyond prostatic capsule or into corpus cavernosum or into bladder neck (as extra-prostatic extension)
- T4   Invasion of other adjacent organs (including bladder)

Urethra (male or female)

T1   Invasion of subepithelial connective tissue
T2   Invasion of corpus spongiosum or prostate or periurethral muscle (including female)
T3   Invasion beyond prostatic capsule or into corpus cavernosum or bladder neck (including female) or anterior vagina
T4   Invasion of other adjacent organs

Regional lymph nodes

Inguinal and pelvic lymph nodes.

- NX   Regional lymph nodes cannot be assessed
- N0   No regional lymph node metastasis
- N1   Metastasis in a single lymph node ≤2 cm in greatest dimension
- N2   Metastasis in a single lymph node >2 cm, or multiple lymph nodes

Metastases

- MX   Distant metastases cannot be assessed
- M0   No distant metastases
- M1   Distant metastases

References

1 World Health Organization Classification of Tumours. Pathology and Genetics of Tumours of the Urinary System and Male Genital Organs. Lyon: IACR Press, 2004.

2 Epstein JI. The new World Health Organization/International Society of Urological Pathology (WHO/ISUP) classification for TA, T1 bladder tumors. Is it an improvement? *Crit Rev Oncol Hematol* 2003; **47**:83–9.

3 *TNM Classification of Malignant Tumours*, 6th edn. New York: Wiley–Liss, 2002.

4 Smits G, Schaafsma E, Kiemeney L, Caris C, Debruyne F, Witjes JA. Microstaging of pT1 transitional cell carcinoma of the bladder: identification of subgroups with distinct risks of progression. *Urology* 1998; **52**:1009–13.

Management of non-muscle invasive TCC

Transurethral resection of bladder tumour (TURBT)

The diagnostic role of TURBT has been discussed in Chapter 3, 📖 p. 114. Therapeutically, a visually complete tumour resection is adequate treatment for 70% of newly presenting patients with Ta/T1 superficial disease. The remaining 30% of patients experience early recurrence, 15% with upstaging. Photodynamic cystoscopy (using 5-aminolevulate or hexaminolevulate to induce tumour fluorescence under blue light) suggests that some tumours, including high-grade lesions and carcinoma *in situ*, may be incompletely resected or 'missed' by white light cystoscopy. Patients with non-invasive disease may be given adjuvant intravesical treatment for reduced recurrence rates (see below). Complications, including bleeding, sepsis, bladder perforation, incomplete resection, and urethral stricture, are uncommon.

Follow-up after TURBT

Review cystoscopy is usually done at 3 months. In some cases earlier re-resection is indicated. If the 3 month cystoscopy demonstrates recurrence, 70% of patients will recur further, and these will continue with cystoscopy every 3 months until there is either no recurrence or indication for additional treatment. The optimal schedule for surveillance after negative cystoscopy is controversial, but is usually based on the risk of recurrence and progression, assessed from the initial and 3-month cystoscopic and histological findings. Transurethral cystodiathermy or laser vaporization are accepted alternative procedures for ablating small superficial recurrences where histological assessment is not required. There is no accepted protocol for upper tract surveillance for patients with a history of bladder TCC, although some urologists recommend IVU every 2 years, particularly in high-risk disease.

Patients at low, intermediate and high risk for recurrence or progression are defined by EORTC risk tables.[1] Stage progression eventually occurs in around 40% of those with G3 disease or CIS. Younger patients may be offered primary radical cystectomy, and others considered for intravesical BCG therapy that has been shown to reduce recurrence and progression rates. Early re-resection (within a few weeks) to detect incomplete resection or understaging may be indicated in selected cases, particularly when muscle is not included in the resected specimen. Patients with recurrent multifocal G1/2 or Ta/1 TCC may also be offered adjuvant intravesical treatment (see 📖 p. 208).

Table 4.1 summarizes the management of bladder cancer stage by stage.

Table 4.1 A summary of the management of bladder cancer

Histology	Risk of recurrence post-TURBT	Risk of stage progression	Further treatment	Urological follow-up
G1/2, Ta/1 TCC	30%	10–15%	Single-dose intravesical chemotherapy	Review cystoscopies, commencing at 3 months
Persistent multi-focal recurrent G1/2, Ta/1	70%+	10–15%	Intravesical chemotherapy ×6 weekly doses	Review cystoscopies, commencing at 3 months
G3, T1 TCC	80%	40%	Intravesical BCG ×6 weekly doses	Review cystoscopies, commencing 6–12 weeks
CIS (carcinoma *in situ*, severe intra-epithelial dysplasia)	80%	40%	Intravesical BCG ×6 weekly doses ± maintenance	Cystoscopies + biopsy and cytology commencing at 3 months
pT2/3, N0, M0 TCC, SCC or adeno-carcinoma	Usually TUR is incomplete	NA	Radical cystectomy, radiotherapy (TCC) or palliative TURBT (unfit)	Cystoscopies if bladder is preserved. Urethral washings for cytology
T4 or metastatic TCC, SCC or adeno-carcinoma	Usually TUR is incomplete	NA	Systemic chemotherapy. Multidisciplinary team symptom palliation	Palliative treatment for local bladder symptoms

Non-invasive TCC: adjuvant intravesical chemotherapy

- Intravesical chemotherapy (e.g. mitomycin C (MMC) 40 mg in 50 mL saline) is used for G1–2, Ta, or T1 tumours and recurrent multifocal TCC. MMC is an antibiotic chemotherapeutic agent that inhibits DNA synthesis. In experimental studies, it may cause regression of small papillary TCC, and so it should be cytotoxic for microscopic residual disease post-TURBT. It significantly (>40%) reduces the likelihood of tumour recurrence compared with TURBT alone, but has never been shown to prevent progression to muscle invasion and has no impact on survival. It is used either as a single dose within 24 hr of first TURBT, or weekly for 6 weeks commencing up to 2 weeks post-TURBT. It is administered via a urethral catheter and held in the bladder for 1 hr.
  - Toxicity of MMC: 15% of patients report transient filling-type LUTS. Occasionally a rash develops on the genitals or palms of the hands, requiring treatment to be stopped. Systemic toxicity is rare with MMC.
- Other intravesical chemotherapeutic agents sometimes used as an alternative to MMC include doxorubicin and epirubicin.

Non-invasive TCC: adjuvant intravesical BCG

Bacille Calmette-Guérin (BCG) is an attenuated strain of *Mycobacterium bovis*. Commercially available strains include Pasteur, Connaught, and Tice. It acts by stimulating the immune response against urothelial tumour cells through upregulation of cytokines such as IL-6 and IL-8 in the bladder wall.

BCG is given as a 6-week course for G2/3 TCC and CIS, starting at least 2 weeks post-TURBT. It is administered via a urethral catheter (80 mg in 50 mL saline) and retained in the bladder for 1 hr. BCG produces complete responses in 60–70% of patients, compared with TURBT alone; 30% do not respond, and 30% of responders relapse within 5 years. It is more effective than MMC for prophylactic treatment of G1/2 and Ta/1 TCC, but is not often used (except as second-line occasionally) because of the additional toxicity. Two studies have suggested that BCG may delay tumour progression to muscle invasion.

BCG causes irritative symptoms related to cystitis, sometimes with haematuria, in nearly all patients. Low-grade fever with myalgia may occur in 25%. UTI contributes to this morbidity, requiring conventional antibiotic therapy, and BCG installations may need to be revised to avoid possible impact of antibiotics (particularly quinolones) on its bacteriological activity. Up to 6% of patients develop a high persistent fever, and occasionally systemic BCG disease may develop (BCGosis). These complications require prompt diagnosis and treatment with antituberculous therapy, usually isoniazid and pyridoxine for up to 6 months, but standard triple therapy (rifampicin, isoniazid, and ethambutol) is necessary in critically ill patients. Granulomatous prostatitis is not uncommon, but unless symptomatic does not require specific treatment. Epididymo-orchitis is a rare complication which may be difficult to distinguish from other differential diagnoses.

Contraindications to intravesical BCG include:
• Immuno-suppressed patients.
• Pregnant or lactating women.
• Patients with haematological malignancy.
• Traumatic catheterization or haematuria.
• Intolerance of therapy.

Cystoscopy too early after BCG can look alarming because of the generalized inflammatory response. Review cystoscopy and biopsy is generally undertaken 6 weeks after BCG to assess residual, persistent, or recurrent tumour; changes of chronic granulomatous inflammation may still be present at this time. Following a complete response, maintenance therapy is generally recommended (e.g. six-monthly treatments for 3 years) and is probably necessary for its efficacy in preventing progression. Nevertheless, careful surveillance is required in view of the adverse prognosis associated with disease recurrence or insidious stage progression. Where an initial induction course of BCG fails to eliminate urothelial disease, more radical therapy may be offered as an alternative to a second induction course of BCG. After initial failure, ~50% of patients will respond to a second course.

Reference

1 Sylvester RJ, van Der Meijden AP, Oosterlinck W, Witjes JA, Bouffioux C, Denis *et al.* Predicting recurrence and progression in individual patients with stage Ta T1 bladder cancer using EORTC risk tables: a combined analysis of 2596 patients from seven EORTC trials. *Eur Urol* 2006; **49**(3): 466–5.

Management of muscle-invasive bladder Cancer: stages T2–T4a

Without definitive treatment, 5-year survival of muscle invasive TCC of the bladder is 3%. In the absence of prospective randomized trials comparing the surgical and non-surgical treatments, the options for a patient with newly diagnosed confined muscle-invasive bladder cancer are as follows.

- Bladder preserving:
  - Radical transurethral resection of bladder tumour (TURBT) with systemic chemotherapy (few data, not mainstream).
  - Palliative TURBT ± palliative radiotherapy (RT): for elderly/unfit patients.
  - Partial cystectomy ± lymphadenectomy ± systemic chemotherapy.
  - TURBT plus definitive RT: can be combined with systemic neo-adjuvant/adjuvant chemotherapy (chemoradiation). SCC and adenocarcinoma are seldom radiosensitive.
- Radical cystectomy with:
  - External urinary diversion (via ileal or other intestinal conduit).
  - Ureterosigmoidostomy urinary diversion.
  - Orthotopic bladder reconstruction (to urethra).
  - Continent urinary diversion with Mitrofanoff catheterizable stoma or diversion to rectosigmoid pouch.
  - ± Chemotherapy: some evidence of benefit for neo-adjuvant chemotherapy.
  - ± Neo-adjuvant RT: no evidence of benefit.

Radical cystectomy with urinary diversion

This is the most effective primary treatment for muscle-invasive TCC, SCC, and adenocarcinoma, and can be used as salvage or palliative treatment if RT has failed. It is also a treatment for G3T1 TCC and CIS refractory to BCG. The operation carries significant morbidity and occasional mortality, and should be offered in the context of multidisciplinary care including a urological surgeon, an oncologist, a cancer specialist nurse, and a stomatherapist or continence advisor.

Salvage radical cystectomy is technically a more difficult and more morbid procedure. Relatively few patients who have failed primary RT are suitable for this as a secondary procedure, because of either poor physical fitness or a low probability of curable (i.e. non-metastatic) disease.

Efficacy of radical cystectomy with lymphadenectomy

Five-year overall survival rates are as follows:

- Stage pT1/CIS   75–90%
- Stage pT2   65–85%
- Stage pT3/4   30–50%
- Stage pN1–2   20–35%
- Salvage pT0   70%
- Salvage pT1   50%
- Salvage pT2/3a   25%

Invasive bladder cancer: radical radiotherapy

Radical external beam radiotherapy (RT) is a good option for treating muscle-invasive (pT2/3/4) TCC in patients who are unfit or unwilling to undergo cystectomy, but who still wish to have the chance of cure. The 5-year survival rates are inferior to those of surgery, but the bladder is preserved and the complications are less significant. Typically, a total dose of 60–70 Gy is administered in 30 fractions over 6 weeks. Higher-grade tumours tend to do less well, perhaps because of the undetected presence of disease outside the field of irradiation. Beyond this, prediction of RT response remains difficult, relying on follow-up cystoscopy and biopsy. CIS, SCC, and adenocarcinoma are poorly sensitive to RT.

There may be a small benefit in the use of neo-adjuvant or adjuvant cisplatin-based combination chemotherapy with RT in locally advanced (pT3b/4) disease.

Complications

Complications occur in 70% of patients; they are self-limiting in 90% of cases. These include radiation cystitis (filling LUTS haematuria and dysuria) and proctitis (diarrhoea and rectal bleeding). These effects usually last only a few months. Refractory radiation cystitis and haematuria may rarely require desperate measures such as intravesical alum, formalin, hyperbaric oxygen, bilateral internal iliac artery embolization, or even palliative cystectomy.

Efficacy of RT

Five-year survival rates are as follows:

- Stage T1   35%
- Stages T2   40%
- Stage T3a   35%
- Stage T3b,T4   20%
- Stage TxN1–2   7%

If disease persists or recurs, salvage cystectomy may still be successful in appropriately-selected patients; 5-year survival rates are 30–50%. Otherwise, cytotoxic chemotherapy and palliative measures may be considered.

Muscle-invasive bladder cancer: management of locally advanced bladder cancer (pT3b/4)

Many patients treated with primary cystectomy or RT with curative intent succumb to metastatic disease due to incomplete tumour excision or micrometastases. At this stage, the 5-year survival is only 5–10%. There is interest in augmenting primary treatment in an effort to improve outcomes.

Neo-adjuvant RT

Randomized studies have suggested improvements in local control using RT prior to cystectomy, but no survival benefit has been demonstrated.

Adjuvant RT

The rationale for post-cystectomy RT is that patients with proven residual or nodal disease may benefit from loco-regional treatment. However, it leads to unacceptably high morbidity and has no demonstrable advantages. Post-treatment bowel obstruction occurs 4.5 times more commonly in RT patients.

Adjuvant cystectomy

Two studies have demonstrated an improvement in local control and a survival advantage when treating locally advanced disease with cystectomy after RT, compared with RT alone. However, this treatment strategy does not happen in current UK practice, probably because of the increased morbidity of surgery in this setting.

Neo-adjuvant chemotherapy

Neo-adjuvant chemotherapy can downstage the disease and treat micro-metastases prior to definitive treatment with radical cystectomy or RT. A recent meta-analysis has suggested that a 5% survival advantage can be gained with the use of cisplatin-based combination chemotherapy.

Adjuvant chemotherapy

The rationale for post-cystectomy chemotherapy is that patients with proven residual or nodal disease may benefit from systemic treatment. Trials have been hampered by protocol problems, surgical complications interfering with treatment, and difficulty in assessing response in the absence of measurable disease. However, two of four studies of cisplatin-based regimes have shown a survival benefit of almost 2 years in the treated groups.

Chemoradiation

Recognizing the benefit of neo-adjuvant chemotherapy, the possibility that radiation may consolidate treatment of primary disease offers a bladder-sparing strategy whereby cystectomy is reserved for incomplete tumour response or recurrence. The feasibility of this approach and its oncological efficacy compared with primary cystectomy requires evaluation in clinical trials.

Metastatic bladder cancer

Systemic chemotherapy

Systemic cisplatin-based chemotherapy can be worthwhile in patients with measurable or symptomatic diffuse metastatic disease. Combination therapy is more effective than single-agent treatment. A complete response is seen in 20% of patients given methotrexate, vinblastine, adriamycin, and cisplatin (MVAC), although 20% pf patients develop neutropenia and very occasionally death from sepsis. Long-term disease-free survival is rare. Most UK centres use cisplatin, methotrexate, and vinblastine (CMV). Gemcitobine, a relatively new antimetabolite agent, has been used alone and in combination with cisplatin, with complete responses reported in 25–40% of patients. Another new class of agents, the taxanes paclitaxel and docetaxel, are microtubule disassembly inhibitors. Responses range from 25% to 80% using these agents alone or in combination.

Radiotherapy

Roles for RT include palliation of metastatic pain (30 Gy) and, spinal cord compression, ureteric obstruction, haematuria, and symptomatic primary disease (40–50 Gy). Ureteric obstruction may be relieved by percutaneous nephrostomy and antegrade stenting. Involvement of a palliative care team is essential.

Surgery

Surgery is effective for control of primary tumour. Simultaneous lympha-dectomy may sometimes contribute to cure when low-volume metastatic disease can be completely removed (see radical cystectomy, 📖 p. 224) Surgery has no role in overall oncological management in the presence of extensive lymphatic or distant metastases, other than urinary diversion with or without a palliative cystectomy. These palliative procedures may be considered where there is a need to improve the quality of remaining life, and a reasonable prospect for benefit and advantage over other forms of management.

Partial cystectomy, ureteric re-implantation, psoas hitch, and Boari flap

Partial cystectomy

Indications

Partial cystectomy is uncommonly performed for primary bladder pathology. It may be carried out for a solitary tumour in an otherwise normal bladder where the tumour cannot be cleared by endoscopic resection, is not associated with multifocal pathology, and (usually) is not located close to the trigone.[1-5] Occasionally, an isolated tumour in a diverticulum may be removed by partial cystectomy; and urachal carcinoma can be treated by extended partial cystectomy (including the urachus and umbilicus).[6] Other neoplastic indications include small squamous cancers (which are neither multifocal nor typically radiosensitive) and benign bladder tumours. Primary adenocarcinoma is usually inadequately treated by partial cystectomy, as it often has an aggressive course, not least because of a tendency to present late and infiltrate extensively beneath the urothelium and beyond the apparent limits of macroscopic disease. Partial cystectomy may be performed for extrinsic pathology that has invaded the bladder from adjacent structures (such as colon or female reproductive organs) or (more rarely) metastasized to the bladder.[4,7,8]

Partial cystectomy has a limited place in the management of primary bladder malignant disease because of the multifocality of transitional cell carcinoma, the risks of tumour seeding at operation, and the potential for leaving microscopic disease in adjacent tissue or its field of lymphatic drainage. Partial cystectomy can be combined with bilateral pelvic lymph node dissection (□ p. 229), still representing a less extensive procedure than radical cystectomy, retaining bladder function and providing prognostic pathological staging to guide further management. Nevertheless, radical cystectomy with lymphadenectomy provides the most reliable clearance of tumour and its lymphatic drainage,[4] and, with urinary tract reconstruction, even so-called favourable localized malignant tumours may be better treated this way.

Operative preparation

Prior to partial cystectomy, the patient and pathology will have been carefully assessed, and the bladder evaluated radiologically and by cystoscopy. Anti-thrombotic stockings, intermittent calf compression boots, low molecular weight heparin, and antibiotic prophylaxis should be used in accordance with local guidelines. Blood should be cross-matched.

The lower abdominal skin should be shaved and prepped with suitable antiseptic solution. Cystoscopy may be repeated before the patient is positioned supine on the operating table. With the mid-table hinge at level of umbilicus, the table is flexed to improve pelvic exposure, and levelled so that the abdomen is parallel to the floor. A urethral catheter is placed within the sterile field as there will be a need for intra-operative re-catheterization. The bladder is partially filled with water or tumoricidal solution.

Incision

With a midline lower abdominal, Pfannelsteil, or suprapubic V incision, a transperitoneal, retropubic, or combined approach can be made, exposing the peritoneal and/or extra-peritoneal surfaces of bladder. The urachus is excised when indicated, in continuity with the umbilicus and bladder dome (see cystectomy, ⌑ p. 224). From the brim of the 'false' pelvis, the peritoneum runs, like a sheet, across the true pelvic organs from the external iliac vessels (laterally), covering the dome of the bladder and female pelvic organs (medially) and anterior surface of the rectum (posteriorly), with the vas deferens or round ligament on its subperitoneal aspect. By dividing this peritoneal 'bridge' lateral to the bladder and anterior to the internal iliac trunk, where it can be referred to as the superior hypogastric wing, the peritoneal and retropubic spaces are brought into continuity, and good access to the posterolateral recesses of the retropubic space is gained. The bladder can be mobilized further by division of the superior vesical artery and dissection of the lateral pedicle (see cystectomy, ⌑ p. 224). Dissection of the distal ureter is described under nephro-ureterectomy (⌑ p. 197). Before opening the bladder, packs should be placed to expose and separate the bladder from the abdominal cavity and the edges of the surgical incision.

The cystotomy is facilitated by prior placement of stay sutures. These define the edges of the proposed opening and assist in its later closure. They should be placed, with the bladder distended, adjacent to the proposed circumferential incision around the tumour with a margin of normal bladder (traditionally 3 cm). Mark the proposed cystotomy with electrocautery. Incision of the bladder wall is then deepened holding the stay sutures on traction. An antero-inferior cystotomy incision should be directed cranially through the bladder wall, as a caudally directed incision tends to dissect within the bladder wall and cause additional bleeding. Once the bladder mucosa is opened, a sucker is used to minimize fluid spillage. The bladder incision is completed, having identified the ureteric orifices to avoid their injury. A small ureteric catheter (5F) can be placed through one or both ureteric orifice(s), particularly where these are close to the line of tumour resection. If it is necessary to include a ureteric orifice with partial resection of the trigone, the trigone must be mobilized (see nephro-ureterectomy, 📖 p. 196) and ureter reimplanted (see below). If appropriate, a bladder neck resection can be combined with prostatic enucleation, but such a procedure would not usually be performed with malignant pathology.

Close the bladder in two layers. Interrupted figure-of-eight stitches with a strong absorbable suture (e.g. 0 Vicryl) are haemostatic and ensure mucosal apposition as well as secure deep muscle closure. Watertight closure is reinforced with an overlying continuous layer including the external deep muscle and its overlying fascial layer (e.g. 2–0 Vicryl).

Place a catheter of sufficiently large calibre that will minimize the likelihood of blockage (i.e. at least 18 or 20Fr) via the urethra into the bladder. An additional suprapubic balloon catheter or Malecot catheter may sometimes be used, unless oncologically contraindicated, to ensure bladder drainage in the event of urethral catheter blockage or for through-and-through irrigation. Catheters must be placed and their balloons tested prior to bladder closure, subsequently taking care during bladder closure to avoid their injury with a needle. A suprapubic catheter should be placed through a small cystotomy (rather than the bladder incision): a diathermy point is used to cut through the bladder wall between two stay sutures held on traction, using forceps to pick up the deeper bladder layers. An extravesical retropubic drain should be placed in case of urinary leak.

Ureteric re-implantation to bladder

Ureteric re-implantation into the bladder is necessary after excision of the distal ureter (distal ureterectomy), transection of the distal ureter, or injury to the distal ureter that is not amenable to stenting and repair. Other indications include lower ureteric stricture, particularly when endoscopic management and stenting has either failed or is not feasible, or for vesico-ureteric reflux associated with symptoms or complications. When planning reimplantation, consideration should be given to bladder pathology and function, and need for a non-refluxing or refluxing an anastomosis. Ureteric re-implantation may be combined with a psoas hitch procedure or Boari flap (see below) to minimize tension on the anastomosis and compensate for loss of ureteric length. In some cases uretero-ureterostomy may be an alternative procedure; this avoids operating within the pelvis and retains a physiological vesico-ureteric junction, but potential complications may involve the contralateral renal unit (Fig. 4.12). With long ureteric defects an ileal or appendicular interposition, a Yang–Monti ileal tube or renal auto-transplantation can restore continuity between the renal pelvis or upper ureter and the bladder, without involving the contralateral renal unit.[9–15]

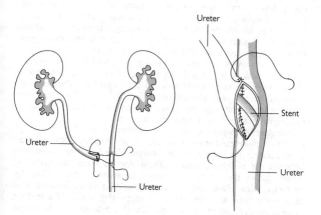

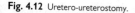

Fig. 4.12 Uretero-ureterostomy.

The ureter must always be dissected with care and manipulated gently, particularly when it is already diseased, to avoid further compromise of its vascular supply with the risk of subsequent ureteric or anastomotic stricture. This includes avoiding damage to vessels supplying the ureter, as well as the intramural adventitial plexus itself. Ureteric drainage is ensured by avoiding ureteric kinking, and planning an appropriate site for uretero-neocystotomy which will not obstruct the ureter or neo-vesicoureteric junction with bladder filling and emptying. A stay suture in the distal ureteric wall minimizes direct handling of the ureter and facilitates its manipulation. The ureter should be mobilized and trimmed according to the optimal length for reconstruction, and then spatulated. Ureteric re-implantation can be combined with a psoas hitch (see below) to avoid tension on the anastomosis, particularly when some ureteric length has been lost.

For a direct uretero-neocystotomy, a tunnelled non-refluxing anastomosis is usually constructed. Open the anterior bladder wall between stay sutures. Identify the site for uretero-neocystotomy on the postero-lateral extra-peritoneal surface of the bladder, and make a direct (stab) through the bladder wall with the diathermy point, Draw the ureter into the bladder with its stay. Make a submucosal tunnel with the jaws of a right-angled clamp, in line with the extravesical ureter; its length should be four times the ureteric width, with a distal opening at the site of the proposed internal neovesico-ureteric orifice (Fig. 4.13a). Bring the ureter from the bladder through this tunnel and back into the bladder, without twisting or tension, by gentle traction on the stay.

Complete the neovesico-ureteric anastomosis with 4–0 or 5–0 Vicryl. Place two interrupted anastomotic sutures which include detrusor muscle to stabilize the ureter at its distal margin. Place four additional sutures between the bladder mucosa (without detrusor) and the spatulated ureter. Suture the extravesical ureteric adventitia to the bladder for additional support with one or two longitudinal sutures. Secure a stent or ureteric catheter across the anastomosis (Fig. 4.13b). If a ureteric catheter is used, this can be brought through the bladder and body wall, and retained by an extravesical suture.

Alternatively, the ureter can be reimplanted with a non-refluxing anastomosis from the external aspect of the bladder, similar to the procedure described by Lich et al.[16] and by Gregoir and Van Regenmorter (Fig. 4.14).[17] Incise the external bladder surface through muscle to but not through the mucosa for 3 cm. Develop the adjacent detrusor as two lateral flaps such that the ureter can be laid along the incision without kinking. Open the mucosa at the distal end of this incision for the internal uretero-neocystotomy anastomosis. Approximate the two external bladder flaps over the ureter (thereby tunnelled) and close the tunnel with a 3–0 Vicryl suture. As previously described, place a stent within the ureter, and secure the ureter to the detrusor at the distal end of its tunnel and the extravesical ureter to the external aspect of the bladder.

Sometimes a direct refluxing uretero-neocystotomy is appropriate, particularly when the need for subsequent uretero-renoscopy (e.g. for upper tract surveillance) is anticipated. This is carried out intravesically or extravesically, anastomosing the spatulated ureter to the bladder mucosa with fine absorbable sutures, deeper stabilising sutures and a JJ stent or secured ureteric catheter, according to the principles previously described.

The bladder should be closed and drained using the standard technique, described for partial cystectomy (📖 p. 214).

(a)

(b)

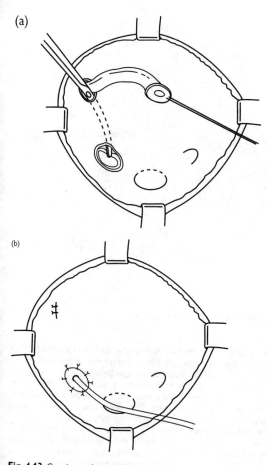

Fig. 4.13 Creating a submucosal tunnel for a non-refluxing ureteric reimplantation.

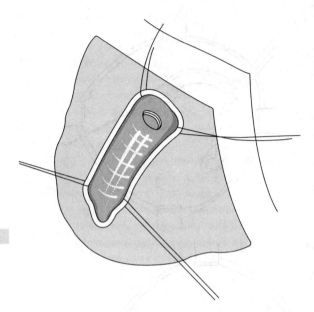

Fig. 4.14 Lich-Gregoir ureteric reimplantation.

Psoas hitch

A psoas hitch procedure enables a normal bladder to be mobilized above and lateral to the iliac vessels.[18,19] It is carried out extra-peritoneally. The contralateral superior vesical artery can be ligated and divided to increase bladder mobility; this anteromedial branch of the internal iliac artery is identified as it crosses the ureter in the lateral pedicle or poster-olateral limit of the retropubic space. The psoas hitch can be combined with ipsilateral renal mobilization to bridge a ureteric defect.[20]

Make an oblique incision across the broadest aspect of the anterior bladder wall, perpendicular to the axis of the bladder hitch; the incision should be sufficiently wide for the proposed cranial mobilization of the bladder (Fig. 4.15). The bladder hitch is usually made to the psoas minor tendon. It is most important to ensure that the tendon is correctly identi-fied and not in fact a nerve trunk. Alternatively, the hitch is made to the psoas major fascia, ensuring that the sutures are placed without injury to the genito-femoral and femoral nerves that pass through and emerge from the psoas muscle. The position of the bladder for the hitch is assessed with a finger inside the fundus of the opened bladder, checking for adequate mobilization to anastomose the ureter without tension.

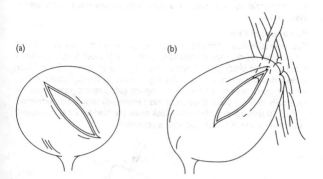

Fig. 4.15 Psoas hitch to psoas minor tendon or psoas major with ureteric reimplantation.

Place a series of three to six hitch sutures parallel with the femoral nerve. An absorbable suture such as 0 PDS can be used to maintain the position until eventually secured by fibrosis and avoid the risks associated with suture erosion into the urinary tract.

The site for ureteric re-implantation should be identified at the apex of the mobilized bladder; it should be stable and not liable to kinking. The spatulated ureter is then re-implanted as previously described; a tunnelled non-refluxing anastomosis of spatulated ureter is usually made. However, if ureteroscopic monitoring of the ipsilateral ureter is anticipated, a non-refluxing anastomosis should be constructed. A ureteric catheter (5–8Fr) should be secured across the anastomosis.

Close the transverse bladder incision longitudinally, and leave an extravesical retropubic drain (see partial cystectomy above).

Boari flap

A Boari flap enables the proximal or mid-ureter to be re-implanted across a longer ureteric defect than is possible by a psoas hitch alone.[21] The base of a bladder flap should be planned such that the posteriorly based convex flap can be rotated to receive the ureteric re-implantation.

Use stay sutures to delineate and manipulate the bladder flap, particularly in view of the tendency of the flap musculature to contract following bladder incision. Place the stay sutures at each base and the apex of the proposed flap incision. The base of the flap must be kept sufficiently broad to maintain adequate vascularization.

Division of the contralateral superior vesical artery (see above) increases bladder mobility. A psoas hitch can also be carried out to avoid anastomotic tension.[22]

The spatulated ureter is re-implanted into the apex of the flap, as described for psoas hitch (Fig. 4.16). Close the bladder flap as a tunnel, in linear continuity with bladder closure, using the standard two-layer bladder closure technique. Place a suprapubic and/or urethral catheter, and a retroperitoneal drain in case of urinary leak, as described under partial cystectomy.

Post-operative care

Post-operative instructions should be given to ensure that any extravesical retroperitoneal drainage is reported, as this would often herald unrecognized catheter blockage and urinary leak. By 5 days, provided that clear urine is draining and extravesical drainage is minimal, the suprapubic catheter and drain can be removed A cystogram (and ureterogram where an externally draining ureteric catheter has been used) should be performed at 7 to 10 days to exclude urinary leak from the bladder or vesicovaginal fistula before the remaining catheter is removed.

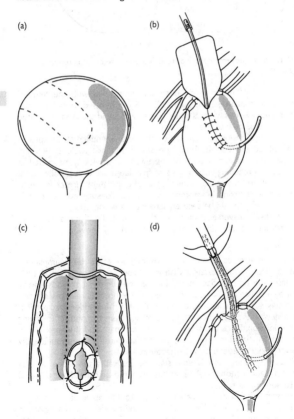

Fig. 4.16 Boari flap with ureteric reimplantation.

Late complications

After partial cystectomy the functional capacity of the bladder tends to be reduced, but usually it adapts to accommodate an adequate volume. Late complications of ureteric reimplantation include obstruction due to ureteric kinking, ischaemia or extrinsic compression within its submucosal tunnel. Other complications relate to stone formation secondary to urinary obstruction or non-absorbable suture material within or adjacent to the urinary tract. Adverse oncological effects relate to tumour implantation or local tumour dissemination.

References

1 Dandekar NP, Tongaonkar FIB, Dalal AV, Kulkarni SN. Partial cystectomy for invasive bladder cancer. *J Surg Oncol* 1995; **60**:24–9.

2 Holzbeierlein JM, Lopez-Corona E, Bochner BH et al. Partial cystectomy: a contemporary review of the Memorial Sloan-Kettering Cancer Center experience and recommendations for patient selection. *J Urol* 2004; **172**:878–81.

3 Kaneti J. Partial cystectomy in the management of bladder carcinoma. *Eur Urol* 1986; **12**:249–52.

4 Novick AC, Stewart BH. Partial cystectomy in the treatment of primary and secondary carcinoma of the bladder. *J Urol* 1976; **116**:570–4.

5 Utz DC, Schmitz SE, Fugelso PD, Farrow G. A clinico-pathologic evaluation of partial cystectomy for carcinoma of the urinary bladder. *Cancer* 1973; **32**:1075–7.

6 Herr HW. Urachal carcinoma: the case for extended partial cystectomy. *J Urol* 1994; **151(2)**:365–366.

7 Fujisawa M, Nakamura T, Ohno M et al. Surgical management of the urinary tract in patients with locally advanced colorectal cancer. *Urology* 2002; **60**:983–7.

8 Weinstein RP, Grob BM, Pachter EM, Soloway S, Fair WR. Partial cystectomy during radical surgery for nonurological malignancy. *J Urol* 2001; **166**:79–81.

9 Goodwin WE, Winter CC, TURNER RD. Replacement of the ureter by small intestine: clinical application and results of the ileal ureter. *J Urol* 1959; **81**:406–18.

10 Olsson CA. Ileal ureter and renal autotransplantation. *Urol Clin North Am* 1983; **10**:685–97.

11 Ali-El-Dein B, Ghoneim MA. Bridging long ureteral defects using the Yang-Monti principle. *J Urol* 2003; **169**:1074–7.

12 Matlaga BR, Shah OD, Hart LJ, Assimos DG. Ileal ureter substitution: a contemporary series. *Urology* 2003; **62**:998–1001.

13 Waldner M, Hertle L, Roth S. Ileal ureteral substitution in reconstructive urological surgery: is an antireflux procedure necessary? *J Urol* 1999; **162**:323–6.

14 Antonelli A, Zani D, Dotti P, Tralce L, Simeone C, Cunico SC. Use of the appendix as ureteral substitute in a patient with a single kidney affected by relapsing upper urinary tract carcinoma. *ScientificWorld Journal* 2005; **5**:276–9.

15 Chung BI, Hamawy KJ, Zinman LN, Libertino JA. The use of bowel for ureteral replacement for complex ureteral reconstruction: long-term results. *J Urol* 2006; **175**:179–83.

16 Lich R Jr, Howerton LW Jr, Goode LS, Davis LA. The uretero-vesical junction of the newborn. *J Urol* 1964; **92**:436–8.

17 Gregoir W, Van Regemorter G. [Congenital vesico-ureteral reflux.] *Urol Int* 1964; **18**:122–36.

18 Warwick RT, Worth PH. The psoas bladder-hitch procedure for the replacement of the lower third of the ureter. *Br J Urol* 1969; **41**:701–9.

19 Riedmiller H, Becht E, Hertle L, Jacobi G, Hohenfellner R. Psoas-hitch ureteroneocystostomy: experience with 181 cases. *Eur Urol* 1984; **10**:145–50.

20 Mathews R, Marshall FF. Versatility of the adult psoas hitch ureteral re-implantation. *J Urol* 1997; **158**:2078–82.

21 Olsson CA, Norlen LJ. Combined Boari bladder flap-psoas bladder hitch procedure in ureteral replacement. *Scand J Urol Nephrol* 1986; **20**:279–84.

22 Kishev SV. Indications for combined psoas-bladder hitch procedure with Boari vesical flap. *Urology* 1975; **6**:447–52.

Radical cystectomy

Radical cystectomy in the male includes *en bloc* removal of the bladder, distal ureters, prostate, membranous urethra, seminal vesicles, distal vasa deferentia, with adjacent connective tissue, their lymphatic drainage, and regional lymph nodes. The entire urethra can be included in the block dissection for simultaneous total urethrectomy. In the female, radical cystectomy includes removal of the bladder, usually with the urethra, adjacent vagina, uterus, Fallopian tubes, round ligaments, ovaries, surrounding connective tissue, lymphatic drainage, and regional lymph nodes, (referred to also as anterior exenteration). The surgical techniques are well described in the literature, along with various modifications necessary for urinary tract reconstruction and/or preservation of sexual function.[1–3]

Oncological indications for radical cystectomy include muscle invasive transitional cell carcinoma (stage T2 at least), particularly in the absence of clinical metastases. It is a mainstay treatment for localised high-grade and organ-confined invasive bladder cancer. Radical cystectomy is also indicated for high-grade non-muscle-invasive stages (stages pTa, pT1) or carcinoma *in situ* (stage pTis) where the pathology is extensive, multifocal, and/or associated with features indicating moderate or high risk of progression. Therefore indications also include failed endoscopic control or recurrence after intravesical therapy.[4] Cystectomy may be performed for recurrent malignancy following radiotherapy (as 'salvage' cystectomy) or for bladder complications following (or related to) previous treatment (such as contracted bladder, persistent haematuria, etc). It is carried out with curative or palliative intent. Radical cystectomy is also indicated for primary bladder tumours of non-transitional cell types, including squamous cell carcinoma, adenocarcinoma, and sarcoma. Pelvic lymphadenectomy is routinely performed with radical cystectomy, removing all regional lymphatic tissue in the field of tumour drainage, for tumour staging, and prognostic assessment that may guide future management. Lymphadenectomy may have potential therapeutic benefit in some cases where low-volume disease has metastasized within, but not beyond, the removed regional nodes (see pelvic node dissection, p. 229). Urinary diversion is required, by either urinary conduit or reconstruction of a continent reservoir.

Radical cystectomy with pelvic lymphadenectomy provides optimal opportunity for control of local disease, preventing pelvic recurrence and offering cure. It provides accurate pathological staging to guide further management and therapeutic intervention. Clinical understaging demonstrated by subsequent pathological examination may overestimate prognosis, and the unsuspected presence or development of distant metastases, even in patients with apparently non-muscle-invasive tumour, reflects the aggressive and life-threatening potential of this disease.

In male patients, urethrectomy may be recommended at the time of radical cystectomy. Specific indications include diffuse carcinoma *in situ* of the bladder, multifocal bladder tumour, tumour involving the bladder neck, prostate, or urethra. These considerations must therefore be assessed by prior endoscopy, biopsy, and/or peri-operative frozen section. When orthotopic reconstruction is planned, frozen section of the urethral margin is sent peroperatively where a positive margin would alter the need for urethrectomy and type of surgical reconstruction. However, the significance of positive prostatic biopsies or a positive urethral margin for recurrence after orthotopic reconstruction in otherwise well-selected patients is controversial.[5] When urethrectomy is not carried out, surveillance urethroscopy can be carried out on a six-monthly basis, particularly in patients with multifocal carcinoma *in situ*. Alternatively, in patients who have had urinary diversion, interval urethrectomy may be offered where extensive carcinoma *in situ* or multifocal malignancy is present in the cystectomy specimen, or in the event of urethral recurrence.

In female patients, urethrectomy is routinely carried out with radical cystectomy (as part of anterior exenteration) unless orthotopic reconstruction is to be performed. Orthotopic reconstruction should not usually be offered when multifocal carcinoma *in situ* is present, when invasive transitional cell carcinoma involves the trigone, bladder neck, or urethra; at surgery, frozen section examination of the bladder neck or proximal urethra showing malignancy at the surgical margin may contraindicate orthotopic reconstruction.[6,7]

Neo-adjuvant cisplatin-based chemotherapy has been shown in meta-analysis to improve 3-year survival in stages T2–T4a bladder cancer. The improvement is small (absolute difference 5–8%, Hazard ratio (HR) 0.8–0.85) but statistically significant.[8,9] Patients who do not have neo-adjuvant chemotherapy may be offered adjuvant therapy, according to local practice, taking into consideration operative and histopathological findings including pathological stage. However, evidence for any benefit is lacking.[10]

Clinical staging

The extent of local, regional, and metastatic disease must be assessed by formal staging investigations, including bimanual examination under anaesthesia, endoscopy, and CT scan of the pelvis, abdomen, and chest. Abnormal clinical, biochemical, and radiological findings must be fully investigated, including their potential to represent metastatic disease. In the presence of skeletal symptoms, raised alkaline phosphatase or raised calcium, bone scintigraphy should be undertaken. Adequate biopsy material must be taken for diagnosis and sufficient histopathological staging necessary for therapeutic planning in the context of other clinical staging assessments. This may include biopsy of radiologically suspected distant metastases, such as in the liver or lung. CT provides valuable structural imaging for treatment planning, but has limited accuracy for evaluating the pathological extent of the primary disease, metastatic lymphadenopathy, or ensuring subsequent metastasis-free survival after radical cystectomy.[11] Radical cystectomy with lymphadenectomy offers the most accurate pathological staging of the local and regional disease.

Operative considerations
Treatment planning and patient preparation

The bladder tumour will have previously been fully evaluated clinically (including urethroscopy, cystoscopy, and examination under anaesthesia), and radiologically (including assessment of the upper urinary tracts for hydronephrosis, synchronous tumour, intercurrent pathology, and renal function where necessary). Sufficient biopsies for histological assessment of muscle invasion and the extent of carcinoma *in situ* are essential. Photodynamic cystoscopy with hexaminolaevulinate has been shown to improve detection of bladder tumours and carcinoma *in situ* for targeting biopsies and more accurate disease mapping.[12,13] Prostatic urothelium can be assessed for carcinoma *in situ* by cold-cup biopsies. To assess prostatic stromal invasion and for staging prostatic urothelial malignancy, resect para-collicular cores of tissue from the bladder neck to verumontanum bilaterally; this is necessary where findings will influence need for urethrectomy and/or options for reconstruction.

The patient must be carefully counselled for a urinary stoma and potential options for reconstruction, based on prior medical investigations and assessment of the individual patient's suitability (see 📖 p. 254 on reconstruction). The stoma therapist has an essential role in informing and preparing the patient, as well as guiding management. Proposed cutaneous stoma sites must be assessed, and their practicality rehearsed with the patient wearing an external appliance. The patient must be well informed about the use and care of any stomas that may be constructed.

The fitness of the patient, pre-existing disease, and cardiorespiratory function may require specific assessment and optimization before radical cystectomy can be recommended. Any implications of previous surgery or radiotherapy, comorbidities, and individual anatomical variations, particularly the possibility of duplex ureters, must be taken into account in surgical planning. Urinary tract infection should be treated, and renal function optimized by appropriate relief of ureteric or bladder outflow obstruction and adequate hydration. Enteral or parenteral feeding may be considered, for the pre- and/or post-operative period.[14]

Operative preparation
Optimum and alternative sites for proposed cutaneous stomas must be marked preoperatively. Bowel preparation (mechanical and/or antibacterial), dietary restriction, and enema, with intravenous crystalloid fluid replacement, are used according to local guidelines and needs of the individual patient. Thrombo-embolic prophylaxis should be used in accordance with local guidelines and anticipated epidural anaesthesia. Anti-thrombotic stockings must be fitted and worn. Antibiotic prophylaxis should follow local protocols. Blood must be cross-matched and available in the operating theatre, according to local transfusion practice and the pre-operative haemoglobin level. Written informed consent for surgery must be obtained.

Patient positioning
The surgeon is always responsible for the appropriate and safe positioning of the patient on the operating table. The patient lies supine, with the mid-table hinge at the level of umbilicus and then flexed to increase pelvic exposure. When urethrectomy is required, provision for perineal access is necessary; the legs may be placed on individual articulating table extensions which allow for abduction, or in stirrups for the Lloyd-Davies position. When using the Lloyd-Davies or modified lithotomy position, use of hip flexion should be minimized because of the associated increase in

anterior compartment pressure and risk of lower limb anterior compartment syndrome, depending on the height and duration of elevation.[15–17] A means of repositioning the legs during surgery is advantageous for minimizing the duration of elevation. When carrying out bladder reconstruction after cystectomy, the patient must be positioned supine. Intermittent calf compression boots should be used. Careful attention must be paid to padding of potential pressure points and avoidance of contact between the patient and metalwork around the operating table. The table should be tilted so that the abdomen is level with the floor, and lowered to a height comfortable for the surgeon. Operating lights should be arranged and focused for abdominal and pelvic illumination; additionally, the surgeon may choose to wear a headlamp. The previously prepared skin mark for the stoma site may need to be reinforced (e.g. with a needle scratch). A nasogastric tube should be positioned unlesss a gastrostomy is to be constructed.

The abdominal skin should be shaved and prepped from the nipples to mid-thighs, including the genitalia. In the male patient, this will include the perineum if perineal urethrectomy is to be carried out. In the female, the perineum and vagina are always prepped (with aqueous antiseptic solution). A 20Fr urethral catheter should be inserted after sterile drapes are placed around the operative field, and positioned to drain by gravity. An inadequately sized catheter may fail to drain adequately as a result of blockage from blood clot, debris, or tumour within the bladder, and consequently restrict surgical access within the pelvis.

Incision and opening of the anterior abdominal wall

The right-handed surgeon will usually begin the operation standing on the left side of the patient. When planning the abdominal incision, consideration must be given to site and type of stoma (non-continent or Mitrofanoff). For non-continent diversion, a stoma site overlying the rectus muscle should be selected with sufficient margin from skin creases, scars, bony prominences and belt line to allow the circumferential application of a stoma appliance.

Usually a midline abdominal incision is made from the pubic symphysis, around the umbilicus contralateral to the proposed stoma, and for sufficient length to provide the required exposure. The subcutaneous fat and midline linea alba are incised in the line of the skin incision. If an umbilical Mitrofanoff stoma is to be constructed, sufficient margin (2–3 cm) must be allowed from the umbilicus. A transverse abdominal incision may be used for the patient who is particularly obese or who has had lower abdominal irradiation.

Divide the anterior rectus fascia below the linea semilunaris, the connective tissue attachments between the rectus muscles, and their attachment to underlying transversalis fascia on each side. The posterior rectus sheath is divided in front of the transversalis fascia above the linea semilunaris, in the midline towards and around the umbilicus. Formally incise the transversalis fascia with scissors in the midline deep to the rectus muscles, from the symphysis to just below umbilicus, thereby opening the retropubic space. The proximal extent of the urachal remnant is identified adjacent to the umbilicus, and the peritoneum opened on each side (where the extra-peritoneal fat is quite loose and thin). Double-clamp the urachus adjacent to the umbilicus, divide the urachus between the clamps, and ligate the two ends. Use scissors to incise the peritoneum alongside the urachal lateral margins medial to the inferior epigastric vessels (forming the lateral umbilical ligaments) and parallel to the more medial obliterated umbilical arteries. This peritoneal incision is guided by a relatively thin line of the extra-peritoneal fat towards, but medial to, the internal inguinal ring. Pelvic exposure can be maximized by dividing the medial attachment of the rectus muscles to the symphysis pubis (and re-attaching them with abdominal closure).

The surgeon must now assess the tumour and abdominal contents for tumour spread, the presence of other intra-abdominal pathology, and local operability. This specifically includes evaluation of bladder, pelvis, lymph nodes, bowel, and mesentery in relation to tumour resectability and options for reconstruction or diversion. Unless there are contraindications to continuing surgery, intraperitoneal adhesions are divided and a gastrostomy may be constructed (if preferred in place of naso-gastric intubation) for post-operative drainage.

Mobilization of the bowel

Bowel mobilization begins with the caecum and ascending colon. Incise the peritoneum just medial to the white line of Toldt, lateral to the peritoneal reflection from the bowel, using scissors or diathermy. This incision is extended medially around the caecum and distal small bowel mesentery, allowing the small bowel and ascending colon to be mobilized from the retroperitoneum, as far as the duodenum if necessary, for reconstruction and subsequent packing. If the right colon is to be used for reconstruction, mobilization must include the hepatic flexure, taking great care to not compromise vascular connections.

Mobilize the sigmoid colon by incising the peritoneum lateral to its mesentery, and immediately medial to the white line of its peritoneal reflection from the posterior abdominal wall. This facilitates subsequent retraction of the sigmoid mesentery, as well as forming a wide window for the left ureter to cross the midline. Mobilization follows a plane within the base of the mesentery, across the underlying sacral promontory and iliac vessels as far as the aortic bifurcation and inferior mesenteric artery. The descending colon can be further mobilized as necessary for exposure, with retraction and packing. The abdominal viscera are now packed into the epigastrium and away from the operative field.

Placement of retractor and packing of abdominal viscera

Prepare rolled large moist abdominal packs for packing the bowel, and deploy them according to preference. For instance, one large wet-pack, folded into three and rolled along the 1/3 axis, is positioned in each paracolic gutter. A third similarly prepared pack is laid transversely caudal to the small bowel and between the distal limits of the two paracolic gutters. Finally, a fourth fully opened pack is placed loosely over the bowel and assembled packs are placed across the width of the open abdomen. This package can then be held in a midline malleable blade retractor with four additional blades for circumferential retraction of the abdominal wall against a ring retractor.

Division of peritoneum

The distal limits of the anterior peritoneal incisions are now extended infero-laterally with scissors towards the false pelvis and hence the peritoneal incisions in the posterior abdominal wall, guided by the external iliac artery and gonadal vessels. (Alternatively, with a finger between the peritoneum and underlying iliopsoas fascia, the pelvic peritoneum can be lifted and divided.) This pelvic peritoneal incision should be made just lateral to the external iliac artery, in preparation for pelvic lymph node dissection. In the female, extend the incision lateral to the ovarian vessels that will be later divided at the level of the common iliac vessels (unless one or both ovaries are to be preserved). In the male, extend the peritoneal incision medial to the spermatic vessels, so that later they can be retracted laterally and preserved. The gonadal vessels also contribute to the vascular supply of the retroperitoneal ureter.

Division of the vas deferens or round ligament

The vas deferens or round ligament of the uterus will be identified just beneath and adherent to the pelvic peritoneum, crossing the line of the peritoneal incision before traversing the external iliac artery. The vasa deferentia begin their subperitoneal course emerging from the internal inguinal ring lateral to the external iliac vessels; they then cross these vessels, continuing in a plane between the bladder and peritoneum, and finally take a posterior and caudal course over the back of the bladder in front of the rectovesical pouch. Ligate the vasa where they cross under the incision of the pelvic peritoneum. The round ligaments emerge similarly from the internal inguinal ring and course within the anterior leaf of the broad ligament to the junction of the body and fundus of the uterus. The round ligaments are ligated and divided with the peritoneal incision, unless their full lengths are to be used for vaginal support of an orthotopic neobladder for which they are ligated close to the uterus. In the female undergoing anterior exenteration without ovarian sparing, the gonadal vessels are ligated and divided where they cross the iliac vessels.

Mobilization of distal ureters

Expose the pelvic ureter at or just cephalad to the bifurcation of the common iliac arteries and trace its retroperitoneal course proximally (having mobilized the sigmoid colon and caecum). A tagged sloop should be placed around each ureter in its pelvic segment. Mobilize the ureter proximally, avoiding damage to its adventitial wall and preserving vascular branches from the common iliac artery contributing to its blood supply. Care should also be taken to avoid damage to the gonadal vessels, which also provide vascular connections. The ureter should not be mobilized more than necessary for distal excision and reconstruction (see below).

Pelvic lymph node dissection

The importance of lymphadenectomy arises from removal of regional lymphatic vessels and nodal tissue, and thereby small isolated metastatic deposits that otherwise may give rise to metastatic recurrence.[18–20] Some patients with small metastatic lymph node deposits appear to be cured by lymphadenectomy, but survival advantage has not been prospectively demonstrated.[21,22] Lymphadenectomy provides additional pathological staging information which may influence adjuvant treatment and subsequent follow-up. The reliability of staging relates to the number of nodes removed and the extent of lymphadenectomy, with prognosis also depending on the number of negative nodes and a concept of lymph node density.[23,24] At cystectomy, dissection of the hypogastric vessels and lateral bladder pedicles is facilitated by prior lymphatic clearance. With bulky bladder tumours and limited surgical exposure, lymphadenectomy may need to be carried out after removal of the bladder.

The sentinel zone of lymphatic drainage from the bladder constitutes the pelvic lymph nodes below the common iliac bifurcation. Lymphatic tissue in this region must be cleared by meticulous dissection. The dissection extends from the femoral canal and circumflex iliac vein distally to the bifurcation of the common iliac artery proximally (Fig. 4.17). Some surgeons extend the lymphatic dissection alongside the common iliac vessels to the aortic bifurcation for any additional staging and potential therapeutic benefit that may be gained.

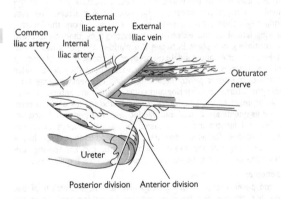

Fig. 4.17 Pelvic lymphadenectomy (left): dissection of the internal iliac artery, its branches, external iliac vessels and obturator nerve.

Lymphadenectomy may not be justified where salvage cystectomy is to be carried out after previous pelvic radiation, particularly where this would further increase the heightened morbidity of surgery in this setting or risk major vascular injury. Where nerve-sparing cystectomy is to be carried out, lymphadenectomy should not extend proximal to the iliac bifurcation to avoid damage to autonomic fibres passing across the common iliac vessels.

Lymphadenectomy requires meticulous technique and is facilitated by appropriate retraction. This requires lateral retraction (that in the male should include the spermatic vessels) and vertical elevation of the ring retractor above the external inguinal ring to expose the distal external iliac lymphatic chain.

Identify and preserve the genito-femoral nerve (and its variable branch) lateral to the external iliac artery; small branches behind the external iliac artery should be sacrificed. Lymphatic and fibro-fatty tissue is released from the psoas muscle and its fascia along a line lateral to and parallel with the common and external iliac arteries. By dividing the adventitia of these arteries, and thereby their lateral attachments to this lymphatic package, an avascular plane of dissection can be followed *lateral* to the iliac vessels into the true pelvis. Similar division of adventitial attachments to the external iliac vein and dissecting directly on the obturator internus muscle enables the lymphatic tissue to be retracted medially. Proceed with this dissection lateral to the iliac vein into the obturator fossa where the obturator nerve must be identified before cutting in its vicinity. Where meticulous clearance is carried out, formal ligation of the obturator vessels safely avoids their bleeding and retracting during the subsequent surgical dissection.

Dissect the lymphatic package from the femoral canal. At this anatomical limit, the lymphatic tissue is clipped and divided. The lymphatic package, including the obturator and external iliac nodes, is thereby released en *bloc*, and this can be further released proximally, lateral to the common iliac artery, and posteromedially from around the internal iliac trunk, which is thereby skeletalized. As this dissection proceeds into the true pelvis, the named branches of the internal iliac trunk can be clearly identified. Lymphatic tissue lateral to the common and external iliac arteries is freed and passed medially under these large vessels. Clip carefully and divide the posterior attachments of the lymphatic package which pass behind and below the internal iliac trunk, as this margin can be the source of troublesome venous bleeding.

Cysto-prostatectomy
Dissection of the superior vesical artery, distal ureter, and lateral bladder pedicle

The lateral and posterior bladder pedicles consist of fibrovascular tissue, connecting the base of the bladder to the lateral pelvic sidewalls. They are closely related to the ureters and include vascular and neural connections to pelvic structures in front of the rectum (Fig. 4.18). Below the base of the bladder, they become continuous with the posterolateral fascial attachments of the prostate and neurovascular bundles therein.

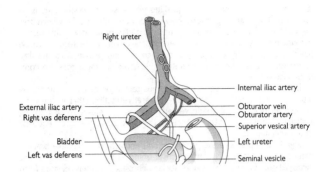

Fig. 4.18 Superior vesical artery and vas deferens crossing the ureter: these structures are the first components of the lateral pedicle to be encountered and divided.

Above and adjacent to the base of the prostate, the bladder pedicles are represented by thick condensed fibrovascular structures and best understood by dissecting the fascial layers that separate the adjacent viscera. The pedicles can thereby be separated into diverging lateral and posterior components for vascular control and division. Dissection of the lateral bladder pedicle is aided by prior dissection of the pelvic lymph nodes, exposing the branches of the internal iliac trunks and the pelvic sidewall.

Retract the bladder with a swab held in the left hand. The superior vesical artery is usually easily identified as the first anterior visceral branch of the anterior hypogastric trunk. Dissect this vessel clear of adjacent tissue, ligate it, and divide it at its origin. Other branches of the hypogastic trunk can be individually dissected, ligated or clipped, and divided in front of the posterior bladder pedicle (Fig. 4.19). In the female, the ureter is crossed by the uterine artery, which is also ligated and divided. The Ligasure™ device provides a good method of haemostasis and facilitates the dissection. With counter-traction on the bladder, a finger can be passed immediately behind the anterior hypogastric branches and in front of the posterior pedicle towards the undersurface of the endopelvic fascia. This manoeuvre may facilitate the dissection, particularly when normal tissue planes have been obliterated (e.g. after radiotherapy). The distal limit of the dissection is the inferior vesical vein, just above the endopelvic fascia. The posterior (deep) limit of this dissection does not need to be extended behind the hypogastric trunk (i.e. posterolaterally leading into the pararectal spaces).

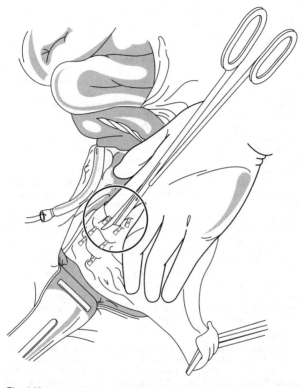

Fig. 4.19 Division of the lateral bladder pedicle is facilitated by prior dissection of the internal iliac trunk, and retraction of the bladder with the left hand.

Release the ureter from the lateral aspect of the bladder by dividing its overlying fascial layer crossing from the bladder to the lateral pelvic sidewall below the level of the anterior hypogastric vessels. This dissection is aided by medial retraction on the bladder with the left hand. Opening this plane allows the ureter to be traced distally, and completes the lateral dissection of the bladder. Contributions from the hypogastric plexus to the bladder and prostatic neurovascular bundles remain undisturbed inferomedial to the ureter within the posterior pedicle, which is tethered posterolateral to the seminal vesicles. After ensuring haemostasis, small packs are placed in the dissection bed lateral to the bladder while attention turned to the pouch of Douglas.

Dissection of the pouch of Douglas and the rectovesical space

Blunt finger dissection immediately posteromedial to the ureters opens a surgical avascular plane in front of the rectum (Fig. 4.20). This space extends below the peritoneal reflection of the pouch of Douglas, behind the seminal vesicles and the anterior layer of Denonvillier's fascia, and medial to the posterior pedicle and its neurovascular attachments (Fig. 4.21). This plane is easily extended across the midline beneath the peritoneum. The peritoneum is then lifted in clamps and divided, thereby opening the roof of the pouch of Douglas.

Using a swab for anterior traction on the bladder and counter-traction on the rectosigmoid, the rectovesical space can usually be developed under direct vision towards the prostatic apex. When there is infiltrative or inflammatory pelvic disease, fibrosis, previous radiotherapy, or previous surgery, or the normal tissue plane does not open readily, sharp dissection (rather than blunt or blind finger dissection) must be used.

Alternatively, the peritoneum of the pouch of Douglas is held in tissue clamps and opened with scissors at its deep extent. The rectovesical space must be developed *behind* the seminal vesicles and thereby between the layers of Denonvillier's fascia. As this dissection continues distally, the attachment of the posterior layer of Denonvillier's fascia must also be opened (with scissors) where it stretches from the front of the rectum to the prostate. This enables the prostatic apex to be reached. If the rectovesical space is mistakenly developed from the plane in front of seminal vesicles or vas deferens, or in front of the anterior layer of Denonvillier's fascia, the surgical space cannot be opened beyond the seminal vesicles. Dissection within the incorrect plane must be re-commenced from the pouch of Douglas at a more distal level, as re-directing the dissection from an incorrect rectovesical plane in a posterior direction risks rectal injury.

Division of ureters

Ligate the ureters proximal and distal to the site of their proposed transection, and then divide them between the ligatures. The level of transection will depend on pathological considerations including tumour cell type, presence and extent of carcinoma *in situ*, and length of ureter required for reconstruction. With multifocal transitional cell carcinoma and/or previous carcinoma *in situ*, frozen section of the distal ureter is required if negative resection margins are to be ensured; the ureteric resection margin may then be taken proximal to the level of positive frozen section until a negative margin is confirmed. The merit or otherwise of a negative frozen-section ureteric resection margin is controversial, and not all surgeons agree on the pathological and therapeutic advantage of a negative margin, not least because of tumour multifocality. The technique of

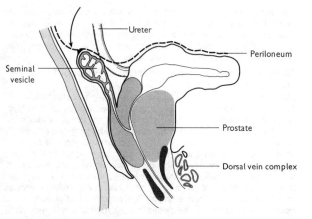

Fig. 4.20 Surgical planes for radical cystoprostatectomy.

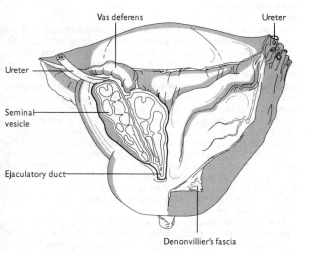

Fig. 4.21 The anatomical relationships of the vas deferens, seminal vesicle and distal ureter to the posterior bladder pedicle.

diversion or reconstruction needs to accommodate the available ureteric length. For squamous cell carcinoma, the full length of ureter may be preserved. Injury to the vessels supplying the ureter, direct injury to the ureter, kinking, and redundant ureteric length must be avoided. Trim excess ureteric length at a later stage of the operation.

Division of the endopelvic fascia, pubo-prostatic ligaments, and dorsal venous complex

Diathermy the superficial dorsal vein, open the endopelvic fascia, and divide the pubo-prostatic ligaments, as described for radical prostatectomy. The prostate is then fixed at its apex by the dorsal venous complex, the urethra, the posterior aspect of the external sphincter, and the lateral para-urethral pillars (of Walsh). The prostate is also held by lateral fascial attachments (containing the neurovascular bundles) to the pelvic sidewall. Transfix and divide the dorsal venous complex, and secure haemostasis. Variations in technique include partial division of the pubo-prostatic ligaments, and bunching of the dorsal venous complex with an angled Babcock clamp before ligation. The attachment of pubo-prostatic ligaments to prostate must be divided at some stage to ensure removal of all apical prostatic tissue.

Dissection of the posterior bladder pedicle, prostate pedicle, and membranous urethra

Non-nerve sparing in the male

The operation then proceeds with further antegrade dissection of the remaining attachments of the bladder and prostate. In this approach, clamp and divide the posterolateral vesical pedicles containing vascular and autonomic attachments to the bladder base and prostate. Then dissect and divide the lateral attachments of the prostate: first, the lateral pelvic fascial attachments to periprostatic fascia, and then the remaining attachments of the prostate apex, taking care to avoid rectal injury. The posterolateral pedicles can be controlled between the jaws of curved clamps, placed under vision, and divided. A second pair of clamps may be used if necessary to reach the base of the seminal vesicles, or alternatively, the Ligasure™ device may be useful in this position. After division of the (clamped) posterior pedicle, the posterior pedicle attachment to the pelvic sidewall can be transfixed and under-run. Thus wider posterolateral surgical margins are gained than is possible with a nerve-preserving technique. Some surgeons defer ligation of the dorsal venous complex until antegrade mobilization of the prostate is completed. Then proceed to urethral division (see below).

As an additional complementary manoeuvre for mobilizing a particularly fixed prostate, the posterior rectoprostatic space can be brought into continuity with the retropubic space by dissection immediately lateral to the apex of the prostate, having previously opened the endopelvic fascia (Fig. 4.22). At this para-apical position, the prostatic attachments to the sidewall are predominantly fascial rather than vascular. This technique defines a surgical plane under the lateral and posterior pedicle of the prostate and bladder which may be valuable for vascular control when normal anatomical planes have been obliterated. The pedicles are then readily clamped and divided.

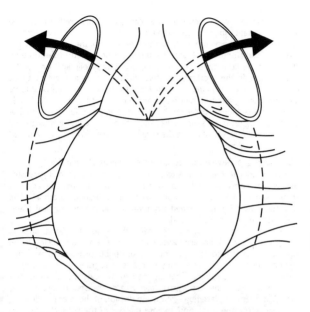

Fig. 4.22 Route for establishing continuity between the surgical rectovesical plane and the endopelvic space (opened by prior incision of the endopelvic fascia lateral to the prostate.

Alternatively, the bladder and prostate can be mobilized by retrograde mobilization of the prostate. Incise the superficial lateral fascial attachments of the prostate to the pelvic sidewall (as described for radical prostatectomy). Divide the urethra (see below) and, with cephalad traction on the clamped catheter, release the apex of the prostate to enter the surgical plane behind Denonvillier's fascia, thereby establishing continuity with the rectovesical space. Thus the lower limits of the lateral and posterior pedicles are clearly identified. The bladder is held by these remaining pedicles, which are clamped and divided, allowing removal of the cystoprostatectomy specimen.

Unless urethrectomy or orthotopic reconstruction is to be performed, the urethra is divided as follows. Apply cephalad traction to the specimen to stretch the membranous urethra into the pelvis and dissect off its rectal attachments. Clamp the membranous urethra and divide it distal to the clamp, with the catheter *in situ*. A segment of membranous urethra can thereby be excised with the cystoprostatectomy specimen.

If orthotopic reconstruction is to be carried out, the urethra is opened at the prostatic apex. Traction on the catheter will prevent tumour spillage. After opening the anterior three-quarters of the urethral circumference, four anterior and lateral sutures can be placed in the urethral stump for the later anastomosis (using 2–0 polyglycolic acid on a UR-6 needle). Divide the urethral catheter, enabling its distal segment to be brought into the pelvis and clamped. Place the final two posterior sutures after completing the urethral division and removal of the specimen. Divide remaining attachments between the prostate and posterior sphincter. The urethral margin can be sent for frozen-section histological examination if the margin status will influence the surgical plan (see 🔲 p. 224 and p. 254 on reconstruction).

Nerve-sparing in the male: dissection of the neurovascular bundles
A nerve-sparing technique aims to preserve the branches of the hypogastric plexus that converge on the prostatic neuro-vascular bundles adjacent to the seminal vesicles and course to the membranous urethra.[25] This dissection must be approached from within the correct surgical plane, and diathermy must not be used.

For the standard retrograde approach, the endopelvic fascia, apex of the prostate, and urethra are dissected first and the neurovascular bundles released as described for open radical retropubic prostatectomy. Some surgeons begin radical cystectomy with this retrograde dissection, particularly when nerve sparing. Thereby the neurovascular bundles and their connections from the hypogastric plexus are released, before bladder mobilization is completed by ligation and division of the lateral pedicles.

For an antegrade dissection, expose the tips of the seminal vesicles at the base of the bladder (i.e. *within* the enclosing fascia of the vesicles); this requires sharp dissection under vision and anterior retraction of the bladder. Gently retract the seminal vesicles from the plane of the hypogastric plexus (i.e. medially), and release them from the medial aspect of the vesicoprostato-pelvic fascia. As dissection of the seminal vesicles proceeds, the pedicle anterior to the vesicles, (i.e. adjacent to the bladder base and prostate) can be progressively divided, in a more ventral plane than with the non-nerve sparing technique, against ligaclips (avoiding clamps and diathermy). The neurovascular connections then fall backwards, retaining their connections to Denonvillier's fascia (posteriorly) and the lateral pelvic fascia. This plane of dissection cannot advance beyond the caudal limit (base) of the seminal vesicles, where the neurovascular bundles come to lie immediately adjacent to the prostate. At the base of the seminal vesicles, the bundles are tethered closely to the prostate by vascular branches and surrounding condensing planes of fascia. At this point, the bundles are particularly vulnerable to surgical injury and must be carefully released before dividing more distal lateral fascial attachments of the prostate.

Antegrade release of the neurovascular bundles then proceeds from the base of the seminal vesicles to the apex of the prostate. Here, the neurovascular bundles run adjacent to the prostate (below the seminal vesicles) and must be released from the anterolateral fascial connections of the prostate. The endopelvic fascia must be opened first, the dorsal vein ligated, and the underlying superficial fascial layer running over the prostate to rectum divided in front of the bundles. Occasional vascular branches between the bundles and prostate must be clipped and divided. Antegrade nerve preservation with a laparoscopic or robotic approach may be facilitated by creating the so-called veil of Aphrodite by releasing the prostatic fascia anteromedial to the bundles (📖 see radical prostatectomy, p. 274).

At the apex of the prostate, the previously straight course of neurovascular bundles may be interrupted by an upward and medial course over the apex of the prostate. At this point, the bundles are tethered to the prostate surface by vascular connections and overlying fascia above the prostato-urethral junction. Manouevres to release the bundles which do not allow for this deviation in their course at the prostatic apex will damage their continuity. The bundles must be released alongside their medial aspect by dividing the overlying prostatic fascia; this is inevitably behind the urethra, where both urethra and prostate are relatively immobile. Therefore this requires prior division of the urethra for adequate access, as for the retrograde dissection. Distal to the prostato-urethral junction, the bundles continue posterolateral to the posterior aspect of the external sphincter, from which they can be separated by the jaws of a right-angled clamp to complete safely the division and release of the sphincter.

Once the cystectomy specimen is removed, haemostasis is secured and the pelvis is packed.

Anterior exenteration

The classical anterior exenteration in the female includes *en bloc* removal of the bladder, distal ureters, uterus, Fallopian tubes, ovaries, anterior vaginal wall, and urethra, with their common lymphatic drainage.

Dissection of the ovarian pedicle, distal ureter, and lateral bladder pedicle in the female

Where the ovaries are to be removed, divide the ovarian pedicles where they cross the iliac vessels. As the ureter is followed distally, it follows a somewhat more lateral course than in the male, passing in front of the posterior uterosacral ligaments and then adjacent to the cervix within facial coverings. Within the lateral bladder pedicle, the uterine artery can be individually identified, ligated, and divided, and can be followed crossing the ureter. Ligate the dorsal vein of the clitoris before proceeding with the vaginal or bladder neck dissection.

Dissection of the pouch of Douglas and the rectovaginal space

In the pouch of Douglas, the peritoneum is reflected from the rectum to the posterior vaginal wall. The uterosacral ligaments limit the lateral extent of the pouch of Douglas, and represent the equivalent of the male posterior pedicle, containing branches of the hypogastric plexus and also providing support for the uterus and vagina. A figure-of-eight stay suture in the body of the uterus (or an Allis clamp) facilitates anterior traction.

Incise the peritoneum in the pouch of Douglas to give surgical access to the posterior vagina (Fig. 4.23). Dissect along the posterior vaginal wall, mobilizing sufficient length for later vaginal reconstruction. The uterosacral ligaments are then easily identified. Place tissue clamps on the posterolateral vagina just behind the cervix. This can be facilitated by manipulating a Betidine-soaked swab-stick in the vagina. Open the posterior vaginal wall in the midline between the clamps. The posterolateral fornices of the vagina and their fascial attachment can be clamped in the line of vaginal division for traction. Haemostasis is facilitated by suture transfixion and a running suture along the paravaginal tissue.

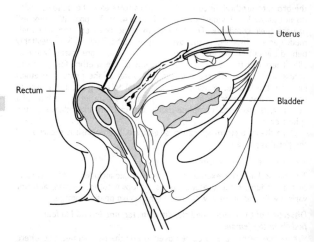

Fig. 4.23 Opening the posterior vaginal wall: incision close to the posterior aspect of the cervix is facilitated by a swab on a stick at the vaginal vault

Non-nerve sparing in the female

Opening the endopelvic fascia and urethrectomy

Proceed by dividing the paravaginal tissues close to the vaginal wall in a line towards the bladder neck and urethra, using diathermy, Ligasure™, or ligation (Fig. 4.24). The endopelvic fascia must be opened before the bladder neck and para-urethral dissection. Having exposed the anterolateral vaginal wall, incise it with a diathermy point towards the bladder neck. Continue this incision caudally alongside urethra, then around the urethral meatus to include complete urethrectomy *en bloc* with the surgical specimen. Alternatvely, the peri-urethral dissection can be carried out or assisted from the perineum.

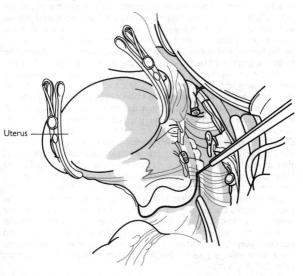

Uterus

Fig. 4.24 The anterolateral vaginal incision is extended anteriorly, then alongside the urethra, to include a strip of anterior vaginal wall with the urethra on the surgical specimen (anterior exenteration).

Nerve-sparing in the female
Division of the urethra without opening the endopelvic fascia
If the urethra (with its nerve supply) is to be preserved, a nerve-sparing dissection of the bladder neck and proximal urethra is required. The anterior endopelvic fascia supporting the bladder neck must also be preserved. The urethra should be divided just distal to the bladder neck, and up to 1 cm of proximal urethra may be excised.[6,26]

Open the posterior vaginal wall in the midline behind the cervix, as previously described. Place clamps on the inferior flap of the opened posterior vaginal wall, and with these apply posterior traction against anterior counter-traction on the bladder. The anterior vaginal wall can then be seen and is incised under the bladder base from within the vagina (Fig. 4.25). Incise the anterior vaginal wall cephalad to the posterior vaginal wall incision so that the subsequent vaginal closure suture line does not impinge on the future urethral anastomosis. Then with posterior traction on Kocker or Allis clamps holding the *anterior* vaginal wall, dissect the bladder trigone and bladder neck from the underlying vagina. The paravaginal tissues remain well defined and undisturbed, and the autonomic nerves passing within this tissue alongside the vagina and bladder neck to the urethra are preserved. Incise the vaginal wall by joining the posterior and anterior vaginal incisions, without disturbing the lateral vaginal wall and its adjacent para-vaginal tissue. The balloon of the Foley catheter indicates the position of the trigone and the cysto-urethral junction. Dissect the bladder neck from surrounding tissues after ligating the dorsal vein, circumferentially exposing the urethra below the bladder base; alternatively, in a retrograde dissection, this manouevre is performed prior to the bladder dissection. Place a vessel loop behind the urethra at the level of the bladder neck for traction to facilitate nerve-sparing dissection of the vagina from the bladder. Finally, using a scapel, incise the anterior urethra transversely, lift out the catheter, and place the anterior urethral anastomotic sutures before completing the posterior urethral incision and removing the surgical specimen. Use a clamp on the divided catheter, keeping its balloon inflated, and gentle traction to prevent any tumour spillage (see 📖 female orthotopic bladder reconstruction, 📖 p. 254) (Fig. 4.26).

Oncological considerations may present reasonable grounds for preserving the uterus (with the ovaries) in women of childbearing age, (e.g. non-multifocal, non-invasive or minimally invasive tumours not involving the bladder base). When appropriate, the bladder can be dissected from the uterus and anterior vaginal wall.

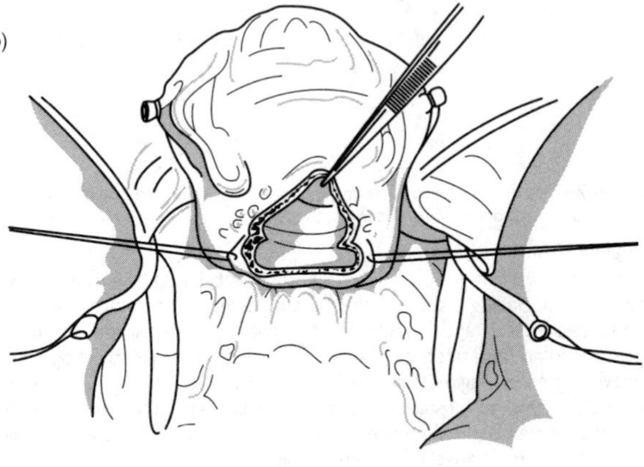

Fig. 4.25 Incision of the anterior vaginal wall behind the bladder for subsequent retrovesical dissection to the bladder neck and orthotopic bladder reconstruction.

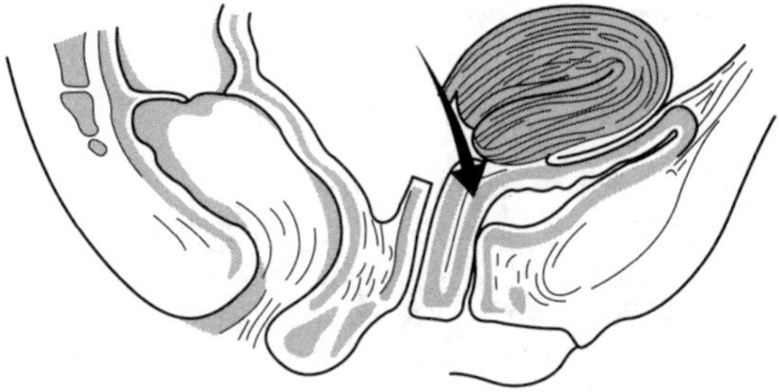

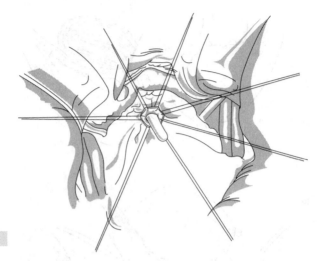

Fig. 4.26 Preservation of the anterior endopelvic fascia and urethral innervation for orthotopic bladder reconstruction in the female

Vaginal closure
Close the vagina with an 0 Vicryl suture, bringing the lateral walls together, beginning distally at the introital defect. This suture line can be continued to the apex (vault), or the apex can be turned down as a posterior flap (facilitated by prior dissection of the rectovesical pouch) to provide greater vaginal girth. Following extensive resection, the vagina may be augmented, usually using a bowel segment, alternatively peritoneum or omentum. A Betidine-soaked vaginal pack is placed in the vagina for 24 hr postoperatively for haemostasis.

Preparation for abdominal closure
Peritoneal lavage facilitates identification of bleeding vessels, and peritoneal toilet. In cases where an ovary is preserved, it must be anchored to prevent subsequent torsion. Ileal conduit and alternative reconstruction are described elsewhere. An open lateral intraperitoneal space should be closed to prevent internal herniation. Adjacent suture lines should be separated, for which omentum can be used. The omentum can be mobilized extensively on its left gastro-epiploic arcade, and hence made to reach the pelvis. A pelvic drain must be placed and secured; the number and position of additional drains depends on the reconstruction carried out (see p. 261). The abdominal viscera should be replaced, with the omentum overlying unless deployed in the pelvis. The abdomen is closed with a standard technique.

Male urethrectomy (see also 📖 p. 312)

When urethrectomy is carried out at the time of cysto-prostatectomy, the urethra should not be divided; the cysto-prostato-urethrectomy specimen should be dissected and removed en bloc. Urethrectomy is usually done via a midline perineal incision behind the scrotum, dividing skin, subcutaneous tissue, and bulbospongiosus muscle. Adequate lighting and retraction with a self-retaining retractor are necessary. The urethral catheter is easily palpated and will guide the dissection of the urethra from the corpus cavernosum. Alternatively, a pre-pubic technique can be used, avoiding perineal exposure.[27]

Having made a midline perineal approach onto the urethra, open the bulbospongiosus muscle in the midline to expose the corpus spongiosum itself. Dissect circumferentially around the corpus spongiosum and pass a wet nylon ribbon around it to facilitate its manipulation. Traction during the dissection everts the penis, allowing the penile urethra and the corpus spongiosum to be dissected distally to the corona. Control vascular branches to surrounding structures with diathermy. The distal urethra is dissected to the fossa navicularis where it can be divided; alternatively, the fossa navicularis can be dissected sharply from the external meatus. Begin the dissection of the bulbar urethra from the pelvic floor in front of the urethra, keeping behind the ligated dorsal vein. Having released the anterior bulbar urethra, continuity is established with the pelvic dissection. Continue with posterolateral dissection of the bulbar urethra where the bulbar arteries should be controlled by ligation before their division. The bulbar arteries are short and have a tendency to retract into surrounding tissues if not ligated before their division. This dissection completes the urethral mobilization, retaining continuity with the membranous and prostatic urethra. The bulbospongiosus muscle, subcutaneous tissue and skin should be closed in layers with absorbable sutures. Drain the deep perineal space either with a corrugated drain through the perineal skin or with a suction drain through the external meatus.

Cystectomy: early post-operative care

Post-operative care following radical cystectomy requires particular attention to fluid, haemodynamic and biochemical shifts, and consequent physiological derangement. Owing to third-space losses, fluid requirements may be substantial, particularly in the first 48 hr, and careful monitoring of fluid requirement and renal function is mandatory. Very occasionally, secondary bleeding may be potentially life-threatening and require laparotomy. Cardiac and pulmonary function must be monitored, with attention to bronchial toilet. Patients should expect early ambulation, and sufficient analgesia. Following cystectomy with a cutaneous urinary conduit, the pelvic drain can usually be removed after 4 or 5 days, where drainage is less than 100 cc on consecutive days.

Summary of post- cystectomy care

• Many patients will spend the first 24 hr in the HDU or ITU depending on local ward expertise.
• Daily clinical evaluation: inspect the wound (and stoma if present), monitor blood count and creatinine/electrolytes.

- Broad-spectrum antimicrobial prophylaxis and thrombo-embolic prophylaxis with TED stockings, pneumatic calf compression, and subcutaneous heparin.
- Mobilization after 24 hr (ideally).
- Chest physiotherapy and adequate analgesia, especially in smokers and patients with chest comorbidity.
- Restrict oral intake until bowel sounds are present; consider parenteral nutrition in the presence of GI complications.
- Drains are usually sited in the pelvis and near the uretero-diversion anastamosis, and may include ureteric catheters passing from the renal pelves through the diversion and exiting percutaneously, and a catheter draining a neobladder exiting urethrally or suprapubically.
- Most patients stay in hospital for 10–14 days.

Outcomes

The oncological benefit of radical cystectomy is well documented.[11,19,28–31] Outcomes are adversely affected by the tumour type, stage, and grade, as well as by patient comorbidity. Concerns with prostate-sparing cystectomy (preserving sexual function) include the multifocality of transitional cell carcinoma, more limited lymphatic clearance, adverse prognosis associated with prostatic involvement, and coexisting prostatic adenocarcinoma.[32]

The overall early complication rate is around 10–15%, with a mortality around 2%.[28,31,33,34] Reconstruction inevitably adds to the overall incidence of complications, and later need for revisional surgery. Late complications relate to the type of diversion or reconstruction. These are discussed on 📖 p. 262.

References

1 Skinner DG. Technique of radical cystectomy. *Urol Clin N Am* 1981; **8**:353–66.
2 Montie JE. Radical cystectomy in women. In: Graham SD, Jr, Glenn JF, eds. *Glenn's Urologic Surgery*. Philadelphia: Lippincott–Williams & Wilkins, **1998**:195–203.
3 Ghoneim MA. Radical cystectomy in men. In: Graham SD, Jr, Glenn JF, eds. *Glenn's Urologic Surgery*. Philadelphia: Lippincott–Williams & Wilkins, **1998**:187–94.
4 Oosterlinck W. Guidelines on diagnosis and treatment of superficial bladder cancer. *Minerva Urol Nefrol* 2004; **56**:65–72.
5 Stein JP, Clark P, Miranda G, Cai J, Groshen S, Skinner DG. Urethral tumor recurrence following cystectomy and urinary diversion: clinical and pathological characteristics in 768 male patients. *J Urol* 2005; **173**:1163–8.
6 Stenzl A, Draxl H, Posch B, Colleselli K, Falk M, Bartsch G. The risk of urethral tumors in female bladder cancer: can the urethra be used for orthotopic reconstruction of the lower urinary tract? *J Urol* 1995; **153**:950–5.
7 Stein JP, Esrig D, Freeman JA *et al.* Prospective pathologic analysis of female cystectomy specimens: risk factors for orthotopic diversion in women. *Urology* 1998; **51**:951–5.
8 Vale C. Neo-adjuvant chemotherapy in invasive bladder cancer: a systematic review and meta-analysis. *Lancet* 2003; **361**:1927–34.
9 Sherif A, Holmberg L, Rintala E *et al.* Neo-adjuvant cisplatinum based combination chemotherapy in patients with invasive bladder cancer: a combined analysis of two Nordic studies. *Eur Urol* 2004; **45**:297–303.

10 Pectasides D, Pectasides M, Nikolaou M. Adjuvant and neo-adjuvant chemotherapy in muscle invasive bladder cancer: literature review. *Eur Urol* 2005; **48**:60–7.

11 Pagano F, Bassi P, Galetti TP et al. Results of contemporary radical cystectomy for invasive bladder cancer: a clinicopathological study with an emphasis on the inadequacy of the tumor, nodes and metastases classification. *J Urol* 1991; **145**:45–50.

12 Zaak D, Hungerhuber E, Schneede P et al. Role of 5-aminolevulinic acid in the detection of urothelial premalignant lesions. *Cancer* 2002; **95**:1234–8.

13 De Dominicis C, Liberti M, Perugia G et al. Role of 5-aminolevulinic acid in the diagnosis and treatment of superficial bladder cancer: improvement in diagnostic sensitivity. *Urology* 2001; **57**:1059–62.

14 Jain S, Simms MS, Mellon JK. Management of the gastrointestinal tract at the time of cystectomy. *Urol Int* 2006; **77**:1–5.

15 Crinnion JN, Marino A, Grace PA, Abel P. Compartment syndrome: a very rare but potentially lethal complication of prolonged pelvic surgery. *Br J Urol* 1996; **77**:750–1.

16 Chase J, Harford F, Pinzur MS, Zussman M. Intra-operative lower extremity compartment pressures in lithotomy-positioned patients. *Dis Colon Rectum* 2000; **43**:678–80.

17 Simms MS, Terry TR. Well leg compartment syndrome after pelvic and perineal surgery in the lithotomy position. *Postgrad Med J* 2005; **81**:534–6.

18 Skinner DG. Management of invasive bladder cancer: a meticulous pelvic node dissection can make a difference. *J Urol* 1982; **128**:34–6.

19 Lerner SP, Skinner DG, Lieskovsky G et al. The rationale for en bloc pelvic lymph node dissection for bladder cancer patients with nodal metastases: long term results. *J Urol* 1993; **149**:758–65.

20 Vieweg J, Whitmore WFJ, Herr HW et al. The role of pelvic lymphadenectomy and radical cystectomy for lymph node positive bladder cancer. The Memorial Sloan–Kettering Cancer Center experience. *Cancer* 1994; **73**:3020–8.

21 Abol-Enein H, El Baz M, Abd El-Hameed MA, Abdel-Latif M, Ghoneim MA. Lymph node involvement in patients with bladder cancer treated with radical cystectomy: a pathoanatomical study--a single center experience. *J Urol* 2004; **172**:1818–21.

22 Ghoneim MA, Abol-Enein H. Lymphadenectomy with cystectomy: is it necessary and what is its extent? *Eur Urol* 2004; **46**:457–61.

23 Stein JP. Lymphadenectomy in bladder cancer: how high is 'high enough'? *Urol Oncol* 2006; **24**:349–55.

24 Kassouf W, Leibovici D, Munsell MF, Dinney CP, Grossman HB, Kamat AM. Evaluation of the relevance of lymph node density in a contemporary series of patients undergoing radical cystectomy. *J Urol* 2006; **176**:53–7.

25 Schlegel PN, Walsh PC. Neuroanatomical approach to radical cystoprostatectomy with preservation of sexual function. *J Urol* 1987; **138**:1402–6.

26 Colleselli K, Stenzl A, Eder R, Strasser H, Poisel S, Bartsch G. The female urethral sphincter: a morphological and topographical study. *J Urol* 1998; **160**:49–54.

27 Van Poppel H, Baert L. Innovative technique for urethrectomy. prepubic technique and results in 41 patients. *Prog Clin Biol Res* 1991; **370**:147–50.

28 Ghoneim MA, el Mekresh MM, el Baz MA, El Attar IA, Ashamallah A. Radical cystectomy for carcinoma of the bladder: critical evaluation of the results in 1026 cases. *J Urol* 1997; **158**:393–9.

29 Frazier HA, Robertson JE, Dodge RK et al. The value of pathologic factors in predicting cancer-specific survival among patients treated with radical cystectomy for transitional cell carcinoma of the bladder and prostate. *Cancer* 1993; **71**:3993–4013.

30 Skinner DG, Crawford ED, Kaufman JJ. Complications of radical cystectomy for carcinoma of the bladder. *J Urol* 1980; **123**:640–3.

31 Stein JP, Lieskovsky G, Cote R et al. Radical cystectomy in the treatment of invasive bladder cancer: long-term results in 1054 patients. *J Clin Oncol* 2001; **19**:666–75.

32 Vallancien G, Abou EF, Cathelineau X, Baumert H, Fromont G, Guillonneau B. Cystectomy with prostate sparing for bladder cancer in 100 patients: 10-year experience. *J Urol* 2002; **168**:2413–7.

33 Studer UE, Danuser H, Merz VW, Springer JP, Zingg EJ. Experience in 100 patients with an ileal low pressure bladder substitute combined with an afferent tubular isoperistaltic segment. *J Urol* 1995; **154**:49–56.

34 Konety BR, Dhawan V, Allareddy V, Joslyn SA. Impact of hospital and surgeon volume on in-hospital mortality from radical cystectomy: data from the health care utilization project. *J Urol* 2005; **173**:1695–1700.

Ileal loop urinary diversion

The ileum is the ideal bowel segment for surface conduit diversion after radical cystectomy. When ileum is not available or suitable, a colonic segment (usually transverse colon, occasionally sigmoid colon) or a jejunal segment (least ideal) can be used.[1,2] Alternative ureteric diversion procedures include cutaneous ureterostomy (particularly with a large or dilated ureter), uretero-ureterostomy, and pyelostomy. Ileal loop urinary diversion is described below.

An ileal segment should be carefully selected. Ensure that the ileocolic artery and its right colonic branch will remain intact, as these supply the distal ileum and right colon. Identify arcades supplying a 12–15 cm length of ileum ~12 cm proximal to ileocaecal valve. The appropriate length can be verified by stretching the ileal segment between the sacral promontory and the stoma site. This segment is then easily manipulated with Babcock clamps placed at its proposed ends. Divide the peritoneal surfaces of the mesentery along two incision lines that will isolate a vascular supply from two branches from the ileocolic arcades to the chosen segment. Then ligate and divide small mesenteric vessels within this incision; mosquito forceps can be used to clamp these vessels prior to division, if preferred. After dividing the bowel at each end of the segment, ileal continuity is restored using a standard small bowel anastomotic technique. Most urological surgeons avoid using bowel clamps. The isolated segment should be cleaned and wrapped until the conduit is to be prepared.

Examine the isolated loop to ensure its viability, particularly at its two ends. Ensure that the proximal and distal ends are correctly oriented, and that the segment is not twisted on its mesentery. Excise redundant fat at the distal end to facilitate construction of the stoma.

Creating a stoma

Before preparing the stoma site, use Lane's tissue forceps on the midline abdominal fascia to ensure its alignment with skin. The stoma skin defect can be made by circumferential incision, or cut tangentially holding the stoma site upwards in Lane's tissue forceps. Excise the subcutaneous fat as a cylinder in line with the skin incision, maintaining haemostasis, using Langenbeck retractors, scissors, forceps, and diathermy. Create a cruciform incision in the anterior rectus fascia. Absorbable sutures (2–0 Vicryl) can then be placed at the apex of each triangle for subsequent fixation to the conduit. Bluntly create a hole in the rectus muscle, avoiding the inferior epigastric vessels, and open the underlying peritoneum. Pass a finger through the abdominal wall defect and dilate with two fingers. At each stage, anatomical alignment through the abdominal wall must be maintained.

Pass the bowel segment through the abdominal wall defect, ensuring its correct orientation. This is done by passing Babcock forceps through the abdominal wall defect, and grasping the terminal end of the conduit. The segment is fixed to the triangles previously made in the anterior rectus fascia with the preplaced sutures. The distal conduit is everted, using Babcock forceps, and its edge is fixed to adjacent serosa of conduit and skin, with interrupted circumferential sutures (2–0 Vicryl). It is often easier to evert the distal conduit *before* bringing it though the abdominal wall. Similarly, the conduit is more easily adjusted by constructing the stoma *before* the uretero-ileal anastomosis.

The ureters should have been previously mobilized sufficiently for the proposed anastomosis, and distal ligation of the ureters allows them to dilate. Each ureter should now be trimmed to the appropriate length to avoid redundancy or kinking, and spatulated. A stay suture in the distal ureteric edge facilitates manipulation, although care must be taken that the ureter does not then twist. For an ileal conduit, the left ureter is conventionally passed behind the sigmoid mesentery below level of inferior mesenteric artery. However, some surgeons pass the ureter above it, to ensure that the ureter is not kinked by this vessel or by other tissue attachments or bands. Vascular branches to the ureter must be preserved wherever possible; these supply a longitudinal vascular plexus within the ureteric adventitia that is easily damaged by inappropriate or excessive surgical manipulation.

Uretero-ileal anastomoses

A refluxing uretero-ileal anastomosis is generally performed. This facilitates radiological monitoring of the upper urinary tract, and may reduce the risk of anastomotic stricture. Sufficient spatulation of the ureter (usually 1–1.5 cm) and care with suture placement (particularly at the apex of the spatulation) are also important to minimize the risk of luminal narrowing or stricture. The edges of the spatulated ureters should correspond in length to the bowel edge to which they will be sutured. A fine absorbable suture should be used, such as 4–0 or 5–0 Vicryl on a non-cutting needle.

The most commonly used anastomotic configurations are those described by Wallace[3,4] and Bricker (Figs. 4.27, 4.28).[5] Both allow urinary reflux. Wallace conformations include ureters sutured together as they lie parallel to one another (Wallace 66), or opposite one another (Wallace 69), or sutured together along both the anterior and posterior walls as a Y for an end ureteroloopostomy (📖 Fig. 4.27). Stays joining the proximal and distal ends of the spatulation help support the ureters while a continuous suture is run between opposing edges.

In a Bricker anastomosis, each ureter is spatulated and implanted separately into the conduit (advantageous in the rare event of tumour recurrence at one anastomosis). A full-thickness plug at the re-implantation site is excised from the bowel wall using scissors by excising the serosa and picking up the underlying mucosa with forceps. Place interrupted sutures to appose all layers of the bowel to ureter, and complete the anastomosis with bowel serosal sutures to the ureter. If desired, a non-refluxing nipple anastomosis can be constructed and similarly implanted.

Each ureteral anastomosis should be supported with a ureteric catheter or infant feeding tube—ideally, a catheter with proximal side-holes. It is generally easier to perform the uretero-ileal anastomosis with ureters already intubated. The catheters should be secured with an absorbable suture placed parallel to the long axis of the ureter (4–0 Vicryl or Vicryl rapide). Devascularization and narrowing of the ureteric circumference must be avoided. The completed anastomosis can be covered with peritoneum, and the lateral space between the conduit and posterolateral abdominal wall closed with a Vicryl suture. The small bowel, caecum and colon should be replaced in their normal anatomic configuration.

A 20F Robinson tube drain with side-holes should be placed in the pelvis. It should not be immediately adjacent to the uretero-ileal anastomosis, as this may encourage anastomotic leak and delay healing.

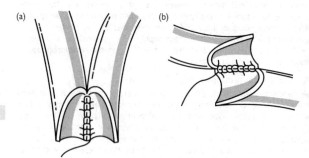

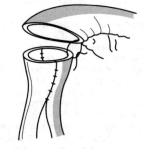

Fig. 4.27 (a) Wallace 66, (b) Wallace 69 and (c) Wallace Y anastomoses.

(a)

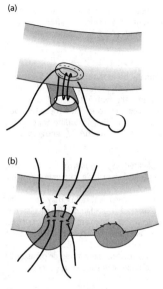

(b)

Fig. 4.28 Bricker ureterointestinal anastomoses.

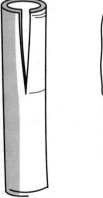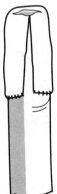

Fig. 4.29 Split nipple.

Post-operative care

The pelvic drain can usually be removed at 4–5 days unless there is high output (>100cc/24 hrs). Ureteric stents are removed after 14 days, provided that no urinary leak is suspected. (Also, see cystectomy: early postoperative care)

Follow-up

Serum creatinine and U&E should initially be monitored every 3 months. The upper urinary tract should be imaged periodically, usually after 6 weeks with ultrasound, and then annually with ultrasound and plain radiography. Additional imaging may be required to exclude metachronous malignancy, calculus, and absence of obstruction, including loopogram where the anastomoses are refluxing, IVU, CT, and MAG3 renography.

Late complications[6-10]

Ureteric anastomosis may be complicated by stenosis, hydronephrosis, and renal obstruction. Other complications include recurrent urinary infection and pyelonephritis, which may relate to ureteric obstruction or urinary stasis within a redundant loop.[9] Uretero-ileal reflux may be associated with mild ureteric dilatation. Several of these factors (particularly in combination) may also contribute to renal deterioration and calculus formation.[10] Metabolic complications are uncommon, but may include vitamin B_{12} deficiency and hyperchloraemic acidosis.[11,12] Stomal complications include stenosis, with or without obstruction, peristomal or parastomal herniae, and peristomal skin reactions to urine, adhesives, or appliances.

References

1 Golimbu M, Morales P. Jejunal conduits: technique and complications. *J Urol* 1975; **113**:787–95.
2 Morales P, Golimbu M. Colonic urinary diversion: 10 years of experience. *J Urol* 1975; **113**:302–7.
3 Wallace DM. Ureteric diversion using a conduit: a simplified technique. *Br J Urol* 1966; **38**:522–7.
4 Wallace DM. Ileal conduit. *Br J Urol* 1967; **39**:681–6.
5 Bricker EM. Bladder substitution after pelvic exenteration. *Surg Gynecol Obstet* 1950; **30**:1511.
6 Sullivan JW, Grabstald H, Whitmore WF, Jr. Complications of ureteroileal conduit with radical cystectomy: review of 336 cases. *J Urol* 1980; **124**:797–801.
7 Schmidt JD, Hawtrey CE, Flocks RH, Culp DA. Complications, results and problems of ileal conduit diversions. *J Urol* 1973; **109**:210–6.
8 Engel RM. Complications of bilateral uretero-ileo-cutaneous urinary diversion: a review of 208 cases. *J Urol* 1969; **101**:508–12.
9 Pitts WR, Jr., Muecke EC. A 20-year experience with ileal conduits: the fate of the kidneys. *J Urol* 1979; **122**:154–7.
10 Dretler SP. The pathogenesis of urinary tract calculi occurring after ileal conduit diversion. I. Clinical study. II. Conduit study. III. Prevention. *J Urol* 1973; **109**:204–9.
11 Elder DD, Moisey CU, Rees RW. A long-term follow-up of the colonic conduit operation in children. *Br J Urol* 1979; **51**:462–5.
12 Kosko JW, Kursh ED, Resnick MI. Metabolic complications of urologic intestinal substitutes. *Urol Clin North Am* 1986; **13**:193–200.

Bladder reconstruction

Bladder reconstruction after radical cystectomy can be offered in many situations, after considering clinical and individual circumstances. Construction of a continent urinary reservoir provides an alternative to a urostomy bag. An orthotopic neobladder permits volitional urethral voiding, but when the urethra is not available, or unsuitable, alternative reconstruction can be offered. This includes a urinary reservoir with a catheterizable stoma and conduit, or a rectosigmoid pouch for peranal voiding. Reconstruction itself does not appear to have an adverse impact on clinical outcomes in the event of tumour recurrence.[1]

Surgical reconstruction must not compromise aspects of oncological control. Radical extirpation of cancer can be compromised by inappropriate preservation of the urethra, bladder neck, prostate, and pelvic nerves for otherwise laudable aims of preserving urethral voiding and sexual function. This concern underlines the importance of careful tumour assessment before considering the technical aspects of reconstruction.

Pre-operative assessment of the availability and suitability of healthy bowel for reservoir reconstruction is essential. This includes consideration of bowel, hepatic, renal, and ureteric function as well as any underlying disease. Bladder reconstruction may exacerbate hepatic or renal insufficiency, and it is generally recommended that GFR should be ≥50 mL/min and serum creatinine <150 mmol/L. Reconstruction from bowel necessarily incurs loss of normal GI tract and potential functional disturbance, with metabolic sequelae from the exposure of GI segments to urine. These and other complications are discussed elsewhere in more detail. Older age does not preclude the need for radical treatment of bladder cancer or for reconstruction after cystectomy, other than through the specific medical considerations and general fitness of the individual patient for such surgery. However, sphincter weakness associated with older age may contribute to post-operative incontinence following orthotopic reconstruction.

The specialist nurse with experience of urological reconstructive surgery has an essential role in the pre-operative instruction and assessment of the patient, making vital contributions to ultimate outcomes and technical success of the surgical procedure. The suitability of the patient for alternative reconstructive procedures must be assessed, and the care and function of alternative configurations explained to the individual for informed decision-making. Potential stoma sites need to be evaluated and the patient should become familiar with any specific necessary skills (e.g. urethral self-catheterization) before surgery.

The patient must be well informed and well motivated. He or she must be able and willing to carry out self-catheterization when necessary, either urethrally (the innervated natural conduit) or through a Mitrofanoff channel (a reconstructed conduit), unless a rectal reservoir is proposed.[2,3] If an orthotopic substitution is contemplated specific assessments are required to assure suitability of the urethra (its integrity and absence of disease), its competence (sphincter function), and the feasibility of urethral self-catheterization (urethral sensitivity, individual capability). Supravesical diversion to a rectal reservoir avoids a stoma and the need for self-catheterization; however, the ability of the anal sphincter to maintain liquid stool continence during daily activity must be tested. Patients undergoing any form of urinary tract reconstruction must accept the importance of clinical follow-up and monitoring in their future care, as well as the not infrequent need for revisional surgery (up to 50% by 10 years). The possibility that reconstruction may prove unfeasible at operation with the necessity for cutaneous diversion must also be understood.

Many techniques of constructing a bladder reservoir are described. They differ according to the bowel segment(s) used, the type of ureteric re-implantation (sometimes incorporating an afferent limb to the reservoir), the construction of the reservoir itself, and the configuration of the outflow conduit. This chapter does not attempt to describe the detail of surgical techniques or review the many named and established procedures that have been adopted (or adapted) in the practice of individual urological departments. It does however, address the surgical principles of bladder reconstruction.

Ureters and the afferent connection

Ureteric re-implantation into the reconstructed reservoir (or its afferent limb) must take into account the anatomy of the ureters, including their length, wall thickness, and diameter. The importance of preventing urinary reflux for prevention of renal complications is strongly debated, and this relates also to the type of reservoir (see below).

Ureterosigmoidostomy is now rarely carried out but remains of considerable historical importance because of well-recognized adverse sequelae. Long-term complications include renal deterioration, particularly with the refluxing ureterosigmoid anastomosis that preceded the non-refluxing Leadbetter–Clarke and Goodwin techniques[4,5] (Figs. 4.30, 4.31).

Anti-reflux mechanisms protect the kidneys against supraphysiological hydrostatic pressure, bacterial reflux, and particularly the combination of reflux and infection. Reflux into the ureter can be prevented by creating a functional valve at the reservoir inflow, either as a ureteric tunnel or as an afferent nipple. Alternatively, reflux can be prevented by connecting the ureters to an afferent 'chimney' of sufficient length for intra-abdominal pressure to provide an effective anti-reflux mechanism.[6]

Having considered the configuration of the ureteric implantation required for the proposed lower urinary tract reconstruction, further manipulation of the ureters is deferred until the reservoir has been constructed (see below).

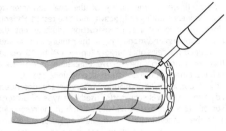

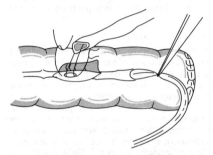

Fig. 4.30 Leadbetter-Clarke ureterosigmoidostomy.

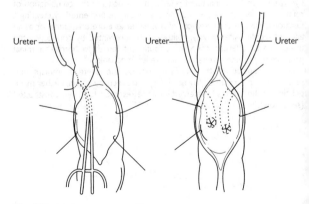

Fig. 4.31 Goodwin ureterosigmoidostomy.

Urinary reservoirs

Reservoirs are constructed either as either an orthotopic substitution (anastomosed to an innervated functional urethra) or a continent diversion, requiring a Mitrofanoff channel to be constructed as a catheterizable continent outflow conduit.[2,3] Alternatively, a rectal reservoirs is used, either without augmentation or with augmentation (including rectosigmoid reconfiguration). For example, the Mainz II rectosigmoid pouch functionally separates the faecal stream from the urinary reservoir, but allows both urine and faeces to be passed through the anus.[7]

Reservoirs are usually constructed from small bowel, large bowel, or both; very occasionally stomach may be used. The segments and length of bowel are selected according to the particular reservoir and necessary afferent/efferent chimney(s), tunnels or conduits to be constructed. In addition to the pre-operative assessments, peri-operative considerations include the availability and suitability of the bowel, the pattern of mesenteric vascular arcades, and bowel mobility on its mesentery (particularly for orthotopic reconstruction).

The selected bowel segments are fully mobilized along the root of their mesentery. The required length of bowel is measured along the mesenteric border. Systemic pharmacological agents causing smooth muscle contraction should be avoided. In isolating a bowel segment, the proximal mesenteric incision should be short, to maintain good vascularization through multiple branches of the ileocolic vessels; the distal mesenteric incision is longer and will cross a major terminal arcade without division of the main ileocolic trunk. Short releasing incisions may be made in the distal cut edge of mesentery to increase mobility.

The bowel to be reconstructed is then isolated. Contamination of the operative field is avoided with towels or open packs. Bowel clamps are generally avoided. Staples and non-absorbable sutures must never be used in the urinary tract. After dividing the bowel and restoring intestinal continuity, the mesenteric defect must be repaired. Where isolated afferent or efferent tunnels are to be used, these segments are now measured and prepared. For the construction of some reservoirs, the ends of the isolated loop are closed with a running suture. The isolated bowel is then ready to be fashioned into a reservoir.

With an ever-growing number of conformations for bladder reconstruction described, quality of life outcome with alternative techniques has not been shown to differ, but familiarity with several reconstructive techniques is essential. Ileal reservoirs illustrated in Fig. 4.32 include those named after Studer,[8] Hautmann (Ileal-W),[9] also the ileal-W with serous lined extramural valves (Mansoura),[10,11] hemi-Kock,[12] and its T-pouch modification.[13] The Mainz I ileocolonic reconstruction[14] and Mainz II rectosigmoid pouch are also shown (Fig. 4.32).

Detubularization (i.e. longitudinal division of the bowel segment, with double folding) effectively reduces the hydrostatic pressures that would otherwise arise within the reconstructed reservoir due to peristalsis. The small bowel is incised along its antimesenteric border and the large bowel along a taenia. This manoeuvre can be facilitated by placing stay sutures holding the bowel in the proposed reservoir conformation, and then incising the bowel wall longitudinally over a large (e.g. 22Fr) catheter. The mucosa of the opened bowel is then cleaned. With the bowel plate supported in its correct conformation by stay sutures, the adjacent bowel edges are sutured together, thereby fashioning the posterior wall of the reservoir. Reconstruction proceeds with construction of afferent and/or efferent segment(s) (as required), followed by ureteric implantation, and finally reservoir closure.

The ureters are trimmed to the correct length, holding the reservoir (with any afferent segment) in its final position; they should be laid in position without kinking or tension and spatulated. Each anastomosis is supported by a ureteric stent or catheter. Tapering of a thickened or dilated ureter for a tunnelled anastomosis risks ischaemia and its complications. The ureteric stents are then brought out through the reservoir wall (and not a suture line), sometimes tunnelled for a short distance within the mesentery, and secured within the reservoir or ureter and to the external wall of the reservoir.

Care is taken to ensure that the reservoir is continent, suture lines are watertight, there is no tension on the ureters or mesentery, no compromise to vascular supply, and no potential for torsion or kinking. The reservoir should be filled and tested with saline or air. Later, it will be sutured in to its correct position and orientation to supporting structures.

(a)

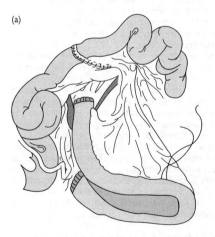

Fig. 4.32 Bladder reconstruction after (a) Studer neobladder.

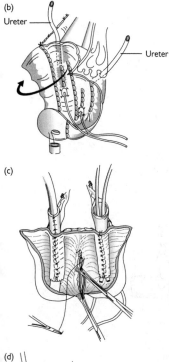

(b)
Ureter

Ureter

(c)

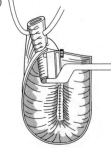

(d)

Fig. 4.32 (*Contd.*) Bladder reconstruction after (b) Hautman Ileal W, (c) Ileal neobladder with serous lined extramural valves (Mansoura), (d) Hemi-Kock pouch.

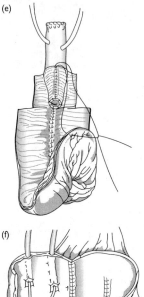

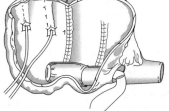

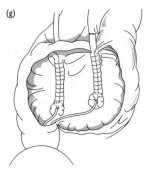

Fig. 4.32 (*Contd.*) Bladder reconstruction after (e) T-pouch, (f) Ileocolonic (Mainz) pouch, (g) Mainz II rectosigmoid pouch.

The outflow conduit

Where non-orthopic reconstruction is carried out, an efferent Mitrofanoff conduit is constructed usually from appendix or a small bowel segment. It must provide a suitable lumen for catheterization, and must be tunnelled to ensure continence. The Mitrofanoff stoma is positioned to be non-obtrusive, usually below the belt line or at the umbilicus. The Mitrofanoff conduit should be straight and easily catheterized.

For an orthotopic reservoir, an outlet is made at the most dependent part of the reservoir as assessed in its correct pelvic position. The outlet can be made in a suture line, although many surgeons prefer to make a new opening and separate the reservoir suture line from the urethral anastomosis. The mucosa of the outlet may sometimes be everted prior to urethral anastomosis. An outflow 'funnel' should never be used, as its tendency to kink will obstruct voiding. The anastomosis of the reservoir to the urethra is completed over a large soft urethral catheter (e.g. 22Fr silicone).

Hypercontinence sometimes prevents normal voiding in female patients having orthotopic substitution. Factors contributing to hypercontinence may include preservation of bladder neck and proximal urethra, denervation of the urethra (preventing normal bladder neck opening), and posterior prolapse of the neobladder causing angulation at the junction between the urethra and neobladder.[15,16] Therefore, during prior cystectomy, care must be taken to excise the bladder neck and proximal urethra, preserve the distal two-thirds of the urethra and its innervation,[17] and ensure that the neobladder is supported in its correct final position. Measures to secure the reservoir position include suturing the round ligaments to the lateral vaginal vaults, reattaching the peritoneum of the pouch of Douglas to the posterior vagina, bringing the omentum into the pelvis behind the bladder, and securing the anterior wall of the reservoir to the adjacent abdominal wall.[16] It is important that the suture lines closing the vaginal stump are not directly adjacent to the urethro-neobladder anastomosis, and are separated by suture fixation of available omentum and posterior peritoneum.

Tubes and drains

Irrespective of the type of reconstruction, each ureter and its anastomosis must be stented with a ureteric catheter. Usually these catheters are passed proximally up the ureters to the kidney and distally through the bladder and body wall, and secured extravesically to the bladder. A 22Fr catheter can be placed in the urethra, or a somewhat smaller catheter (e.g. 16Fr) in a Mitrofanoff conduit; in addition a large suprapubic tube (e.g. 20Fr) is placed into the reservoir and secured to its peritoneal surface. The bladder will thereby be drained through both a suprapubic tube and a catheter in the outflow channel. The reservoir is fixed in position to the anterior abdominal wall. Surgical drains and catheters are secured to the skin. A rectal reservoir will be drained with a large rectal tube (e.g. 24Fr), secured to the peri-anal skin.

Post-operative management

In addition to all the considerations in the care of the post-cystectomy patient, there is additional potential for metabolic complications, anastomotic leak, and their consequences. Patency of all tubes and drains must be ensured with saline flushes and washouts. Bladder lavage should be carried out every 6 hr. The sequence of supra-pubic catheter and drain removal will reflect the type of reconstruction and local institution practice. Bladder drainage is usually maintained for 3–6 weeks. At least one of the intra-abdominal drains should remain *in situ* for at least 10 days to establish a tract in case of delayed urinary leak. A pouchogram is performed before removing the bladder catheter, and retrograde ureterograms via the ureteric catheters may be carried out if there is concern about persistent urinary leak. Sepsis or infection must be detected promptly and treated.

After removal of reservoir catheters, the patient with orthotopic reconstruction should be instructed in voiding. For men, voiding should begin in the sitting position, using pelvic floor relaxation and avoiding undue straining. Patients with a Mitrofanoff stoma will carry out clean intermittent catheterization. Voiding or self-catheterization should be attempted every 2 hr then at a gradually increasing interval to bring the functional bladder capacity to around 500 mL. Bladder emptying should be assessed by ultrasound and initially also by catheterization. The patients must void at least once during the night, and set an alarm clock to do so. Maintaining adequate fluid intake (2–3 L) is essential, and body weight should be monitored. Diet should contain sufficient salt and bicarbonate supplement (2–6 g/day) may be required, monitored by serum electrolytes, bicarbonate, and chloride. Otherwise, metabolic acidosis may become symptomatic with lethargy, malaise, nausea, and epigastric discomfort. Bladder lavage may be necessary to evacuate mucus, particularly in the early months following surgery. Continence may be acquired more efficaciously with appropriate pelvic floor exercises, sphincter exercises, and supervision. The upper tracts are evaluated by ultrasound or IVU within 3 months.

Late complications of bladder reconstruction

The type of bladder reconstruction impacts reservoir pressure, capacity (from a given segment length), propensity to infection and performance. It also has varying consequences for GI function. The development and degree of metabolic complications specifically reflect the intestinal segments used (Table 4.2) and renal function.[18,19] Preservation and long-term protection of renal function is of paramount importance, therefore the choice of bowel segment sets the scene for long-term outcome and potential for long-term complications.

Overall continence rates of 85–90% are achieved. Enuresis with daytime continence may require timed voiding at night. Mucus production can sometimes be troublesome, causing outflow obstruction, predisposing to infection and calculi; it may require periodic bladder washouts and/or intermittent self-catheterization. Bladder rupture (either spontanous or traumatic) may present with signs of urinary peritonitis or as an intra-abdominal collection. After continent urinary diversion, the Mitrofanoff conduit may develop stricture or become leaky, requiring surgical revision.

Careful follow-up is required to ensure that specific factors contributing to renal deterioration are identified early and treated. Urinary infection must be treated promptly. Asymptomatic bacteriuria should be treated in patients with orthotopic reconstruction, but is to be expected in patients who intermittently self-catheterize and treatment of these individuals results in bacterial resistance. The significance of asymptomatic bacteriuria relates to renal function, particularly with refluxing ureters and high reservoir pressures, as well as predisposing to urinary tract infection and its complications. Recurrent urinary tract infection, pyelonephritis, high urinary pressure, and reflux contribute to renal scarring and deterioration in renal function, exemplified following ureterosigmoidostomy. Mucus production, incomplete reservoir emptying, and stone formation also predispose to reservoir infection. Renal complications may be exacerbated by obstruction due to stricture of the lower ureter or its anastomosis, upper tract calculus, or metachronous upper tract malignancy.

Metabolic complications of bladder substitution relate to the segment of bowel used, its surface area, and therefrom the duration of urinary exposure as well as renal reserve. Hyperchloraemic acidosis, and its clinical sequelae, were first described in relation to ureterosigmoidostomy.[20–23] Similar metabolic derangement may follow where ileum and/or colon are incorporated in a urinary reservoir, and can be prevented by bicarbonate salt replacement and adequate fluid intake. The pattern of fluid and electrolyte imbalance which may develop following urinary tract reconstruction reflects the segment of GI tract exposed to urine (Table 4.2).[19] Systemic complications of chronic metabolic derangement and acidosis include osteomalacia, osteoporosis, nutritional deficit, and growth retardation in children. Urinary stone formation is related to metabolic changes, infection, obstruction, mucus production, and particularly urinary exposure to foreign suture or staple materials.[24,25] Loss of the ileocaecal valve (with ileocolonic segments) may be associated with diarrhoea, bile acid malabsorption, hyperoxaluria, cholelithiasis, and increased tendency to vitamin B_{12} deficiency.

Malignant transformation is associated with exposing bowel to urine or to the mixing of urine with faeces within the bowel lumen.[26,27] This well-recognized complication with ureteric re-implantation into the sigmoid colon can also develop in reservoirs constructed from isolated bowel segments that are exposed only to urine. The risk relates to the length of follow-up, and the malignancy tends to develop at the urothelial–enteric anastomosis but can also develop in the enteric mucosa. Adenocarcinoma is the most common, and transitional cell carcinoma or squamous cell carcinoma also arise. In view of this significant risk, annual cystoscopy should be performed after 5 years. Following orthotopic reconstruction for transitional cell tumour, metachronous tumour may occasionally develop in the urethra;[28,29] the upper tracts should be surveyed periodically regardless of the type of reconstruction. The development of malignancy necessitates further surgery for oncological control, with revision of the reconstruction or urinary diversion.

Table 4.2 Electrolyte disturbance with reservoirs incorporating alternative intestinal segments

Stomach	Hypochloraemic alkalosis
Jejunum	Hyponatraemic, hypochoraemic, hyperkalaemic, acidosis
Ileum/colon	Hyperchloraemic acidosis

References

1 Tefilli MV, Gheiler EL, Tiguert R et al. Urinary diversion-related outcome in patients with pelvic recurrence after radical cystectomy for bladder cancer. *Urology* 1999; **53**:999–1004.
2 Mitrofanoff P. [Trans-appendicular continent cystostomy in the management of the neurogenic bladder]. *Chir Pediatr* 1980; **21**:297–305.
3 Monti PR, Lara RC, Dutra MA, de Carvalho JR. New techniques for construction of efferent conduits based on the Mitrofanoff principle. *Urology* 1997; **49**:112–15.

4 Clarke BG, Leadbetter WF. Ureterosigmoidostomy collective review of results in 2897 reported cases. *J Urol* 1955; **73**:999–1008.

5 Goodwin WE, Harris AP, Kaufman JJ, Beal JM. Open transcolonic ureterointestinal anastomosis: a new approach. *Surg Gynecol Obstet* 1953; **97**:295.

6 Ghoneim MA. Ureterointestinal anastomosis in continent urinary diversion: an antirefluxing procedure--is it necessary? *Tech Urol* 2001; **7**:203–8.

7 Fisch M, Wammack R, Hohenfellner R. The sigma rectum pouch (Mainz pouch II). *World J Urol* 1996; **14**:68–72.

8 Studer UE, Burkhard FC, Schumacher M, Kessler TM, Thoeny H, Fleischmann A *et al.* Twenty years experience with an ileal orthotopic low pressure bladder substitute--lessons to be learned. *J Urol* 2006; **176**:161–6.

9 Hautmann RE, Egghart G, Frohneberg D, Miller K. The ileal neobladder. *J Urol* 1988; **139**:39–42.

10 Abol-Enein H, Salem M, Mesbah A *et al.* Continent cutaneous ileal pouch using the serous lined extramural valves: the Mansoura experience in more than 100 patients. *J Urol* 2004; **172**:588–91.

11 Abol-Enein H, Ghoneim MA. Functional results of orthotopic ileal neobladder with serous-lined extramural ureteral re-implantation: experience with 450 patients. *J Urol* 2001; **165**:1427–32.

12 Boyd SD, Lieskovsky G, Skinner DG. Kock pouch bladder replacement. *Urol Clin N Am* 1991; **18**:641–8.

13 Stein JP, Dunn MD, Quek ML, Miranda G, Skinner DG. The orthotopic T pouch ileal neobladder: experience with 209 patients. *J Urol* 2004; **172**:584–7.

14 Thüroff JW, Alken P, Engelmann U, Riedmiller H, Jacobi GH, Hohenfellner R. The Mainz pouch (mixed augmentation ileum 'n zecum) for bladder augmentation and continent urinary diversion. *Eur Urol* 1985; **11**:152–60.

15 Stenzl A, Colleselli K, Poisel S, Feichtinger H, Pontasch H, Bartsch G. Rationale and technique of nerve sparing radical cystectomy before an orthotopic neobladder procedure in women. *J Urol* 1995; **154**:2044–9.

16 Ali-El-Dein B, Gomha M, Ghoneim MA. Critical evaluation of the problem of chronic urinary retention after orthotopic bladder substitution in women. *J Urol* 2002; **168**:587–92.

17 Colleselli K, Stenzl A, Eder R, Strasser H, Poisel S, Bartsch G. The female urethral sphincter: a morphological and topographical study. *J Urol* 1998; **160**:49–54.

18 Golimbu M, Morales P. Jejunal conduits: technique and complications. *J Urol* 1975; **113**:787–95.

19 Kosko JW, Kursh ED, Resnick MI. Metabolic complications of urologic intestinal substitutes. *Urol Clin North Am* 1986; **13**:193–200.

20 Ferris DO, Odel HM. Electrolyte pattern of the blood after bilateral ureterosigmoidostomy. *J Am Med Assoc* 1950; **142**:634–41.

21 Odel HM, Ferris DO, Priestley JT. Further observations on the electrolyte pattern of the blood after bilateral ureterosigmoidostomy. *J Urol* 1951; **65**:1013–20.

22 Hall MC, Koch MO, McDougal WS. Metabolic consequences of urinary diversion through intestinal segments. *Urol Clin North Am* 1991; **18**:725–35.

23 Gerharz EW, Turner WH, Kalble T, Woodhouse CR. Metabolic and functional consequences of urinary reconstruction with bowel. *BJU Int* 2003; **91**:143–9.

24 Dretler SP. The pathogenesis of urinary tract calculi occurring after ileal conduit diversion. I. Clinical study. II. Conduit study. III. Prevention. *J Urol* 1973; **109**:204–9.

25 Skinner DG, Lieskovsky G, Boyd SD. Continuing experience with the continent ileal reservoir (Kock pouch) as an alternative to cutaneous urinary diversion: an update after 250 cases. *J Urol* 1987; **137**:1140–5.

26 Husmann DA, Spence HM. Current status of tumor of the bowel following ureterosigmoidostomy: a review. *J Urol* 1990; **144**:607–10.

27 Filmer RB, Spencer JR. Malignancies in bladder augmentations and intestinal conduits. *J Urol* 1990; **143**:671–8.

28 Akkad T, Gozzi C, Deibl M, *et al.* Tumor recurrence in the remnant urothelium of females undergoing radical cystectomy for transitional cell carcinoma of the bladder: long-term results from a single center. *J Urol* 2006; **175**:1268–71.

29 Stein JP, Clark P, Miranda G, Cai J, Groshen S, Skinner DG. Urethral tumor recurrence following cystectomy and urinary diversion: clinical and pathological characteristics in 768 male patients. *J Urol* 2005; **173**:1163–8.

Prostate adenocarcinoma: pathology and staging

Prostate cancer is graded by the Gleason grading system, which was first described by Gleason and Mellinger[1] in 1974. Recent modifications have been recommended for consistency and reproducibility among pathologists.

A sum score between 2 (least aggressive) and 10 (most aggressive) is derived from the sum of the two most common Gleason patterns (graded from 1 to 5) in biopsy or surgical specimens. Primary and secondary grades are given (e.g. 3+4); where there is no secondary grade, the primary grade is designated as both the primary and secondary grade (e.g. 3+3). Occasionally, a tertiary score may be given where this is of higher grade than the primary and secondary grades.

Pathology and pre-malignant lesions

Two histological diagnoses associated with prostate cancer represent either pre-malignant or peri-malignant lesions. They are prostatic intra-epithelial neoplasia and atypical small acinar proliferation.

Prostatic intra-epithelial neoplasia (PIN)

PIN consists of architecturally benign prostatic acini and ducts lined by cytologically atypical cells. The basal cell layer is present, although the basement membrane may be fragmented. PIN was formerly known as ductal dysplasia or reported by pathologists as 'suspicious for cancer.' PIN was classified into low-grade (mild) and high-grade (moderate to severe) forms, based on the presence of prominent nucleoli. Subsequently pathologists have agreed to report only high-grade PIN, since low-grade PIN reporting is very subjective and has no prognostic value. On the other hand, high-grade PIN is believed to be a precursor for intermediate or high-grade prostate cancer and it's finding in sextant peripheral zone prostate biopsies was formerly associated with a 30–40% prediction of prostate cancer at subsequent biopsy. However, with the widespread use of more extensive biopsy protocols, the significance of isolated high-grade PIN has become less clear.

High-grade PIN is reported in 5–10% of prostate needle biopsies. It does not appear to affect the serum PSA value. The site of the PIN is not necessarily indicative of the site of subsequently diagnosed cancer, nor is PIN always present in a prostate containing a cancer. Currently it is recommended that repeat or interval systematic biopsies should be performed if isolated high-grade PIN is reported on needle biopsy or TURP, giving consideration to the extent of sampling and other clinical factors which may indicate missed cancer.[2]

Atypical small acinar proliferation (ASAP)

This is another histopathological prostatic lesion which pathologists report on needle biopsies as 'suspicious for cancer.' The acini are small and are lined with cytologically abnormal epithelial cells. The columnar cells have prominent nuclei containing nucleoli, while the basal layer may be focally absent. The basement membrane is intact. Similar to PIN, studies have shown that ASAP in needle biopsy predicts cancer at subsequent biopsy in >40% of cases.[3] Currently it is recommended that repeat systematic biopsies should be performed if isolated ASAP is reported on needle biopsy or TURP.

2002 TNM (tumour, node, metastasis) classification for adenocarcinoma of prostate[4]

The T category is based on clinical examination, imaging, endoscopy, biopsy, and biochemical tests. The N category is based on clinical examination or imaging. The M category is based on clinical examination, imaging, skeletal studies, and biochemical tests.

Primary tumour

- TX   Primary tumour cannot be assessed
- T0   No evidence of primary tumour
- T1   Clinically inapparent tumour, not palpable or visible by imaging
- T1a   Tumour (non-palpable) as incidental histological finding at transurethral resection of prostate in ≤5% of tissue resected
- T1b   Tumour (non-palpable) as incidental histological finding at transurethral resection of prostate in >5% of tissue resected
- T1c   Tumour (non-palpable) identified by needle biopsy (for elevated serum PSA), includes bilateral non-palpable tumour on needle biopsy
- T2   Tumour confined within prostate (including prostatic apex, prostate capsule) that is either palpable or visible on imaging, or (with p-prefix) demonstrated in radical prostatectomy specimen
- T2a   Tumour involving half of one lobe or less
- T2b   Tumour involving more than half of one lobe but not both lobes
- T2c   Tumour involving both lobes
- T3   Tumour extends through prostatic capsule
- T3a   Extra-capsular extension
- T3b   Seminal vesicle(s) invasion
- T4   Tumour fixed or invades adjacent structures: bladder neck, external sphincter, rectum, levator muscles, pelvic wall

Regional lymph nodes

Pelvic lymph nodes below bifurcation of common iliac arteries.

- NX   Regional lymph nodes cannot be assessed
- N0   No regional lymph node metastases
- N1   Regional lymph node metastases within true pelvis, below common iliac artery bifurcation, either unilateral or bilateral

Metastases

- MX   Distant metastases cannot be assessed
- M0   No distant metastases
- M1a   Non-regional lymph node metastasis
- M1b   Bone(s) metastasis
- M1c   Other site(s) of metastasis

References

1 Gleason DF, Mellinger GT. Prediction of prognosis for prostatic adenocarcinoma by combined histological grading and clinical staging. *J Urol* 1974; **111**:58–64.
2 Lefkowitz GK, Taneja SS, Brown J, Melamed J, Lepor H. Follow-up interval prostate biopsy 3 years after diagnosis of high grade prostatic intraepithelial neoplasia is associated with high likelihood of prostate cancer, independent of change in prostate specific antigen levels. *J Urol* 2002; **168**:1415–18.
3 Chan TY, Epstein JI. Follow-up of atypical prostate needle biopsies suspicious for cancer. *Urology* 1999; **53**:351–5.
4 *TNM Classification of Malignant Tumours*, 6th edn. New York: Wiley–Liss, 2002.

Prostate cancer: transrectal ultrasonography and biopsies

Prostate cancer: transrectal ultrasonography and biopsies

The diagnosis of prostate cancer is made most commonly with needle biopsy guided by transrectal ultrasonography (TRUS). TRUS provides imaging of the prostate and seminal vesicles using a 7.5 mHZ biplane intra-rectal probe measuring ~1.5 cm in diameter. Most patients find the procedure uncomfortable, and some find it painful. It takes ~5 min and is performed on an outpatient basis with or without some form of anaesthetic. Among various anaesthetic techniques available, ultrasound-guided peri-prostatic injection of local anaesthetic is the most commonly used. A DRE precedes insertion of the probe. If biopsies are planned, rectal wall cleansing with antiseptic may be done. Broad-spectrum antimicrobials are given before and after the procedure.

TRUS can image the outline of the prostate, cysts, abscesses, and calcifications within the prostate. Hypoechoic and hyperechoic lesions in the peripheral zone may be due to prostate cancer or inflammatory conditions, but most prostate cancers are isoechoic and not 'seen'.

Indications for TRUS alone

- Accurate measurement of prostate volume.
- Male infertility with azospermia, to look for seminal vesicle and ejaculatory duct obstruction due to calculus or Mullerian cyst.
- Suspected prostatic abscess (can be drained by percutaneous needle aspiration).
- Investigation of chronic pelvic pain, looking for prostatic cyst or calculi.

Indications for TRUS with biopsies

- An abnormal DRE and/or an elevated PSA (exceptions include very elderly men with massively elevated PSA and abnormal DRE, or those in whom a TURP is indicated for BOO with severe LUTS/retention where histology will be obtained).
- Previous biopsies showing isolated PIN or ASAP.
- Previous biopsies normal, but PSA rising or DRE abnormal.
- To confirm viable prostate cancer following a treatment if further treatment is being considered.

Biopsy protocol

6–12 18FG trucut needle biopsies are taken in a systematic fashion to include any palpable or sonographic target lesion. The traditional sextant protocol (a parasagittal base, mid-gland and apex from each side) has been superseded by 8, 10, or 12 biopsies, adding samples from the far lateral peripheral zones. Studies have demonstrated that these extra biopsies detect up to 15% more cancers. Additional biopsies of each transition zone may be taken if a transition zone cancer is suspected, or if a patient is undergoing repeat biopsies because of a rising PSA. Seminal vesicle biopsies are undertaken occasionally, particularly for cancer staging where the vesicles appear abnormal on DRE, TRUS, or MRI, but such staging can be unreliable and thereby has limited clinical utility.

Complications of prostatic biopsy
- Occasional vaso-vagal 'fainting' immediately after the procedure.
- 0.5% risk of septicaemia, which may be life-threatening.
- 0.5% risk of significant rectal bleeding.
- Probable mild haemospermia or haematuria, 3–6 weeks.

Note

It is not safe to biopsy a warfarinized patient; biopsying patients on low-dose aspirin remains controversial, but is not at present considered unsafe.[1] Other anti-platelet drugs (e.g. clopidogrel) are usually stopped for 10 days prior to biopsy.

It is important that the patient appreciates that negative biopsies do not exclude the possibility of prostate cancer, and that a positive result will not necessarily result in the recommendation of immediate treatment.

Prostate cancer may also be diagnosed by TURP histology or clinically (without histology) in certain circumstances. For example, it could be viewed as unnecessarily invasive to biopsy a frail symptomatic patient with a craggy hard prostate and a PSA >100 ng/mL prior to commencing hormone therapy.

Reference

1 Masood J, Hafeez A, Calleary, Barua JM. Aspirin use and transrectal ultrasonography guided prostate biopsy: a national survey. *BJU Int* 2007; **99**:965–6.

Management of localized prostate cancer: watchful waiting

More men die with prostate cancer than because of it, owing to the increasing incidence of the disease with advancing age and the slow progression of early-stage disease. Therefore, with advancing age, the threat of early-stage prostate cancer is frequently overtaken by competing causes of mortality. The mortality of prostate cancer is invariably associated with metastases, whereas, in its early stages, prostate cancer is generally asymptomatic. Therefore the clinical significance of early-stage prostate cancer relates principally to its potential to reduce life expectancy against competing causes of death, and its biological potential for progression.[1] This forms the basis for 'watchful waiting' (WW) as a management option for men with non-metastatic prostatic cancer, particularly those having limited life-expectancy and/or low-risk disease. With WW, therapeutic intervention is deferred until progression or symptoms arise, thus avoiding treatment-related side-effects. However, careful clinical monitoring (with PSA, clinical examination, etc.) is necessary because of the risk of asymptomatic stage progression.

The risks of developing metastatic disease and of death due to prostate cancer after 10–15 years of WW can be considered using published data, according to biopsy grade (Table 4.3).

Selection of patients for watchful waiting

Watchful waiting is the best option for patients with clinically localized prostate cancer and:
- Gleason score 2–4 disease (in which the results of the more aggressive treatments described below are no better) any age.
- Gleason score 5 and 6 disease where age >75 years, or age <75 years where low-volume disease is predicted by DRE, serum PSA, biopsy, and imaging.
- Significant comorbidity and/or life expectancy considered <10 years.
- Stage T1a disease with normal PSA (only 17% T1a will progress compared with 68% with T1b; however, transrectal needle biopsy should be considered to assess residual prostatic malignancy, particularly where life expectancy may be >10 years).
- Serum PSA level and PSA kinetics should be taken into consideration, based on age and disease risk.

Watchful waiting protocols

Most men with localized prostate cancer on WW are seen every 6 months for clinical history, examination including a DRE, and a serum PSA test. If the disease progresses during follow-up, further staging investigations and appropriate palliative treatment (e.g. anti-androgen or androgen deprivation therapy) are recommended. The threshold for treatment was traditionally when symptoms and signs of advanced disease appeared, e.g. back pain and metastases on bone scan. Treatment (with androgen deprivation) should be recommended upon development of distant metastases, particularly bone metastases, and therefore WW

Table 4.3 Natural history of localized prostate cancer managed with no initial treatment in the pre-PSA era[2]

Biopsy grade	% risk of metastasis (10 years)	% risk of prostate cancer death (15 years)	Estimated lost years of life
2–4	19	4–7	<1
5	42	6–11	4
6	42	18–30	4
7	42	42–70	5
8–10	74	56–87	6–8

Table 4.4 Natural history of screen detected prostate cancer[3]

Biopsy grade	% risk of prostate cancer death managed conservatively (15 years)	% survival benefit from curative treatment, aged 55–59 years (15 year)
<7	0–2	0
7	9–31	12
8–10	28–72	26

should include periodic bone scans. The evidence of benefit with earlier use of hormone therapy, the use of PSA (for disease monitoring and PSA kinetics for risk assessment), and the involvement of patient choice has driven earlier thresholds for treatment. Hence, an asymptomatic patient with a rising PSA may choose to treat his disease and accept therapeutic side-effects, or to maintain his current quality of life while leaving the disease untreated.

A more intensive form of WW is termed 'active surveillance.'[4] This is aimed at younger men with low-volume moderate-grade disease who might be considered for, but wish to avoid (or defer), curative treatment. These men are seen with PSA every 3 months and may undergo annual repeat biopsy to detect PSA progression and/or upgrading. Evidence of progression may prompt aggressive treatment. This strategy may reduce over-treatment but there is a risk that aggressive disease may progress beyond a curative stage during the period of observation. The balance of these risks reflects patient selection. Careful assessment of the individual patient and his involvement in informed decision-making are essential.

References

1 Albertsen PC, Hanley JA, Fine J. 20-year outcomes following conservative management of clinically localized prostate cancer. *JAMA* 2005; **293**:2095–101.

2 Albertsen PC, Hanley JA, Gleason DF, Barry MJ. Competing risk analysis of men aged 55 to 74 years at diagnosis managed conservatively for clinically localized prostate cancer. *JAMA* 1998; **280**:975–80.

3 Parker C, Muston D, Melia J, Moss S, Dearnaley D. A model of the natural history of screen-detected prostate cancer, and the effect of radical treatment on overall survival. *Br J Cancer* 2006; **94**:1361–8.

4 Klotz L. Active surveillance versus radical treatment for favorable-risk localized prostate cancer. *Curr Treat Options Oncol* 2006; **7**:355–62.

Radical prostatectomy

Radical prostatectomy includes total removal of the prostate, seminal vesicles, and distal vasa deferentia, with a margin of surrounding connective tissue, and urethrovesical reconstruction. The surgical margin may be only a millimetre or so from the prostatic capsule, and wide excision of one or both neurovascular bundles may be performed in some cases to ensure negative margins. The intent of surgery is to achieve negative surgical margins, undetectable PSA following surgery, and cure, with minimum impact on morbidity.[1]

Lymphadenectomy may be performed for pathological staging and to provide additional prognostic information.[2] The therapeutic value of lymphadenectomy is controversial, but some patients with low-volume nodal metastatic disease may have extended disease-free survival; adjuvant hormone therapy may be indicated for those with high-risk disease.[3-6] Neo-adjuvant hormone therapy reduces tumour stage and the positive margin rate, but no effect on PSA recurrence has been demonstrated.[7,8]

Indications

Radical prostatectomy is usually performed for clinically localized prostate cancer, with curative intent.[9] Where cure is not achieved, symptoms of locally advanced disease may be averted. Radical prostatectomy is occasionally carried out as a salvage procedure for biochemical recurrence after radical radiotherapy where there is no evidence of regional or distant metastatic disease. For this indication, additional surgical morbidity may be anticipated. Some surgeons have advocated radical prostatectomy without curative intent for control of symptoms associated with locally advanced disease. Here, we describe the anatomic retropubic radical prostatectomy, and the reader is referred to other texts for discussion of its surgical modifications and for a description of radical perineal prostatectomy.[10]

Patient preparation

The tumour will have been diagnosed histologically, and assessed by digital rectal examination, serum PSA, and additional staging investigations according to local guidelines. A bone scan is recommended for patients with any suspicion for bone metastases, including bone symptoms, abnormal alkaline phosphatase or calcium, high-grade tumour (Gleason pattern ≥ 4 or sum score ≥ 8), PSA >10 ng/mL, or clinical suspicion of extraprostatic extension. An MRI scan of the prostate and pelvis may be carried out where additional staging and assessment of the primary tumour is required for therapeutic decisions or treatment planning.

Operative preparation

The abdominal skin, including the genitalia and proximal thighs, should be shaved and prepped with suitable antiseptic solution. A 16Fr urethral catheter should be inserted after sterile drapes are placed around the operative field. Anti-thrombotic stockings, intermittent calf compression boots, low molecular weight heparin, and antibiotic prophylaxis should be used in accordance with local guidelines. Cross-matched blood should be available.

Patient position

The patient lies supine on the operating table, with the mid-table hinge at the level of umbilicus. The hinge may then be flexed to increase pelvic exposure. Careful attention must be paid to padding of potential pressure points and avoidance of contact between the patient and metalwork around the operating table. The table should be levelled so that the abdomen is flat, and adjusted to a height comfortable for the surgeon. Operating lights should be arranged and focused for abdominal and pelvic illumination. The surgeon may choose to wear a headlamp.

Incision

Most surgeons use a lower abdominal midline incision. The length of the incision may vary according to the exposure required, extending cranially from the pubic symphysis as a short mini-laparotomy incision or as far as the umbilicus. Some surgeons use a Pfannenstiel incision.

For the midline approach, incise skin and subcutaneous fat in the midline from the pubic symphysis to a point just below the umbilicus. Incise the linea alba in the same line, and separate the medial edges of the two rectus muscles.

Opening the retropubic space

Divide the median connective tissue attachments of the rectus muscles. Below the linea semilunaris, cut any loose attachments between the recti and underlying transversalis fascia. Divide the posterior rectus sheath at the upper segment of the wound, after insinuating a finger between it and transversalis fascia. Formally divide the transversus fascia with scissors in the line of the abdominal incision to expose the fatty tissue of the retropubic space. By finger dissection, open the retropubic space from within the transversalis fascia, reflecting fat laterally from the parietal surface of the peritoneum. The space will open, exposing the external iliac vein.

Obturator lymph node dissection

This may be omitted in patients with low risk of lymph node metastases. In other patients with relatively high risk of lymph node metastases, where the presence or absence of nodal metastases would influence treatment decisions, lymph node dissection may be carried out prior to definitive treatment as a primary staging procedure.

Histopathological assessment of pelvic lymph nodes provides potentially valuable prognostic and staging information. Frozen section may fail to detect nodal metastasis subsequently identified in paraffin sections, particularly in low-volume metastatic disease. The therapeutic value of lymph node dissection is controversial,[11–14] and therefore, not surprisingly, the optimal extent of lymph node dissection is unknown, particularly in terms of its prognostic and therapeutic value. The uncertain advantages of extended lymphatic clearance should be considered against its potential morbidity and the increase in operative time.[15]

Reflect the peritoneum upwards by finger dissection, lifting the vas as it crosses the iliac vessels and courses towards its paravesical fascial plane. Lifting the vas creates a pocket beneath it which admits the tip of a narrow curved retractor for cranial retraction. The bladder is then retracted medially with a second broader retractor. For pelvic exposure, it is obvious but important to ensure that the bladder is fully drained by the urethral catheter.

Using non-toothed forceps, pick up the adventitia overlying the external iliac vein, thereby separating it from the vein wall, and incise the adventitia with scissors. This incision is extended along the length of the vein. Having raised the advential layer as a flap, separate the connective and lymphatic tissue from the vein, following the vein wall inferiorly onto the muscle of the pelvic side wall. Sweep the fat and lymph tissue medially away from the pelvic side wall, continuing this dissection distally from just below the iliac bifurcation towards the femoral canal. Identify the obturator nerve before ligating and dividing the lymphatic chain at the femoral canal. Use of ligaclips may reduce the risk of lymphocele. This distal limit may require careful dissection to identify and control aberrant blood vessels which otherwise bleed and retract. Dissect the lymphatic package proximally from the obturator nerve towards the ureter and internal iliac artery. This is accomplished easily with forceps and the aid of a sucker; a Babcock clamp is useful for manipulating the lymphatic package during its dissection.

Division of the endopelvic fascia and pubo-prostatic ligaments

Open the endopelvic fascia with scissors and divide it lateral to the prostate, keeping close to the pelvic side wall. There may be a relatively thin or fenestrated defect just lateral to the pubo-prostatic ligaments which can be opened relatively easily to begin this incision. Be wary of small vessels perforating the pelvic floor just beneath the fascia which require the judicious application of small ligaclip before their division. Anteriorly, the endopelvic fascial incision is continuous with the lateral aspect of the pubo-prostatic ligaments. These pyramidal ligaments may be divided at their midpoint between the pubis and prostate, but the urethral component must *not* be divided. Trim the ligaments from their lateral aspect to the level of the prostate apex; this will improve exposure during division of the dorsal venous complex later. The distal limit of the pubo-prostatic incision is judged by identification of the prostatic apex visually or by palpation. During their incision, the deeper aspects of the pubo-prostatic ligaments are exposed by applying appropriate backward pressure on the anterior surface of the prostate with a swab-stick. The infra-prostatic component of the ligament is preserved for pubic support of the proximal membranous urethra. It is not necessary to dissect a urethral stump (Fig. 4.33).

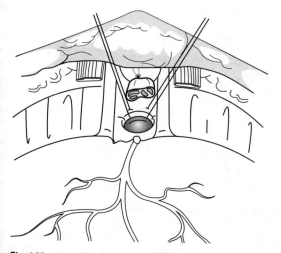

Fig. 4.33 Incision of the endopelvic fascia and opening of urethra.

Division of the dorsal venous complex

The dorsal venous complex must now be ligated with a needle-mounted absorbable suture (e.g. 3–0 or 2–0 according to needle preference). A curved needle is held in a long needle long holder, and passed from right to left under the venous complex.[16] This ligature can be combined with suture anchorage of the dorsal venous complex to the pubic periosteum, as described by Walsh,[1] to maintain urethral support previously provided by the (now divided) prostate component of the pubo-prostatic ligaments. The ligature can then be tied, securing the complex and restoring urethral position (Fig. 4.34). Manoeuvres that bunch the dorsal venous complex may displace the apical neurovascular bundles anteriorly risking subsequent injury, or further compromise the external sphincter on dividing the dorsal venous complex.

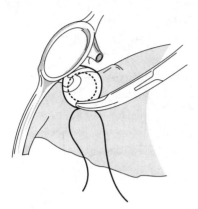

Fig. 4.34 Ligation of the dorsal venous complex after division of the puboprostatic ligaments.

Divide the dorsal venous complex under vision (with scissors or blade on a long handle), using the swab-stick on the anterior prostate to control prostatic displacement and back-bleeding. As the complex is released from the prostate, its horseshoe-shaped anterior attachment is displayed. If the complex is divided too distal or too far from the anterior prostate, or the incision is deepened without following the slope of the anterior prostate, the apex will not be exposed at the base of the horseshoe, as it should. If the dorsal complex is released correctly, the proximal urethra will be reached at the prostatic apex.[17]

Division of the urethra

When the anterior surface of the prostato-urethral junction is revealed, gently separate the lateral walls of the urethra (medially) from the lateral pillars of the external sphincter. Complete haemostasis of the divided distal edge of the dorsal venous complex, using the needle suture already secured to this complex, preserving its inverted U-shaped margin in front of the urethra. Control back-bleeding with a continuous running suture (e.g. 3–0 Vicryl) along the horseshoe-shaped reflection of the divided dorsal complex on the anterior prostate.

Open the urethra at the prostatic apex with scissors, exposing the urethral catheter, and divide the anterior two-thirds of the proximal urethra immediately below the prostatic apex (Fig. 4.35). Deflate the urethral catheter balloon and bring the catheter tip into the membranous urethra. Interrupted anastomotic sutures can be placed circumferentially into the urethral edge at this time. Most surgeons employ six sutures. 3–0 monocryl is suitable, because of its absorptive and handling properties. If

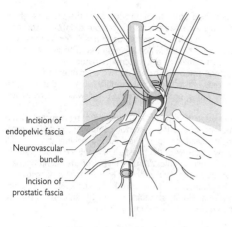

Incision of endopelvic fascia

Neurovascular bundle

Incision of prostatic fascia

Fig. 4.35 Division of the anterior urethral wall and placement of anastomotic sutures.

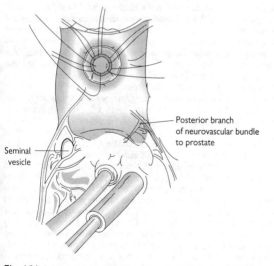

Posterior branch of neurovascular bundle to prostate

Seminal vesicle

Fig. 4.36 Release of the prostate from the neurovascular bundle, beginning at the prostatic apex.

the needles are all passed through the urethra from the patient's left to right, the needles of the left-sided sutures (placed out-to-in) will used later to complete the anastomosis, whereas a Mayo needle or sutures with double-ended needles will be needed on the right side. The sutures should pick up the urethral urothelium and external striated muscle to avoid damage to the urethral smooth muscle. The two ends of each suture are placed in artery forceps, which in turn are carefully laid around the surgical wound and covered with a protective sterile towel while the operation continues.

The posterior urethra is divided after passing a right-angled clamp between its posterior wall and the posterior component of the external sphincter. The right-angled clamp is then passed behind the external sphincter, just below the apex of the prostate, and thence into a plane in front of the neurovascular bundles. With the jaws of the clamp opened, the dorsal component can be divided precisely, from lateral to medial on each side, using the blade of a long-handled knife. The apex of the prostate is thereby released with its glandular margin, minimizing the risks of apical incision or compromise of urethral sphincter.[18]

Mobilization of the prostate and seminal vesicles with neurovascular bundle preservation[19,20]

Divide the lateral pelvic fascia from the bladder neck, in a distal direction, along a line medial to the reflection of this fascia onto the lateral surface of the prostate. This is carried out by running the jaws of a right-angled clamp under the fascial layer, lifting and cutting the fascia with scissors between the jaws. Repeat this on the contralateral side; the prostate can then be rotated freely from side to side. Feel the groove for the neurovascular bundle posterolaterally, and a second groove behind this which separates the rectum from the prostate.

Divide the anterior and medial fascial attachments of the neurovascular bundles. This dissection begins at the apex with a fine right-angled clamp, where opening the space between the two neurovascular bundles (inferiorly) and the prostatic apex (superiorly) defines the correct surgical plane behind the posterior layer of Denonvillier's fascia. Particular care is necessary to identify and release the bundles where their course may deviate over the surface of the apical prostate. Having correctly opened the space behind Denonvillier's fascia, release the bundles by retrograde dissection, again using a right-angled clamp to lift the fascial attachments between the bundles and the prostate, and rotating the gland laterally as necessary with a swab-stick (Fig. 4.37). Use ligaclips on small vascular attachments, particularly at the prostatic apex, where the bundles may pass over the prostate surface, and at the base of the seminal vesicles. Diathermy may damage the neurovascular bundles and should be avoided.

Having released the apex of the prostate in a retrograde direction as far as the base of the seminal vesicles, divide the midline attachment (behind the prostate) of the posterior layer of Denonvillier's fascia to the rectum. The lateral fascial attachments near the base of the seminal vesicles may be quite dense, and their release requires careful consideration of the neurovascular bundles contained therein. Ligate any vascular branches at this point with a ligaclip, before proceeding to release the seminal vesicles from the neurovascular bundles in a retrograde direction. Divide the posterior layer of Denonvillier's fascia close to the apices of the seminal vesicles, thereby directly exposing the vesicles. At this point, remaining anterolateral attachments (the prostatic pedicle) can be safely divided again in retrograde fashion (the bundles are already released posteriorly). By applying ligaclips and dividing the pedicle progressively from the front and working proximally, the lateral aspect of the bladder neck is reached.

The seminal vesicles can be safely dissected after their fascial attachments to the prostate are released and the space in front of the posterior layer of Denonvillier's has been formally opened. Their dissection at this stage will allow the bladder neck to be approached from behind. Alternatively, the anterior bladder neck can be opened and the seminal vesicles approached from the front. Vascular lateral attachments of the bladder neck are ligaclipped and divided. The space between the bladder and seminal vesicles (underneath the trigone) should then be defined with a right-angled clamp before dividing the posterior bladder neck in front of the ureteric orifices. Care should be taken to ensure that residual prostate (including any median lobe) is not left attached to the trigone, especially when preserving the bladder neck. The vasa are identified in the midline, ligaclipped, and divided. The seminal vesicles are dissected free, if this has not been previously completed. Care should be taken to identify and clip the artery to the tip of seminal vesicle. Residual posterolateral prostatic attachments are divided, and the prostate removed.

When a neurovascular bundle is to be formally excised, it is divided at the prostatic apex at the initial apical dissection. A ligaclip may be used if bleeding obscures the subsequent dissection; otherwise is not necessary. Divide the lateral pelvic fascia lateral to the prostate and in front of the rectum, and more cranially alongside the seminal vesicle (Fig. 4.37). The bundle with its adjacent fascia is left on the prostate and the adjacent seminal vesicle.

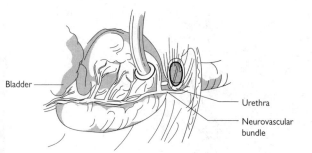

Bladder

Urethra

Neurovascular bundle

Fig. 4.37 Wide excision of the right neurovascular bundle.

Bladder neck reconstruction and urethral anastomosis

A tennis-racket reconstruction is used to reduce a large bladder neck defect. This is not required if the bladder neck has been preserved. Bladder neck preservation has not been shown to influence long-term continence outcomes. The posterior aspect of the bladder defect is closed in a sagital line with a continuous absorbable suture (e.g. 3–0 Vicryl) running anteriorly from a terminal stay, knotted on the bladder exterior. A tennis-racket reconstruction creates a bladder opening approximately the size of the index finger for anastomosis to the urethra (Fig. 4.38). Evert the bladder urothelium of the reconstructed bladder neck using absorbable interrupted sutures (4–0 Vicryl). Check pelvic haemostasis at this stage; lavage may help identify bleeding points. A bladder washout should be carried out to evacuate clots.

The urethral anastomosis is then completed in a parachute fashion. Pass the pre-placed urethral sutures through the reconstructed bladder neck, from inside to outside, beginning posteriorly and working anteriorly. (If sutures with double-ended needles have not been used, a Mayo needle is required on the right side). Once these sutures are positioned, pass an 18 or 20Fr silastic catheter (having tested the balloon) from the external meatus, across the urethrovesical defect (without tangling it in the sutures), and through the reconstructed bladder neck. Level the operating table, remove the retractors, and draw the bladder down into the pelvis. Withdraw any slack of each of the sutures, and check apposition of the bladder neck to the urethra. Check that the catheter's antegrade travel is unimpeded and the catheter tip is correctly positioned in the bladder before inflating the catheter balloon with ~10 cc sterile water. Tie the sutures sequentially, pushing each knot throw down alongside the urethrovesical junction with the index finger, beginning anteriorly and leaving the (weakest) posterior suture for last. A final bladder washout through the catheter should be done to ensure that residual clots are evacuated.

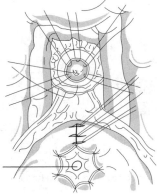

Everted bladder mucosa

Fig. 4.38 Reconstruction of the bladder neck.

Drains

Place drains alongside the pelvic dissection in case of lymphatic or urinary leakage. The drains should not lie immediately adjacent to the anastomosis where they would encourage urinary leakage.

Post-operative care

Early mobilization and chest physiotherapy are essential for prompt rehabilitation and to minimize risks associated with thrombo-embolism and atelectasis. Early mobilization will also contribute to lower analgesic usage and minimizing adverse effects of opiates on GI motility. Intravenous opiate patient-controlled analgesia is sufficient for the first 12–24 hr until mobilization has begun; thereafter an oral opiate in combination with paracetamol usually suffices. Light diet may be commenced the morning following surgery, unless there has been concern relating to post-operative haemorrhage. A Dulcolax suppository is often helpful in relieving colicky abdominal pain on the second day (unless there is concern about a rectal injury). Haemoglobin, fluid, and electrolyte balance must be monitored, with due attention also paid to thrombo-embolism prophylaxis, antibiotic prophylaxis, GI function, individual comorbidity, urinary drainage per catheter, and pelvic drain output. Bladder washouts are necessary if clots of blood or debris are seen or if blockage to urinary drainage is suspected.

Outcomes

Indicators of long-term outcomes include pathological stage, whole tumour Gleason grade, and surgical margin status.[21–30] Although negative margins may relate to better oncological outcomes, the majority of well-selected patients with a microscopic positive margin do not develop biochemical recurrence in the absence of additional adverse risk factors.[31,32] However, survival advantage over deferred treatment may not be realized for many years,[33] and the proportion of men who will benefit decreases with advancing age because of comorbidity and competing causes of mortality.

Late complications

Late complications include erectile dysfunction, anastomotic stricture, and incontinence. Erectile failure is reported in 29–100% patients undergoing radical prostatectomy. It is related to pre-operative erectile function, patient age, tumour stage, and nerve preservation. Phosphodiesterase inhibitors can be used to promote early return of erectile function, and contribute to the quality of erections, but are unlikely to influence long-term erectile failure following neurovascular bundle injury or resection. Persistent erectile failure can be managed by intracaversonal injection of alprostadil, vacuum pump therapy, or a penile prosthesis.

Stress incontinence (mild, 4–50%; severe, 0–15%) usually reflects external sphincter weakness, and may be aggravated by bladder instability. Early incontinence may be improved by physiotherapy, and pelvic floor exercises. Attention to fluid intake and diet are important, and antimuscarinic agents may be supportive until urinary control is regained. Biofeedback and pelvic floor electrical stimulation may also be useful in individual cases. For persistent incontinence (i.e. 1–2 years post surgery where no further improvement can be anticipated), a peri-urethral bulking agent, a urethral sling, or (more definitively) artificial urinary sphincter placement may be considered.[3,4]

It is important to recognize urinary tract infection and anastomotic stricture as causes of voiding difficulties and incontinence. Anastomotic strictures are reported in up to 10% of cases. Most can be treated by dilatation or endoscopic incision, with due care to avoid sphincteric injury. Clean intermittent self-catheterization may reduce recurrent stricture formation. Recurrent strictures may be more definitively managed by endoscopic resection. Surgical interventions for anastomotic distraction stricture and for recurrent stricture associated with persistent incontinence are particularly challenging, and the management of these patients requires expertise in reconstructive procedures.

Radical prostatectomy provides the opportunity for durable cancer-free survival and cure, and following a successful operation, excellent quality of life is restored in the majority of patients by 1 year, an important principle in the recommendation for surgery.

References

1 Walsh PC. Anatomic radical prostatectomy: evolution of the surgical technique. *J Urol* 1998; **160**:2418–24.

2 Burkhard FC, Bader P, Schneider E, Markwalder R, Studer UE. Reliability of preoperative values to determine the need for lymphadenectomy in patients with prostate cancer and meticulous lymph node dissection. *Eur Urol* 2002; **42**:84–90.

3 Messing EM, Manola J, Yao J et al. Immediate versus deferred androgen deprivation treatment in patients with node-positive prostate cancer after radical prostatectomy and pelvic lymphadenectomy. *Lancet Oncol* 2006; **7**:472–9.

4 Medical Research Council Prostate Cancer Working Party Investigators Group. Immediate versus deferred treatment for advanced prostatic cancer: initial results of the Medical Research Council Trial. *Br J Urol* 1997; **79**:235–46.

5 Studer UE, Whelan P, Albrecht W et al. Immediate or deferred androgen deprivation for patients with prostate cancer not suitable for local treatment with curative intent: European Organization for Research and Treatment of Cancer (EORTC) Trial 30891. *J Clin Oncol* 2006; **24**:1868–76.

6 McLeod DG, Iversen P, See WA, Morris T, Armstrong J, Wirth MP. Bicalutamide 150 mg plus standard care vs standard care alone for early prostate cancer. *BJU Int* 2006; **97**:247–54.

7 Soloway MS, Sharifi R, Wajsman Z, McLeod D, Wood DPJ, Puras-Baez A. Randomized prospective study comparing radical prostatectomy alone versus radical prostatectomy preceded by androgen blockade in clinical stage B2 (T2bNxM0) prostate cancer. The Lupron Depot Neoadjuvant Prostate Cancer Study Group. *J Urol* 1995; **154**:424–8.

8 Soloway MS, Pareek K, Sharifi R et al. Neo-adjuvant androgen ablation before radical prostatectomy in cT2bNxMo prostate cancer: 5-year results. J Urol 2002; 167:112–16.

9 Aus G, Abbou CC, Bolla M et al. EAU guidelines on prostate cancer. Eur Urol 2005; 48:546–51.

10 Kirby RS, Partin AW, Feneley MR, Parsons JK, eds. Prostate Cancer: Principles and Practice. London: Taylor & Francis, 2005.

11 Joslyn SA, Konety BR. Impact of extent of lymphadenectomy on survival after radical prostatectomy for prostate cancer. Urology 2006; 68:121–5.

12 Pagliarulo V, Hawes D, Brands FH, et al. Detection of occult lymph node metastases in locally advanced node-negative prostate cancer. J Clin Oncol 2006; 24:2735–42.

13 Bader P, Burkhard FC, Markwalder R, Studer UE. Disease progression and survival of patients with positive lymph nodes after radical prostatectomy. Is there a chance of cure? J Urol 2003; 169:849–54.

14 Masterson TA, Bianco FJ, Jr., Vickers AJ et al. The association between total and positive lymph node counts, and disease progression in clinically localized prostate cancer. J Urol 2006; 175:1320–4.

15 McLaughlin AP, Saltzstein SI, McCollough DL, Gittes RF. Prostatic carcinoma incidence and location of unsuspected lymphatic metastases. J Urol 1976; 115:89–94.

16 Reiner WG, Walsh PC. An anatomical approach to the surgical management of the dorsal vein and Santorini's plexus during radical retropubic surgery. J Urol 1979; 121:198–200.

17 Myers RP, Goellner JR, Cahill DR. Prostate shape, external striated urethral sphincter and radical prostatectomy: the apical dissection. J Urol 1987; 138:543–50.

18 Narayan P, Konety B, Aslam K, Aboseif S, Blumenfeld W, Tanagho E. Neuroanatomy of the external urethral sphincter: implications for urinary continence preservation during radical prostate surgery. J Urol 1995; 153:337–41.

20 Walsh PC, Donker PJ. Impotence following radical prostatectomy: insight into etiology and prevention. J Urol 1982; 128:492–7.

21 Walsh PC, Lepor H, Eggleston JC. Radical prostatectomy with preservation of sexual function: anatomical and pathological considerations. Prostate 1983; 4:473–85.

22 Pound CR, Partin AW, Eisenberger MA, Chan DW, Pearson JD, Walsh PC. Natural history of progression after PSA elevation following radical prostatectomy. JAMA 1999; 281:1591–7.

23 Epstein JI, Partin AW, Sauvageot J, Walsh PC. Prediction of progression following radical prostatectomy: a multivariate analysis of 721 men with long-term follow-up. Am J Surg Pathol 1996; 20:286–92.

24 Swindle P, Eastham JA, Ohori M et al. Do margins matter? The prognostic significance of positive surgical margins in radical prostatectomy specimens. J Urol 2005; 174:903–7.

25 Karakiewicz PI, Eastham JA, Graefen M et al. Prognostic impact of positive surgical margins in surgically treated prostate cancer: multi-institutional assessment of 5831 patients. Urology 2005; 66:1245–50.

26 Ohori M, Wheeler TM, Kattan MW, Goto Y, Scardino PT. Prognostic significance of positive surgical margins in radical prostatectomy specimens. J Urol 1995; 154:1818–24.

27 Bastian PJ, Gonzalgo ML, Aronson WJ et al. Clinical and pathologic outcome after radical prostatectomy for prostate cancer patients with a preoperative Gleason sum of 8 to 10. Cancer 2006; 107:1265–72.

28 Stamey TA, McNeal JE, Yemoto CM, Sigal BM, Johnstone IM. Biological determinants of cancer progression in men with prostate cancer. JAMA 1999; 281:1395–1400.

29 Palisaar RJ, Graefen M, Karakiewicz PI et al. Assessment of clinical and pathologic characteristics predisposing to disease recurrence following radical prostatectomy in men with pathologically organ-confined prostate cancer. Eur Urol 2002; 41:155–61.

30 Mian BM, Troncoso P, Okihara K et al. Outcome of patients with Gleason score 8 or higher prostate cancer following radical prostatectomy alone. J Urol 2002; 167:1675–80.

31 Porter CR, Kodama K, Gibbons RP et al. 25-year prostate cancer control and survival outcomes: a 40-year radical prostatectomy single institution series. J Urol 2006; 176:569–74.

32 Vis AN, Schroder FH, van der Kwast TH. The actual value of the surgical margin status as a predictor of disease progression in men with early prostate cancer. Eur Urol 2006; 50:258–65.

33 Simon MA, Kim S, Soloway MS. Prostate specific antigen recurrence rates are low after radical retropubic prostatectomy and positive margins. J Urol 2006; 175:140–4.

34 Bill-Axelson A, Holmberg L, Ruutu M et al. Radical prostatectomy versus watchful waiting in early prostate cancer. N Engl J Med 2005; 352:1977–84.

35 Urinary incontinence. In: Kirby RS, Partin AW, Feneley MR, Parsons JK, eds. London: Taylor & Francis, 2005.

Minimally invasive therapeutic alternatives to radical prostatectomy

There is growing interest in minimally invasive therapeutic alternatives to radical prostatectomy.

Brachytherapy

The efficacy of radiation therapy is well established. The oncological outcomes and side-effects relate very significantly to radiation dose and technique. Brachytherapy uses radioactive seeds to deliver higher radiation doses to the prostate than is possible with external beam radiotherapy alone, without necessarily increasing the side-effects.

Brachytherapy techniques include low-dose-rate brachytherapy (LDR) with permanent implantation of multiple radioactive seeds, and high-dose-rate brachytherapy (HDR) with a single radioactive source and computer-controlled afterloading.[1,2] The placement of multiple seeds (for LDR) or the single-source control (HDR afterloading) is calculated to provide the prescribed radiation dose and distribution. Radioactive seeds are delivered transperineally through needles/tubes positioned under general anaesthesia through a template grid, with TRUS guidance and direct endoscopic assessment to exclude endoluminal seed deployment or needle displacement. Brachytherapy techniques can be combined with external beam radiotherapy for higher radiation doses or wider tissue delivery. Neo-adjuvant and adjuvant hormone therapy may be given to reduce volume for radiation exposure as well as for improved oncological control. Brachytherapy is generally contraindicated by moderate or severe urinary symptoms, bladder outflow obstruction, or large prostate volume. Previous transurethral resection of the prostate may impair secure seed placement (often considered a contraindication) and increase the risk of complications, particularly in relation to the urethra and external sphincter function.

Cryotherapy and high-intensity focussed ultrasound

Minimally invasive tissue-ablative technologies have attracted interest, including cryotherapy and high-intensity focused ultrasound (HIFU).[3] Currently the clinical indications and long-term outcomes for these technologies are not well defined, but they offer the technological opportunity for local treatment, principally for biochemical failure after radiotherapy treatment failure (salvage), with the possibility of repeated treatments.

Cryotherapy uses a sequence of freeze–thaw cycles to induce tissue necrosis. Multiple needle probes are placed in the target tissue through an extracorporeal perineal template. Ice-balls are created around the needle tips by heat exchange, monitored by TRUS imaging. The technical principles of cryotherapy are considered further in the discussion of its renal applications (📖 p. 190). HIFU causes tissue destruction by explosive vaporization. Contraindications include prostatic calcification, which may limit ultrasound transmission, and large prostate volume. The optimal setting for these treatments and long-term outcomes require further investigation in research trials.

Future developments

The therapeutic effects of minimally invasive technology causing tumour (and normal tissue) necrosis appear promising. Patient follow-up demonstrates PSA response, prostate volume and/or prostate tumour reduction (on imaging and biopsy), and the feasibility of repeat treatment.[4] However, ablative minimally invasive therapies must be considered investigational, particularly for treatment of primary disease. For any primary therapy, concern relates to the long-term oncological benefit and treatment-related morbidity.

Any local therapy for prostate cancer is likely to have some (adverse) effects on normal structures adjacent to the limit of oncological efficacy. These adverse effects can be controlled and minimized according to the treatment modality and precision of the technique (extra-prostatic therapeutic spill necessary to ensure adequate treatment of the entire prostate also brings additional morbidity). Acute side-effects of minimally invasive therapies include inflammation, swelling, prostatitis, voiding difficulty, and exacerbation of previous voiding symptoms. Dose-related side-effects which affect the neurovascular bundles, urethra, bladder neck, external sphincter, and rectal mucosa are associated with longer-term complications. Such concerns have driven considerable technical refinements, particularly in the field of radiation therapy, reducing morbidity without loss of oncological effectiveness.

In the hands of experts, established definitive treatments for early-stage prostate cancer achieve low overall morbidity. Unfortunately, widely reported potential complications and their morbidity may dominate individual therapeutic decisions. There is a tendency for such decisions to be guided by the potential for complications, particularly where the differences in oncological outcome between alternative modalities and implications of therapeutic failure are poorly understood. In the future, it is possible (or likely) that certain advantages can be ensured by minimal invasive technology, demonstrable by favourable comparison with standard surgical and radiation techniques. However, such considerations may be of subsidiary importance compared with wider health-care issues arising from screening and treatment of screen-detected cancer. These concerns relate to case selection for treatment, risk and consequences of over-treatment, and the assessment and management of treatment failure. If, in the future, diagnostic markers were able to distinguish life-threatening cancers at a curable stage, alternative treatments could be compared more effectively according to oncological outcome.

References

1 Acher PL, Morris SL, Popert RJ, Perry MJ, Potters L, Beaney RP. Permanent prostate brachytherapy: a century of technical evolution. *Prostate Cancer Prostatic Dis* 2006; **9**:215–20.

2 Hoskin PJ, Bownes P. Innovative technologies in radiation therapy: brachytherapy. *Semin Radiat Oncol* 2006; **16**:209–17.

3 Aus G. Current status of HIFU and cryotherapy in prostate cancer: a review. *Eur Urol* 2006; **50**:927–34.

4 Petraki CD, Sfikas CP. Histopathological changes induced by therapies in the benign prostate and prostate adenocarcinoma. *Histol Histopathol* 2007; **22**:107–18.

Per-operative and early post-operative complications of urological cancer surgery

Per-operative complications

Haemorrhage and vascular injury

Mobilization and resection of large and extensive retroperitoneal tumours demands meticulous care for precise identification of major vessels. The position and course of the inferior vena cava, the renal veins, and other major vascular structures can be substantially and surprisingly displaced, associated with risk of misidentification and injury. When dissecting around and behind major vessels for placement of sloops, care should be taken to identify posterior branches (particularly venous tributaries). Sloops greatly facilitate manipulation of vascular structures during surgical dissection, as well as providing ready control. When dividing larger vessels, they should be doubly ligated with a sufficient gap between ligatures.

Even a small vascular injury from major retroperitoneal and pelvic veins may give rise to alarming bleeding. The source of such bleeding may be difficult to identify, and requires good illumination, retraction, suction, and surgical assistance. Initially, bleeding should be arrested with pressure, using either a finger or a pack. Sometimes light compression with one or two small swabs achieves haemostasis while the operation proceeds, and these swabs can be removed later without the need for any vascular suturing. Timed pressure for 10 min may similarly stop or reduce venous bleeding. This also provides time to prepare additional vascular instruments and sutures, transfer blood for transfusion to the operating room, and prepare for necessary resuscitative measures. By slowly rolling the swab back and forth, the site of the defect can be uncovered and visually assessed. With the defect covered, a vascular suture (such as 5–0 prolene) can be placed in the vessel wall and tied at one end, and, as the swab is rolled, a continuous suture can be run until the defect is closed. Alternatively, a defect (such as in the vena cava, external or common iliac vein) may be exposed and isolated by proximal and distal pressure or vascular clamps, and thereby sutured under vision. Blind clamping may cause additional injury and must be avoided. Vascular clamps can be placed either parallel to the long axis of a major vein, or transversely proximal and distal to the defect. Bleeding from an injury to a tributary of a major vein can be difficult to localize as a result of both antegrade and retrograde bleeding from the respective ends of the defect.

Where a solitary right renal vein has been injured, ligation will prevent renal perfusion and effectively necessitate nephrectomy. Since the left renal vein has several tributaries along its longer length, this vessel can be ligated without severely compromising renal function if repair is not feasible. Bleeding from the dorsal venous complex can be difficult to control until the entire structure has been completely released from the prostate and urethra; it can then be controlled by suture ligation.

Bleeding from the adrenal bed is best controlled by suture ligation. A small splenic capsular injury can often be controlled with haemostatic material and pressure, whereas a large or persistently bleeding injury may require splenectomy. After nephrectomy, an open adrenal vein is the occasional cause of delayed haemorrhage and necessitates re-exploration. Bleeding from the wound can similarly present as delayed haemorrhage. Secondary, bleeding from the ligated renal pedicles is very rare.

Surgical viseral injuries

The risk of injury to intra-abdominal organs (including colon bowel, duodenum, spleen, etc.) can often be reduced by their adequate exposure and mobilization prior to dissection of a major tumour mass. During a flank nephrectomy, it may be safer to open the peritoneum to reflect the colon, duodenum (right side), or duodenojeunal flexure (left side), rather than to attempt tumour resection and risk hidden visceral or vascular injury. Where colonic involvement is anticipated, pre-operative bowel preparation should be used. Colonic injury or resection may require a defunctioning ileostomy or colostomy according to the degree of contamination and bowel preparation.

During operations involving or adjacent to the distal ureter and bladder trigone, attention to surgical technique will usually avoid ureteric injury and consequent obstruction. When performing a psoas hitch, genito-femoral or femoral nerve injury should be avoided by careful placement of sutures parallel to the course of the nerves.

With a flank incision where the pleura is not formally opened, but a small tear is incurred, this injury can usually be repaired with an absorbable suture (e.g. 2–0 Vicryl), closing the defect after re-expanding the lung. A rubber catheter can be placed through the defect with the distal end in a receiver of water to evacuate air from the pleural space while the tear is closed; once the tear is closed, the catheter is removed. A chest drain will be required for larger pleural defects and thoracoabdominal incisions. If a retroperitoneal drain is required where there is the possibility that it may communicate with (and therefore cause) a pneumothorax, it should be attached to an underwater seal. A post-operative chest X-ray will also be required.

Rectal injury

Rectal injury is an uncommon complication during cystoprostatectomy or radical prostatectomy (<1%), and even less common in female anterior exenteration.[1,2] Previous pelvic irradiation or surgery significantly increases the risk, and particular care is required in these circumstances. Per-operative recognition of the injury is essential to prevent serious peri-operative complications from sepsis and fistula. At cystoprostatectomy, rectal injury tends to occur when the incorrect recto-prostatic plane is entered, usually because the dissection has been commenced too anteriorly from the recto-vesical pouch. Rectal injury may also occur when the correct plane is not dissected sufficiently distal (i.e. does not reach the prostatic apex), the rectum is tethered, and a distally directed incision enters the rectal lumen. At radical prostatectomy or retrograde cystoprostatectomy, rectal injury tends to occur at the prostatic apex, particularly when there is extensive apical tumour or fibrosis. The rectal injury can be closed in two continuous layers (2–0 monocril), and an omental flap created and sutured over the repaired defect. The region must be thoroughly cleaned with irrigation, and broad-spectrum antibiotics initiated. An anal dilatation should be carried out at the end of the procedure. Where there is a substantial injury, extensive contamination, or previous radiation, a defunctioning temporary colostomy should be created.

Post-operative care

The general principles of post-operative care are described in Chapter 1. The importance of nursing care, analgesia, early mobilization, and post-operative physiotherapy for prevention of complications cannot be overestimated. Judicious use of opiate analgesia involves attention to bowel function, including use of suppositories as necessary. Fluid and electrolyte balance must be monitored, with provision for metabolic and nutritional requirements, parenterally or orally as necessary. Continued attention must be paid to thrombo-embolism prophylaxis, antibiotic prophylaxis, prompt diagnosis and treatment of infection, and careful monitoring of pre-existing comorbidity. Care must be taken with placement of drains and catheters; maintaining their free drainage will minimize the risk of complications that may arise from urinary leak or from urinary or lymphatic collections. Normal diet may be resumed once GI function has resumed, demonstrated by normal bowel sounds and passage of flatus per rectum.

Early post-operative complications

Complications and mortality following major urological surgery relate to surgical technique and peri-operative care as well as to patient comorbidity and tumour-related factors.[3–5] The importance of case volume and experience has been emphasized for surgical centres as well as for individual surgeons.[6,7] Mortality rates should be low (<1% for radical prostatectomy and <3% for radical cystectomy), based on large series from centres of excellence. Complications should be identified early and wherever possible prevented.

Post-operative haemorrhage

Post-operative intra-abdominal bleeding after oncological surgery is a major surgical complication which must be identified early to avert disaster. Unrecognized bleeding incurs a substantial risk for additional complications, multi-organ failure, and death. A high level of suspicion for bleeding must be maintained in the early post-operative period, based on monitoring for clinical signs of bleeding and factors that may potentially disguise its clinical manifestation, including the development of systemic or organ-specific complications. A CT scan may be useful in situations where the diagnosis is uncertain, provided that it does not delay a necessary laparotomy. Haemorrhage following nephron-sparing surgery may be controlled by selective arterial embolization, thereby avoiding laparotomy and possibility of nephrectomy. Where pelvic bleeding following radical prostatectomy can be managed conservatively, observational reports suggest that re-exploration may be preferable and reduce subsequent morbidity.[8,9] Laparotomy must be performed early where there are clinical signs of persistent bleeding despite initial adequate resuscitation.

Urinary leak and fistulae

Urinary leak may be suspected where there is persistent high-volume drain output, and diagnosed by measuring the concentration of sodium (low) and creatinine (high) in the drain fluid, or by a radiological contrast study (when necessary). Where significant urinary leak is suspected, it will generally settle without additional intervention, provided that anatomical continuity is ensured and the necessary stents, catheters, and drains are unobstructed and secured in their correct position. Drains should be left in position to prevent urinoma or infective collection until the leak settles or a tract is established.

Occasionally, presentation of urinary leak is delayed, with signs of sepsis and/or renal impairment, and will be associated with urinary ascites, urinoma, or fistula. An undrained urinary collection can be drained externally by radiologically guided percutaneous drainage. Internal stenting across the leak and proximal and distal external drainage are also required, and may allow complete resolution with healing. Antibiotics should be used, guided by microbiological examination. Ongoing leak may be due to unrecognized duplex ureter or distraction of a ureteric implantation, and should be managed by the same principles until surgical re-implantation. A persistent urinary fistula requires surgical repair; provided that it is well drained, the repair can be delayed until 3 months.

Other complications

Wound complications include haematoma, infection, dehiscence, and hernia. Other septic complications include pneumonia, urinary tract infection, septicaemia, and intra-abdominal abscess. Local or systemic infection requires treatment with appropriate parenteral antibiotics, guided by microbiological investigation. Localized collections, including wound haematoma, wound abscess, and intra-abdominal abscess require drainage. Septic collections may raise the possibility of additional underlying complications, such as bowel injury or urinary leak, which must be considered. Wound dehiscence requires immediate exploration with excision of devitalized tissue, wound lavage, mass closure of the abdominal wall with interrupted monofilament absorbable sutures (such as PDS, as a figure-of-eight); subcutaneous drain, and skin closure (if possible) with interrupted sutures.

Gastrointestinal function

The development of complications after major surgery, particularly those compromising GI function, may give rise to the need for nutritional support. This need must be addressed early in view of a catabolic metabolic status. Ileus can sometimes be prolonged, and occasionally laparotomy is necessary for mechanical obstruction or intra-abdominal complications (including closed loop or ischaemia), and must be considered where GI function has not returned within the first 10 days. Mechanical obstruction should be diagnosed early by gastrograffin follow-through and requires urgent laparotomy. Enterocutaneous fistula without septic complications may settle with conservative management, but otherwise requires surgical repair, with drainage and bowel defunctioning as necessary.[10]

Acute colonic pseudo-obstruction (Ogilvie's syndrome) may occasionally develop following pelvic surgery, and is associated with failure to pass flatus and proximal colonic distension.[11] This should be recognized early with a plain abdominal X-ray and where prompt resolution fails to occur with conservative measures, colonoscopic decompression may be required.

Thrombo-embolism

Thrombo-embolism can be a sudden fatal event in the first few weeks following major surgery, particularly in patients with malignant disease and after pelvic surgery. It may occur despite prophylactic measures and in the absence of other operative or post-operative complications. The possibility of deep venous thrombosis and non-fatal embolism must be recognized early and treated with full anticoagulation.

Ureteric stricture

Ureteric stricture and ureteric anastomotic stenosis may develop early (i.e. within weeks of surgery), presenting with hydronephrosis or its complications. Obstruction can be diagnosed with a radio-isotope dynamic renogram and defined further by radiological contrast study (such as IVU or antegrade ureterogram).

Strictures of the ureter and its anastomosis can sometimes be treated by minimally invasive interventions such as balloon dilatation or cold knife or laser incision, followed by a period of stenting (4–6 weeks). Where such measures have failed, re-operation with excision of the diseased ureter and neo-implantation must be considered as a definitive alternative to long-term stenting; both requiring careful monitoring of renal function.[12–15]

Erectile dysfunction following non-nerve-sparing pelvic surgery

With non-nerve-sparing pelvic surgery, erectile dysfunction should be considered as a surgical inevitability rather than a complication. Resulting erectile dysfunction can be managed by intracaversonal alprostadil injection, a vacuum pump, or a penile prosthesis. Nerve sparing may preserve sexual function and contribute to sphincter function in both sexes.

References

1 Flechner SM, Spaulding JT. Management of rectal injury during cystectomy. *Urology* 1982; **19**:143–7.

2 Borland RN, Walsh PC. The management of rectal injury during radical retropubic prostatectomy. *J Urol* 1992; **147**:905–7.

3 Novotny V, Hakenberg OW, Wiessner D et al. Perioperative complications of radical cystectomy in a contemporary series. *Eur Urol* 2007; **51**:397–402.

4 Quek ML, Stein JP, Daneshmand S et al. A critical analysis of perioperative mortality from radical cystectomy. *J Urol* 2006; **175**:886–9.

5 Lepor H, Kaci L. Contemporary evaluation of operative parameters and complications related to open radical retropubic prostatectomy. *Urology* 2003; **62**:702–6.

6 Bianco FJ, Jr, Riedel ER, Begg CB, Kattan MW, Scardino PT. Variations among high volume surgeons in the rate of complications after radical prostatectomy: further evidence that technique matters. *J Urol* 2005; **173**:2099–103.

7 Birkmeyer JD, Siewers AE, Finlayson EV et al. Hospital volume and surgical mortality in the United States. *N Engl J Med* 2002; **346**:1128–37.

8 Hedican SP, Walsh PC. Postoperative bleeding following radical retropubic prostatectomy. *J Urol* 1994; **152**:1181–3.

9 Kaufman JD, Lepor H. Reoperation versus observation in men with major bleeding after radical retropubic prostatectomy. *Urology* 2005; **66**:561–5.

10 Draus JM Jr., Huss SA, Harty NJ, Cheadle WG, Larson GM. Enterocutaneous fistula: are treatments improving? 2006; **9**:361–8.

11 Tack J. Acute colonic pseudo-obstruction (Ogilvie's syndrome). *Curr Treat Options Gastroenterol* 2006; **9**:361–8.

12 Rapp DE, Laven BA, Steinberg GD, Gerber GS. Percutaneous placement of permanent metal stents for treatment of ureteroenteric anastomotic strictures. *J Endourol* 2004; **18**:677–81.

13 Laven BA, O'Connor RC, Gerber GS, Steinberg GD. Long-term results of endoureterotomy and open surgical revision for the management of ureteroenteric strictures after urinary diversion. *J Urol* 2003; **170**:1226–30.

14 DiMarco DS, LeRoy AJ, Thieling S, Bergstralh EJ, Segura JW. Long-term results of treatment for ureteroenteric strictures. *Urology* 2001; **58**:909–13.

15 Ravery V, de la Taille A, Hoffmann P et al. Balloon catheter dilatation in the treatment of ureteral and ureteroenteric stricture. *J Endourol* 1998; **12**:335–40.

Testicular cancer

Pathology

The testes contain seminiferous tubules (comprised of spermatogenic cells and supporting Sertoli cells) and stroma (containing interstitial Leydig cells which produce the testosterone necessary for spermatogenesis). Germ cell tumours (GCTs) are those which arise from the spermatogenic cells. Tumours may also arise from the non-spermatogenic cells (Sertoli and Leydig cells), the epididymis, and cord structures. GCTs account for 90–95% of testicular tumours. They are classified depending on the cell types that they contain (Table 4.5). GCTs arise from pluripotent stem cells. They are composed of cells of five main types based on cellular morphology: seminoma, teratoma, yolk sac tumours, embryonal cell carcinoma, choriocarcinoma. A tumour may contain a pure population of one of these cell types but more than 50% of GCTs contain more than one type of cell (mixed GCTs). The cell type is frequently predictive of tumour behaviour and response to treatment. For treatment planning, GCTs are broadly subdivided into seminomas and non-seminomatous GCTs (NSGCTs).

Carcinoma *in situ* (CIS) of the testis (synonymous with intra-tubular germ cell neoplasia (ITGCN)) is defined by the presence of atypical intratubular germ cells. CIS is considered to be a precursor of all GCTs other than spermatocytic seminoma. Of men with CIS, 10% per annum will develop invasive testicular cancer. The incidence of CIS in the general population is 0.8%, but it is much more common in men with cryptorchidism (3%), contralateral testicular cancer (5%), infertility (1.1%), and testicular atrophy with a history of contralateral testicular cancer (30%).[1] CIS is found throughout an affected testis; a small random biopsy is sufficient to establish its presence.

Testicular cancer usually spreads predictably to draining nodes (with the exception of choriocarcinoma). Lymph vessels in the spermatic cord drain medially to retroperitoneal nodes. The right testis drains first to inter-aortocaval nodes at L2. The left testis drains first to para-aortic nodes in a region defined by the aorta medially, the ureter laterally, the left renal vein superiorly, and the inferior mesenteric artery inferiorly. Spread from one side of the retroperitoneum to the other occurs most commonly from right to left (following the direction of lymph flow). Subsequent drainage from the primary retroperitoneal nodes may be cephalad to the thoracic duct and supraclavicular nodes or caudally to pelvic or inguinal nodes. Spread to extra-nodal sites may occur because of direct communication of lymphatic channels with the intravascular space (e.g. thoracic duct into subclavian vein) or because the primary tumour breaches the tunica albuginea and invades the vessels of the epididymis or cord.

Staging

The existence of several different staging systems has confused the issue of staging testicular cancers. The 1997 American Joint Committee on Cancer (AJCC) TNM system (Table 4.6) is an internationally agreed consensus.

Table 4.5 WHO Classification of germ cell tumours of the testis[2]

Precursor lesions	ITGCN/CIS
Tumours of one histological type	Seminoma
	Spermatocytic seminoma
	Embryonal carcinoma
	Yolk sac tumour
	Polyembryona
	Trophoblastic tumour
	Pure choriocarcinoma
	Choriocarcinoma with other cell types
	Placental site implantation tumour
	Teratoma
	Mature
	Immature
	Teratoma with malignant areas

Tumours of more than one histological subtype (specify percentage volume of each component)

Table 4.6 AJCC 1997 TNM staging of testicular tumours

TX	Primary tumour cannot be assessed (e.g. no orchidectomy performed)
T0	No evidence of primary tumour (e.g. only scar in testis)
Tis	CIS/ITGCN
T1	Tumour confined to testis/epididymis, no lymphovascular invasion
T2	Tumour confined to testis/epididymis with lymphovascular invasion or tumour through tunica albuginea
T3	Tumour involves cord
T4	Tumour involves scrotum
NX	Regional nodes cannot be assessed
N0	No nodal metastases
N1	Single or multiple involved nodes with no nodal mass >2 cm in diameter
N2	Single or multiple involved nodes with a nodal mass >2 cm but <5 cm in diameter
N3	Lymph node mass >5 cm in diameter
M0	No distant metastases
M1	Non-regional nodal metastases or pulmonary metastases
M2	Non-pulmonary visceral metastases

Serum markers

The existence of serum markers for testicular cancer greatly facilitates treatment. The level of tumour markers is valuable in determining prognosis at diagnosis and during treatment.

- α-Fetoprotein (AFP) is produced normally by yolk sac cells during gestation. It is also produced by yolk sac cells in GCTs and hepatocellular tumours. (AFP levels may also be elevated in other primary malignancies including pancreatic, gastric and bronchogenic carcinomas). AFP has a half life of 5–7 days.
- Human chorionic gonadotrophin (hCG) is produced by syncitiotrophoblast cells of the placenta. hCG is comprised of two subunits (α and β); the β subunit is routinely measured. βhCG levels are elevated in pregnancy and in the presence of various tumours (breast, renal, gastric, hepatobiliary). The half life of βhCG is 24 hr. Elevated levels of βhCG are found in all patients with choriocarcinoma and about 50% of patients with embryonal carcinoma. βhCG is also elevated in the 5% of cases of seminoma that contain syncitiotrophoblast cells.

Overall either AFP or βhCG is elevated in 90% of cases of NSGCT. AFP is elevated in 50–70% and βHCG in 40–60%. AFP and βHCG should be measure prior to orchiectomy. Whilst elevation of these markers postorchiectomy may be spurious, it is generally taken as evidence of metastatic disease. Unfortunately, the converse may not hold true: normalization of markers after treatment for systemic disease may not be indicative of complete response.

- Lactate dehydrogenase (LDH) is a non-specific marker elevated in some patients with seminoma. It is of limited value, but when produced by seminoma the level of LDH can correlate with the overall bulk of the disease.
- PLAP (placental alkaline phosphatase) is elevated in the presence of some seminomas but its poor sensitivity and specificity limits its routine clinical application.

Anatomical considerations in surgery for testicular cancer

The lymphatic drainage of the epididymis is to external iliac nodes. If the primary tumour breaches the tough tunica albuginea, then these nodes may be involved. Further invasion into the scrotum may be associated with inguinal lymphadenopathy.

The autonomic nerves that control emission and ejaculation of semen may be damaged during retroperitoneal lymphadenectomy. Emission (the deposition of semen in the urethra prior to ejaculation) is sympathetically mediated. Ejaculation (the antegrade propulsion of semen) is a complex process mediated by autonomic and somatic nerves. Bladder neck closure is sympathetically mediated, relaxation of the external urethral sphincter is parasympathetically mediated, and contraction of the bulbocavernosus muscle is somatically mediated via the pudendal nerve. The sympathetic outflow from the cord is from cord segments T12 to L3. These nerves gather into the sympathetic chain which runs in the paravertebral space medial to the psoas and dorsal to the great vessels. They coalesce in the superior hypogastric plexus anterior to the aortic bifurcation at L5. From here the right and left hypogastric nerves pass into the pelvic plexuses. The pelvic plexuses are situated on the lateral aspect of the rectum, bladder, prostate, and vesicles, and they provide autonomic innervation to these organs. Damage to the superior hypogastric plexus causes loss of emission and ejaculation.

Surgical management of testicular cancer

The treatment of testicular cancer is multimodal, involving surgery, radiotherapy, and chemotherapy. Which treatments are used, and in what order, depends on the histological type of the tumour, the degree of spread, the level of tumour markers, and the preferences of the treating institution. The reader is directed to general urological texts for more detail on these issues.

Radical inguinal orchiectomy (see Chapter 9 (scrotal surgery)) almost always forms part of the treatment of testicular cancer. If serum markers are elevated prior to orchiectomy, they should be measured on a weekly basis in the post-operative period.

Retroperitoneal lymph node dissection (RPLND)

RPLND is used in the management of testicular cancer in three main settings.

- Prophylactic node dissection in patients prophyly with NSGCT confined to the testis (i.e. with no radiological features of spread to the retroperitoneum and with no involved nodes found during the RPLND). RPLND in this context is called RPLND-I. (This approach is more common in the USA. In Europe, stage 1 NSGCT is more likely to be managed by surveillance, radiotherapy, or chemotherapy).
- Resection of (low-volume) retroperitoneal nodes in NSGCT as part of the initial therapy. RPLND in this context is known as RPLND-II. RPLND-II is performed when low volume disease has been identified on clinical staging or when involved nodes are discovered during RPLND-I (i.e. ~20–30% of cases clinical stage I disease).
- Resection of post-chemotherapy or post-RPLND-I/RPLND-II masses following primary treatment of metastatic NSGCT or metastatic seminoma. RPLND in this context is called RPLND-III.

RPLND-I

When RPLND is performed in this context it is usually a modified RPLND. In a non-modified or standard RPLND, the aim is to excise all the retroperitoneal lymphoid tissue. A modified, template, or nerve-sparing RPLND is less extensive and aims to excise lymphoid tissue most likely to harbour metastatic disease. The templates reflect the known lymphatic drainage of each testis. Modified RPLND aims to spare the autonomic nerves controlling emission and ejaculation by removal of nodal tissue from around the post-ganglionic fibres. In experienced hands preservation of ejaculation has been reported in 100% of patients.[3]

The boundaries of dissection for RPLND-I for right-sided primary tumours are shown in Fig. 4.39. The dissection extends from the right renal hilum along the right ureter to the point where it crosses the right common iliac artery. Dissection then proceeds superiorly along the common iliac and aorta (to the right of the origin of the inferior mesenteric artery) to the left renal artery and back to the right renal hilum. These landmarks define the outline of the dissection. It is important that lymphoid tissue is excised from behind the great vessels (30% of all involved nodes are behind the IVC/aorta); to do this lumbar arteries and veins must be divided.

The boundaries of dissection for RPLND-I for left-sided tumours are shown in Fig. 4.40. Note that the template does not cross the midline (because left to right spread is rare). The dissection begins at the junction of the left renal vein with the IVC and continues inferiorly down the right-hand border of the aorta to the level of the inferior mesenteric artery. The dissection then crosses to the left of the aorta and continues to the point where the left common iliac artery is crossed by the ureter before turning superiorly to follow the medial border of the left ureter back to the left renal vein.

RPLND-II
The surgical margins are more extensive than in RPLND-I. Specifically, the dissection is usually bilateral, and extends below the origin of the inferior mesenteric artery and above the renal arteries.

RPLND-III
RPLND-III involves a complete bilateral RPLND together with resection of any lymph node masses. Occasionally the surgery is very extensive (e.g. going above the renal vessels to the diaphragm or into the mediastinum, or resection of segments of the great vessels and replacement with prosthetic grafts).

Bilateral trans-abdominal RPLND
A trans-abdominal approach using a midline incision is adequate for most cases. A midline incision can be curved in to the ninth or tenth intercostal space if it becomes necessary to enter the chest. A thoraco-abdominal incision at the outset is an alternative approach.

The first part of the surgery aims to achieve adequate exposure of the retroperitoneum. The second part of the operation is the lymph node dissection itself. A non-modified bilateral RPLND is described here but for RPLND-I the templates can me modified as described above.

Exposure of the retroperitoneum
Make a midline incision from the xiphisternum to the pubis. Open the peritoneum. Divide the falciform ligament to allow upward displacement of the liver. Hold the wound open with a self-retaining retractor (e.g. Balfour) placed at each end of the wound. Inspect and palpate the intra-abdominal organs and the retroperitoneum to establish the extent of the disease and to assess resectability. Reflect the greater omentum and the transverse colon superiorly on the chest and protect them with moist packs. Reflect the small bowel to the right side of the abdomen. Incise the posterior peritoneum medial to the inferior mesenteric vein and extend this incision superiorly to the ligament of Treitz and then to the duodenal–jejunal junction to allow cephalad mobilization of the fourth

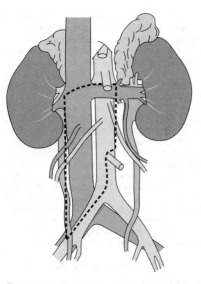

Fig. 4.39 RPLND-I template for right-sided tumours.

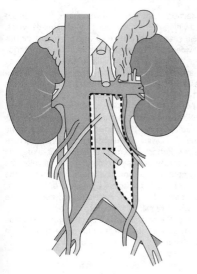

Fig. 4.40 RPLND-I template for left-sided tumours.

part of the duodenum and the head of the pancreas (Fig. 4.41). Extend the incision inferiorly to the caecum and then around the base of the caecum to the right paracolic gutter. Continue up the avascular plane lateral to the right colon to the foramen of Winslow and in doing so mobilize the hepatic flexure. Reflect the small bowel, caecum, and right colon superiorly, place in a bowel bag, and lay on the chest wall. This manoeuvre will require careful division of attachments between the infero-posterior surfaces of the duodenum and pancreas and the supero-anterior surface of the left renal vein (Fig. 4.42). Ensure that the superior mesenteric artery has been identified and that it is not compromised by excessive tension or by injudicious placement of retractors. To achieve adequate exposure of the left renal hilum, develop a plane lateral to the left gonadal vein and medial to the inferior mesenteric vein (Fig. 4.43). Several lymphatic trunks may be encountered here and these should be clipped and divided. It may also be necessary to tie and divide the inferior mesenteric vein. The retroperitoneal space should now be exposed (Fig. 4.44) from the suprahilar areas bilaterally to the bifurcation of the great vessels inferiorly. Identify the renal vessels and ureters and the pancreas to minimize the chance of damaging them subsequently. Place sloops around the ureters and gently retract them laterally; the lateral extent of the dissection is defined by the medial border of the ureters. Be cognisant of some common anatomical variations; there are accessory renal arteries in one in five people and a retro-aortic left renal vein in 2–3%.

Lymph node dissection: the split and role technique (Fig. 4.45)

Begin the lymph node dissection at the left renal vein, lifting off lymphoid tissue and exposing and dividing the left adrenal and left gonadal veins. Beware a short lumbar vein entering the left renal vein posteriorly; if this is present, it should be divided. Work medially and expose the anterior surface of the aorta. Divide the adrenal and gonadal arteries. Continue to the right to the anterior aspect of the IVC at the level of the left renal vein. Lift the tissue of the anterior of the IVC and use scissors to enter a plane right on the vessel surface. Develop this incision inferiorly over the anterior surface of the IVC. Ligate and divide the right gonadal vein. With a split in the lymphoid tissue along the anterior surface of the IVC, roll the leaflets of tissue laterally (right) and medially (left) to clear the anterolateral surfaces of the IVC. Divide any lumbar veins that are encountered during this manoeuvre. Perform a similar anterior split along the surface of the aorta to the bifurcation of the common iliacs. Develop the right and left leaflets of lymphatic tissue on the anterior surface of the aorta and roll them off the surface of the aorta. Ligate and divide lumbar arteries as they are encountered. The great vessels should now be free from the lymphoid tissue which remains attached to the posterior body wall and renal arteries. Dissect the renal arteries from the lymphoid tissue and release the lymphoid mass from its attachments to the psoas fascia and the anterior spinous ligament.

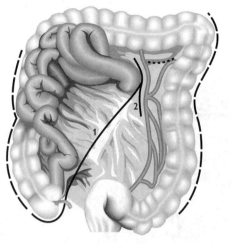

Fig. 4.41 Incision of the posterior parietal peritoneum.

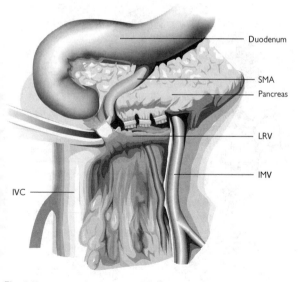

Fig. 4.42 Division of the attachments of the duodenum and pancreas.

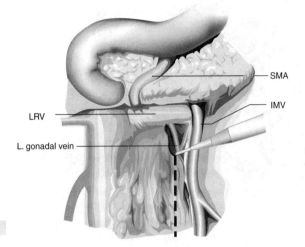

Fig. 4.43 Development of the left leaf of posterior peritoneum.

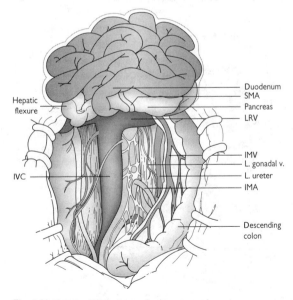

Fig. 4.44 The retroperitoneal space has been exposed.

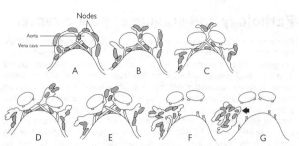

Fig. 4.45 The split and roll technique.

Irrigate and inspect the operative site. Ensure haemo- and lymphostasis. Tack down the posterior peritoneum with 3–0 absorbable sutures to prevent bowel adhering to the great vessels when it is returned to the abdomen. Inspect the mesentery and bowel for signs of vascular damage/compromise.

Nerve sparing

The sympathetic chain runs longitudinally on either side of the spine. On the right, the chain is posterior to the IVC and its post-ganglionic fibres run anterior to the aorta to the hypogastric plexus on the anterior surface of the aorta at the level of the bifurcation. On the left, the chain is lateral and posterior to the lateral aorta and post-ganglionic fibres run obliquely posterolateral to the aorta to reach the hypogastric plexus. Given this anatomy, the post-ganglionic fibres from the right side are not vulnerable to damage during the anterior split manoeuvre on the IVC, but they are vulnerable during the split along the anterior surface of the aorta. During a nerve-preserving procedure, the post-ganglionic sympathetic trunks (especially those from L3 and L4 which are believed to be most valuable in preserving ejaculation) should be identified, dissected free from lymph tissue, and isolated with vessel sloops.

Really useful aside

Use ties rather than clips to control vessels on the surface of the IVC/aorta. Clips are too easily dislodged during subsequent dissection.

References

1 Harland SJ, Cook PA, Fossa SD et al. Intratubular germ cell neoplasia of the contralateral testis in testicular cancer: defining a high risk group. *J Urol* 1998; **160**:1353–7.

2 Mostofi FK, Sesterhenn IA, Sobin LH: Histological typing of testes tumors. In: *World Health Organization: International Histological Typing of Tumors*, 2nd edn. Berlin: Springer-Verlag, 1998.

3 Foster RS, McNulty A, Rubin LR et al. The fertility of patients with clinical stage I testis cancer managed by nerve sparing retroperitoneal lymph node dissection. *J Urol* 1994; **152**:1139–43.

Pathology and staging of penile cancer

Penile cancer is a rare malignancy (0.1–1/100 000 in Europe and the USA, 19/100 000 in South America and Asia): 48% of primary tumours are on the glans, 21% on the prepuce, 9% on both the glans and the prepuce, 6% in the coronal sulcus, and <2% on the shaft. More than 95% of penile carcinomas are squamous cell cancers, 3% are mesenchymal tumours (Kaposi's sarcoma, angiosarcoma), and 1–2% are metastases from other primaries (e.g. renal, prostate). Risk factors for penile cancer include poor hygiene, phimosis, and infection with human papilloma virus (HPV), especially HPV16 and HPV18. There are a number of conditions of the penis including penile horn, Bowenoid papulosis, leukoplakia, lichen sclerosus et atrophicus (LSA) (balanitis xerotica obliterans (BXO)). Erythroplasia of Queryat and Bowen's disease are considered to represent penile intra-epithelial neoplasia (PIN). Penile cancer exhibits a variable growth pattern (classic, verrucous, superficial spreading). Tumours are graded G1 (most differentiated) to G3 (poorly differentiated). The staging of penile cancer is according to the TNM system (Table 4.7).

Table 4.7 Staging of penile cancer

Primary tumour	
Tx	Cannot be assessed
T0	No evidence of primary
Tis	CIS
Ta	Non-invasive verrucous
T1	Invades subepithelial connective tissue
T2	Invades spongiosum or cavernosum
T3	Invades urethra or prostate
T4	Invades other adjacent structures
Nodes	
Nx	Cannot be assessed
N0	No evidence of nodes
N1	Single inguinal node
N2	More than one inguinal node
N3	Deep inguinal or pelvic nodes
Metastases	
Mx	Cannot be assessed
M0	No evidence
M1	Distant metastases

Surgical treatment of penile cancer

Treatment of the primary lesion

Biopsy to confirm the diagnosis

The diagnosis must be confirmed by biopsy. This also allows determination of the tumour grade and depth of invasion. If the prepuce is too tight to allow retraction, circumcision (or a dorsal slit) may be necessary to allow access to a suspicious palpable lesion. Take a wedge biopsy from the edge of the lesion (so that normal tissue is also included in the specimen) with a 15 blade. A piece of tissue 5–10 mm long by a few millimetres wide will usually suffice. Close the incision with a few 4–0 absorbable sutures.

Partial penectomy

After partial penectomy there must be sufficient penile stump for the man to be able to hold and direct the penis to allow him to void standing up. The minimum that should be left to preserve adequate function is usually 3–4 cm. If this length of penis cannot be left, a total penectomy and perineal urethrostomy should be performed (see below). The length of the stump depends on the amount of normal tissue resected proximal to the tumour to achieve negative margins. A 2 cm resection margin has been considered standard practice when resecting the primary lesion. This convention has been challenged recently and 5–10 mm or less may be adequate.[1,2]

Technique

Position the patient supine, prep, and drape, and cover the lesion with a condom or glove sutured to the penile skin proximal to the tumour so that the stump will not be contaminated with tumour cells. Elevate and squeeze the penis to empty it of blood and apply a tourniquet to the base using a Penrose drain secured with an artery forcep. Draw circumferentially with a skin marker around the shaft at a point 2 cm proximal to the lesion. Cut through the skin and divide and ligate the dorsal neurovascular bundle. Cut through the tunica albuginea and corporal bodies from dorsally to ventrally with a knife. Take not to damage the urethra. The ends of the cavernosal arteries are usually obvious in the centre of the corporal bodies. Grasp them with a fine artery forcep and tie with a 3–0 absorbable tie. If you cannot see the arteries, temporary release of the tourniquet will bring them into view. Divide the urethra 1 cm distal to the level of resection of the corporal bodies and spatulate it for a few millimetres on the dorsal and ventral surface. Close the ends of the corpora using 2–0 sutures placed transversely: pick up the lateral edge of one corpus, the middle septum, and the lateral edge of the contralateral corpus with each suture. Release the tourniquet and check for haemostasis. Do not worry about bleeding from the urethral stump; this is usually controlled when fashioning the neo-meatus. Close the skin vertically beginning ventrally. Drape the skin around the urethra and use 4–0 absorbable sutures to stitch the urethra to the penile skin. Take full-thickness bites of the urethra including the mucosa. Dorsal to the urethra, stitch the edges of penile skin together to leave a vertical suture line. Insert a urethral catheter and leave it for a minimum of 10 days.

Alternative technique

Some surgeons prefer to leave a longer ventral skin flap and to fold this up over the stump. Excise an ellipse of skin in the ventral flap for the urethra to protrude through. Close the skin transversely with interrupted sutures on the dorsum of the stump. Place some proximal sutures superficially through the outer (adventitial) surface of the urethra where it emerges through the ventral flap and stitch it to the edges of the skin ellipse. Spatulate the urethra dorsally and ventrally as described above and evert the urethra by taking full-thickness bites through the mucosa and stitching it down to the skin edge.

Total penectomy

Isolate the lesion with a glove or condom as described above. Mark a circumferential incision around the base of the penis with a pen and extend it dorsally and ventrally in the midline over 2 cm in each direction. Make the skin cut and then pull the penis ventrally to tension the dorsal structures. Sharply divide the suspensory ligament. Clip and divide the superficial and deep vessels and tie them with 3–0 ties. Flip the penis dorsally to place the ventral surface on tension. Cut Buck's fascia transversely at the base of the penis and dissect the urethra free from the corporal bodies. Make sure that the urethra is separate from the corporal bodies over a few centimetres (slide a right-angled forceps behind it). Divide the urethra approximately at mid-shaft level (you need enough length to create the perineal urethrostomy (see below). If in doubt about urethral involvement, send a frozen section. Place a stay suture through the urethral stump. Place the divided urethra on gentle traction towards the perineum and sharply dissect the dorsal surface of the urethra from the corporal bodies. Place a heavy artery forceps across the crus of each corpora close to the inferior pubic rami. Divide the corpora and close the ends with interrupted 3–0 sutures. Divide any remaining attachments and remove the specimen. Mark and excise a skin ellipse (about 1 cm long) in the middle of the perineal skin. Tunnel subcutaneously with a curved artery forceps from the perineum through the scrotum until the tip emerges in the penectomy wound. Grasp the end of the urethral stay suture and gently pull the urethra through. Excise any excess urethra and spatulate the urethra dorsally over a few millimetres. Take full-thickness bites of the urethra and suture it to the skin with interrupted 3–0 sutures. Close the scrotal wound transversely.

Penis-preserving treatment (non-surgical)

If the primary tumour is in a low-risk group (pTis, pTaG1–2, pT1G1–2), a penis preserving strategy should be considered. Penis-preserving treatments may be non-surgical or surgical. Non-surgical treatments include laser ablation (Nd:YAG or CO_2), topical 5-FU, cryoablation, external beam radiotherapy, and interstitial brachytherapy. Penile cancer is a rare tumour and few institutions have large numbers of patients. Consequently there are very few comparative studies of these non-surgical treatments in the literature. Overall, non-surgical penis-preserving strategies have a local recurrence rate of 10–20%.

Penis preserving treatment (surgical)

Although partial and total penectomy have been the mainstay of penile cancer surgery for many years, there has been recent advocacy of less mutilating (penis preserving) strategies. These newer techniques are described briefly here.

Glans resurfacing

Watkin[3] has developed this technique for CIS and Ta/T1 disease. They have yet to publish full details of the procedure, but essentially it involves removal of the glans epithelium and subepithelial connective tissue in quadrants to expose the underlying corpus spongiosum. Frozen sections are taken to ensure adequate margins before 'resurfacing' the glans with split skin graft.

Glansectomy and reconstruction

This new technique is used for tumours confined to the glans and prepuce; up to 80% of invasive penile cancers can be treated in this way. Watkin has reported a series of 39 patients, none of whom had recurrent disease at 24 months.[3] A tourniquet is placed around the base of the penis using a Penrose drain wrapped twice around the shaft and secured with artery forceps. Incise the distal shaft skin circumferentially to Buck's fascia. Develop this plane distally, lifting the glans cap from the distal limit of the corpora (Fig. 4.46). Divide the urethra at the undersurface of the glans cap, leaving it a little longer than the corpora. Send frozen sections from the distal urethral margin and from the tunica albuginea at the tips of the corpora. Spatulate the urethra for a few millimetres ventrally. Suture the urethra to the tunica over the corporal heads to create a neo-meatus. Use interrupted 4–0 absorbable sutures and try to evert the urethral mucosa as you do this. Suture the shaft skin to the tunica at a point 2 cm proximal to the end of the corpora. Harvest a split-skin graft (e.g. from the inner thigh using a dermatome or a Humby knife). Drape the graft over the corpora and trim it to size, remembering to preserve an opening for the neo-meatus. Suture the graft to the tunica adjacent to the distal limit of the shaft skin and to the neo-meatus using interrupted 4–0 absorbable sutures. Quilt the graft down on to the corpora using 4–0 silk (Fig. 4.47). Insert a urethral catheter. Dress with paraffin gauze and loose dressing swabs. Keep the patient on bed rest for 5 days before the dressings are taken down.

Distal corporectomy and reconstruction

This technique is used if there is clearly involvement of the distal corpora or if the frozen sections are positive during a glansectomy. The corpora are resected until frozen sections are clear. The urethral meatus is fashioned as described above. The shaft skin is dissected free from the shaft as far proximally as possible to prevent subsequent shortening. Extra apparent penile length can be gained by dividing the suspensory ligaments of the penis. The exposed corporal bodies are covered with a split-skin graft.

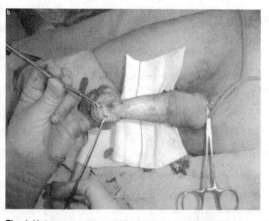

Fig. 4.46 Raising the glans cap. Reproduced with permission from Pietrzak, Corbishley, and Watkin, Organ sparing surgery for invasive penile cancer: early follow-up data. *B J Urol Int*, Blackwell, 2004; **94**:1253–7.

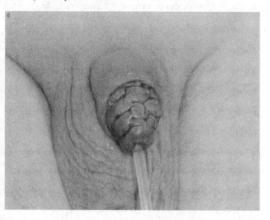

Fig. 4.47 Quilting the skin graft. Reproduced with permission from Pietrzak, Corbishley, and Watkin, Organ sparing surgery for invasive penile cancer: early follow-up data. *B J Urol Int*, Blackwell, 2004; **94**:1253–7.

References

1 Agrawal A, Pai D, Ananthakrishnan N, Smile SR, Ratnakar C. The histological extent of the local spread of carcinoma of the penis and its therapeutic implications. *BJU Int* 2000; **85**:299–301.
2 Hoffman MA, Renshaw AA, Loughlin KR. Squamous cell carcinoma of the penis and microscopic pathologic margins: how much margin is needed for local cure? *Cancer* 1999; **85**:1565–8.
3 Pietrzak P, Corbishley C, Watkin N. Organ-sparing surgery for invasive penile cancer: early follow-up data. *BJU Int* 2004; **94**:1253–7.

Paratesticular tumours

Non-germ cell primary testicular tumours

Non-germ cell tumours of the testis account for 5–10% of testicular neoplasms. This group includes Leydig cell tumours, Sertoli cell tumours, gonadoblastoma, mesenchymal tumours (fibromas, leiomyomas, angiomas), epidermoid tumours, and adenocarcinomas of the rete testis. The initial treatment for all of these tumours is radical inguinal orchidectomy (indeed, it is often only after orchidectomy that the diagnosis is made).

Epididymal tumours

Masses within the epididymis that do not transilluminate or are solid on ultrasound are likely to be epididymal neoplasms. They are usually painless. They occur typically in the second or third decade but can present at any age. Most of these masses are confined to the epididymis but can also involve the tunica albuginea or the cord. Epididymal tumours are nearly always benign adenomas (adenomatoid tumours of the epididymis).[1] Malignant primary epididymal neoplasms are very rare. Surgery for solid epididymal masses should be via an inguinal approach with control of the cord before delivery of the testis. Biopsy and analysis of a frozen section can be used to differentiate benign from malignant epididymal tumours intra-operatively. The former can be excised with preservation of the testis whilst the latter should be managed by orchidectomy.[2]

References

1 Folpe AL, Weiss SW. Paratesticular soft tissue neoplasms. *Semin Diagn Pathol* 2000; **17**:307–18.
2 Goldstein M, Waterhouse K. When to use the Chevassu maneuver during exploration of intrascrotal masses. *J Urol* 1983; **130**:1199–200.

Urethral cancer

Urethral cancer in the male

Pathology

Urethral cancer in the male is rare. Risk factors include urethral stricture disease, sexually transmitted diseases (especially HPV) for SCCs, and urethritis. The majority (80%) of male urethral cancers are SCCs, 15% are TCC, and the remainder are adenocarcinomas or poorly differentiated tumours. The histology depends to an extent on the location of the tumour (Fig. 4.48). Urethral cancers spread directly into adjacent structures or to regional nodes (the anterior urethra drains to inguinal nodes and the posterior urethra to pelvic nodes). Invasion into adjacent structures is more common with posterior urethral tumours than with anterior tumours.

Treatment

Whatever the site of the tumour, surgical excision is the treatment of choice. Superficial tumours of the distal urethra can be managed by transurethral resection. More extensive tumours of the distal urethra should be managed by partial or total penectomy.

Tumours of the bulbomembranous urethra are rarely manageable by transurethral resection or by segmental excision and primary anastamosis; the disease is usually too advanced. In most cases total penectomy and radical cystoprostatectomy (together with pelvic node dissection) is the treatment of choice. The specimen is usually removed *en bloc*.

Isolated primary tumours of the prostatic urethra are rare; most cases of prostatic urethral carcinoma are associated with TCC elsewhere. Differentiation from prostatic adenocarcinoma can be difficult. Isolated superficial tumours of the prostatic urethra may be amenable to trans-urethral resection but most are best managed by cytsoprostatectomy.

Urethrectomy may also be indicated after cystoprostatectomy for TCC of the bladder. This is elective either because the risk of urethral recurrence is high (e.g. patients with involvement of the prostatic urethra or those where the urethral resection margin is positive for TCC or CIS) or because there is evidence of urethral recurrence on surveillance ure-throscopy or urethral washings.

Urethrectomy: surgical technique

When urethrectomy is performed as part of a cystoprostatectomy the procedure is as for cystectomy up to division of the pubo-prostatic ligaments and mobilization of the prostate.

The patient is placed in the lithotomy position. Insert a urethral catheter to the limit of the urethral stump and secure it to the glans. An inverted U-shaped incision (Fig. 4.49) gives excellent access to the urethra, but a midline incision (which can be converted to a Mercedes Benz incision by extending it posterolaterally on either side) is favoured by some surgeons. Divide the skin, subcutaneous tissue, and bulbocavernosus in the midline to expose the corpus spongiosum of the bulbar urethra. Use a ring

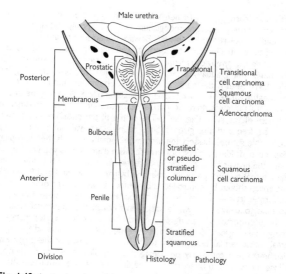

Fig. 4.48 Anatomic regions of the male urethra.

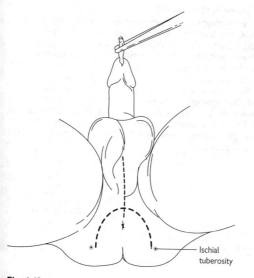

Fig. 4.49 An inverted U-shaped incision.

retractor such as a Turner–Warwick ring or a Lone Star ring retractor. Free the corpus spongiosum circumferentially and sling it with a broad tape or rubber drain tube. Beware the arteries to the bulb which should be controlled and divided (Fig. 4.50). Follow the urethra distally separating the spongiosus from the corpora carvernosa. As you do this the penis will gradually invert until you reach the base of the glans (Fig. 4.51). Return the penis to its normal orientation and circumscribe the meatus with a knife, extending this incision bilaterally along the under surface of the glans. Join the two limbs of this incision just proximal to the base of the glans (Fig. 4.52). The whole of the distal urethra should now be free and the glans should be repaired with interrupted 2–0 absorbable sutures. Dissect the urethra proximally towards the urogenital diaphragm, dividing the bulbocavernosus with diathermy as you go. As you reach the urogenital diaphragm, enlarge the hiatus. Urethral branches from the internal pudendal arteries enter the bulbar urethra at 4 and 8 o'clock and these should be controlled and divided. If the urethrectomy is being performed at the same time as a cystoprostatectomy, it should now be possible to deliver the whole specimen through the abdominal wound. If the urethrectomy is being performed after a previous cystoprostatectomy, take great care when traversing the urogenital diaphragm. Small intestine may be adherent to the superior surface of the urogenital diaphragm and can easily be damaged by injudicious use of diathermy. Close the wound in layers over a tube drain taking care with haemostasis and apply a pressure dressing.

Urethral cancer in the female

Urethral cancer is several times more common in females than in males. Presentation is with bleeding, frequency, discharge, or a palpable mass. Disease is often advanced at presentation and invasion into vagina, vulva, or bladder is not uncommon. As in the male the anterior urethra drains to inguinal nodes and the posterior urethra to pelvic nodes. The more proximal the tumour the more likely it is to be high grade and invasive. SCC is the most common histological type. For small superficial well-differentiated distal tumours it may be possible to achieve control with a distal urethrectomy and spatulation of the remaining urethra to the vaginal wall. For all other tumours cure is usually only achievable with urethrectomy and anterior exenteration together with total or subtotal vaginectomy (📖 p. 239).

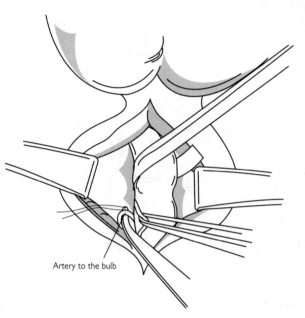

Artery to the bulb

Fig. 4.50 Arteries to the bulb.

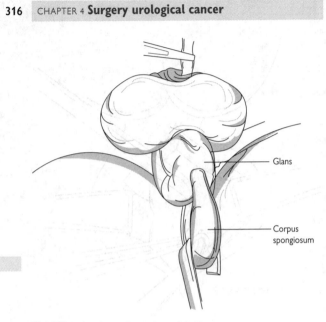

Fig. 4.51 Inverted penis showing base of the glans.

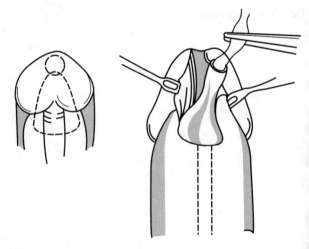

Fig. 4.52 Incision of meatus and glans.

Laparoscopic urological surgery

General principles

Laparoscopy has been a relatively recent development in the treatment of urological pathology.

History

- 1991 First laparoscopic nephrectomy (Clayman, USA).[1]
- 1991 First laparoscopic nephro-ureterectomy (Clayman, USA).[2]
- 1991 First laparoscopic pelvic lymphadenectomy (Schuessler, USA).[3]
- 1992 First laparoscopic cystectomy (Parra, USA).[4]
- 1993 First laparoscopic pyeloplasty (Schuessler, USA).[5]
- 1997 First laparoscopic radical prostatectomy (Schuessler, USA).[6]

Some of these procedures have clear benefits, but some do not, although may prove to with time. A surgeon must recognize his or her limitations with these procedures, and more complex cases may need additional support from more experienced laparoscopic urologists.

- Appropriate patient selection is essential and each case should be treated on its merits, with careful consideration of each patient's expectations.
- Pain, though less, does occur and requires post-operative analgesia and convalescence.
- General anaesthesia is required and patients not suitable (e.g. those with severe cardiopulmonary disease) will not be able to undergo laparoscopy.
- Patients with mild to moderate chronic obstructive pulmonary disease may struggle to compensate for the hypercarbia associated with insufflation, and the insufflation pressures may need to be reduced.[7]
- Laparoscopy is contraindicated in patients with severely dilated bowel from functional or obstructive ileus, uncorrected coagulopathy, untreated infection, or hypovolaemic shock.[8]
- Care needs to be taken in patients who have had previous retro- or transperitoneal surgery. Adhesions are more likely and an open-access approach is recommended. Obese patients can present problems with trocar placement, masked anatomic landmarks, and difficulty acquiring an adequate intra-abdominal pressure, thereby limiting the workspace.
- Informed consent must be obtained with discussion of all complications, ideally quoting the surgeon's own experience.
  Patient preparation is discussed in relation to each procedure.

Basic laparoscopic equipment

Video systems[9]

The laparoscopic image is created by combining a laparoscope with a video system. The video system consists of a video camera, a light cable, a light source, a video processor (often referred to as the camera control unit (CCU)), and a video display (monitor).

Laparoscopes usually have a 0° or 30° lens and are 10 mm in size (range 2.7–12 mm). Larger laparoscopes give a wider field of vision, better optical resolution, and a brighter image. The camera is locked to the eyepiece in its correct position with 0° laparoscopes, whilst with 30° laparoscopes it is loosely attached so that it can rotate. The camera assistant needs to hold the camera in the true upright position whilst rotating the laparoscope to allow a wider and more complete field of vision. This is especially helpful around vascular structures. However, inexperienced camera assistants can easily disorientate the view with 30° laparoscopes, with potentially disastrous effects on correct identification of anatomy.

The camera head contains charge-coupled devices (CCDs) composed of minute photoelectrical elements (pixels) arranged in a rectangular grid, allowing image acquisition. Reflected light from the surgical field is focused on the pixels by the endoscope lens system, producing an electronic response from the pixels which is transmitted by wire to the video processor for conversion to a video signal.

Video cameras contain either one CCD or three CCDs—one-chip and three-chip cameras, respectively. Three-chip cameras provide higher resolution and better colour reproduction. Video processors are usually designed to accept input from either a one-chip or a three-chip camera, but not both; however, there are exceptions.

Video monitors are available in two sizes (13 or 19 inches). Higher resolution images are obtained with the smaller screens. One monitor will suffice with pelvic procedures, whilst two are needed with upper tract surgery to allow clear views to surgeons, assistants, scrub nurses, and the anaesthetist.

Insufflation system

Insufflation is required to achieve satisfactory working space in either the peritoneum or retroperitoneum. Usually CO_2 is used via tubing attached to the initial hasson port or veress needle. Flow is initially at 1 L/min to assess safe entry and can then be increased to high flow (20–40 L/min). Accumulation of CO_2 in the blood can be dangerous in patients with chronic respiratory disease, and helium has been used as an alternative insufflation gas.

Laparoscopic trocars

Numerous disposable and reusable trocars are available in various sizes (2, 5, 10, 12, and 15 mm) (Fig. 5.1). The trocar tip can be bladed or blunt. The larger ports (10, 12, and 15 mm) have a valve or reducer system to allow the passage of smaller instruments without gas leakage. Longer trocars are available for morbidly obese patients.

Hand pieces

A huge range of these exist, both reusable and disposable, and the choice is very individual (Fig. 5.2).

Grasping instruments

These instruments are traumatic or atraumatic, locking or unlocking, single or double action, and come in various sizes (2–12 mm). Reusable instruments are modular, allowing attachment of different tips to different handles with varying shaft lengths.

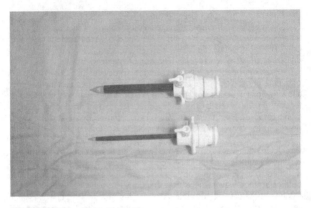

Fig. 5.1 12 mm and 5 mm disposable ports.

Cutting instruments
Straight or curved scissors are available with attachment for electrosurgical leads to deliver monopolar diathermy. Coagulation is set at 30–55 W and cutting at 35 W. The J hook can also be used to dissect through tissues using monpolar diathermy and is very precise around vascular structures. Bipolar devices which will coagulate the tissue, which then needs to be cut with another device, also exist.

Needle holders
There are many of these, and the surgeon needs to try each out and select his or her preference. Numerous devices have also been developed to facilitate both intra- and extracorporeal suturing. These may help the novice laparoscopist, but we believe that freehand intracorporeal suturing allows the greatest flexibility and versatility.

High-energy dissectors
Numerous devices (e.g. Harmonic, LigaSure, hydrodissector, argon beam) have been introduced for laparoscopic tissue cutting and haemostasis. Ultrasonic energy allows tissue cutting and coagulation at lower temperatures (50–100°C), thus reducing scatter and charring. It is potentially financially restrictive. LigaSure seals vessels ≤7 mm in diameter and reduces charring.[10]

The argon beam coagulator is good for haemostasis on superficial bleeding surfaces such as liver, spleen, kidney, and muscle. There is no forward scatter from this device but it can cause a very rapid rise in intra-abdominal pressure. One of the trocars should be continuously vented to avoid this.[11]

(a)

(b)

(c)

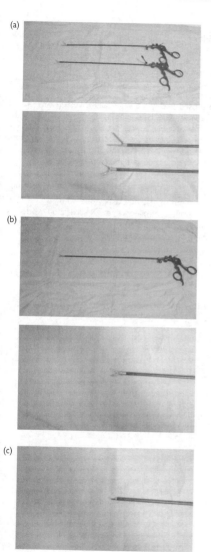

Fig. 5.2 (a) Laparoscopic grasping instruments, (b) Laparoscopic scissors, (c) Laparoscopic J hook.

Clips and staplers

These devices are vital for controlling medium- and large-calibre vessels. The clips are made from titanium or plastic and may or may not interlock. The titanium clips are applied through manual or self-loading applicators and need to be evenly spaced and non-crossing when applied. The interlocking plastic clips allow visualization of complete encirclement of the vessel and are our preferred method (Fig. 5.3).

Endoscopic staples are used mainly for large-calibre vessels such as the renal vein. They are of a linear GIA type applying six rows of staples and cutting between rows 3 and 4. Newer devices can also reticulate and articulate, allowing a greater range of angles for application. Different cartridge sizes (30, 45, and 60 mm) and heights (2, 2.5, and 3 mm) are available. The staples can not be applied over clips and care must be taken here.

Aspiration and irrigation instruments

There are a variety of these devices, both reusable and disposable. The aspirator is a 5- or 10-mm metal or plastic tube with suction controlled via a stopcock or spring-controlled valve. The irrigation works via the same mechanism. The usual irrigant is normal saline or Ringer's solution and may need to be delivered under pressure (Fig. 5.4).

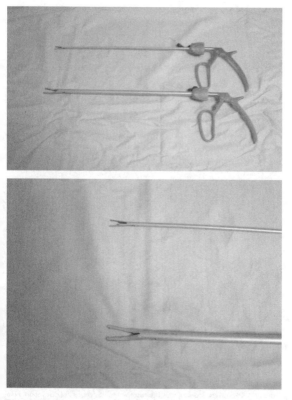

Fig. 5.3 Laparoscopic clip appliers.

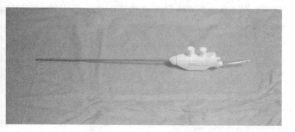

Fig. 5.4 Laparoscopic aspirator.

References

1 Clayman RV, Kavoussi LR, Soper NJ et al. Laparoscopic nephrectomy: initial case report. *J Urol* 1991; **146**:278–82.

2 Clayman RV, Kavoussi LR, Soper NJ et al. Laparoscopic nephroureterectomy:initial case report. *J Laparoendosc Surgery* 1991; **1**:343–9.

3 Scheussler WW, Vancaillie TG, Reich H et al. Transperitoneal endosurgical lymphadenectomy in patients with localized prostate cancer. *J Urol* 1991; **145**:988–91.

4 Parra RO, Andrus CH, Jones JP et al. Laparoscopic cystectomy: initial report on a new treatment for retained bladder. *J Urol* 1992; **148**:1140–4.

5 Schuessler WW, Grune MT, Tecuanhuey LV et al. Laparoscopic dismembered pyeloplasty. *J Urol* 1993; **150**:1795–9.

6 Scheussler WW, Schulam PG, Clayman RV et al. Laparoscopic radical prostatectomy:initial short term experience. *Urology* 1997; **50**:854–7.

7 Monk TG, Weldon BC. Anaesthetic considerations for laparoscopic surgery. *J Endourol* 1992; **6**:89.

8 Capelouto CC, Kavoussi LR. Complications of laparoscopic surgery. *Urology* 1993; **42**:2–12.

9 Bromwich E, Sullivan ME, Keoghane SR. Surgical video systems. *Urol News* 2005; **10**:13–16.

10 Romano F, Caprotti R, Franciosi C et al. The use of LigaSure during paediatric laparoscopic nephrectomy:a preliminary report. *Paediatr Surg Int* 2003; **19**:721–4.

11 Kwon AH, Matsui Y, Inui H et al. Laparoscopic treatment using an argon beam coagulator for nonparasitic liver cysts. *Am J Surg* 2003; **185**:273–7.

Laparoscopic access

Accessing the space to perform the relevant laparoscopic procedure is fundamental to a successful outcome. If this step is not achieved correctly, problems ranging from air leakage and a subsequently inadequate operating space to trocar injuries can lead to a disastrous attempt at laparoscopic surgery and possible early conversion. Both open and closed access techniques have been described for transperitoneal approaches.

Open access (Hasson technique)[1]

This is our preferred approach. Make a 2.5 cm incision at the position of the laparoscope port site. Continue the incision down through the various abdominal wall layers. Place two 0 PDS stay sutures into the rectus fascia, which aids closure at the end of the procedure, particularly in obese patients, and can improve the seal around the port. On reaching the peritoneum, grasp it with a right angle, palpate to check that no bowel has been caught, and open sharply. Introduce a finger into the peritoneal cavity to check correct positioning.

Obtaining an air-tight seal is now critical to prevent insufflation leakage. Insert a Hasson blunt-tip cannula into the peritoneal cavity and secure with the previously placed fascial sutures. Alternatively, a blunt-tip balloon cannula can be used, which allows the abdominal wall to be cinched between an inflated balloon and sponge on the cannula. This provides an excellent seal.

Closed access using a Veress needle[2]

Place a Veress needle percutaneously into the peritoneal cavity, again via the laparoscope port site. The Veress needle is metallic and has a retractable protective blunt tip. The blunt tip retracts when the tip of the Veress needle presses against a tough structure such as the fascia, exposing the sharp edge of the needle. Once the needle passes through the abdominal wall and into the peritoneal cavity, the blunt tip is deployed, protecting the abdominal viscera. The cannula is hollow which allows peritoneal insufflation.

Two distinct sensations of giving way are described during passage of the needle, one at the level of the external oblique/rectus fascia and the second at the transversalis fascia/peritoneum. Once through these layers, the needle is aspirated to rule out blood or bowel contents and correct placement is further confirmed by injecting a small volume of saline and watching the meniscus drop rapidly. A final confirmation is achieved by observing a low intra-abdominal pressure after initiating insufflation at a low flow (1 L/min). Once confirmed, the insufflation rate can be increased to a maximum (40 L/min). When the abdomen is maximally inflated (intra-abdominal pressure 15–20 mmHg) the first trocar is placed, via a generous skin incision (to minimize skin gripping on the trocar).

With pelvic laparoscopic procedures, the bladder needs to be emptied, the patient placed in a Trendelenburg tilt, and the needle directed towards the pelvis to avoid injury to the great vessels.

Once the primary port has been placed the additional trocars are placed under laparoscopic visualization, minimizing inadvertent vascular or visceral injury.

Retroperitoneal access is usually via an open technique.[3] Make the initial incision just below the tip of the 12th rib. Incise the skin, subcutaneous layer, and external oblique fascia with scissors or diathermy. Separate the fibres of the internal oblique and transverses bluntly with Langebeck retractors, revealing the thoracolumbar fascia. Divide the fascia sharply and enter the retroperitoneum. Fat oftens pouts when the fascia is incised and to confirm that the retroperitoneum has been entered a finger is inserted and the psoas palpated posteriorly and the lower pole kidney superiorly.

Numerous devices can now be used to develop the working space. A 22Fr silicone catheter with the middle finger of a surgical glove attached is an inexpensive and, in our view, effective way of dilating the retroperitoneal space.[4] Up to 500–600 mL of saline or air can easily be introduced via a bladder syringe. Although visualization of the dilatation is not possible, we have not found this to be a problem. Alternatives include the PDB balloon dilator. This allows visualization and positioning of the balloon to precisely dilate the space between the posterior abdominal wall and the kidney. The balloon is dilated up to 800 mL incrementally.

Insert a 10 mm blunt tip balloon trocar through the incision to provide a good seal and minimize gas leak. This is even more important in the retroperitoneum, where there is generally a more limited working space.

References

1 Hassan HM. A modified instrument and method for laparoscopy. *Am J Obstet Gynaecol* 1971; **110**:886–7.

2 Florio G, Silvestro C, Polito DS. Periumbilical Veress needle pneumoperitoneum:technique and results. *Chir Ital* 2003; **55**:51–4.

3 Gill IS, Rassweiler JJ. Retroperitoneoscopic renal surgery:our approach. *Urology* 1999; **54**:734–8

4 Gaur DD. Laparoscopic operative retroperitoneoscopy: use of a new device. *J Urol* 1992; **148**:1137–9.

Basic laparoscopic skills

Skills development is a steadily progressive acquisition of surgical dexterity and spatial orientation. It is now necessary for surgeons to be able to practice new procedures repeatedly until judged to be proficient without endangering patients. The complex surgical psychomotor skills needed for laparoscopy are part innate and part learned from extensive and repetitive practice.

Recommendations for acquiring basic laparoscopic skills have involved one of the following.

• Attending basic skills courses followed by live animal courses and then incorporating a mentor into the training when the operation is being performed in patients.
• Undergoing a laparoscopic fellowship.

Aspects of both these approaches have been shown to reduce surgeons' learning curves. However, none have been able to guarantee competency. Tools to assess competency are not yet in place and need to be developed as soon as possible.

A significant additional problem is the lack of an easy laparoscopic urological procedure to allow for repetitive practice. This problem may be overcome by simulation, including bench models, animal simulation, and cadaveric simulation. Developments are awaited here.

Laparoscopic simple nephrectomy

Following the first description of of a laparoscopic nephrectomy by Clayman et al.,[1] numerous centres have reported results for laparoscopic simple nephrectomy over the last 10 years.[2–6] The procedure has been established as safe, with additional improved outcomes of reduced analgesic requirements, improved cosmesis, reduced hospital stay and shorter convalescence at home. Thus this approach is now an accepted technique and is considered by some to be the gold standard of treatment.

The operation has been described via the retroperitoneal route, the transperitoneal route, or hand assisted.[2–6] None of these approaches has been shown to be superior to the others, with the possible exception of reduced operating time for the retroperitoneal or hand-assisted routes. Therefore choice of approach tends to be dictated by the surgeon preference, although previous surgery may contraindicate one route. Ideally, the surgeon should be comfortable with both retroperitoneal or transperitoneal approaches.

Indications
- Poorly functioning or non-functioning kidneys.
- Occasionally due to chronic renal pain.

Absolute contraindications
- Severe chronic obstructive pulmonary disease.
- Active peritonitis.
- Intestinal obstruction.
- Bleeding diathesis.
- Abdominal wall infections.
- Malignant ascites.

The above contraindications apply to all the techniques described subsequently in this chapter.

Relative contraindications
- Previous abdominal/retroperitoneal surgery.
- Large staghorn calculi.
- Organomegaly (transperitoneal).
- Aortic/iliac aneurysms.
- Ascites (transperitoneal).
- Morbid obesity (transperitoneal).
- Severe diaphragmatic hernia (transperitoneal).
- Prior inguinal hernia repair (extraperitoneal).

Immediate pre-operative preparation
- Informed consent. Ideally, this should take the surgeon's results into consideration including access injuries, transfusion rates, and conversion rates.
- Patient's side marked and signed by the surgeon.
- Patient imaging on screen in theatre.
- Prophylactic IV antibiotics: gentamicin 240 mg + cefuroxime 1.5 g at induction plus three post-operative doses of cefuroxime 750 mg.

- Prophylactic heparinization: unfractionated heparin 5000 IU twice daily or fractionated heparin once daily until discharge. There is some controversy with regard to this approach as compression boots may provide a similar level of protection against thrombosis with fewer haemorrhagic events.
- Shave in theatre.
- Catheterize the patient (12–14Ch catheter).

Patient positioning

- Transperitoneal approach: flank (lateral decubitus position) with the affected side upwards. It is not absolutely necessary to break the table, although some prefer a small break to open up the area under the 12th rib. It is vital to pad soft tissues and bony sites carefully to minimize the risk of neuropraxia. Particular attention should be paid to the downside shoulder (axillary roll and posterior back support), and the hip, knee, and ankle (we prefer a pillow between the legs, buttock support posteriorly and gel ankle supports). Body warming devices and compression boots are also recommended. This position is the same for transperitoneal radical nephrectomy.
- Retroperitoneal approach: flank position with table broken so that lumbar support is raised to maximum height. Similar attention to padding as for the transperitoneal approach. Exactly the same position is adopted for retroperitoneal radical nephrectomy or pyeloplasty.

Operative technique

Transperitoneal

We recommend the open technique (Hasson technique) for initial port placement (port 1). A closed technique using a Veress needle has been described, but this carries a 4% complication rate. CO_2 insufflation is delivered at low flow and the laparoscope inserted into the port to check correct positioning. The intra-abdominal contents are inspected to exclude inadvertent injury, especially to the bowel. Insert the three other working ports (ports 2–4) under vision (Fig. 5.5).

Mobilize the colon (ascending on right, descending on left) by incising the line of Toldt and then reflect it medially. Incise a second layer between the bowel mesentery and Gerota's fascia; this allows peeling between these two layers. On the right the duodenum will come into view and is Kocherized medially to reveal the anterior surface of the IVC. Then identify the ureter inferior to the lower pole of the kidney as this allows a safe approach to the renal pedicle by following the ureter and gonadal vein superiorly (remember that the gonadal vein inserts into the IVC on the right and into the renal vein on the left). Traction on the ureter facilitates this dissection. Incise Gerota's fascia over the lower pole and extend superiorly to the upper pole. The kidney can then be dissected out easily with further care around the pedicles. It is not usually necessary to divide the posterior hepatic ligament (on the right) or the splenocolic ligament (on the left) for simple nephrectomy. Dissection of these tissues can be performed with a combination of scissors, heat (uni- or bipolar diathermy, harmonic scalpel, LigaSure), and blunt dissection using the sucker tip or Johann's forceps.

(a)

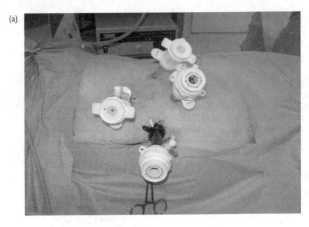

(b)

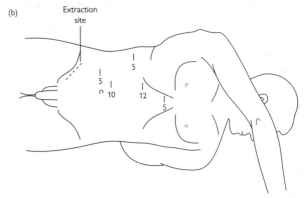

Fig. 5.5 Port positions for transperitoneal laparoscopic (a) left or; (b) right/simple/radical/partial nephrectomy, nephroureterectomy or pyeloplasty.

Clip the gonadal vein and divide it (although this is not absolutely necessary on the right). Similarly, the adrenal vein may require division. Dissect out the renal vein, taking care to watch for lumbar branches posteriorly. The renal artery can usually be seen at this point and should be carefully dissected out, ideally removing all surrounding connective tissues. Clip the artery with Hem-O-Loks, metal clips, or stapling devices (e.g. endo GIA stapler via a 12 mm port). We prefer Hem-O-Lok clips with a minimum of three on the proximal end and then division of the artery. Observe the kidney to see ischaemia indicating a single renal artery, but if it does not beware of further arteries. Clip the vein with large or extra-large Hem-O-Loks or stapling devices. The kidney will normally dissect out easily. Beware of upper or lower pole vessels. Divide the ureter and then remove the kidney in an entrapment sac (e.g. Lapsac, Endocatch, Endopouch). As the kidney may require morcellation, the Lapsac, which is stronger, is preferred for simple nephrectomy. Bring the entrapment device out via one of the 12 mm port sites. Small atrophic kidneys will often come out whole, but larger kidneys will require either morcellation or cutting with scissors and removal piecemeal. Check haemostasis with the CO_2 insufflation at low pressures (5 mmHg).

A tube drain may be required if there is concern regarding infection or breach of kidney tissue, leading to urine spillage. Close the fascia of the larger port sites ($\geq$10 mm) with 0 PDS on a J needle, as risk of hernia exists.

Retroperitoneal

Make an open incision just anterior and inferior to the tip of the 12th rib. Incise the abdominal wall and the transversalis fascia. Fat often appears on incision of the transversalis fascia to reveal the para-renal space. Develop the space with a finger or balloon dilatation. Place the other three ports with digital guidance or under laparoscopic vision as shown (Fig. 5.6). After insufflation it is necessary to identify the psoas muscle. If this is not done, it is easy to incise what appears to be Gerota's fascia superiorly and end up intraperitoneally. Incise Gerota's fascia just above the psoas muscle in a transverse direction. Place a retractor under the upper leaf of Gerota's fascia and dissect through the peri-renal fat. The kidney will become evident and should be dissected out from the peri-renal fat. The ureter can be identified medially in the operative field and divided. With the kidney mobile, place a retractor with its leaves open under the kidney and elevate. This puts the renal pedicle under tension and allows easier dissection of the renal vein(s) and artery(ies). Use blunt dissection and careful heat to strip out the vessels and then clip or staple as discussed above. The adrenal may be separated from the kidney already, but check that this is the case and if not dissect it away from the kidney. Check haemostasis as above, and place the kidney in an entrapment sac and remove in the same way as transperitoneally. Fascial closure is less important as hernias should not be a risk.

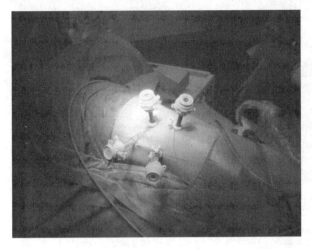

Fig. 5.6 Port positions for retroperitoneal laparoscopic right simple/radical/partial nephrectomy, nephroureterectomy or pyeloplasty.

Outcomes and complications[2–6]

Average operative duration is 3 hr. Major complications are seen in 2% of cases and minor complications in 15%. Hospital stay is 4 days and convalescence 16 weeks. These are generally up to half those seen in open cases and analgesic requirements are significantly less in the laparoscopic cohort. Conversion rates are approximately 5%. No significant differences in outcome are seen between the retroperitoneal and transperitoneal routes. Despite mainly retrospective studies, this is now considered the gold standard approach to simple nephrectomy.

References

1 Clayman RV, Kavoussi LR, Soper NJ et al. Laparoscopic nephrectomy:initial case report. J Urol 1991; **146**:278–82.
2 Kerbl K, Clayman RV, McDougall EM et al. Transperitoneal nephrectomy for benign disease of the kidney: a comparison of laparoscopic and open techniques. Urology 1994; **43**:607–12.
3 Parra RO, Marceliano G, Perez J et al. Comparison between standard flank versus laparoscopic nephrectomy for benign renal disease. J Urol 1995; **153**:1171–4.
4 Doublet JD, Barreto HS, Degremont AC et al. Retroperitoneal nephrectomy:comparison of laparoscopy with open surgery. World J Surg 1996; **20**:713–6.
5 Fornara P, Doehn C, Jocham D. Nonrandomized comparison of open flank versus laparoscopic nephrectomy in 249 patients with benign renal disease. Eur Urol 2001; **40**:24–31.
6 Gill IS, Kavoussi LR, Clayman RV et al. Complications of laparoscopic nephrectomy in 185 patients: a multi-institutional review. J Urol 1995; **154**:479–83.

Laparoscopic renal cyst deroofing/excision

Renal cystic disease is a common finding either incidentally or radiographically (33% of 60-year-olds). Most are asymptomatic, In the small number in whom symptoms (pain, palpable mass) or complications (bleeding, hypertension, infection or collecting system obstruction) develop, laparoscopic surgery either trans- or retroperitoneally is now an option.

Indications
- Symptomatic simple renal cyst(s).
- Peri-pelvic or para-pelvic renal cysts causing obstruction/pain/stone formation.
- Autosomal dominant polycystic kidney disease (ADPKD) with complications.

Immediate pre-operative preparation
- Informed consent. Ideally, this should take the surgeon's results into consideration including access injuries, success rates, and conversion rates.
- Patient's side marked and signed by the surgeon.
- Prophylactic heparinization: unfractionated heparin 5000 IU single dose at induction.
- Shave in theatre.
- Catheterize patient (12–14Ch catheter).

Patient positioning
- Transperitoneal approach: flank (lateral decubitus position) with the affected side upwards. It is not absolutely necessary to break the table, although some prefer a small break in the table to open up the area under the 12th rib. It is vital to pad soft tissues and bony sites carefully to minimize the risk of neuropraxia. Particular attention should be paid to the downside shoulder (axillary roll and posterior back support), and the hip, knee, and ankle (we prefer a pillow between the legs, buttock support posteriorly and gel ankle supports). Body warming devices and compression boots are also recommended. This position is the same for transperitoneal simple/radical nephrectomy.
- Retroperitoneal approach: flank position with table broken so that lumbar support is raised to maximum height. Similar attention to padding as for transperitoneal approach.

Operative technique

Transperitoneal

The initial port placement and dissection are the same as for transperitoneal simple nephrectomy except that an 11 cm port replaces the 12 cm port. Only three ports are required initially (ports 1–3). Mobilize the ascending (right) or descending (left) colon and reflect medially; alternatively, a trans-mesocolon route can be adopted. Anterior, medial, or lateral simple cysts are usually obvious at this stage; posterior simple cysts will require mobilization of the lateral attachments of the kidney. Dissect Gerota's fascia and peri-nephric fat off the cyst. Puncture the cyst with scissors or a hook, drain the fluid and send for cytology. Elevate the cyst wall and treat as follows.

- Complete excision if a good plane of cleavage is possible.
- Near-complete excision if complete excision is not possible; this is often best done with a harmonic scalpel or LigaSure device.
- Marsupializing the cyst wall after deroofing ± tacking peri-nephric fat into the remaining cavity.

With peri-pelvic or para-pelvic cysts, the collecting system and/or renal vessels may be splayed over the cyst(s). A ureteric catheter can aid in identification of the ureter and renal pelvis. Identify the renal vessels and dissect out very carefully. Once the cyst is identified, perform incomplete excision or marsupialization. Aggressive dissection should be avoided as the cyst(s) lie deep into the renal sinus. Peri-pelvic fat can be tacked into the cavity. Inject methylene blue up the ureteric catheter to check for pelvicalyceal leak.

In ADPKD, Gerota's fascia and any peri-nephric fat is dissected off the posterior, polar, lateral, and anterior surfaces. The cysts are obvious: the walls of larger cysts are excised with diathermy scissors or the harmonic scalpel; smaller cysts can simply be punctured with a diathermy hook.

The transperitoneal approach carries the advantages of space and easier approach to anteromedial amd para-pelvic cysts.

Retroperitoneal

The initial port placement is the same as for retroperitoneal laparoscopic simple nephrectomy. The approach to dealing with the various cysts is then the same as for the transperitoneal description. The retroperitoneal approach has the advantages of easier access to posterior placed cysts and prevents spillage of renal cyst fluid into the peritoneal cavity.

Outcomes and complications

- Most simple cysts treated laparoscopically have been large (6–20 cm) and approached via the transperitoneal route. Operating times of 52–147 min have been reported and hospital stays of 2–5 days. Minor complications are low (0–3.5%) and recurrences uncommon (0–5%).[1-5]
- There are limited published data on peri-pelvic cysts.[6,7] Operating times are long (170–338 min) but complications have not been reported and hospital stay is short (2–2.75 days). Recurrence has been seen in 10%.
- In ADPKD long-term (2 years) relief of pain has been reported in 57–60%.[1,8] Stabilization of renal function was seen in 84% at more than 2 years and hypertension improved in three different studies. This has important implications for delaying renal replacement therapy.

Longer-term follow up of laparoscopic treatment of various kinds of renal cysts is needed, but it looks a promising prospect.

References

1 Hemal AK, Gupta NP, Rajeev NP *et al.* Retroperitoneoscopic management of infected cysts in adult polycystic kidney disease. *Urol Int* 1999; **62**:40–3.

2 Consonni P, Nava L, Scattani V *et al.* Percutaneous echo-guided drainage and sclerotherapy of symptomatic renal cysts: critical comparison with laparoscopic treatment. *Arch Ital Urol Androl* 1996; **68**:27–30.

3 Santiago L, Yamaguchi R, Kaswick J *et al.* Laparoscopic management of indeterminate renal cysts. *Urology* 1998; **52**:379–83.

4 Gill IS, Clayman RV, Albala DM. Retroperitoneal and pelvic extraperitoneal laparoscopy: an international perspective. *Urology* 1998; **52**:566–71.

5 Fahlenkamp D, Rassweiler J, Fornara P *et al.* Complications of laparoscopic procedures in urology: experience with 2407 procedures at 4 German centres. *J Urol* 1999; **162**:765–70.

6 Hemal AK, Aron M, Gupta NP *et al.* The role of retroperitoneoscopy in the management of renal and adrenal pathology. *BJU Int* 1999; **83**:929–36.

7 Hoenig DM, McDougall EM, Shalhav AL *et al.* Laparoscopic ablation of peripelvic cysts. *J Urol* 1997; **158**:1345–8.

8 Dunn M, McDougall EM, Clayman RV. Laparoscopic cyst marsupialization for patients with autosomal dominant polycystic kidney disease. *J Endourol* 1999; **13**:A1225.

Laparoscopic dismembered pyeloplasty

Reconstructive techniques followed quickly after ablative procedures in urological laparoscopy. A variety of pyeloplasty techniques were initially described, although the consensus now appears to be that a dismembered pyeloplasty is the technique of choice.[1-8] Controversy still exists with respect to crossing vessels and the need for transposition. Laparoscopic pyeloplasty is now an accepted technique, with some authors stating that it should be the standard of care in expert hands.[6] Both retro- and transperitoneal approaches have been described.

Indications
- Symptomatic PUJ obstruction.
- Urinary tract infections/stones.
- Progressive renal deterioration.
- Causal hypertension (rarely).
- Impaired renal function in a solitary kidney or bilateral disease.

Relative contraindications
- Previous surgery.
- Renal inflammation.

Immediate pre-operative preparation
- Informed consent. Ideally, this should take the surgeon's results into consideration including access injuries, success rates, and conversion rates.
- Patient's side marked and signed by the surgeon.
- Patient imaging on screen in theatre.
- Prophylactic antibiotics: gentamicin 240 mg + cefuroxime 1.5 g at induction plus three post-operative doses of cefuroxime (750 mg).
- Prophylactic heparinization : unfractionated heparin 5000 IU twice daily or fractionated heparin once daily until discharge. There is some controversy with regard to this approach as compression boots may provide a similar level of protection against thrombosis with fewer haemorrhagic events.
- Shave in theatre.
- Initial cystoscopy, retrograde pyelogram, and JJ stent insertion (6Fr, 28 cm) on affected side. We prefer to do this as a final check for stones and stricture as these can alter the surgery required. The stent can be placed antegrade during laparoscopy, but we do it at cystoscopy to be certain of its position and aid in ureteric identification in difficult cases during the laparoscopic pyeloplasty. The stent is 28Fr as this allows the J at the renal end to lie well above the anastomosis and not potentially cantilever on it, leading to urine leak and loosening of sutures.
- Catheterize patient (12–14Ch catheter).

Patient positioning
- Transperitoneal and retroperitoneal approaches: as for laparoscopic simple nephrectomy.

Operative technique

Transperitoneal

The initial port placement and dissection are the same as for transperitoneal simple nephrectomy except that an 11 cm port replaces the 12 cm port. Identify the proximal ureter lying on the psoas with the gonadal vein in close proximity. Dissect out the proximal ureter, being careful not to skeletonise it too much and risk devascularization. Continue the dissection proximally to the pelvi-ureteric junction and the pelvis. If a crossing vessel is seen, it will normally lie on the medial aspect of the pelvi-ureteric junction. We prefer to transpose the pelvis and ureter if a vessel is found. If this is the case, the crossing vessel needs to be dissected out and freed from the peri-pelvic tissue. The pelvis also needs to be mobilized to allow a tension-free anastomosis. Then incise the pelvi-ureteric junction, carefully avoiding cutting the stent. Spatulate the pelvis and ureter at opposing sides. Pelvic reduction can be performed, although this is not absolutely necessary. Transpose the pelvis and ureter and perform an interrupted 4–0 Vicryl anastomosis intracorporeally. We prefer this to a running suture which is potentially more ischaemic; if the suture loosens the whole anastomosis can be affected.

Irrigate the operative site with normal saline and place a tube drain to lie close to but not on the anastomosis and brought out via one of the port sites.

Wound closure is as for simple nephrectomy.

Remove the catheter on day 2 post-operatively. If there is no further significant drainage from the tube drain in the next 24 hr, remove this on day 3, the day of discharge.

The patient returns for a flexible cystoscopy and removal of the JJ stent 4 weeks post-operatively. A MAG3 renogram is performed 3 months post-operatively.

Retroperitoneal

The initial port placement and dissection are the same as for retroperitoneal simple nephrectomy except that an 11 cm port replaces the 12 cm port.

Open Gerota's fascia near the psoas transversely. Retract the cut upper leaflet of Gerota's fascia superiorly using a fan retractor and sweep the peri-nephric fat superiorly and inferiorly to reveal the kidney. Mobilize the lower pole of the kidney and then retract superiorly. Dissect the tissue lying inferior to the lower pole carefully by blunt dissection, revealing the renal pelvis and ureter. The same steps as transperitoneally are followed at this stage with the same post-operative care.

Outcomes and complications[1–8]

Complication rates are low at 5%. Conversion rates are around 5%, although they appear to improve with experience. Success rates based on symptoms and renograms post-operatively are around 94%, comparable to open pyeloplasty results. Mean duration of surgery is 2.5 hr and mean hospital stay is 3 days. These results are all comparable with open pyeloplasty and certainly provide a better cosmetic outcome. Transposition adds 30 min to the procedure, and there appear to be no significant differences related to the approach. However, this is a relatively difficult procedure laparoscopically, and currently the reproducibility of the initial results from centres of excellence is not clear.

References

1 Schuessler WW, Grune MT, Tecuanhuey LV et al. Laparoscopic dismembered pyeloplasty. J Urol 1993; **150**:1795–9.

2 Kavoussi LR, Peters CA. Laparoscopic pyeloplasty. J Urol 1993; **150**:1891–4.

3 Janetschek G, Peschel R, Altarac S et al. Laparoscopic and retroperitoneoscopic repair of ureteropelvic junction obstruction. Urology 1996; **47**:311–16.

4 Moore RG, Averch TD, Schulman PG et al. Laparoscopic pyeloplasty:experience with the initial 30 cases. J Urol 1997; **157**:459–62.

5 Bauer JJ, Bishoff JT, Moore RG et al. Laparoscopic versus open pyeloplasty:assessment of objective and subjective outcome. J Urol 1999; **162**:692–5.

6 Moon DA, El-Shazly MA, Chang CM, Gianduzzo TR, Eden CG. Laparoscopic pyeloplasty: evolution of a new gold standard. Urology 2006; **67**:932–6.

7 Davenport K, Minervini A, Timoney AG, Keeley FX Jr. Our experience with retroperitoneal and transperitoneal laparoscopic pyeloplasty for pelvi-ureteric junction obstruction. Eur Urol 2005; **48**:973–7.

8 Inagaki T, Rha KH, Ong AM, Kavoussi LR, Jarrett TW. Laparoscopic pyeloplasty:current status. BJU Int. 2005; **95**(Suppl 2):102–5.

Laparoscopic ureterolithotomy

Most ureteric stones can be managed by minimally invasive techniques, such as extracorporeal lithotripsy, percutaneous nephrolithotomy, or ureteroscopy. However, occasionally large impacted ureteric stones cannot be treated by any of the above techniques and are managed by laparoscopic removal.

Indications
- Impacted ureteric stones refractory to other minimally invasive treatments.

Immediate pre-operative preparation
- Informed consent. Ideally, this should take the surgeon's results into consideration including access injuries, success rates, and conversion rates.
- Patient's side marked and signed by the surgeon.
- Patient imaging on screen in theatre.
- Prophylactic antibiotics: gentamicin 240 mg + cefuroxime 1.5 g at induction plus three post-operative doses of cefuroxime 750 mg.
- Prophylactic heparinization: unfractionated heparin 5000 IU twice daily or fractionated heparin once daily until discharge. There is some controversy with regard to this approach as compression boots may provide a similar level of protection against thrombosis with fewer haemorrhagic events.
- Shave in theatre.

Patient positioning
- Retroperitoneal approach: flank position as for retroperitoneal pyeloplasty.

Operative technique
Retroperitoneal
Make an open incision just anterior and inferior to the tip of the 12th rib. Incise the abdominal wall and the transversalis fascia. Fat often appears on incision of the transversalis fascia to reveal the para-renal space. Develop the space with a finger or balloon dilatation. Place two other ports with digital guidance or under laparoscopic vision as shown (Fig. 5.6). After insufflation, identify the psoas muscle. Then identify the ureter anterior to the psoas and dissect it out. Further confirmation is achieved by visualizing ureteric peristalsis. The stone can be identified by a bulge in the ureter. It is wise to place a loop proximal to the stone and tent the ureter at this point to prevent proximal migration of the stone. Then incise the ureter with scissors, an endoknife, or diathermy. Remove the stone by leverage, ureteric angling, a grasper, or compression. Place the stone in the cut finger of a disposable glove and retrieve via one of the port sites. Close the ureter with 4–0 Vicryl interrupted sutures. This may not always be possible because of inflammation, and the ureter can be left open over a stent to heal by secondary intention. Place a 20Fr Robinson drain in the retroperitoneal space and close the wounds in standard fashion.

Transperitoneal route

The transperitoneal route can be used, but we do not recommend it because urine leak in the peritoneal cavity is best avoided.

Outcomes and complications[1-3]

This approach has been shown to have significant advantages of reduced analgesia, hospital stay, convalescence, and cosmesis over Open uretero-lithotomy. Operative times are similar to the open approach.

References

1 Goel A, Hemal AK. Upper and mid-ureteric stones: a prospective unrandomized comparison of retroperitoneoscopic and open ureterolithotomy. *BJU Int* 2001; **88**:679–82.
2 Skrepetis K, Doumas K, Siafakas I *et al.* Laparoscopic versus open ureterolithotomy. *Eur Urol* 2001; **40**:32–7.
3 Gaur DD, Trivedi S, Prabhudesal HR *et al.* Laparoscopic ureterolithotomy: technical considerations and long-term follow up. *BJU Int* 2002; **89**:339–43.

Laparoscopic varicocoelectomy

Indications

- Recurrent varicocoele.
- Bilateral varicocoeles.

Immediate pre-operative preparation

- Informed consent: this should include the surgeon's results.
- Patient's side marked and signed by the surgeon.
- Prophylactic heparinization: unfractionated heparin 5000 IU at induction of anaesthesia.
- Cefuroxime 1.5 g IV at induction.
- Shave in theatre.
- Catheterize patient (12–14Ch catheter).

Patient positioning

- Transperitoneal approach: patient is placed in dorsal supine position. The arms are padded and fixed alongside the body using Inco pads. This gives the surgeon more space in which to move. The legs are spread at the hip joints with a 25–30° angle. The TV monitor is placed at the leg end of the patient. The surgeon stands at the contralateral side with the assistant on the ipsilateral side of the varicocoele.
  With unilateral cases transperitoneally, the side to be operated on can be raised laterally. This allows the bowel to fall away from the gonadal vessels and the vas.
- Retroperitoneal approach: the same position is adopted as for the transperitoneal route.

Operative technique

Transperitoneal

Make a transverse subumbilical incision and deepen down to the peritoneum. Open the peritoneum and insert a 10 mm Hasson port with sliding foam seal under direct vision. The pneumoperitoneum is created, the laparoscope is inserted, and two 5 mm ports are placed under laparoscopic vision 2 inches inferior and lateral to the umbilical port. Carefully identify the pelvic anatomy and the vas and gonadal vessels. Traction on the ipsilateral testicle can help if there is doubt about the spermatic cord. Lift the peritoneum overlying the spermatic cord with laparoscopic forceps and incise with scissors or harmonic scalpel, creating a T-shaped peritoneotomy. Visualize the spermatic vessels (it is wise to use a laparoscopic Doppler probe to confirm the position of the spermatic artery(s)). The spermatic veins are then cleared off the cord and can be clipped or coagulated and cut with the harmonic scalpel or LigaSure. The integrity of the spermatic artery should be rechecked. Using clips has the potential advantage of removing them (Wek-Loks) if the Doppler arterial signal is lost. Haemostasis is checked at lower insufflation pressures (5 mmHg). Repeat the procedure on the other side if bilateral treatment is required. On the left side it is sometimes necessary to mobilize the sigmoid colon when adhesions are present to expose the spermatic cord. Care should be taken as there can be sigmoid diverticulae present which extend more laterally than is initially appreciated.

Extraperitoneal

Make a 2 cm incision two finger-breadths above the iliac crest within Petit's (lumbar) triangle. This triangle is bordered by latissimus dorsi, external oblique, and the iliac crest. Open the layers bluntly through the transversus abdominus and into the retroperitoneal space. Place a pre-peritoneal balloon dilator and check the position with a laparoscope. If satisfactory, fill the dilator to 1000 mL and observe displacement of the peritoneum medially. The spermatic vessels lie antero-inferiorly and the psoas muscle posteriorly. Scrotal retraction of the testis will confirm the location of the spermatic cord. Place a Hasson type sheath or Tyco structural balloon trocar and secure with the stay sutures. Two 10 mm ports are then placed under vision into the lower quadrant. Use sharp and blunt dissection to isolate the spermatic vessels. The laparoscopic Doppler can be used to distinguish the artery from the vein. Doubly clip the gonadal veins. Recheck the artery for patency with the Doppler probe. Check haemostasis at 5 mmHg and close the port sites in standard fashion.

Outcomes and complications[1–3]

- Successful outcomes are achieved in 83–98% of cases.
- Operative times vary from 15 to 82 min, and most can be done as day case procedures.
- Minor complications such as haematoma, hydrocoele, and testicular atrophy are rarely reported.

References

1 Miersch WDE, Schoeneich G, Winter P et al. Laparoscopic varicocoelectomy:indication, technique and surgical results. Br J Urol 1995; **76**:636–8.
2 Hirsch IH, Abdel-Meguid TA, Gomella LG. Postsurgical outcomes assessment following varicocoele ligation:laparoscopic versus subinguinal approach. Urology 1998; **51**:810–15.
3 Cohen RC. Laparoscopic varicocoelectomy with preservation of the testicular artery in adolescents. J Paed Surg 2001; **36**:394–6.

Laparoscopic radical nephrectomy

Similar benefits for laparoscopic radical nephrectomy in terms of reduced analgesic requirements, improved cosmesis, reduced hospital stay, and shorter convalescence at home compared with the open approach have also been demonstrated.[1–9] More importantly, 5-year cancer specific survival rates are equivalent to the open nephrectomy results.[10] Consequently, this is now an accepted technique and considered by some to be the gold standard of treatment for pT1-3b renal cell carcinomas (excluding IVC involvement). Retroperitoneal routes, transperitoneal routes, and hand-assisted approaches have been described.[1–9]

Indications
- pT1-3b renal cell carcinomas.

Relative contraindications
- Previous surgery.
- IVC involvement with tumour.
- Large tumours (>10 cm), especially retroperitoneal approach.
- Renal inflammation.

Immediate pre-operative preparation
- Informed consent. Ideally, this should take the surgeon's results into consideration including access injuries, transfusion rates, and conversion rates.
- Patient's side marked and signed by the surgeon.
- Patient imaging on screen in theatre.
- Prophylactic antibiotics: cefuroxime 1.5 g at induction.
- Prophylactic heparinization: unfractionated heparin 5000 IU twice daily or fractionated heparin once daily until discharge and/or compression boots.
- Shave in theatre.
- Catheterize patient (12–14Ch catheter).

Patient positioning
- Transperitoneal and retroperitoneal approaches: as for simple nephrectomy.

Operative technique
Transperitoneal
The same initial approach as the transperitoneal simple nephrectomy is adopted. Gerota's fascia is not incised and needs to be dissected round. On the right, incise the posterior hepatic ligament. On the left, incise the spleno-colic ligament at the splenic flexure and then, with great care, release the splenorenal peritoneal attachments to mobilize the spleen off the upper pole of Gerota.

From the inferior pole with traction on the ureter it is usually very easy to sweep Gerota's fascia off the psoas muscle with blunt dissection all the way to the upper pole, taking care to avoid the renal pedicle medially. The renal pedicle is then dealt with in the same way as for transperitoneal simple nephrectomy. On the left, care needs to be taken with the pancreas which can be draped over the pedicle or be very close to the kidney superior to the pedicle. The crux of this is getting in the right plane at the pedicle or superior to the pedicle, when the pancreas can usually be retracted medially easily.

Adrenalectomy is increasingly controversial and may only be required if a metastasis is seen on the pre-operative CT urogram. If it is to be performed, the adrenal vein needs to be identified. This is usually straightforward on the left, coming off the left renal vein, but on the right it can be high up coming off the inferior vena cava. If the adrenal is to be left *in situ*, the plane between kidney and adrenal needs to be developed which can be done with a combination of heat and blunt dissection ± clips.

Then detach the upper pole kidney. This can be facilitated by gentle retraction on the liver/spleen superiorly and the upper pole inferiorly. Divide the tissues with a combination of heat and blunt dissection. Clip ligate the ureter and divide the remaining tissue (beware the gonadal vein in this tissue, which should be clipped). Divide the remaining tissue attached to the lateral aspect of Gerota's fascia.

Specimen entrapment is via one of the laparoscopic sacs. (Currently, we prefer the Endocatch 15 mm bag). We do not advocate specimen morcellation because of concerns about tumour spillage, inexact pathological assessment, and no clear benefit in recovery). Extract the bagged specimen via a low muscle-splitting incision in the right or left iliac fossa (This usually is 6 or 7 cm long). Check haemostasis prior to extraction as for simple nephrectomy.

Wash all wounds with aqueous Bethidine (might reduce port site metastases) and close the fascia with 0 PDS (two layers for the iliac incision). We do not use tube drainage for radical nephrectomy.

Retroperitoneal

Access as for retroperitoneal simple nephrectomy. The initial dissection involves opening up the plane between Gerota's fascia and the psoas muscle. Gerota's fascia can usually be swept off the psoas easily. The assistant needs to place a closed retractor in this plane and raise the kidney superiorly. This is vital to access the pedicle safely. On the left, the renal artery will be encountered very quickly; on the right, the inferior vena cava may be seen first. Then identify the ureter and gonadal vein inferiorly and expose. Retrograde dissection will reveal the renal vein. Clip or staple the vessels as previously discussed. Mobilize the kidney posteriorly; the superior aspect can also be freed bluntly off the diaphragm. If adrenalectomy is being performed, the adrenal vein should be clipped during renal pedicle dissection. Anterior dissection between Gerota's fascia and the peritoneum is then performed, followed by mobilization of the lower pole.

Clip-ligate and divide the ureter. Retrieve the specimen with an Endocatch bag via a similar iliac incision to the transperitoneal approach. Iodine toilet and 0 PDS fascial closure, as previously discussed, with no tube drainage.

Outcomes and complications[1-10]

- Major complications have been reported in 3–5% of cases and minor complications in 25%.
- The retroperitoneal approach is associated with a shorter operating time (mean 2 hr) compared with the transperitoneal approach (2.5 hr).
- Risks of ileus are probably greater in the transperitoneal approach, but no other significant differences have been shown and surgeon preference should probably dictate the route taken.
- Compared with open radical nephrectomy, there is a 67% reduction in analgesia, 29% reduction in hospital stay, 10% fewer complications, and 73% less convalescence time.
- Five-year oncological efficacy appears comparable to open nephrectomy. No clear increased risk of port site metastases.
- Cost benefits are difficult to assess as they depend on the healthcare system involved, variable cost of disposables, and inability to cost reduced convalescence and community healthcare.

References

1 Barrett PH, Fentie DD, Taranger LA. Laparoscopic radical nephrectomy with morcellation for renal cell carcinoma: Saskatoon experience. *Urology* 1998; **52**:23–8.
2 Ono Y, Kinukawa T, Hattori R. Laparoscopic radical nephrectomy for renal cell carcinoma: a 5 yr experience. *Urology* 1999; **53**:280–6.
3 Dunn MD, Portis AJ, Shalhav AL *et al.* Laparoscopic versus open radical nephrectomy: a 9-year experience. *J Urol* 2000; **164**:1153–9.
4 Janetschek G, al-Zachrani H, Vrabec G *et al.* Laparoscopic tumour nephrectomy. *Urologe* 2002; **A41**:101–6.
5 McDougall E, Clayman RV, Elashry OM. Laparoscopic radical nephrectomy for renal tumour: the Washington University experience. *J Urol* 1996; **155**:1180–5.
6 Abbou CC, Cicco A, Gasman D *et al.* Retroperitoneal laparoscopic versus open radical nephrectomy. *J Urol* 1999; **161**:1776–80.
7 Gill IS, Schweizer D, Hobart MG *et al.* Retroperitoneal laparoscopic radical nephrectomy:the Cleveland experience. *J Urol* 2000; **163**:1665–70.
8 Stifelman MD, Sosa RE, Shichman SJ. Hand-assisted laparoscopy in urology. *Rev Urol* 2001; **3**:63–71.
9 Nelson CP, Wolf JS. Comparison of hand assisted versus standard laparoscopic radical nephrectomy for suspected renal cell carcinoma. *J Urol* 2002; **167**:1989–94.
10 Portis AJ, Yan Y, Landman J *et al.* Long-term follow-up after laparoscopic radical nephrectomy. *J Urol* 2002; **167**:1257–62.

Laparoscopic partial nephrectomy

Several institutions of excellence have described the feasibility of laparoscopic partial nephrectomy.[1–7] Attempts have been made to duplicate the techniques of open nephron-sparing surgery. At present, short-term data are available only from a very small number of centres.[1–7]

Indications
- pT1a renal cell carcinoma.
- Benign conditions damaging polar parts of the kidney (e.g. nephrolithiasis).

Relative contraindications
- Previous surgery.
- Renal inflammation.
- Intra-renal tumours.

Immediate pre-operative preparation
- Informed consent. Ideally, this should take the surgeon's results into consideration including access injuries, transfusion rates, and conversion rates.
- Patient's side marked and signed by the surgeon.
- Patient imaging on screen in theatre.
- Prophylactic antibiotics: cefuroxime 1.5 g at induction.
- Prophylactic heparinization : unfractionated heparin 5000 IU twice daily or fractionated heparin once daily until discharge and/or compression boots.
- Shave in theatre.
- Cystoscopic insertion of open-ended ureteral catheter to renal pelvis of affected kidney.
- Catheterize patient (12–14Ch catheter).

Patient positioning
- Transperitoneal and retroperitoneal approaches: as for simple nephrectomy.

Operative technique
Transperitoneal[8]
The same initial approach as for transperitoneal radical nephrectomy is adopted. Dissect out the ureter and renal hilar vessels initially. It is important to know where the proximal ureter lies to avoid injury. Dissect Gerota's fascia off the renal surface where the tumour is located. For posterior tumours, the layer between Gerota's fascia and the lumbar aponeurosis posterolaterally needs to be incised. This allows medial rotation of the kidney through 180° and direct access to the tumour. Dissect the peri-nephric fat off the kidney adjacent to but not directly over the tumour down to the renal capsule. When there is difficulty identifying the tumour or its margins intra-operative laparoscopic ultrasound can be used.

Techniques to create cold ischaemia have been described: using ice slush in a bag preplaced intra- or retro-peritoneally and entrapping the kidney, or instilling cold Hartmann's solution via an arterial catheter placed pre-operatively in the renal artery via the femoral artery.

These techniques have not been universally adopted and most partial nephrectomies have been performed under warm ischaemia with laparoscopic occlusion of the renal artery ± vein.

Initially a 5 mm margin of healthy tissue is demarcated with diathermy scissors. The artery ± vein is then occluded with a laparoscopic Satinsky, laparoscopic bulldogs, or a tourniquet.

Resect the tumour with cold endoscopic shears or bipolar diathermy. Suture bleeding vessels in the base of the kidney with 4–0 Vicryl. Inject methylene blue via the ureteral catheter to check the integrity of the collecting system. Any breach is oversewn with 4–0 Vicryl. Close the parenchyma over a surgical bolster using 3–0 prolene. Interrupted sutures can be placed through a running suture with LaproTy clips or Wek-Lok clips placed at each capsular throw of the suture. This has the potential to reduce the warm ischaemia time.

Revascularize the kidney and observe haemostasis at low insufflation pressures (5 mmHg). Various haemostatic agents (Floseal, Tisseel) have been placed in the resection plane to control haemostasis. Currently, it is advised to use these as an option in combination with the bolster and suturing, but not in isolation.

Intra-operative surgical margin status can be assessed using laparoscopic visualization of the partial nephrectomy bed. If doubt persists, deep tumour bed biopsies can be sent for frozen section. If concern still remains following these it is safest to proceed with a laparoscopic radical nephrectomy.

Remove the specimen in one of the extraction bags described. Place a drain (20 Robinson or similar) adjacent to the remaining kidney (typically removed when drainage is minimal i.e. <50 mL or urine extravasation is excluded). If the kidney has been mobilized laterally for a posterior tumour it is advisable to suture the intact Gerota's fascia to the lateral peritoneal attachments to prevent kidney rotation and potential torsion or nephroptosis. Close the ports in standard fashion.

Retroperitoneal[9]

Access is as for retroperitoneal radical nephrectomy. The initial dissection involves opening up the plane between Gerota's fascia and the psoas muscle. Gerota's fascia can usually be swept off the psoas easily. The assistant then places a closed retractor in this plane and raises the kidney superiorly. This is vital to access the pedicle safely. On the left, the renal artery will be encountered very quickly; on the right, the inferior vena cava may be seen first. Identify the ureter and gonadal vein inferiorly and expose. Retrograde dissection will then reveal the renal vein. Dissect Gerota's fascia off the renal surface as in the transperitoneal approach and then follow the same technique.

Outcomes and complications[1-7]

- Complications have been reported in up to 21% of cases.
- Urine leak has been seen in up to 10% of cases.
- Mean warm ischaemia time of 27 min and mean operative duration of 2–3.2 hr.
- Mean blood loss of 120–708 mL (using different techniques to control bleeding).
- Mean hospital stay of 2–5.8 days.
- Risks of ileus are probably greater in the transperitoneal group, and duration of operation is longer.
- The position of the tumour should probably dictate the approach, with polar or posterolateral masses easier from a retroperitoneal approach and anterior and medial tumors best suited to a transperitoneal approach.[9]
- Three-year oncological efficacy appears comparable to open partial nephrectomy.[10] No clear increased risk of port site metastases.

This procedure is technically very difficult laparoscopically. Cancer data are immature at present, and it is not clear whether the results from a few centres of excellence can easily be transferred to other centres.

References

1 Janetschek G, Jeschke K, Peschel R et al. Laparoscopic surgery for stage T1 renal cell carcinoma: radical nephrectomy and wedge resection. Eur Urol 2000; **38**:131–8.

2 Harmon WJ, Kavoussi LR, Bishoff JT. Laparoscopic nephron-sparing surgery for solid renal masses using the ultrasonic shears. Urology 2000; **56**:754–9.

3 Rassweiler JJ, Abbou C, Janetschek G et al. Laparoscopic partial nephrectomy. The European experience. Urol Clin North Am 2000; **27**:721–36.

4 Guillonneau B, Bermudez H, Gholami S et al. Laparoscopic partial nephrectomy for renal tumour:single centre experience comparing clamping and no clamping techniques of the renal vasculature. J Urol 2003; **169**:483–6.

5 Kim FJ, Rha KH, Fernandez F et al. Laparoscopic radical versus partial nephrectomy: assessment of complications. J Urol 2003; **170**:408–11.

6 Simon SD, Ferrigni RG, Novicki DE et al. Mayo clinic Scottsdale experience with laparoscopic nephron sparing surgery for renal tumours. J Urol 2003; **169**:2059–62.

7 Gill IS, Matin SF, Desai MM et al. Comparative analysis of laparoscopic versus open partial nephrectomy for renal tumours in 200 patients. J Urol 2003; **170**:64–8.

8 Gill IS, Desai MM, Kaouk JH et al. Laparoscopic partial nephrectomy for renal tumour: duplicating open surgical techniques. J Urol 2002; **167**:469–75.

9 Ng CS, Gill IS, Ramani AP et al. Transperitoneal versus retroperitoneal laparoscopic partial nephrectomy:patient selection and perioperative outcomes. J Urol 2005; **174**:846–9.

10 Moinzadeh A, Gill IS, Finelli A et al. Laparoscopic partial nephrectomy: 3 year follow-up. J Urol 2006; **175**:459–62.

Laparoscopic nephro-ureterectomy

The standard treatment for upper urinary tract transitional cell carcinoma is open nephro-ureterectomy. Endoscopic treatment of small superficial tumours and segmental ureteric resection are alternative options in selected cases. The incision(s) used with the open approach are associated with significant morbidity. Numerous centres of excellence have reported their experience with transperitoneal,[1–10] retroperitoneal laparoscopic,[8, 11–14] and hand-assisted nephro-ureterectomy.[15–21]

Indications
- Upper tract transitional cell carcinoma.
- Poorly functioning/non-functioning kidneys secondary to reflux with ongoing pain or urinary infections.

Relative contraindications
- Previous surgery.
- Renal inflammation.

Immediate pre-operative preparation
- As for laparoscopic radical nephrectomy.

Patient positioning
- Transperitoneal and retroperitoneal approaches: as for simple nephrectomy.

Operative technique
Controversy still exists about the need to perform a radical rather than a simple nephrectomy for the nephrectomy part of this procedure. The nephrectomy part of the procedure follows exactly the same steps as for simple or radical nephrectomy (transperitoneal or retroperitoneal). We advise early clipping of the ureter distal to the tumour to minimize tumour seeding into the more distal urinary tract prior to nephrectomy. Dissect the ureter distally to the bladder. There are usually ureteric arterial branches which require clipping proximally.

The management of the distal ureter is controversial. Numerous techniques, including open surgery, the 'pluck' procedure, extravesical stapling, and ureteric intussusception, have been described.

Open surgery
This is reliable and advised in distal ureteric tumours and previous pelvic radiotherapy. It can compromise the contralateral ureter and occasionally there is inadequate total distal resection. We recommend this technique as the extraction of the kidney can be performed through an iliac fossa incision, and the distal ureteric resection can then be carried out through the same incision, usually without difficulty. The patient does not have to be repositioned.

Pluck procedure

Dissect the ureteric orifice and intramural ureter endoscopically using a loop or Collins knife.[22,23] This can be done before or after the laparoscopic nephrectomy. The latter may decrease the risk of tumour seeding. Two variations on the standard pluck procedure have been described.

- Balloon occlusion involves initial placement of a ureteric catheter endoscopically prior to the dissection of the ureter.[16] Once the ureter is free endoscopically the catheter is replaced with a balloon catheter (7Fr) with the balloon inflated distal to the tumour. The ureter is then plucked laparoscopically after the nephrectomy.
- Transvesical ligation involves placing two transvesical needlescopic instruments suprapubically into the bladder under endoscopic vision.[24] The intravesical ureter is dissected out and freed, and then an Endoloop is passed down one of the needlescopic tracts and cinched down, occluding the ureter. The patient is then repositioned for the laparoscopic part of the operation.

Extravesical stapling

The distal ureter at the bladder is stapled during the laparoscopic technique. One centre recommends cystoscopy and resection of the intramural ureter until the staples are seen.[17]

Intussusception

The laparoscopic nephrectomy is performed first with clipping or tying of the proximal ureter and then sectioning the ureter distal to the clip/tie.[13] Dissect out the upper portion of the distal ureter. Place a Chevassu catheter cystoscopically into the relevant ureter, and place a further tie/clip around the ureter and catheter below the catheter bulb. The catheter is then pulled out under cystoscopic vision, invaginating the ureter. Resect the intramural ureter and extract cystoscopically. It is not possible to perform this technique in the 10% of cases requiring open conversion.[13] Other complications have been described in 10% of cases: catheter breakage, failure to progress with the ureter, anchorage of the pelvic ureter, and urethral stricture.

Outcomes and complications[1–20]

- The usual laparoscopic benefits of reduced morbidity, hospital stay, and convalescence have been demonstrated.
- Operative time is 2.6–7.3 hr.
- Complications were reported in up to 48% of cases, and conversion in up to 18%. Most importantly, cancer efficacy data have revealed bladder recurrence in up to 48%, local recurrence in up to 15%, and distant metastases in 5–18%. However, these data are immature with maximum follow-up at 3 years.

Clearly the cancer efficacy data need to mature before we can consider the laparoscopic approach to be a standard of care and how the distal ureter is best managed. There does not appear to be any significant difference between the transperitoneal, retroperitoneal, or hand-assissted approach in these outcome parameters.

References

1 Kerbl K, Clayman R, McDougall E et al. Laparoscopic nephroureterectomy:evaluation of first clinical series. Eur Urol 1993; **23**:431–6.

2 McDougall EM, Clayman RV, Elashry O. Laparoscopic nephroureterectomy for upper tract transitional cell cancer:the Washington University experience. J Urol 1995; **154**:975–9.

3 Keeley FX, Jr, Tolley DA. Laparoscopic nephroureterectomy:making management of upper tract transitional cell carcinoma entirely minimally invasive. J Endourol 1998; **12**:139–41.

4 Shalhav AL, Dunn MD, Portis AJ et al. Laparoscopic nephroureterectomy for upper tract transitional cell cancer: the Washington University experience. J Urol 2000; **163**:1100–4.

5 McNeill SA, Tolley DA. Laparoscopic nephroureterectomy for upper tract transitional cell cancer. Arch Esp Urol 2002; **55**:595–601.

6 Jarret TW, Chan DY, Cadeddu JA et al. Laparoscopic nephroureterectomy for the treatment of transitional cell carcinoma of the upper urinary tract. Urology 2001; **58**:448–53.

7 El Fattouh HA, Rassweiler JJ, Schulze M et al. Laparoscopic radical nephroureterectomy:results of a international multicentre study. Eur Urol 2002; **42**:447–52.

8 Gill IS, Sung GT, Hobart MG et al. Laparoscopic radical nephroureterectomy for upper tract transitional cell carcinoma: the Cleveland clinic experience. J Urol 2000; **164**:1513–22.

9 Klinger HC, Lodde M, Pycha A et al. Modified laparoscopic nephroureterectomy for treatment of upper urinary tract transitional cell cancer is not associated with an increased risk of tumour recurrence. Eur Urol 2003; **44**:442–7.

10 Valdivia JG, Sanchez JM, Regojo O et al. Nefroureterectomia laparoscopica en tumores de urotelia alto. Arch Esp Urol 2004; **57**:319–24.

11 Salomon L, Hoznek A, Cicco A et al. Retroperitoneoscopic nephroureterectomy for renal pelvic tumours with a single iliac incision. J Urol 1999; **161**:541–4.

12 Goel A, Hemal AK, Gupta NP. Retroperitoneal radical nephrectomy and nephroureterectomy and comparison with open surgery. World J Urol 2002; **20**:219–23.

13 Matsui Y, Ohara H, Ichioka K et al. Retroperitoneoscopy-assisted total nephroureterectomy for upper urinary tract transitional cell carcinoma. Urology 2002; **60**:1010–15.

14 Yoshino Y, Ono Y, Hattori R et al. Retroperitoneoscopic nephroureterectomy for transitional cell carcinoma of the renal pelvis and ureter: Nagoya experience. Urology 2003; **61**:533–8.

15 Stifelman MD, Sosa RE, Andrade A et al. Hand-assisted laparoscopic nephroureterectomy for treatment of transitional cell carcinoma of the upper urinary tract. Urology 2000; **56**:741–7.

16 Chen J, Chueh SC, Hsu WT et al. Modified approach of hand-assisted laparoscopic nephroureterectomy for treatment of transitional cell carcinoma of the upper urinary tract. Urology 2001; **58**:741–7.

17 Seifman BD, Montie JE, Wolf JS Jr. Prospective comparison between hand-assisted laparoscopic and open surgical nephroureterectomy for urothelial cell carcinoma. Urology 2001; **57**:133–7.

18 Landman J, Lev RY, Bhayani S et al. Comparison of hand assisted and standard laparoscopic radical nephroureterectomy for the management of localised transitional cell carcinoma. J Urol 2002; **167**:2387–91.

19 Uozomi J, Fujiyama C, Meiri H et al. Hand-assisted retroperitoneoscopic nephroureterectomy for upper urinary tract urothelial tumours. J Endourol 2002; **16**:743–7.

20 Chueh SC, Chen J, Hsu WT et al. Hand assisted laparoscopic bilateral nephroureterectomy in 1 session without repositioning patients is facilitated by alternating inflation cuffs. J Urol 2002; **167**:44–7.

21 Kawauchi A, Fujito A, Ukimura O et al. Hand-assisted retroperitoneoscopic nephroureterectomy:comparison with the open procedure. J Urol 2003; **169**:890–4.

22 Abercrombie GF, Eardley I, Payne SR et al. Modified nephroureterectomy: long-term follow up with particular reference to subsequent bladder tumours. Br J Urol 1988; **61**:198–200.

23 Palou J, Caparros J, Orsola A et al. Transurethral resection of the intramural ureter as the first step of nephroureterectomy. J Urol 1995; **154**:43–4.

24 Gill IS, Soble JJ, Miller SD et al. A novel technique for management of the en bloc bladder cuff and distal ureter during laparoscopic nephroureterectomy. J Urol 1999; **161**:430–4.

Laparoscopic pelvic lymph node dissection

This technique is primarily used for accurate staging of prostate cancer. Estimates of lymph node metastases can be made using Partin's tables, although 2–30% of patients with presumed localized disease are found to have lymph node metastases.[1,2] Despite developments in imaging (MRI, CT, ultrasonography, and pelvic scintigraphy), the sensitivity and specificity are too low, and currently laparoscopic pelvic lymph node dissection allows more accurate staging in high-risk prostate cancer compared with MRI or CT.

Indications

- Intermediate to high-risk prostate cancer groups prior to radiotherapy (based on Partin's tables).
- Significantly enlarged pelvic lymph nodes (>8 mm) on imaging in men with known prostate cancer seeking radical treatment.
- Prior to salvage therapy for biopsy-proven recurrent prostate cancer.

Relative contraindications

- Previous pelvic surgery.
- Previous pelvic radiotherapy.
- Pelvic inflammation.

Immediate pre-operative preparation

- Informed consent. Ideally, this should take the surgeon's results into consideration, including access injuries, transfusion rates, and conversion rates.
- Prophylactic heparinization: unfractionated heparin 5000 IU twice daily or fractionated heparin once daily until discharge and/or compression boots.
- Shave in theatre.
- Catheterize patient (12–14Ch catheter).

Patient positioning

Patient is placed in dorsal supine position. The arms are padded and fixed alongside the body using Inco pads. This gives the surgeon more space in which to move. The legs are spread at the hip joints with a 25–30° angle. The TV monitor is placed at the leg end of the patient. The surgeon stands at the contralateral side with the assistant on the ipsilateral side of the lymph node dissection.

Operative technique

Both transperitoneal and extraperitoneal routes have been described. Three ports in a V-shaped configuration (see Fig. 5.7) are sufficient. Two 10–12 mm ports are required for the laparoscope together with a clipping device and retrieval bag. An umbilical port is used for the laparoscope. The two lateral ports are placed about 2 inches inferior and lateral to the umbilicus towards McBurney's point. An additional 5 mm port can be

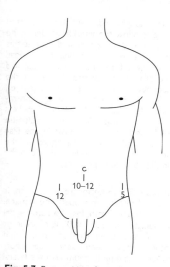

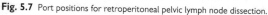

Fig. 5.7 Port positions for retroperitoneal pelvic lymph node dissection.

placed midway between umbilicus and symphysis pubis if tissue retraction is a problem. We advocate an initial open cut-down, as with all laparoscopic procedures, although a Veress needle approach has been used.

Transperitoneal

Place the initial port (10–12 mm) after open cut-down intraperitoneally. The other ports are placed under vision with insufflation (12–15 mmHg). The patient is then placed in a 15–25° Trendelenburg position. Lateral rotation may be helpful to raise the side of the intended lymph node dissection.

Identify the pulsating external iliac artery first. The sigmoid or caecum may be overlying on the left or right, respectively. Mobilize these organs if necessary. Visualize the external iliac vein and artery (vein posterior to artery) and vas deferens. The umbilical ligament lies medial to the vessels. Incise the posterior peritoneal leaf with scissors between the umbilical ligament and external iliac artery extending from the vas deferens cephalad to bifurcation of the common iliac artery cephalad (beware the ureter). Then develop the plane between the medial border of the external iliac vein and the the connective/lymphatic tissue of the obturator packet. This may require initial cutting with scissors. Small vessels and lymphatic channels are often encountered and require bipolar coagulation or clipping. The pubic bone becomes visible laterally, and this plane can be developed easily with blunt dissection. A circumflex vein draining into the external iliac vein is often present here and should be clipped. The plane will lead onto the pubic bone caudally where the node of Cloquet is situated and needs to be taken as part of the package. We advocate clipping all vessels/ lymphatics running into the node to minimize lymphocoele development.

The lymph node packet now has some mobility and needs to be retracted laterally and medially by the assistant to allow the inferior border to be developed. Identify the obturator nerve with its artery and vein at this stage. The nerve is a glistening white structure running cephalad to caudal. Dissect the lymph node packet bluntly off the nerve using cephalad retraction. The packet can now be seen at its superior border at the common iliac bifurcation and the connective tissue needs to be thinned down here using clips as required. Repeat the procedure on the contra-lateral side with the surgeon changing sides. Place the lymph node packets in separate Lapsacs or Endocatch 10 mm bags. Drop the insufflation pressures to 5 mmHg for a careful check for haemostasis in the iliac regions. Desufflate the operating space and retrieve the nodes via the 10–12 mm port. Toilet the port sites with aqueous iodine and close the sheaths with 0 PDS on a J needle in the 10–12 mm port sites.

Extraperitoneal

Make a vertical infra-umbilical incision. The anterior rectus sheath is incised and a finger can then be placed into the retroperitoneal space. Place two stay sutures (0 PDS) in the anterior sheath. Insert a commercial or home-made balloon trocar and insufflate with 500–1000 mL of saline or air. Place a Hasson type sheath or Tyco structural balloon trocar and secure with the stay sutures. The other ports are then placed under vision. Care needs to be taken to avoid traversing the peritoneum with the lateral ports as this will insufflate the peritoneal cavity and collapse the extraperitoneal space. Small peritoneal tears can be closed by suturing or clips.

The posterior peritoneal membrane and colon are not relevant with this approach, and the dissection can start straight on the iliac vessels. The vas deferens is not usually seen either. The procedure is otherwise the same as the transperitoneal approach. At closure the stay sutures are tied to close the anterior rectus sheath, but the other port sites do not strictly require sheath closure as there is no hernia risk.

Outcomes and complications

Studies suggest the usual benefits of laparoscopy in terms of analgesic use, hospital stay, and convalescence.[3–6] The number of lymph nodes removed is higher, although not significantly so, in open dissection. Current series show complication rates of 5.5–12%.[7,8] Complication rates appear to decrease markedly with experience. Earlier studies show rates of 15–33%,[3,5,9,10] which drop significantly after the first 50 cases.[11] The most common complications are lymphocoele, vascular injury, bowel injury, ureteric injury, and lymphoedema. Lymphocoeles appear to be more common in the laparoscopic approach,[12] although there may be some association with prophylactic anticoagulation, extent of dissection,[13] and morbid obesity.[14] The extraperitoneal route shortens the operating time, but appears to have a higher complication rate in terms of conversion and lymphocoeles.[15,16] Some of these results came from earlier studies and are probably not representative of today. One port site recurrence has been reported.[17]

There is controversy about the extent of pelvic lymph node dissection for staging and potentially treating prostate cancer presently. Some authors advocate an extended dissection to include external iliac nodes, hypogastric nodes, and presacral nodes.[18] The rationale for this is that some studies suggest that, in those men with lymph node metastases, up to half are outside the obturator region.[18] Furthermore, they may only be present in other regions (e.g. internal iliac chain). Some groups have also suggested a survival advantage with this extended dissection.[19,20] The complication rates (36%) are significantly higher with an extended dissection though this may decrease with experience.[21] Clearly, a more detailed mapping technique for pathological nodes is needed either to limit the degree of lymph node dissection required for accurate staging or even possibly to avoid the need for it at all. Randomized controlled studies are also required to clarify what benefits, if any, an extended dissection provides in terms of both staging and cancer-specific survival.

References

1 Partin AW, Kattan MW, Subong EN et al. Combination of prostate-specific antigen, clinical stage, and Gleason score to predict pathological stage of localised prostate cancer: a multi-institutional study. *JAMA* 1997; **277**:1445–51.

2 Stamey TA, McNeal JE, Yemoto CM et al. Biological determinants of progression in men with prostate cancer. *JAMA* 1999; **281**:395–400.

3 Winfield HN, Donovan JF, See WA et al. Laparoscopic pelvic lymph node dissection for genitourinary malignancies: indications, techniques and results. *J Endourol* 1992; **6**:103–11.

4 Parra RO, Andrus C, Boullier J. Staging laparoscopic pelvic lymph node dissection: comparison of results with open pelvic lymphadenectomy. *J Urol* 1992; **147**:875–8.

5 Kerbl K, Clayman RV, Petros JA et al. Staging pelvic lymphadenectomy for prostate cancer: a comparison of laparoscopic and open techniques. *J Urol* 1993; **150**:396–8.

6 Herrell DS, Trachtenberg J, Theodorescu D. Staging pelvic lymphadenectomy for localised carcinoma of the prostate: a comparison of 3 surgical techniques. *J Urol* 1997; **157**:1337–9.

7 Vallancien G, Cathelineau X, Baumert H et al. Complications of transperitoneal laparoscopic surgery in urology: review of 1311 procedures at a single centre. *J Urol* 2002; **168**:23–6.

8 Soulie M, Salomon L, Seguin P et al. Multi-institutional study of complications in 1085 laparoscopic urological procedures. *Urology* 2001; **58**:899–903.

9 Scheussler WW, Pharand D, Vancaille TG. Laparoscopic standard pelvic lymph node dissection for carcinoma of the prostate: is it accurate?. *J Urol* 1993; **150**:898–901.

10 Kavoussi LR, Sosa E, Chandoke P et al. Complications of pelvic lymph node dissection. *J Urol* 1993; **149**:322–5.

11 Lang GS, Ruckle HC, Hadley HR et al. One hundred consecutive laparoscopic pelvic lymph node dissections:comparing complications of the first 50 cases to the second 50 cases. *Urology* 1994; **44**:221–5.

12 Solberg A, Angelsen A, Bergan U et al. Frequency of lymphocoeles after open and laparoscopic pelvic lymph node dissection in patients with prostate cancer. *Scand J Urol Nephrol* 2003; **28**:218–21.

13 Stone NN, Stock RG. Laparoscopic pelvic lymph node dissection in the staging of prostate cancer. *Mt Sinai J Med* 1999; **66**:26–30.

14 Mendoza D, Newman RC, Albala D et al. Laparoscopic complications in markedly obese urologic patients (a multi-institutional review). *Urology* 1996; **48**:562–7.

15 Persson BE, Haggman M. Minimally invasive techniques for prostate cancer pelvic lymph node dissection:a randomised trial of trans- and extraperitoneal methods. *J Urol* 1996; **155**:658A.

16 Raboy A, Adler H, Albert P. Extraperitoneal endoscopic pelvic lymph node dissection:a review of 125 patients. *J Urol* 1997; **158**:2202–5.

17 Bangma CH, Kirkels WJ, Chadha S et al. Cutaneous metastasis following laparoscopic pelvic lympadenectomy for prostatic carcinoma. *J Urol* 1995; **153**:1635–6.

18 Bader P, Burkhard FC, Markwalder R et al. Is a limited lymph node dissection an adequate staging procedure for prostate cancer? *J Urol* 2002; **168**:514–18.

19 Bader P, Burkhard FC, Markwalder R et al. Disease progression and survival of patients with positive lymph nodes after radical prostatectomy. Is there a chance of cure? *J Urol* 2003; **169**:849–54.

20 Han M, Partin AW, Pound CR et al. Long-term biochemical disease-free and cancer-specific survival following anatomic radical retropubic prostatectomy: the 15-year Johns Hopkins experience. *Urol Clin North Am* 2001; **28**:555–65.

21 Stone NN, Stock RG, Unger P. Laparoscopic pelvic lymph node dissection for prostate cancer: comparison of the extended and modified techniques. *J Urol* 1997; **158**:1891–4.

Laparoscopic radical prostatectomy

The first description of this procedure in 1992 was followed by reports of the first nine cases from the same group.[1] They concluded that the technique did not provide any advantages over the open approach because of procedural difficulties resulting in very long operating times. However further reports from centres of excellence in France suggested that transperitoneal approach was feasible and safe.[2,3] With experience, variations in approach and surgical refinements were reported such that it is now considered an established technique.[4–12]

Indications
- Organ-confined prostate cancer.

Relative contraindications
- Previous pelvic surgery.
- Previous pelvic radiotherapy.
- Pelvic inflammation.

Immediate pre-operative preparation
- Informed consent. Ideally, this should take the surgeon's results into consideration including access injuries, transfusion rates, positive margin rates, incidence of incontinence and erectile dysfunction, and conversion rates.
- Prophylactic heparinization : unfractionated heparin 5000 IU twice daily or fractionated heparin once daily until discharge and/or compression boots.
- Prophylactic antibiotics: cefuroxime 1.5 g IV single dose at induction of anaesthesia.
- Shave in theatre.
- Catheterize patient (12–14Ch catheter).

Patient positioning
Patient is placed in dorsal supine position with exaggerated Trendelenburg tilt. The arms are padded and fixed alongside the body using Inco pads. The straight legs are abducted and extended at the hip joints with 15° angle (this minimizes the risk of lower limb ischaemia). The patient is secured to the operating table with surgical tape. The TV monitor is placed at the leg end of the patient. The surgeon stands at the patient's left side with the assistant(s) on the right side.

Operative technique
Both transperitoneal[2–5,8–10] and extraperitoneal[6,11,12] routes have been described. Five ports in various configurations have been used. Two 10–12 mm ports are required for the laparoscope and a clipping device and retrieval bag. Use an umbilical port for the laparoscope. The other ports are placed as shown in Fig. 5.8a, b. We advocate an initial open cut-down for the umbilical port, although a Veress needle approach has been used.

Transperitoneal

This approach was described by the pioneering group in Montsouris.[2,10] Seven critical steps have been identified:

- Incision of the posterior vesical peritoneum with dissection of the vas deferens and seminal vesicles, finishing by opening the Denonvilliers fascia.
- Dissection of the space of Retzius with incision of the intrapelvic fascia and selective suture ligation of Santorini's plexus.
- Identification of the bladder neck and seminal vesicle dissection.
- Dissection of the lateral surfaces of the prostate in the intrafascial plane in order to preserve the neurovascular bundles (when indicated).
- Selective dissection of the urethra.
- Extraction of the prostate using a laparoscopic bag.
- The vesico-urethral anastomosis is performed with interrupted or running Vicryl sutures.

Place a urethral Foley catheter and leave a drain in the surgical space.

Extraperitoneal

Make a vertical infra-umbilical incision. Incise the anterior rectus sheath and place a finger into the retroperitoneal space. Place two stay sutures (0 PDS) in the anterior sheath. Insert a commercial or home-made balloon trocar inserted and insufflate with 500–1000 mL of saline or air to dissect a pre-peritoneal workspace. Place a Hasson type sheath or Tyco structural balloon trocar. The foam collar of the Tyco device is cinched onto the skin to create an air-tight seal and secured with the stay sutures. Place the secondary ports (Fig. 5.8) under vision. Care needs to be taken to avoid traversing the peritoneum with the lateral ports as this will insufflate the peritoneal cavity and collapse the extraperitoneal space. Small peritoneal tears can be closed by suturing or clips.

Remove the fat overlying the prostate, incise the endopelvic fascia, and divide the puboprostatic ligaments. Ligate the dorsal vein complex twice using 0 polygalactin suture on a 35 mm half-circle needle. Incise the anterior bladder neck at the vesico-prostatic junction. This junction can be recognized by the point at which the fat is adherent, where a triangle of detrusor muscle fibres is seen, and where the Foley catheter balloon stops when pulled inferiorly.

At this point exchange the Foley catheter for a 18/22Fr urethral sound, which is used to raise the prostate anteriorly. Posterior counter-traction of the anterior bladder neck with the suction cannula facilitates dissection of the posterior bladder neck, and this area is deepened through the anterior layer of the Denonvilliers fascia until the vasa and seminal vesicles are reached. These structures are then dissected out. Bladder neck preservation is attempted when possible. Neurovascular bundle preservation is attempted in potent patients aged ≤70 years with PSA <10 mcg/L and Gleason sum ≤7 if pre-operative biopsies failed to demonstrate perineural invasion and tissue consistency was normal during dissection. If induration is present, the ipsilateral neurovascular bundle is excised. Use titanium clips during dissection of the lateral pedicles and neurovascular bundle to eliminate the risk of thermal injury. If nerve-sparing is not required, the prostatic pedicles can be taken down with a wider margin using thermal devices such as harmonic scalpels (Ethicon, Tyco) or LigaSure (Tyco).

(a)

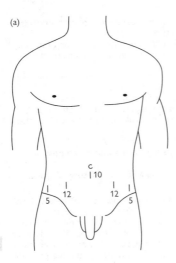

(b)

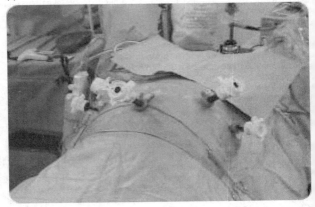

Fig. 5.8 Port positions for retroperitoneal laparoscopic radical prostatectomy.

Divide the dorsal vein complex using scissors and bipolar diathermy sparingly where required. The urethra is divided using scissors. The rectum can come very close to the prostatic apex and it is here that an injury is most likely to occur. Great care is needed at this point and it is often wise to take the tissue down at the apex from different angles with continual reference to the rectal wall. A disposable sigmoidoscope in the rectum can help if this is difficult. Once the prostate is detached, place it in a 10 mm organ retrieval bag. Reconstruct the bladder neck using a posterior racket handle technique with interrupted sutures if there is any disparity between the calibre of the bladder neck and the urethral stump.

Fashion the urethra-vesical anastomosis using interrupted 3-0 polysorb sutures upto a maximum of six. Place the sutures with a 16Fr silicone catheter *in situ*. Alternatively, a continuous anastomosis can be performed using two sutures tied at the posterior midline and run to the anterior border where they are also tied. Fill the bladder with 120 mL saline via the urethral catheter to check anastomosis integrity.

Insert a 20Fr drain through the right iliac fossa 10 mm port before the prostate is removed via the umbilical port site, which may need to be enlarged. Close the wounds in a standard fashion.

Outcomes and complications[3–12]

The major intra-operative complications associated with laparoscopic radical prostatectomy are rectal injury (1.4–2.5%) and haemorrhage (1.2–5%). Rectal injury occurs mainly during apical dissection, and bleeding comes from the dorsal vein complex. Other post-operative complications include thromboemboli (0.1–0.3%), urine leak/urinoma (3–13.6%), recto-urethral fistulae (0.7–0.9%), vesico-cutaneous fistula (0.1–0.2%), ileus (1–3.2%), epigastric vessel injury (≤0.5%), intestinal injury (≤0.1%), anastomotic stricture (≤0.1–0.3%), ureteric injury (≤0.2%), lymphocoele (0.2–0.8%), and urinary retention (0.2–3.5%).

Incontinence and erectile dysfunction rates have suffered from the usual difficulties in assessment. Continence rates have been reported to be >84% and erectile function rates ≥64% for bilateral nerve-sparing and ≥43% in unilateral nerve-sparing.

There appear to be no clear data supporting one route (transperitoneal versus extraperitoneal) over the other.[13] The quality of the surgery depends on the surgeon's experience and standardization of the approach. The extraperitoneal approach may be slightly faster with easier management of minor complications, such as haematoma or urine leak. The extraperitoneal approach can be difficult if there has been a previous hernia mesh repair; the working space is smaller and tension on the vesico-urethral anastomosis can be greater.

Oncological outcomes remain immature. Three-year data have been presented which show comparable outcomes to open radical prostatectomy.[14,15] Positive margin rates are similar in transperitoneal (15%) and extraperitoneal (21%) approaches.[13] Evidence that positive margin rates decrease with surgeon experience is also emerging.[16] Mature cancer data are eagerly awaited.

A steep learning curve is encountered with laparoscopic radical prostatectomy, with many of the major complications occurring in the first 30–50 cases. Optimized training programs are needed to transfer these techniques and minimize the morbidity to our patients.[17]

References

1 Scheussler WW, Schulam PG, Clayman RV et al. Laparoscopic radical prostatectomy: initial short term experience. *Urology* 1997; **50**:854–7.

2 Guillonneau B, Cathelineau X, Barret E et al. Laparoscopic radical prostatectomy: technique and early oncological assessment of 40 operations. *Eur Urol* 1999; **36**:14–20.

3 Abbou CC, Salomon L, Hoznek A et al. Laparoscopic radical prostatectomy:preliminary results. *Urology* 2000; **55**:630–4.

4 Turk I, Deger S, Winkelmann B et al. Laparoscopic radical prostatectomy: technical aspects and experience with 125 cases. *Eur Urol* 2001; **40**:46–52.

5 Rassweiler J, Sentker L, Seemann O et al. Laparoscopic radical prostatectomy with the Heilbronn technique:an analysis of the first 180 cases. *J Urol* 2001; **166**:2101–8.

6 Bollens R, Vanden Bossche M, Roumeguere T et al. Extraperitoneal laparoscopic radical prostatectomy: results after 50 cases. *Eur Urol* 2001; **40**:65–9.

7 Hoznek A, Salomon L, Olsson LE et al. Laparoscopic radical prostatectomy: the Creteil experience. *Eur Urol* 2001; **40**:38–45.

8 Gill IS, Zippe CD. Laparoscopic radical prostatectomy: technique. *Urol Clin North Am* 2001; **28**:423–36.

9 Eden CG, Cahill D, Vass JA et al. Laparoscopic radical prostatectomy: the initial UK series. *BJU Int* 2002; **90**:876–82.

10 Guillonneau B, Cathelineau X, Doublet JD et al. Laparoscopic radical prostatectomy assessment after 550 procedures. *Crit Rev Oncol Haematol* 2002; **43**:123–33.

11 Stolzenburg JU, Do M, Rabenalt R et al. Endoscopic extraperitoneal radical prostatectomy: initial experience after 70 procedures. *J Urol* 2003; **169**:2066–71.

12 Dubernard P, Benchetrit S, Chaffange P et al. Retrograde extraperitoneal laparoscopic prostatectomy (REIP): simplified technique (based on a series of 143 cases). *Prog Urol* 2003; **13**:163–74.

13 Cathelineau X, Cahill D, Widmer H et al. Transperitoneal or extraperitoneal approach for laparoscopic radical prostatectomy:a false debate over a real challenge. *J Urol* 2004; **171**:714–16.

14 Rassweiler J, Schulze M, Teber D et al. Laparoscopic radical prostatectomy with the Heilbronn technique: oncological results in the first 500 patients. *J Urol.* 2005; **173**:761–4.

15 Guillonneau B, el-Fettouh H, Baumert H, Cathelineau X, Doublet JD, Fromont G, Vallancien G. Laparoscopic radical prostatectomy: oncological evaluation after 1000 cases at Montsouris Institute. *J Urol.* 2003; **169**:1261–6.

16 Katz R, Salomon L, Hoznek A et al. Positive surgical margins in laparoscopic radical prostatectomy: the impact of apical dissection, bladder neck remodeling and nerve preservation. *J Urol* 2003; **169**:2049–52.

17 Frede T, Erdogru T, Zukosky D et al. Comparison of training modalities for performing laparoscopic radical prostatectomy: experience with 1000 patients. *J Urol* 2005; **174**:673–8.

Laparoscopic radical cystectomy

Indications
- Organ-confined bladder cancer.
- pT1 G3 disease with multiple recurrences or not responding to intravesical therapy and carcinoma *in situ* not responding to intravesical BCG.

Relative contraindications
- Previous pelvic surgery.
- Previous pelvic radiotherapy.
- Pelvic inflammation.

Immediate pre-operative preparation
- Informed consent. Ideally, this should take the surgeon's results into consideration including access injuries, transfusion rates, positive margin rates, and conversion rates.
- Prophylactic heparinization: unfractionated heparin 5000 IU twice daily or fractionated heparin once daily until discharge and/or compression boots.
- Prophylactic antibiotics: cefuroxime 1.5 g IV and metronidazole 500 mg IV single dose at induction of anaesthesia.
- Shave in theatre.
- Catheterize patient (14–16Ch catheter).

Patient positioning[1]
The patient is positioned in Lloyd-Davies stirrups with the hips straight and the knees bent at 90°. The legs are dressed in anti-embolism stockings and covered with calf compressors. The Velcro of the stirrups is secured using Elastoplast tape, making sure the calves are not compressed. A disposable sigmoidoscope is placed in the rectum and secured with tape. The table is raised into severe Trendelenburg. We do not use any form of shoulder strap to avoid even the slightest risk of brachial plexus injury. All the extremities are checked and padded and a Bear Hugger warming system is placed over the upper half of the patient. The patient is secured to the operating table with surgical tape. The TV monitor is placed at the leg end of the patient. The surgeon stands at the patients left side with the assistant(s) on the right side. Finally, a trestle is placed on the patients left and some padding or foam is placed on the side of the table to protect the surgeon's right leg from the edge of the table.

Operative technique[1]
Use a four-port transperitoneal approach (Fig. 5.9). Establish a pneumoperitoneum by open cut-down and place the first port just *above* the umbilicus. Place the second port two finger-breadths inferiorly and three finger-breadths left laterally to the first port. It is essential to monitor these port placements carefully to avoid damage to the deep inferior epigastric artery. The third port is placed two finger-breadths inferior and two finger-breadths lateral to the second port. These two ports should be

placed soas to allow free cranial movement of the instruments within them. Place the fourth port at McBurney's point on the insufflated abdomen and make the incision at a slight angle to fit in with the appendix incision which it will become (Fig. 5.9). The steps are then as follows.

- **Step 1** Free all adhesions and mobilize the sigmoid colon along the white line of Toldt as high as the lower pole of the kidney. Identify the left ureter in the retroperitoneum as it crosses the bifurcating iliac vessel. Incise the posterior vesical peritoneum over the common iliac arteries, and free the left ureter with a generous surrounding of tissue down to the bladder where it is clipped and cut and the distal end is sent for frozen section. It is easy to strip the ureter of vessels laparoscopically as the view magnifies the peri-ureteric tissue risking ischaemic strictures. Mobilize the caecum and the right ureter, the latter with a generous margin of tissue down to the bladder where it is clipped and cut.

- **Step 2** Open the peritoneum between the two ureteric stumps, joining a line between the vasa, as it recesses between the posterior bladder wall and anterior rectal wall. If this incision is too high it is difficult to dissect the peritoneum from the bladder, and if it is too low, the rectum is too close to the line of dissection. Dissect the vasa deferentia and seminal vesicles out but maintain en bloc with the specimen. Retract the vasa and seminal vesicles superiorly, revealing Denonvilliers fascia which is incised horizontally to expose the prerectal fat. The plane in Denonvilliers fascia contains a little fat and this indicates the correct level for dissection. To facilitate this dissection, the disposable sigmoidoscope can be moved gently to define the rectum clearly. Continue this dissection as far inferiorly and posteriorly to the prostate as is feasibly possible, taking great care to avoid the rectum. If you go too wide you will ruin any chance of nerve-sparing. The vesical and prostatic vascular pedicles are revealed laterally.

- **Step 3** Once the dissection posterior to the prostate has been developed as far as possible, attention is given to developing the bladder pedicles. Open the peritoneum along the external iliac artery up to the internal inguinal ring, usually starting on the right-hand side. Dissect the peritoneum off the external iliac vein and develop a plane medial to the vein heading towards the lateral pelvic wall. Take care to identify the obturator nerve and to leave the obturator lymph nodes in place. If the nodes are dissected at this stage, they tend to obscure the view of the lateral pedicle at a later stage. Open the space of Retzius and gently continue dissection down to the endopelvic fascia. The tissue medial to the space now opened is retracted medially and the bladder pedicle can be transected using the linear stapler (which is very expensive) or a harmonic technology. Care is taken when approaching the inferior aspect of the pedicle to avoid the rectum. The same procedure is followed on the left hand side, again taking care to avoid the rectum or any diverticulae which may be close to the operating field.

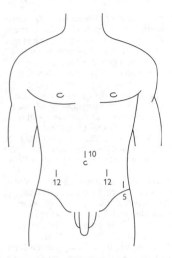

Fig. 5.9 Port positions for retroperitoneal laparoscopic radical cystectomy.

- **Step 4** Attention now moves to the dissection of the anterior bladder wall from the rectus sheath and muscle. Run 200 mL of 2% formal saline into the bladder at this point. This fills the bladder and helps to make it 'hang' dependently from the anterior abdominal wall. The surgeon can use diathermy or ultrasonic technology to free the anterior bladder wall. Incise the peritoneum from the apex of the urachus laterally and inferiorly to the deep inguinal ring. Care is taken to follow the lateral umbilical ligament closely as the inferior epigastric artery lies very close by and a little laterally, and can cause very troublesome bleeding if injured. The entire urachus can be included in this dissection because the camera port is *above* the umbilicus.
- **Step 5** The dissection proceeds under the symphysis pubis and now the bladder can be drained. The superficial dorsal vein can be treated by ultrasonic techniques or diathermy. It must be well secured. Define the endopelvic fascia clearly and incise quite laterally to avoid damaging the dorsal venous complex. Tease the pelvic floor muscles off the prostate lateral aspects using a laparoscopic cotton-tip dissector. Gently incise and free the puboprostatic ligaments so that the prostate is freed and the dorsal vein complex (DVC) is mobilized for capturing in a suture. A 35 mm half circle needle and 0 polygalactin suture are introduced into the abdomen, and the suture is passed behind the DVC from right to left swinging the prostate left to right to clear the field of vision. A good tip is to align the needle under the symphysis and to straighten it a little. The needle pass is directly right to left and *not* 'looping' around the DVC. The suture is pulled through, tied securely, and cut.

- **Step 6** Incise the tissue just proximal to the DVC using diathermy or harmonics to the level of the urethra. It should be noted that this tissue is thicker than is usually appreciated. Care must also be taken to incise perpendicularly here and not to undermine the DVC under the pubic arch. Once the urethra is opened, the catheter is withdrawn and a Weck clip applied to the proximal urethra to prevent any spillage from the bladder. After the posterior urethra is freed from the rectum with a right-angle dissector, it is incised carefully and traction can be applied to free any last tags holding it to the rectum. There are usually two small bands of posterolateral tissue from the prostate and these often include the neurovascular bundles. They can be freed or mobilized and spared if necessary.

- **Step 7** Place the free bladder into a 15 cm catch bag. Introduce this bag via the 12 mm port site on the right of the patient without enlarging the incision. Simply remove the port, extend the tip of the bag about 1 cm to act as an obturator, and guide the bag gently into the abdomen. Open the bag. Lift the bladder and place it inside the bag. Draw the mouth of the bag through the port site, rinse, and tie with 2–0 Vicryl suture to ensure that it is impermeable.

- **Step 8** Lower the pressure of the pneumo-peritoneum to about 5 mmH$_2$O. Check the pelvis thoroughly and secure meticulous haemostasis.

- **Step 9** Perform the lymph node dissection on the right side first and then on the left. The collection of lymph nodes from each side is bagged separately and the strings marked to differentiate the sides. A further haemostatic check is made at this stage.

- **Step 10** Transfer the left ureter to the right side once the lymph node dissection is completed. Snare the left ureter in an Endo-loop tie or fashion a secure slip knot by hand on a 2–0 Vicryl suture cut to a length of 15 cm. Grasp the tip of the tie firmly in an Endo-catch ratcheted grasper. The left lateral edge of the peritoneum on the sigmoid meso-colon is identified at the level of the iliac vessels and the grasper is passed just beneath it. Elevate the sigmoid colon and transfer to the left side. Identify the lateral edge of the peritoneum of the right meso-colon just below the iliac vessels and pass the grasper gently under the meso-colon over the sacral promontory until it exits under the peritoneum on the right-hand side. Firmly grasp the tie and withdraw the grasper with the jaws held slightly open to create a passage for the ureter. Pull the tie through so that it draws the ureter from left to right. Finally, grasp both ureters in the Endo-catch on the right side and place a last grasper on the terminal ileum. The graspers ensure that the ureters and the ileum are easily available once the appendix incision is opened.

- We advocate performing ileal conduits, continent diversions, or neobladders extracorporeally via a small extension of the appendix or via a subumbilical incision (for neobladders) at this stage, as there does not appear to be any clear advantage to doing them laparoscopically. These procedures are described in 📖 Chapter 2. Close the port sites in a routine fashion.

Outcomes and complications[2-9]

- The usual laparoscopic advantages of less pain and earlier mobilization have not yet been shown, mainly because of the small numbers and lack of data at present.
- Peri-operative complications have been reported in 15–17% of laparoscopic radical cystectomies, with a 3–4% re-operation rate. These include mortality (due to disseminated intravascular coagulation), fistulae (Mainz pouch, cutaneous and vaginal), urinary leaks, urinary infections and sepsis, bleeding, ileus, ureteral stenosis, urinary retention, GI bleed, and deep vein thrombosis.
- Oncological outcomes also remain immature. The issue of extended lymph node dissection is also uncertain in terms of the average number of lymph nodes removed laparoscopically.
- A steep learning curve is encountered with laparoscopic radical cystectomy. As with laparoscopic radical prostatectomy, optimized training programmes will be needed if we are to transfer these techniques and minimize the morbidity to our patients.

Currently, there are too many unanswered questions with regard to outcomes in laparoscopic radical cystectomy. Therefore this procedure should be considered developmental and probably be reserved for centres of excellence with experienced laparoscopists.

References

1 Rimington P. Personal communication, 2006.
2 Denewer A, Kotb S, Hussein O et al. Laparoscopic assisted cystectomy and lymphadenectomy for bladder cancer: initial experience. World J Surg 1999; 23:608–11.
3 Gill IS, Kaouk JH, Meraney AM et al. Laparoscopic radical cystectomy and continent orthotopic ileal neobladder performed completely intracorporeally: the initial experience. J Urol 2002; 168:13–18.
4 Goharderakhshan RZ, Kawachi MH, Ramin SA et al. Analysis of complications associated with laparoscopic radical cystectomy. J Urol 2003; 169:339 (abstr DP5).
5 Van Velthoven R, Peltier A, Bar SM et al. Laparoscopic radical cystectomy: pilot study on feasibility. J Endourol 2003; 17:A80.
6 Huang J, Xu KW, Yao YS et al. Laparoscopic radical cystectomy with orthotopic ileal neobladder: report of 33 cases. Chin Med J (Engl) 2005; 118:27–33.
7 Cathelineau X, Arroyo C, Rozet F et al. Laparoscopic assisted radical cystectomy: the Montsouris experience after 84 cases. Eur Urol 2005; 47:780–4.
8 Gerullis H, Kuemmel C, Popken G. Laparoscopic cystectomy with extracorporeal-assisted urinary diversion: experience with 34 patients. Eur Urol 2007; 51:193–8.
9 Castillo OA, Abreu SC, Mariano MB et al. Complications in laparoscopic radical cystectomy: the South American experience with 59 cases. Int Braz J Urol 2006; 32:300–5.

Robotic urological surgery

Telerobotic surgery involves placing a computer between the patient and the surgeon. The surgeon's hand movements are digitized to improve dexterity. The system also has three-dimensional visualization and is intuitive for the surgeon. The Da Vinci Surgical Robotic System (Intuitive Surgical, CA, USA) represents the major technical advance in robotics. It is a master–slave telemanipulation system consisting of a remote console where the operating surgeon (master) controls the robotic surgical arms (slave) via a telerobotic videoscopic link. The surgeon controls the robotic arms with master handles which are located in virtual three-dimensional space below the visual display. Foot controls are used to activate electrocautery, repositioning the master handles and focusing. The master handles also control endoscope selection and the motion-scaling ratio, as well as filtering tremor in the surgeon's hands and arms.

The robotic arm cart holds three or four robotic arms on a central tower. One arm holds the videoscope, whilst the others are used to attach instrument adaptors connected to robotic instrumentation through the trocars. Stereoscopic vision is provided via a 0° or 30° three-dimensional endoscope.

The robotic instruments have both an elbow and a wrist joint, allowing seven degrees of freedom and two degrees of axial rotation mimicking natural motions of open surgery.

Radical prostatectomy is the operation which has been taken up by enthusiastic robotic surgeons. The technique has tended to follow the steps of laparoscopic radical prostatectomy. A small number of centres worldwide have reported their results which appear comparable to laparoscopic series.[1–4]

Robotic surgeons argue that the three-dimensional Da Vinci system is more accurate than the two-dimensional system, seven degrees of freedom are better than four, and lack of tremor is better than the presence of tremor. However, currently none of these have been shown to translate into significantly improved outcomes over standard laparoscopy. The Da Vinci system is also prohibitively expensive, and critical evaluation of this machine is required to clarify its role in urological surgery.

References

1 Menon M, Shrivastava A, Tewari A. Laparoscopic radical prostatectomy: conventional and robotic. *Urology* 2005; **66**(Suppl 5):101–4.

2 Ahlering TE, Skarecky D, Lee D *et al.* Successful transfer of open surgical skills to a laparoscopic environment using a robotic interface:initial experience with laparoscopic radical prostatectomy. *J Urol* 2003; **170**:1738–41.

3 Van Appledorn S, Bouchier-Hayes D, Agarwal D *et al.* Robotic laparoscopic radical prostatectomy setup and procedural techniques after 150 cases. *Urology*. 2006; **67**:364–7.

4 Patel VR, Tully AS, Holmes R *et al.* Robotic radical prostatectomy in the community setting: the learning curve and beyond. Initial 200 cases. *J Urol* 2005; **174**:269–72.

Chapter 6

Stone disease

Kidney stones: treatment options and watchful waiting

The traditional indications for intervention for kidney stones are pain, infection, and obstruction. With the advent of extra-corporeal shock-wave lithotripsy (ESWL) and minimally invasive options such as flexible ureteroscopy and laser fragmentation, the indications for treatment have been broadened to small currently asymptomatic stones which have the potential to increase in size and migrate into the ureter. Haematuria caused by a stone is only very rarely severe or frequent enough to be the only reason to warrant treatment.

Before embarking on treatment of a stone which you think is the cause of the patient's pain or infection, warn them that although you may be able to remove the stone successfully, their pain or infection may persist i.e. the stone may be coincidental to these symptoms. Remember that both urinary tract infections (UTIs) and stones are common in women, and therefore it is not surprising that the two may coexist in the same patient, but be otherwise unrelated. Warn your patient that treatment of kidney stones which are thought to be the cause of recurrent UTIs does not always result in a resolution of these infections.

Options for stone management

Options include watchful waiting, ESWL, flexible ureteroscopy, percutaneous nephrolithotomy (PCNL), open surgery, and medical 'dissolution' therapy.

When to watch and wait and when not to

In the pre-ESWL and pre-ureteroscopy era only stones causing substantial pain, obstruction, or frequent infections were treated, because treatment involved major open surgery. The advent of the minimally invasive treatment options of ESWL, and more recently flexible ureteroscopy and laser fragmentation, have made treatment of small renal stones easier and less morbid. As a consequence, the traditional indications for stone treatment (pain, infection, obstruction) have been broadened to include small asymptomatic stones.

There are two rationales behind treating small asymptomatic stones:
- They have the potential at some future point in time to become symptomatic either as a consequence of migration into the ureter causing ureteric obstruction or by causing chronic loin pain.
- Such stones, while small, are amenable to relatively non-invasive techniques such as ESWL or flexible ureteroscopy and laser treatment. However, if allowed to grow they may move out of the range of effectiveness of these relatively non-invasive techniques and into the realm of treatments which have the potential for substantial morbidity (PCNL or even open stone surgery).

The difficulty for the stone surgeon is that not all small asymptomatic stones will cause problems and therefore treatment of all asymptomatic renal stones would represent substantial over-treatment. Which stones should be treated and which can safely be left alone?

Stones which are definitely *not* suitable for watchful waiting

- Struvite (i.e. infection-related) staghorn calculi will, if untreated, eventually destroy the kidney and are a significant risk to the patient's life. Historical series showed that approximately 30% of patients with staghorn calculi who did not undergo surgical removal died from renal-related causes—renal failure, urosepsis (septicaemia, pyonephrosis, perinephric abscess).[1,2] The combination of a neurogenic bladder and staghorn calculus seems to be particularly associated with a poor outcome.[3] Therefore watchful waiting is not recommended for staghorn calculi unless patient comorbidity is such that surgery would be a higher risk option than watchful waiting (although in practice the relative risk of morbidity and mortality from the stone versus that from the patient's associated comorbidity can be difficult or impossible to quantify).
- Asymptomatic calyceal stones in children, patients with a solitary kidney, and patients in certain professions (e.g. pilots), and women considering pregnancy should be treated.[4]

Asymptomatic calyceal stones which can be observed

As a rule of thumb, active treatment will be more seriously considered for younger patients with larger stones. Thus, one would be inclined to do nothing about a 1 cm symptomless stone in the kidney of a 95-year-old patient. However, a 1 cm stone in a symptomless 20-year-old runs the risk of causing problems (ureteric migration causing ureteric colic, increase in size, pain) over the remaining (many) years of the patient's life.

The natural history of asymptomatic (painless) renal stones

Probability of a symptomatic stone event (Tables 6.1 and 6.2):

- After 1 year 10% of patients have had a symptomatic event.
- After 2 years 20% of patients have had a symptomatic event.
- After 3 years 30% of patients have had a symptomatic event.
- After 4 years 40% of patients have had a symptomatic event.

The cumulative probability of a symptomatic event over a 5-year period is in the order of 50%. Half of these events require intervention (ESWL, ureteroscopy, PCNL), and half do not. Thus a substantial proportion of patients develop symptoms, some requiring surgical intervention, but a substantial proportion do not.

The risk of asymptomatic calyceal stones becoming symptomatic (e.g. pain, symptoms of UTI) and requiring treatment will increase with longer follow-up. When followed for 3–7 years:[5,6]

- 15% pass spontaneously (sudden onset of acute loin pain).
- 15–50% require surgical intervention for pain and/or migration into the ureter (ESWL 8%, ureteroscopy 6%, PCNL 3%).
- 40% remain *in situ*.
- 45% increase in size.

In a contemporary study, asymptomatic calyceal stones which were followed over a 3-year period were more likely to require intervention (surgery or ESWL) or to increase in size or cause pain if they were >4 mm in diameter and were located in a middle or lower pole calyx.[7] The approximate risks (relative to stone size) over 3 years of follow-up of requiring intervention, developing pain or increase in stone size are shown in Table 6.3.

The advice given by the NIH Consensus Conference[8] in 1988 to use ESWL for the management of small (<5 mm) incidentally discovered asymptomatic kidney calculi is controversial. Lingeman et al.[4] stated that the value of 'prophylactic treatment of small stones <5 mm, non-obstructive, asymptomatic stones remains to be determined'. The study by Burgher et al.[7] suggests that asymptomatic stones <5 mm in diameter can certainly develop into painful stones in a substantial proportion (40%) of patients, and that a substantial minority (20%) will require intervention in some form or other.

Table 6.1 Natural history of asymptomatic stones according to stone size

Stone size at initial diagnosis	Number (percentage) of patients experiencing an event
1–2 mm	8 (25%)
3–2 mm	11 (31%)
≥7 mm	12 (41%)
Overall	31 (32%)

Stones followed for >6 months after first identification; mean follow-up 32 months.
Data from Glowacki et al.[6]

Table 6.2 Natural history of asymptomatic stones according to stone number

Number of stones at initial diagnosis	Number (percentage) of patients experiencing an event
1	7 (18%)
2	7 (27%)
≥3	20 (49%)

Table 6.3 Likelihood of asymptomatic calyceal stones requiring intervention when followed over a 3-year period[7]

	<5 mm	5–10 mm	11–15 mm	>15 mm
Requiring intervention	20%	25%	40%	30%
Causing pain	40%	40%	40%	60%
Increasing in size	50%	55%	60%	70%

References

1 Blandy JP, Singh M. The case for a more aggressive approach to staghorn stones. *J Urol* 1976; **115**:505–6.

2 Rous SN, Turner WR. Retrospective study of 95 patients with staghorn calculus disease *J Urol* 1977; **118**:902.

3 Teichmann JM, Long RD, Hulbert JC. Long-term renal fate and prognosis after staghorn calculus management *J Urol* 1995; **153**:1403–7.

4 Lingeman JE, Lifshitz DA, Evan AP. Surgical management of urinary lithiasis. In *Campbell's Urology* 8th edn, ed Walsh PC, Retik AB, Vaughan ED, Wein AJ. Philadelphia, PA: WB Saunders, 2002, pp 3361–451.

5 Hubner WA, Porpaczy P. Treatment of calyceal calculi. *Br J Urol* 1990; **66**:9–11.

6 Glowacki LS, Beecroft ML, Cook RJ *et al.* The natural history of asymptomatic urolithiasis. *J Urol* 1992; **147**:319–21.

7 Burgher A, Beman M, Holtzmann JL, Monga M. Progression of nephrolithiasis: long-term outcomes with observation of asymptomatic calculi *J Endourol* 2004; **18**:534–9.

8 NIH Consensus Conference. Prevention and treatment of kidney stones. *JAMA* 1988; **260**:977–81.

Active treatment options for kidney stones

For some stones the treatment choices are limited to just one or two options. A struvite staghorn calculus can only sensibly be managed by PCNL or open surgery. On the other hand, few surgeons would advocate open surgery for stones <1 cm in diameter. While large stones generally require PCNL or open surgery and small stones are generally treated by ESWL, those ~2 cm in diameter fall into a 'middle ground' where ESWL is less effective at stone clearance, but PCNL seems a little too aggressive. Flexible ureterorenoscopy and laser treatment is an 'in between' option for such stones—more efficient at stone fragmentation than ESWL, but with less morbidity than PCNL.

The most important factor in determining treatment is stone size. Stone location, stone composition and stone number are also important, as are patient-related factors such as age, weight, shape, comorbidity, kidney position (normal versus pelvic), and whether the stone is in a solitary kidney. Of course, patient choice is also a factor. The influence that these various factors have on treatment choice is best considered in the context of stone size.

Small kidney stones: diameter <1 cm

The likelihood of fragmentation with ESWL depends on stone size and location, anatomy of the renal collecting system, presence or absence of hydronephrosis, degree of obesity, and stone composition. As a general rule of thumb, if a stone has failed to disintegrate after three sessions of ESWL consider an alternative form of therapy.

ESWL

This is usually the first line treatment for small stones. Fragmentation and successful clearance of the fragments become less likely with increasing stone size and number. ESWL is most effective for stones <2 cm in diameter in favourable anatomical locations (upper and middle pole calyces). It is less effective for stones >2 cm diameter, stones in the lower pole or a calyceal diverticulum, and stones composed of cystine or calcium oxalate monohydrate (very hard). The great advantage of ESWL is its ease of administration (day-case procedure), the absence of any requirement for general anaesthesia, and its low complication rates. This must be balanced against lower stone-free rates compared with flexible ureterorenoscopy and laser treatment, PCNL, or open surgery as stone burden increases. However, some patients are happy to accept a lower probability of stone clearance because of the minimal morbidity of ESWL.

Stone size and ESWL outcome

Stone-free rates for solitary stones within the kidney following ESWL according to stone diameter are:
- <1 cm 80%
- 1–2 cm 60%
- >2 cm 50%.

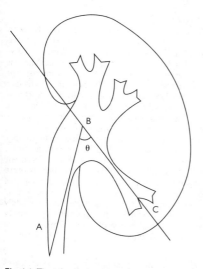

Fig. 6.1 The infundibulopelvic angle.

Stone location and ESWL outcome
Stones within lower pole calyces are less likely to fragment and clear than those in middle and upper pole calyces.[1]

Infundibulopelvic angle, dimensions, and ESWL outcome
The infundibulopelvic angle is the angle between the intersection of the infundibular axis (a line connecting the centre of the renal pelvis with the bottom of the stone-bearing calyx) and the ureteropelvic axis (a line connecting the centre of the pelvis with a point in the upper ureter opposite the lower pole of the kidney) (Fig. 6.1). Small (acute) lower pole infundibulopelvic angles are associated with a lower chance of stone clearance (e.g. 75% chance of clearance with an angle >70° versus 55% chance of clearance with an angle <70°).[2] Similarly, if the infundibular length is >5 cm, stone clearance is less likely.[2]

Some studies have suggested that a long narrow infundibulum is associated with lower stone-free rates post-ESWL,[3–5] but others have found no such association.[6]

Stone composition and ESWL outcome

Some stones are less fragile than others and therefore are less likely to fragment with ESWL. Stone composition, and to some extent stone shape, determines stone fragility. Cystine and calcium oxalate monohydrate stones are particularly hard and respond less well to ESWL. It is reasonable to use ESWL for cystine stones up to 1 cm in diameter, but above this size flexible ureterorenoscopy or PCNL offer more efficient clearance. Stones which have a smooth surface are less likely to fragment than those with irregular margins, whether composed of calcium[7,8] or cystine.[9] Stone-free rates for cystine stones are of the order of 70% for stones <1.5 cm in diameter and 40% for stones >2 cm in diameter.[10]

CT urography provides better density discrimination than plain radiography and is of some value in predicting the likelihood of successful stone fragmentation. Stones with a density <750 HU are more likely to fragment than are those with a density >750 HU.[11] Calcium oxalate monohydrate and calcium mono- and dihydrate stones tend to have high densities, as opposed to calcium oxalate dihydrate stones. Having said this, not all patients with low-density stones achieve stone clearance (approximately 1 in 10 do not), and a substantial proportion of patients with high-density stones become stone free (approximately two-thirds).[11] Thus it is still worthwhile considering ESWL as an option for the latter group of patients.

Lithotripter type

There have been no randomized studies comparing stone-free rates between different lithotripters. In non-randomized studies, rather surprisingly, when it comes to efficacy of stone fragmentation, older (the original Dornier HM3 machine) is better (but there is a higher requirement for analgesia and sedation or general anaesthesia). Less powerful (modern) lithotripters have lower stone-free rates and higher re-treatment rates.

Some patients are so obese that either they cannot safely be accommodated on the lithotripter or the distance between the shock wave head and the stone is greater than the focal point of the lithotripter.

Contraindications for ESWL

ESWL is contraindicated for pregnant women and patients with uncorrected clotting disorders. For pregnant women with renal (as opposed to ureteric) stones, treatment can almost always be deferred until after the baby has been born. For the patient on warfarin, anticoagulation can be stopped for about a week until the INR is normal and ESWL can then commence. The patient will be at risk of a thromboembolic event during this time and the size of this risk must be taken into account. Patients who take warfarin because they have an artificial heart valve are at significant risk of having a stroke while uncoagulated, and you must decide whether the risk of this outweighs the benefits of ESWL. An acceptable alternative option is to 'swap' anticoagulation to intravenous heparin, and to stop the heparin for a brief window to allow ESWL to be safely carried out. Alternatively, keep the patient on their full dose of warfarin and use the flexible ureterorenoscope and laser to fragment the stone. The risk of bleeding secondary to this treatment is probably less than that of a stroke.

Flexible ureterorenoscopy

Where ESWL has failed to achieve stone clearance, flexible ureteroreno-scopy ureteroscopy and laser fragmentation (📖 p. 406) is a very reasonable second-line option. Clearance rates are of the order of 60–90%, depending on stone size and whether the stone is located in the lower pole.

'Grey area' stones: diameter 1–2 cm

Options include ESWL (consider a JJ stent *in situ* for stones of diameter of the order of 2 cm), flexible ureterorenoscopy and laser fragmentation, and PCNL. PCNL gives the best chance of complete stone clearance with a single procedure, but this is achieved at a higher risk of morbidity. Stone-free rates for stones of diameter 1–2 cm are of the order of 60%.

The Lower Pole Study Group multicentre randomized trial of ESWL versus PCNL reported a stone-free rate for lower pole stones >1 cm in diameter of 21% for ESWL and 91% for PCNL.[12] The Lower Pole Study II, which has been designed to determine the effectiveness of flexible uretero-renoscopy for management of lower pole stones, is currently in progress.

Some patients will opt for several sessions of ESWL or flexible uretero-renoscopy and laser treatment, and the possible risk of ultimately requiring PCNL because of failure of ESWL or laser treatment, rather than proceeding with PCNL 'up front'. Some series report fragmentation rates of 50% for stones >2 cm in diameter using flexible ureterorenoscopy and laser treatment, but not all surgeons will be able to achieve such results. Therefore patient preference is an important factor in deciding treatment for middle-ground stones.

Large stones: diameter >2 cm or staghorns

As a rule of thumb, most stones >2 cm in diameter will respond poorly to ESWL (stone-free rates of the order of 50%) and are best treated with PCNL. Staghorn calculi (those occupying the renal pelvis and one or more calyces) can only sensibly be managed by PCNL or open surgery. 'Sandwich' therapy, i.e. PCNL to remove the bulk of the stone, followed by ESWL to attempt clearance of residual fragments, has been used with success for large stone burdens.

Recently, clearance rates with flexible ureterorenoscopy and laser treatment of 75% with a single session and 90% with second-look treatment have been reported for stones >2 cm in diameter.[13]

References

1 Madbouly K, Sheir KZ, ElSobky E. Impact of lower pole renal anatomy on stone clearance after shock wave lithotripsy: fact or fiction? *J Urol* 2001; **165**:1415.

2 Ghoneim IA, Ziada AM, ElKatib SE. Predictive factors of lower calyceal stone clearance after extracorporeal shockwave lithotripsy (ESWL): a focus on the infundibulopelvic angle. *Eur Urol* 2005; **48**:296–302.

3 Elbanasy AM, Shalhav AL, Hoenig DM et al. Lower caliceal stone clearance after shock wave lithotripsy or ureteroscopy. *J Urol* 1998; **159**:676–82.

4 Gupta NP, Singh DV, Hemal AK, Mandal S. Infundibulopelvic anatomy and clearance of inferior caliceal calculi with shock wave lithotripsy. *J Urol* 2000; **163**:24–7.

5 Poulakis V, Dahm P, Witzsch U et al. Prediction of lower pole stone clearance after shock wave lithotripsy using an artificial neural network. *J Urol* 2003;**169**:1250–6.

6 Sorensen CM, Chandoke PS. Is lower pole caliceal anatomy predictive of extracorporeal shock wave lithotripsy success for primary lower pole kidney stones? *J Urol* 2002; **168**:377–82.

7 Dretler SP, Polykoff G. Calcium oxalate stone morphology: fine tuning our therapeutic distinctions. *J Urol* 1996; **155**:823–33.

8 Bon D, Dore B, Irani J, Marroncle M, Aubert J. Radiographic prognostic criteria for extracorporeal shock-wave lithotripsy: a study of 485 patients. *Urology* 1996; **48**:556–61.

9 Bhatta KM, Prien EL Jr, Dretler SP. Cystone calculi rough and smooth: a new clinical distinction. *J Urol* 1989; **142**:937–40.

10 Graff J, Diedrichs W, Schulze H. Long term follow-up in 1003 extracorporeal shock wave lithotripsy patients. *J Urol* 1988; **140**:479–83.

11 Narmada PG, Ansari MS, Kesarvani P et al. Role of computed tomography with no contrast medium enhancement in predicting the outcome of extracorporeal shock wave lithotripsy for urinary calculi. *BJU Int* 2005; **95**:1285–8.

12 Albala DM, Assimos DG, Clayman RV et al. Lower Pole I: a prospective randomized trial of extracorporeal shockwave lithotripsy and percutaneous nephrostolithotomy for lower pole nephrolithiasis. Initial results. *J Urol* 2001; **166**:2072–80.

13 Grasso M, Conlin M, Bagley D. Retrograde ureteropyeloscopic treatment of 2 cm or greater upper urinary tract and minor staghorn calculi. *J Urol* 1998; **160**:346–351.

Clinically insignificant residual fragments

Clinically insignificant residual fragments (CIRFs) are residual fragments of stone ≤4 mm in diameter in an asymptomatic (no pain or haematuria) non-obstructed patient with sterile urine following ESWL.[1] They are described as being clinically insignificant because it is anticipated that they will pass spontaneously without the need for further treatment and will not subsequently develop into a larger stone. Residual stones are defined as particles of stone of diameter ≥5 mm.

Clearly, the incidence of clinically insignificant residual fragments in reported series of ESWL outcomes will be influenced by the sensitivity of the imaging test used to look for them. Most series base their stone-free or clinically insignificant residual fragment rates on KUB X-ray imaging. Those which use CT urography, with its higher sensitivity for detecting stone fragments, will naturally report higher rates of incomplete stone clearance.

CIRFs or residual stones have the potential to act as a nidus for increase in stone size. Their fate (Table 6.4) depends on how long they are followed up, as an event is more likely to occur with longer follow-up. Clearance is less likely to occur in cases with lower pole CIRFs.

It has been suggested that oral potassium citrate can increase the stone-free rate following ESWL.[1–3]

Table 6.4 Fate of CIRFs

Reference	Percentage of patients experiencing growth of CIRFs (percentage requiring further stone treatment)	Mean length of follow-up (years)
Yu et al.[4]	25	6
Candau et al.[5]	35 (20)	3
Osman et al.[6]	20 (20)	5

References

1 Cicerello E, Merlo F, Gambaro G. Effect of alkaline citrate therapy on clearance of residual stone fragments after extracorporeal shock wave lithotripsy in sterile calcium and infection nephrolithiasis patients. *J Urol* 1994; **151**:5–9.

2 Fine KF, Pak CYC, Preminger GM. Effects of medical management and residual fragments on recurrent stone formation following shockwave lithotripsy. *J Urol* 1995; **153**:27–33.

3 Soygür T, Akbay A, Kupeli S. Effect of potassium citrate therapy on stone recurrence and residual fragments after shock wave lithotripsy in lower caliceal calcium oxalate urolithiasis: a randomized controlled trial. *J Endourol* 2002; **16**:149–52.

4 Yu CC, Lee YH, Huang JK et al. Long-term stone regrowth and recurrence rates after extracorporeal shock wave lithotripsy. *Br J Urol* 1993; **72**:688–91.

5 Candau C, Saussine C, Lang H et al. Natural history of residual renal stone fragments after ESWL. *Eur Urol* 2000; **37**:18–22.

6 Osman M, Alfano Y, Kemp S et al. 5 year follow-up of patients with clinically insignificant residual fragments after extracorporeal shockwave lithotripsy. *Eur Urol* 2005; **47**:860–4.

Management of stones in difficult anatomical locations

Caliceal diverticula are non-secretory outpouchings of the renal collecting system which communicate with a calyx by a tight neck. Indications for treating stones in a caliceal diverticula are pain and infection. It can be very difficult to determine if the loin pain complained of by a patient is due to the stone or some other cause. Warn the patient that even successful stone clearance may not stop the pain.

Options for treating stones in caliceal diverticula

- ESWL: pain relief may be achieved in as many as 70–80% of cases despite stone clearance in just 25%.[1]
- Ureterorenoscopy (URS) ± incision of the caliceal neck. Stone clearance averages about 50%, being reasonably good for upper pole caliceal stones and very poor for lower pole.[2]
- PCNL ± incision of the caliceal neck.[3] Stone-free rates of ~80% versus 20% for PCNL and URS (and resolution of pain in 90% versus 40%) have been reported.[3,4]
- Open surgery to excise the stone, ligate the diverticular neck, and marsupialize the diverticulum or excise the diverticulum altogether (historical).
- Laparoscopic stone removal and marsupialization of the diverticulum.

Stones in horseshoe kidneys

Stones are said to occur in 20–60% of horseshoe kidneys and PUJO occurs in 15%.[5] The standard range of general treatment options is still available (ESWL, ureterorenoscopy, PCNL, open surgery).

As a general rule of thumb, try ESWL first, but warn the patient that requirement for re-treatment is high[6] and that progression of treatment to flexible ureterorenoscopy or PCNL is often required.[7] Clearance of stones in the lower pole post-ESWL can be poor because of a very dependent lower pole and the anterior insertion of the ureter at the PUJ (middle and upper pole stone clearance is better). Prone positioning may be required. For the same reason, lower pole access for ureterorenoscopy can be difficult. PCNL can be very effective. A CT should be done to determine whether the stone can be safely approached without damaging adjacent organs.[8]

Stones in renal transplants

The incidence varies considerably, from 0.3% to 3% depending on the series.[9] The presentation is usually one of deterioration in renal function. Anuria can occur. Pain is an uncommon presentation because the kidney has been denervated. The stone has sometimes been present at the time of transplantion. Metabolic causes are common (tertiary hyperparathyroidism, hypercalciuria, hypocitraturia).

Treatment is essentially as for solitary kidneys. Where there is obstruction (worsening renal function, anuria) a percutaneous nephrostomy provides a rapid temporizing method of management. Where there is expertise, JJ stent insertion may be possible, although this can be technically challenging because of the abnormal position of the new ureteric orifice.

The kidney may be shielded anteriorly by overlying bowel and posteriorly by the ilium and therefore both ESWL and PCNL may not be feasible. If there is no overlying bowel, ESWL in the prone position is an option, but fragments may not pass through the vesico-ureteric junction (VUJ) in the way that they would through a 'normal' VUJ. It is sensible to limit ESWL to small (diameter <1 cm) stones.

Retrograde access to the ureter for ureterorenoscopy for larger stones or those which fail to fragment with ESWL is difficult because of the abnormal position of the new ureteric orifice in the dome of the bladder. Placing a guidewire across the new VUJ can be technically very challenging (Fig. 6.2). Antegrade guidewire or stent placement (if technically possible) may make such access easier for the ureteroscopist. Occasionally stricturing of the neo-VUJ is encountered. This can be managed by balloon dilatation, but may require re-implantation of the ureter.

PCNL is reserved for large stones (>2 cm) or those that cannot be treated by or have failed to respond to ESWL or flexible ureterorenoscopy. The superficial position of the transplant kidney can make access relatively easy. However, transplanted kidneys are often encased in a fibrous sheath which makes development of an access track difficult.

Stones in pelvic kidneys

Many of the same issues concerning stone treatment in transplant kidneys apply to the management of stones in the pelvic kidney. PCNL can be impossible because of overlying bowel gas. Laparoscopy is an option.

Stones in kidneys that drain into ileal conduits

Renal stones are more common in patients with ileal conduits (relative urinary stasis, upper tract bacterial colonization and infection) (Fig. 6.3).[10] ESWL, ureterenoscopy, and PCNL are all options. In general terms, ESWL can be used for stones <2 cm in diameter and PCNL for larger stones. Retrograde access can be achieved using very flexible wires and ureteric catheters. Failing a retrograde approach, antegrade placement of a guidewire or JJ stent can make the passage of a flexible ureterorenoscope easier.

Medullary sponge kidney

ESWL for stones in cases of medullary sponge kidney can be useful for pain relief, even in the absence of stone fragmentation.[11]

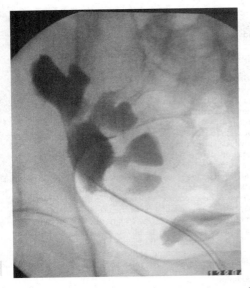

Fig. 6.2 Two guidewires have been negotiated into the ureter of a renal transplant, in preparation for passage of the flexible ureteroscope to allow ablation of a stone in the ureter.

(a)

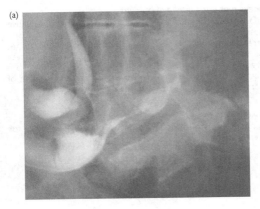

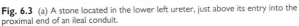

Fig. 6.3 (a) A stone located in the lower left ureter, just above its entry into the proximal end of an ileal conduit.

(b)

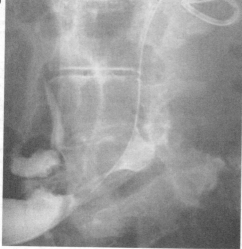

Fig. 6.3 (*Contd.*) (b) A guide wire has been negotiated past the stone to allow antegrade stenting.

References

1 Streem SB, Yost A. Treatment of caliceal diverticular calculi with extracorporeal shock wave lithotripsy: patient selection and extended follow-up. *J Urol* 1992; **148**:1043–6.
2 Chong TW, Bui MH, Fuchs GJ. Calyceal diverticula: ureteroscopic management. *Urol Clin North Am* 2000; **27**:647–54.
3 Shalhav AL, Soble JJ, Nakada SY et al. Long term outcome of caliceal diverticula following percutaneous endosurgical management. *J Urol* 1998; **160**:1635–9.
4 Auge BK, Munver R, Kourambas J et al. Endoscopic management of symptomatic caliceal diverticula: a retrospective comparison of percutaneous nephrolithotripsy and ureteroscopy. *J Endourol* 2002; **16**:557–63.
5 Pitts WR Jr, Muecke EC. Horseshoe kidneys: a 40-year experience. *J Urol* 1975; **113**:743–6.
6 Locke DR, Newman RC, Steinbock GS, Finlayson B. Extracorporeal shock wave lithotripsy in horseshoe kidneys. *Urology* 1990; **31**:407–11.
7 Jones DJ, Wickham JE, Kellett MJ. Percutaneous nephrolithotomy for calculi in horseshoe kidneys. *J Urol* 1991; **145**:481–3.
8 Kunzel KH, Sclocler H, Janetschek G. Arterial blood supply of horseshoe kidneys with special reference to percutaneous lithotripsy. *Urology* 1989; **27**:240–5.
9 Crook T, Keoghane S. Renal transplant lithiasis: rare but time-consuming. *BJU Int* 2005; **95**:931–2.
10 Turk TM, Koleski FC, Albala DM. Incidence of urolithiasis in cystectomy patients after intestinal conduit or continent urinary diversion. *World J Urol* 1999; **17**:305–7.
11 Holmes SA, Eardley I, Corry DA, Nockler I, Whitfield HN. The use of extracorporeal shock-wave lithotripsy for medullary sponge kidney. *Br J Urol* 1992; **70**:352–4.

Medical therapy (dissolution therapy)

Uric acid and cystine stones are potentially suitable for dissolution therapy. Calcium within either stone type reduces the chances of successful dissolution.

Uric acid stones

Urine is frequently supersaturated with uric acid (derived from a purine-rich diet, i.e. animal protein). Fifty per cent of patients who form uric acid stones have gout. The other 50% do so because of a high protein and low fluid intake ('Western lifestyle'). In patients with gout, the risk of developing stones is about 1% per year after the first attack. Therefore most patients with gout do not form uric acid stones, but many patients with uric acid stones have gout.

Uric acid stones form in concentrated *acid* urine. Dissolution therapy is based on hydration, urine alkalinization, allopurinol, and dietary manipulation, the aim being to reduce urinary uric acid saturation. Maintain a high fluid intake (urine output 2–3 L/day), 'alkalinize' the urine to pH 6.5–7 (sodium bicarbonate 650 mg three or four times daily or potassium citrate (30–60 mEq/day, equivalent to 15–30 mL of a postassium citrate solution three or four times daily). In those with hyperuricaemia or urinary uric acid excretion >1200 mg/day, add allopurinol 300–600 mg/day (inhibits conversion of hypoxanthine and xanthine to uric acid). Dissolution of large stones (even staghorn calculi) is possible with this regimen.

Cystine stones

Cystinuria is an inherited kidney and intestinal transepithelial transport defect for the amino acids cystine, ornithine, arginine, and lysine (COAL) leading to excessive urinary excretion of cystine (autosomal recessive inheritance; prevalence of 1 in 700 are homozygous, i.e. both genes are defective; occurs equally in both sexes). Approximately 3% of adult stone formers and 6% of stone-forming children are cystinuric.

Most cystinuric patients excrete about 1 g of cystine per day, which is well above its solubility. Cystine solubility in acid solutions is low (300 mg/L at pH 5, 400 mg/L at pH 7). Patients with cystinuria present with renal calculi, often in their teens or twenties. Cystine stones are relatively radiodense because they contain sulphur atoms. The cyanide nitroprusside test will detect most homozygote stone formers and some heterozygotes (false-positive results occur in the presence of ketones).

Treatment of existing stones and prevention of further stones

The aim is to reduce cystine excretion (dietary restriction of the cystine precursor amino acid methionine and also of sodium intake to <100 mg/day) and to increase the solubility of cystine by alkalinization of the urine to >pH 7.5, maintenance of a high fluid intake, and use of drugs which convert cystine to more soluble compounds. D-Penicillamine, N-acetyl-D-penicillamine, and mercaptopropionylglycine bind to cystine, and the compounds formed are more soluble in urine than is cystine alone. D-Penicillamine has potentially unpleasant and serious side-effects (allergic reactions, nephrotic syndrome, pancytopenia, proteinuria, epidermolysis, thrombocytosis, hypogeusia). Therefore it is reserved for cases where alkalinization therapy and high fluid intake fail to dissolve the stones.

Treatment for failed dissolution therapy

Cystine stones are very hard and therefore are relatively resistant to ESWL. Nonetheless, a substantial proportion of small cystine stones will respond to ESWL. Flexible ureteroscopy (for small) and PCNL (for larger) cystine stones are used where ESWL fragmentation has failed.

Percutaneous dissolution therapy

This procedure has been used for infection stones (10% hemiacidrin solution, acidic pH 3.5–4) and cystine and uric acid stones (THAM solutions (trihydroxymethyl ammonium 0.3–0.6 mmol/L) with pH 8.5–9).[1] Two percutaneous nephrostomy tubes are inserted to enable irrigation and drainage of irrigant fluid, with a JJ stent if the stone burden is large to prevent large fragments generated during the dissolution process from migrating into the ureter. ESWL may be used during the process of irrigation. By generating fragments of stone the surface area exposed to the various chemolytic agents is increased, thus optimizing dissolution. Several weeks may be required for dissolution of a large staghorn, so this is not the simple option that it might appear. This, combined with the cardiotoxicity (cardiac arrest) of the hypermagnesaemia occurring secondary to absorption of magnesium from the hemicidrin solution and the limited experience of using this technique limits the widespread application of this technique of stone treatment.

Reference

1 Tiselius HG, Hellgren E, Anderrson A *et al.* Minimally invasive treatment of infection staghorn stones with shock wave lithotripsy and chemolysis. *Scand J Urol Nephrol* 1999; **33**:286–90.

Fragmentation techniques: extra-corporeal lithotripsy

Extra-corporeal lithotripsy (ESWL) is the technique of focusing externally generated shock waves on a target (the stone). It was first used in humans in 1980.[1] The first commercial lithotripter, the Dornier HM2, was installed in Munich in 1982. ESWL has revolutionized kidney and ureteric stone treatment. Three methods of shock wave generation are commercially available: electrohydraulic, electromagnetic, and piezoelectric.

- *Electrohydraulic* Application of a high-voltage electrical current between two electrodes about 1 mm apart under water causes discharge of a spark. Water around the tip of the electrode is vaporized by the high temperature, resulting in a rapidly expanding gas bubble. The rapid expansion and then the rapid collapse of this bubble generates a shock wave which is focused by a metal reflector shaped as a hemi-ellipsoid. This method was used in the original Dornier HM3 lithotripter.

- *Electromagnetic* Two electrically conducting cylindrical plates are separated by a thin membrane of insulating material. Passage of an electrical current through the plates generates a strong magnetic field between them, the subsequent movement of which generates a shock wave. An 'acoustic' lens is used to focus the shock wave.

- *Piezoelectric* A spherical dish is covered with about 3000 small ceramic elements, each of which expands rapidly when a high voltage is applied across them. This rapid expansion generates a shock wave.

First-generation lithotripter

In the HM3 (Human Model 3) lithotripter shock waves were generated electrohydraulically by discharge of a spark under water. The shock waves were coupled (delivered) to the patient by immersion in a water bath, with an ellipsoid reflector used to focus the shock waves onto the stone. General or spinal anaesthesia was required. The aperture through which the shock waves was delivered was small, thereby 'concentrating' the shock waves. No longer manufactured, although still used in some centres.

Second-generation lithotripters

Designed to be multifunctional and to allow pain-free application of shock waves. Shock-wave generation using non-electrohydraulic methods (electromagnetic and piezoelectric) was introduced in combination with acoustic lenses which allowed the shock waves to be focused. A water cushion system of coupling of shock waves to the patient was introduced, thereby obviating the need to immerse the patient in a bath of water.

Piezoelectric devices have a larger aperture, allowing application of shock waves over a greater surface area. This reduced the pain associated with ESWL, but at the expense of less efficient fragmentation and therefore a greater requirement for re-treatment. These second generation devices introduced ultrasonic localizing systems.

Third generation lithotripters

These combine fluoroscopic and ultrasound stone localizing systems, use larger apertures (to allow pain-free shock-wave treatment), and incorporate all the components of the lithotripter within a single functional unit.

Mechanisms of stone fragmentation by lithotripsy

Shock waves consist of a positive and a negative pressure wave (Fig. 6.4). Stones are fragmented by the following mechanisms.

- Tear and shear forces (by reflection of shock waves at acoustic interfaces) which are believed to initiate stone fragmentation (comminution). The large positive pressure of the shock wave compresses the front of the stone (compressive fracturing). As the pressure wave hits the back of the stone, some of it is reflected and this tends to put the stone under tensile stress (pulling the stone apart).
- Cavitation: secondary shock waves are generated by a process of bubble formation and collapse. Bubble formation is induced by the negative pressure wave of the shock wave. During the negative pressure phase, air within the water surrounding and within the stone expands. As this occurs very rapidly, a shock wave is generated which can fragment the stone. A second shock wave is generated by the collapse of the bubble produced by the cavitation effect. Cavitation is believed to be involved in the final phase of stone disintegration.
- Quasistatic squeezing: literally squeezing of the stone by the shock wave.
- Dynamic fatigue: the evolution (propagation and eventual coalescence) of microcracks within the stone, which are produced by the mechanical stresses of the tear and shear forces and cavitation.

Shock wave energy (rather than peak pressure or rise time of the pressure wave) is believed to be the most important factor in stone fragmentation. Higher focal pressures or peak pressures in some devices have not translated into higher stone-free rates. Energy density is responsible for shock-wave-induced tissue trauma, which is mainly due to cavitation.

Efficacy of ESWL

Renal stones

The likelihood of fragmentation with ESWL depends on stone size and location, anatomy of the renal collecting system, degree of obesity, and stone composition. It is most effective for stones <2 cm in diameter in favourable anatomical locations. It is less effective for stones >2 cm in diameter, in the lower pole (in the majority of studies), in a calyceal diverticulum, and composed of cystine or calcium oxalate monohydrate (very hard).

Stone-free rates for solitary kidney stones are 80% for stones <1 cm in diameter, 60% for stones 1–2 cm in diameter, and 50% for stones >2 cm in diameter. Lower stone-free rates compared with open surgery or PCNL are accepted because of the minimal morbidity of ESWL. In general terms, the re-treatment rate is approximately 5–15% (depending on the published series) with the Dornier HM3 device, 20–35% with newer lithotripters, and 40–60% with 'pain-free' piezoelectric devices.[2]

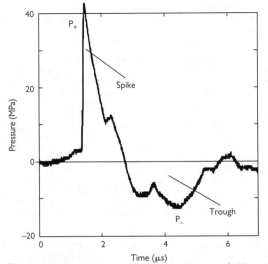

Fig. 6.4 The pressure changes occurring at the focal point of a lithotripter during shock wave application. Reproduced with permission from *Campbell's Urology 8th edition*, Walsh et al, 2002, Elsevier.

Ureteric stones

Stone-free rates for ureteric stones are of the order of 70–75%. The placement of JJ stents prior to ESWL for ureteric stones and the presence/absence of hydronephrosis probably have little impact on stone-free rates.[3]

Which lithotripter is best?

The answer to this question depends on how you define 'best'. There have been no randomized studies comparing stone-free rates between different lithotripters. In non-randomized studies, rather surprisingly, when it comes to efficacy of stone fragmentation, older (the original Dornier HM3 machine) is better, but this must be balanced against a higher requirement for analgesia and sedation or general anaesthesia with the older generation machines. More modern lithotripters have higher peak pressures per shock wave, but the shock wave energy per impulse is lower. Therefore they are less powerful and as a consequence have lower stone-free rates and higher re-treatment rates.

The shock-wave-generating mechanism of electromagnetic lithotripters (lifespan can be as long as a million shock waves) is more durable than that of electrohydraulic lithotripters (lifespan can be as short as 10 000 shock waves). Piezoelectric devices can last as long as 5 million shock waves. Thus the maintenance costs and 'down time' (for replacement of components) is greater for electrohydraulic lithotripters. One additional advantage of electromagnetic lithotripters is a more consistent energy level for each impulse, whereas the energy levels of electrohydraulic lithotripters have a tendency to tail off towards the end of the lifespan of the electrode.

Interval between treatments

There are no clearly defined rules, but as a rule of thumb based on the time to resolution of shock-wave renal contusions (averaging 2 weeks[4]) it seems sensible to allow a period of 10–14 days between ESWL treatments. There is no consensus on the number of shock waves that should be given per treatment session.

Side-effects of ESWL

Effects of ESWL on the kidney and adjacent organs

- Macroscopic haematuria as a direct result of renal parenchymal damage.
- Elevated levels of bilirubin, lactate dehydrogenase, serum glutamic transaminase, and creatinine phosphokinase occuring within 24 hr of treatment and normalizing within 3 months, indicating liver and skeletal muscle damage.
- Gastric or duodenal erosions.
- Damage to the parenchyma of the lung if exposed directly to shock waves.
- Acute pancreatitis (elevated serum amylase).
- Induction of extrasystoles. This led to shock wave delivery being synchronized with the R-wave of the ECG ('gating'). However, it has been demonstrated that ungated shock-wave delivery is safe and ESWL is not contraindicated in patients with an irregular cardiac rhythm.[5]
- Shock-wave-induced renal injury (peri- and intra-renal haematomas and oedema) has been demonstrated (using MRI and radionuclear scanning lithotripter) in approximately two-thirds of patients following ESWL with the Dornier HM3. Peri-renal haematoma formation, if looked for with renal ultrasound or CT, is common.[6] Second-generation lithotripters have also been shown to induce radiologically demonstrable renal injuries. Only rarely is haematoma formation severe enough to necessitate blood transfusion. There is a suggestion that patients with hypertension, diabetics, and those on aspirin may be more prone to haematoma formation following ESWL.
- Renal biopsies done a week after ESWL demonstrate tubular, vascular, and interstitial changes in the zone of the pressure wave.[7]

Acute alterations in renal function after ESWL

- Effective plasma flow, measured by renography, falls in approximately a third of kidneys after ESWL.[8]
- In solitary kidneys there is a significant reduction in glomerular filtration rate 3 months after ESWL.[9]

These changes are thought to be due to a vasoconstrictive response resulting in a fall in RBF and glomerular filtration rate.

Long-term adverse effects of ESWL as a consequence of scar formation within the kidney

Acute renal injuries post-ESWL progress to scar formation,[10] and there is some evidence that this may lead to the development of longer term problems.

Hypertension

In one study 8% of 243 patients who were normotensive at the time of ESWL developed blood pressure changes requiring antihypertensive medication with a mean follow-up of 1.5 years which translated into an annual incidence of hypertension of 5.5%.[11] However, other studies have found no change in blood pressure after ESWL.[12,13]

Decrease in renal function

In patients with a solitary kidney serum creatinine levels were elevated 5 years after ESWL.[14]

Pancreatic injury leading to diabetes

Whether or not ESWL can damage the endocrine components of the pancreas, leading to the later development of diabetes, remains contentious. Most authorities think this unlikely.[15]

Contraindications to ESWL

- Pregnancy, uncorrected blood clotting disorders (including anticoagulation), and renal artery aneurysms[16] are absolute contraindications to ESWL.
- The presence of a pacemaker is *not* a contraindication.

References

1 Chaussy CG, Brendel W, Schmidt E. Extracorporeal induced destruction of kidney stones by shock waves. *Lancet* 1980; **2**:1265.

2 Rassweiler JJ, Tailly GG, Chaussy C. Progress in lithotripter technology. *EAU Update Series* 2005; **3**:17–36.

3 Seitz C, Fajkovic H, Waldert M et al. Extracorporeal shock wave lithotripsy in the treatment of proximal ureteral stones: does the presence and degree of hydronephrosis affect success? *Eur Urol* 2006; **49**:378–83.

4 Villanyi KK, Szekely JG, Farkas LM et al. Short term change sin renal function after extracorporeal shock wave lithotripsy in children. *J Urol* 2001; **166**:222–4.

5 Cass AS. The use of ungating with the Medstone lithotriptor. *J Urol* 1996; **156**:896–8.

6 Knapp PM, Kulb TB, Lingeman JE et al. Extracorporeal shock wave lithotripsy induced perirenal hematomas. *J Urol* 1988; **139**:700–3.

7 Rigatti P, Colombo PR, Centemero A et al. Histological and ultrastructural evaluation of extracorporeal shock wave lithotripsy-induced acute renal lesions: preliminary report. *Eur Urol* 1989; **16**:207–11.

8 Kaude JV, Williams MC, Millner MR et al. Renal morphology and function immediately after extracorporeal shock wave lithotripsy. *Am J Roentgenol* 1985; **145**:305–14.

9 Karlsen SJ, Berg K: Acute changes in renal function following extracorporeal shock wave lithotripsy in patients with a solitary kidney. *J Urol* 1991; **145**:253–6.

10 Lechevallier E, Siles S, Ortega JC et al. Comparison by SPECT of renal scars after extracorporeal shock wave lithotripsy and percutaneous nephrolithotomy. *J Endourol* 1993; **7**:465–7.

11 Lingeman JE, Kulb TB, Newman DM et al. Hypertension following ESWL. *J Urol* 1987; **137**:142.

12 Evan AP, McAteer JA. Current perspectives on shock wave lithotripsy: adverse effects. In *Topics in clinical urology: new developments in the management of urolithiasis*, ed. Lingeman JE, Preminger GM. New York, Igaku-Shion, 1996, pp 3–20.

13 Jewett MAS, Bombardier C, Logan AG, et al. A randomized controlled trial to assess the incidence of new onset hypertension in patients after shock wave lithotripsy for symptomatic renal calculi. *J Urol* 1998; **160**:1241–3.

14 Brito CG, Lingeman JE, Newman DM Long-term follow-up of renal function in ESWL-treated patients with solitary kidney. *J Urol* 1990; **143**:299.

15 Wendt-Nordahl G, Krombach P, Hannak D et al. Prospective evaluation of acute endocrine pancreatic injury as collateral damage of shockwave lithotripsy for upper urinary tract stones. *BJU Int* 2007; **100**:1339–43.

16 Ignatoff JM, Nelson JB. Use of extracorporeal shock wave lithotripsy in a solitary kidney with renal artery aneurysm. *J Urol* 1993; **149**:359–60.

Fragmentation techniques: intra-corporeal techniques of stone fragmentation

Electrohydraulic lithotripsy

Electrohydraulic lithotripsy (EHL) was the first technique developed for intra-corporeal lithotripsy. A high voltage applied across a concentric electrode under water generates a spark. This vaporizes water, and the subsequent expansion and collapse of the gas bubble generates a shock wave. This is an effective form of stone fragmentation. The shock wave is not focused, and so the EHL probe must be applied within 1 mm of the stone to optimize stone fragmentation. EHL has a narrower safety margin than pneumatic, ultrasonic or laser lithotripsy, and should be kept as far away as possible from the wall of the ureter, renal pelvis, or bladder to limit damage to these structures, and at least 2 mm away from the cystoscope, ureteroscope, or nephroscope to prevent lens fracture.

Principal uses
Bladder stones (wider safety margin than in the narrower ureter).

Pneumatic (ballistic) lithotripsy (Fig. 6.5)

A metal projectile contained within the handpiece is propelled backwards and forwards at great speed by bursts of compressed air. It strikes a long thin metal probe at one end of the handpiece at 12 Hz (12 strikes per second) transmitting shock waves to the probe, which, when in contact with a rigid structure such as a stone, fragments the stone. It is used for stone fragmentation in the ureter (using a thin probe to allow insertion down a ureteroscope) or kidney (a thicker probe can be used, with an inbuilt suction device (Lithovac) to remove stone fragments).

Pneumatic lithotripsy is very safe since the excursion of the end of probe is about a millimetre and it bounces off the pliable wall of the ureter. Therefore ureteric perforation is rare. It is also low cost and low maintenance. However, its ballistic effect has a tendency to cause the stone to migrate into the proximal ureter or renal pelvis, where it may be inaccessible for further treatment. The metal probe cannot bend around corners, so it cannot be used for ureteroscopic treatment of stones within the kidney.

Principal uses
Ureteric stone fragmentation; it can be used for fragmentation of intrarenal stones, but ultrasonic fragmentation is more commonly used for such stones.

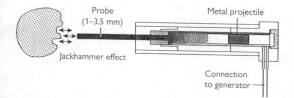

Fig. 6.5 The Lithoclast, a pneumatic lithotripsy device. Reproduced with permission from *Campbell's Urology*, 8th edition, Walsh et al, 2002, Elsevier.

Ultrasonic lithotripsy

An electrical current applied across a piezoceramic plate located in the ultrasound transducer generates ultrasonic waves of a specific frequency (23000–25000 Hz). The ultrasonic energy is transmitted to a hollow metal probe, which in turn is applied to the stone (Fig. 6.6). The stone resonates at high frequency and this causes it to break into small fragments (analogous to an opera singer breaking a glass) which are then sucked out through the centre of the hollow probe. Soft tissues do not resonate when the probe is applied to them, and therefore are not damaged. The high-frequency vibrations of the probe cause a heating effect. While the proximal (transducer) end of the probe can become too hot to touch during continuous application of energy, the distal end (adjacent to the stone and surrounding renal tissues) is cooled by the continuous flow of irrigant.

Principal uses

Ultrasonic lithotripsy is most useful for stone fragmentation in PCNL. The probes vary in size from 3 to 12Ch (10Ch is a common size for PCNL) and can only be used down straight instruments. The smaller diameter probes are solid and have no central suction channel. Avoid allowing the probe to contact the metal of the nephroscope, since this will dissipate energy in the form of heat and reduce the efficacy of stone fragmentation.

Smooth stones and hard stones (uric acid, cystine, calcium oxalate monohydrate) are more difficult to fragment, When fragmenting a smooth stone (e.g. uric acid), aim to drill a hole through the smooth outer surface to expose the inside of the stone.

Laser lithotripsy

Laser stands for light amplification by stimulated emission of radiation. When an atom is stimulated by an external energy source, photons are emitted when electrons drop from a high-energy to a lower-energy orbit. Laser light is coherent (all photons are in phase), collimated (photons travel parallel to each other), and monochromatic (all photons have the same wavelength).

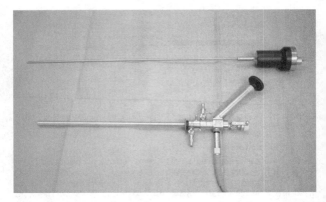

Fig. 6.6 Ultrasonic lithotripsy device. Reproduced with permission from Walsh et al., Campbell's Urology, 8th edn. 2002, Elsevier.

The holmium:yttrium aluminium garnet (Ho:YAG) laser is commonly used in urological surgery. The principal mode of action is a photothermal mechanism, in which light energy is converted to heat causing stone vaporization (the older pulsed dye lasers generated so-called plasma bubbles, the collapse of which led to shock-wave generation and stone fragmentation). The Ho:YAG laser causes minimal shock-wave generation, and consequently there is less risk of stone migration. The laser energy is delivered through quartz fibres which vary in diameter from 200 to 360 microns. The 200 micron fibre is very flexible and can be used to gain access to stones even within the lower pole of the kidney (🕮 2.13, Fig. 6.7), but its small diameter limits delivery of laser energy to the stone and therefore stone fragmentation takes longer. The 360 micron fibres deliver higher energy to the stone, but deflection of the tip of the scope is compromised by the greater rigidity of the fibres. A 270 micron fibre provides reasonable rates of energy delivery without compromising scope flexibility. Pulse energy is of the order of 0.6–1.2 J and pulse rates of 5–15 Hz are used for stone fragmentation.

The zone of thermal injury is limited to 0.5–1 mm from the laser tip. No stone can withstand the heat generated by the Ho:YAG laser. However, laser lithotripsy takes time, because the thin laser fibre must be 'painted' over the surface of the stone to vaporize it.

Discharge of the laser within 2–3 mm of the end of the ureteroscope can fracture the lens. Avoid discharging the laser near guidewires or stone baskets as it can cut through metal.

Principal uses
Fragmentation of ureteric stones and small intra-renal stones (using the flexible ureteroscope); it can also be used for prostatic resection in cases of benign prostatic enlargement (larger diameter fibres are used), urethral and ureteric stricture, and vaporization of urothelial tumours.

Flexible ureterorenoscopy and laser treatment

The development of small calibre ureteroscopes with active deflecting mechanisms and instrument channels, in combination with the development of laser technology, small diameter laser fibres, and stone baskets and graspers, has opened the way for intra-corporeal endoscopic treatment of kidney stones. Access to virtually the entire collecting system is possible with modern instruments. The Ho:YAG laser has a minimal effect on tissues at distances of 2–3 mm from the laser tip and so 'collateral' tissue damage is minimal with this laser type.

The fibre-optic bundles in flexible ureterorenoscopes are the same as those in semi-rigid scopes, only of smaller diameter. Thus image quality and light transmission are not as good as with semi-rigid scopes, but are usually adequate. With modern active secondary deflection ureterorenoscopes, access to most, if not all, parts of the renal collecting system is possible.

The working tip of most current models is of the order of 7–8Ch, and the proximal end of the scope is of the order of 9–10Ch. There is usually at least one working channel of at least 3.6Ch. Behind the actively deflecting tip of the scope is a segment which is more flexible than the rest of the shaft. This section can passively deflect (when the tip is fully actively deflected) by advancing the scope further. This flexible segment allows even more deflection. Flexible ureterorenoscopes which have two actively deflecting segments have recently been developed (e.g. ACMI DUR-8 Elite and Storz Flex-X). Flexible ureterorenoscopes are intrinsically more intricate and are therefore less durable than semi-rigid scopes. On average, major repairs will be required after roughly 15 procedures.

Flexible ureterorenoscopy and laser fragmentation offers an alternative treatment option to ESWL, with the advantage over PCNL of lower morbidity. In some situations (e.g. lower pole stones) it may achieve higher stone-free rates than ESWL (Fig. 6.7). There is also the added appeal that once a stone has been completely destroyed by the laser, one can genuinely say that stone clearance has been achieved. It is likely that many published estimates of stone-free rates after ESWL are over-estimates, since small fragments may not be visible with conventional follow-up imaging (KUB X-ray). These may act as the nidus for future stone recurrence.

Flexible ureteroscopy usually requires a general anaesthetic (few patients will tolerate it with sedation alone) and it is a more complex option than ESWL, with the potential for complications, albeit infrequently. These disadvantages must be balanced against its ability to access areas of the kidney where ESWL is less efficient, or where PCNL cannot reach. It is most suited to stones <2 cm in diameter, although second- or third-look flexible ureteroscopy can achieve good clearance rates for larger stone burdens. It is a particularly appealing option for the solitary kidney where the stone burden is too large for ESWL and where the concern with PCNL is the possibility of heavy bleeding, necessitating (albeit rarely) embolization or even emergency partial nephrectomy.

Table 6.5 Characteristics of some currently available flexible ureteroscopes

Ureteroscope	Tip diameter (Ch (mm))	Shaft diameter (Ch (mm))	Channel size (Ch (mm))	Active deflection down/up
ACMI DUR 8 Elite	6.75 (2.1)	8.6 (2.7)	3.6 (1.2)	175°/185°°[a]
Olympus URF-P3	6.9 (2.2)	8.4 (2.7)	3.6 (1.2)	180°/100°
Storz Flex-X	7.5 (2.4)	8.4 (2.7)	3.6 (1.2)	>300°/>300°
Wolf 7325.172	6.8 (2.2)	7.5 (2.4)	3.6 (1.2)	130°/160°

[a] The ACMI DUR 8 Elite has active secondary deflection of 165°.

Indications

- ESWL failure (probably the most common indication).
- Lower pole stone (reduces likelihood of stone passage post-ESWL as fragments have to pass 'up hill').
- Cystine stones (ESWL is relatively ineffective).
- Obesity such that PCNL access is technically difficult or impossible (nephroscopes may not be long enough to reach the stone) (Fig. 6.8).
- Obesity such that ESWL is technically difficult or impossible. BMI >28 is associated with lower ESWL success rates. Treatment distance may exceed the focal length of lithotripter.
- Musculoskeletal deformities such that stone access by PCNL or ESWL is difficult or impossible (e.g. kyphoscoliosis).
- Stone in a calyceal diverticulum (accessing stones in small diverticulae in upper and anterior calyces is difficult and carries significant risks).
- Stenosis of a calyceal infundibulum or 'tight' angle between renal pelvis and infundibulum. The flexible ureteroscope can negotiate acute angles and the laser can be used to divide the neck of the calyx.
- Bleeding diathesis where reversal of this diathesis, in order to allow PCNL to be performed safely, is potentially dangerous or difficult.
- Horseshoe or pelvic kidney. ESWL fragmentation rates are only 50% in such cases[1] because of difficulties of shock-wave transmission through overlying organs (bowel). PCNL for such kidneys is difficult because of bowel proximity and variable blood supply (blood supply derived from multiple sources).
- Patient preference.

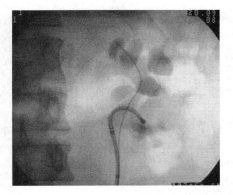

Fig. 6.7 Access to the lower pole of the kidney with a flexible uretrorenoscope.

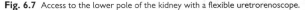

Operative technique

Flexible ureterorenoscopy and laser treatment can be performed with topical urethral local anaesthesia and sedation. However, trying to fragment a moving stone with the laser can be time consuming, and the patient may find it difficult to tolerate a lengthy procedure. Therefore ureteroscopy is most easily performed under general anaesthesia with endotracheal intubation (rather than a laryngeal mask) to allow short periods of suspension of respiration and so stop movement of the kidney and its contained stone.

Pass two guidewires into the renal pelvis using the same technique as described for ureteroscopy for ureteric stones (📖 p. 456). One serves as a safety guidewire and the other assists passage of the flexible ureteroscope up the ureter and into the kidney. The use of the dual-lumen catheter for second guidewire placement also dilates the ureter to help subsequent passage of the flexible ureterorenoscope.

Empty the bladder to prevent 'coiling' of the scope in the bladder. Ureteric access sheaths, which have outer diameters from 10 to 14Ch may facilitate access to the ureter and are particularly useful if it is anticipated that the ureterorenoscope will have to be passed up and down the ureter on multiple occasions (to retrieve fragments of stone) (Fig. 6.9). In addition, access sheaths facilitate the outflow of irrigant fluid from the pelvis of the kidney, thereby maintaining the field of view and decreasing intra-renal pressures. Peel Away access sheaths can be removed by pulling the two wings of the sheath apart.

Pass the scope over the second guidewire. This requires two people: the surgeon holds the shaft of the scope and the assistant applies tension to the guidewire to fix the latter in position without pulling it down and out of the ureter. This allows the scope to progress easily up the ureter. The assistant also ensures that acute angulation of the scope where the handle meets the shaft does not occur. The flexible ureterorenoscope should slide easily up the ureter and into the renal pelvis.

Use normal saline for irrigation. Once in the kidney, turn off the irrigation to avoid over-filling the collecting system. Inject contrast medium (diluted 50:50 with saline) to outline the collecting system so that you can systematically inspect each and every calyx for stones. Avoid undiluted contrast since this can obscure small stones, making them more difficult to localize radiographically. Use a combination of direct vision down the scope and X-ray screening to inspect each calyx, using the active deflection mechanism. Rotation of the scope will be required in order to orient the plane of deflection of the scope into the desired position.

Once the stone has been located, decide whether to fragment it with the laser or whether it is small enough to be removed safely by a stone basket. As a general rule avoid attempting to remove large stones with a basket, as they may very easily become stuck in the ureter. If you encounter resistance during attempted stone removal, stop. Do not attempt to pull the stone out, as this is a recipe for avulsion of the ureter. Dismantle the basket by removing the handle. This allows the scope to be withdrawn over the wire of the basket, so leaving the entrapped stone within the cage of the basket. Re-insert an 'access' guidewire beyond the trapped stone by passing the dual-lumen catheter over the safety guidewire. The ureteroscope (semi-rigid or flexible) can then be advanced up to the stone over the access guidewire and alongside the wire of the basket, and the stone can be fragmented using a laser fibre inserted down the ureterorenoscope. A stone trapped in a basket tends to raise the surgeon's pulse rate somewhat, but as long as you stick to these 'rules' damage to the ureter can be avoided.

The author has never been in the situation of not being able to get back to the stone to fragment it, but if it is not possible to reach the stone with the ureteroscope, there are two options: either proceed immediately to open stone removal, or leave a ureteric catheter or JJ stent in place for 24 hr to allow passive ureteric dilatation and then make a further attempt at ureteroscopic stone fragmentation 24 hr later (leaving a urethral catheter in place to which the wire of the basket can be tapped). The short period of ureteric dilatation may be all that is required to allow safe endoscopic stone removal. This latter approach has the added advantage of allowing you the opportunity to inform the patient what has happened and explain your plan of action, so that they are prepared for an open procedure.

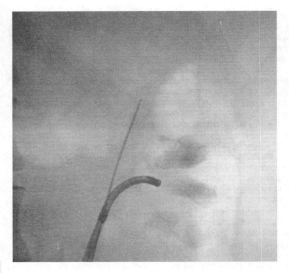

Fig. 6.8 Fragmentation of the staghorn calculus in a patient with gross obesity in whom the nephroscope could not access the collecting system. Complete fragmentation of this large stone was achieved with 3 procedures. Reproduced with permission from Reynard et al, *Oxford Handbook of Urology*, 2006, Oxford University Press.

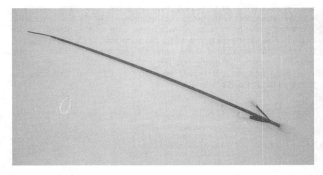

Fig. 6.9 A Peel-Away sheath.

Whenever passing a laser fibre or basket down the instrument channel of the flexible ureterorenoscope, make sure that the scope is straight rather than deflected (confirm by X-ray screening). Passage of instruments, particularly sharp laser fibres, through a deflected scope can damage the lining of the instrument channel, leading to extravasation of irrigant fluid into the optical system of the scope. Fibre diameters of 200, 270, and 365 microns are available. Larger diameter fibres are stiffer and therefore they reduce deflection of the tip of the scope. In most cases we use a 270 micron fibre for stone fragmentation, and a 200 micron fibre when substantial deflection of the scope is required (e.g. for lower pole stone fragmentation). Laser fibres are covered in an outer layer of blue cladding, which allows easier visualization and helps to avoid inadvertent discharge of the laser too close to the end of the scope.

Since the Ho:YAG laser energy is absorbed within 3 mm of water, the tip of the laser fibre must make contact with the stone in order to fragment it. Make sure that you can see the aiming beam (a helium–neon red laser). If you cannot, this indicates a defect (a crack) in the laser fibre at some point along its length. Activation of the laser in this situation could lead to delivery of laser energy within the working elements of the scope, causing irreparable damage.

When applying the laser energy to the stone, aim to paint the surface backwards and forwards so that the stone is slowly and methodically vaporized. Try to avoid breaking it into several large fragments, since these are more mobile than a single large stone and will tend to 'dance' irritatingly in front of you each time the laser is deployed, making effective targeting of the laser onto the stone surface very difficult.

Failure to pass the flexible ureterorenoscope

- Failure to pass the flexible ureterorenoscope following dilatation of the ureter to 10Ch using a dual lumen catheter is influenced by:
  - Ureteroscope size (diameter)—failure to pass a flexible scope occurs in 35% of cases for diameter 9Ch, 8% of cases for 8.6Ch, 5% of cases for 8.4Ch, and 1% of cases for 7.4Ch.[2]
  - Shaft strength.
  - Tip shape.
  - Outer sheath characteristics.
- If you encounter difficulty in passing the scope carry out the following:
  - Ensure that the ureter has been dilated with a 10Ch dual lumen catheter.
  - Pass a semi-rigid ureterorenoscope to dilate the ureteric orifice.
  - Pass an access sheath.
  - Consider balloon dilatation to a maximum of 15Ch.
- If difficulty is still encountered, you have no option other than to place a JJ stent to allow passive dilatation of the ureter, and then to attempt ureteroscopy a few days or weeks later.

Disadvantages and difficulties of flexible ureterorenoscopic stone fragmentation

- Efficacy diminishes as stone burden increases: it simply takes a long time to 'paint' the surface of the stone with laser energy in order to vaporize it.
- A dust-cloud is produced as the stone fragments, and this temporarily obscures the view until it has been washed away by irrigant fluid.
- Stone-free rates for those expert in flexible ureteroscopy are 70–80% for stones <2 cm in diameter and 50% for those >2cm in diameter.[3]
- Approximately 10% of patients will require two or more treatment sessions.

Use of stone baskets with the flexible ureterorenoscope

Laser fragmentation of lower pole stones in particular is technically challenging since the rigidity of the laser fibre limits the deflection of the scope, such that it can be difficult to effectively target the laser onto the stone. In such cases, consider manipulating the stone from the lower pole calyx into a middle or upper pole calyx using a stone basket. This may only improve stone-free rates to a modest degree (90% versus 83% stone free for repositioned stones versus those treated *in situ* in the lower pole), but it certainly makes laser treatment easier.[4]

A zero tip basket can more easily entrap a stone than a basket with a projecting wire end (Fig. 6.10). The major concern when using stone baskets, both in the kidney and the ureter, is the possible problem of being unable to detach the stone once it is engaged within the basket. Don't panic! Gently push the basket, in the 'open' position, back and forth, nudging the stone against the wall of the renal pelvis. Sometimes it will disengage from the basket. If it does not, unscrew the handle of the basket, slide the handle off, and then withdraw the scope from the basket. Reinsert the ureteroscope and use the laser to carefully fragment the stone (avoiding fragmentation of the wires of the basket!) (Fig. 6.11). Once the stone has been broken into smaller pieces, these will drop out of the basket, which can then be removed without avulsing the ureter.

To avoid the hazard of basket entrapment, some surgeons do not use stone baskets, preferring instead to use a tri-radiate grabber to manipulate stones. This is certainly a safer technique, but the amount of grip that can be applied to stones using such delicate grabbers is limited and they tend to disengage almost as soon as they have been trapped.

The use of a ureteral access sheath can make retrieval of multiple fragments of stones, followed by reinsertion of the flexible ureterorenoscope, considerably easier.

The use of routine JJ stenting after flexible ureterorenoscopy for renal calculi is controversial. There is certainly evidence that not all patients need to be stented.[5]

Outcomes

Clearance rates for stones <1 cm in diameter of the order of 60–90%, depending on stone size and whether the stone is lower pole in location, have been reported. For stones >2cm in diameter, clearance rates of 75% with a single session of flexible ureterorenoscopy and laser treatment and 90% with a second-look treatment have been reported.[6]

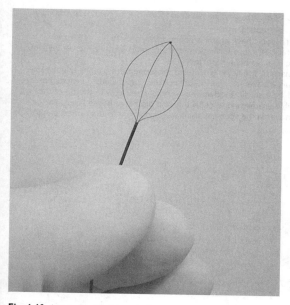

Fig. 6.10 A zero-tip nitinol stone basket.

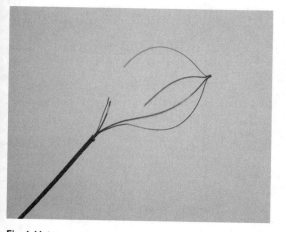

Fig. 6.11 It is possible to cut the wires of a basket with the laser!

Complications and hazards of flexible ureterorenoscopy

- UTI and septicaemia.
- Macroscopic haematuria is common.
- Ureteric stricture formation: stricture rates of the order of 0.5% of patients have been reported.[7-9]
- Damage to the flexible ureterorenoscope necessitating major repair occurs on average after 15 uses of the scope. Causes include passage of sharp laser fibre down the working channel with the tip of the flexible ureteroscope deflected, and discharge of the laser near or even within the scope, causing major damage to the optical system.

References

1 Kupeli B, Isen K, Biri H et al. Extracorporeal shockwave lithotripsy in anomalous kidneys. J Endourol 1999; **13**:39–52.

2 Hudson RG, Conlin MJ, Bagley DH. Ureteric access with flexible ureteroscopes: effect of the size of the ureteroscope. Br J Urol 2005; **95**:1043–4.

3 Dasgupta P Cynk MS, Bultitude MF, Tiptaft RC, Glass JM. Flexible ureterorenoscopy: prospective analysis of the Guy's experience. Ann R Coll Surgeons Engl 2004; **86**:367–370.

4 Auge BK, Dahm P, Wu NZ, Preminger GM. Ureteroscopic management of lower-pole renal calculi: technique of calculus displacement. J Endourol 2001; **15**:835–8.

5 Byrne RR, Auge BK, Kourambas J et al. Routine ureteral stenting is not necessary after ureteroscopy and ureteropyeloscopy: a randomized trail. J Endourol 2002; **16**:9–13.

6 Grasso M, Conlin M, Bagley D. Retrograde ureteropyeloscopic treatment of 2 cm or greater upper urinary tract and minor staghorn calculi. J Urol 1998; **160**:346–51.

7 Sofer M, Watterson JD, Wollin TA et al. Holmium:YAG laser lithotripsy for upper urinary tract calculi in 598 patients. J Urol 2002; **167**:31–4.

8 Harmon WJ, Sershon PD, Blute ML et al. Ureteroscopy: current practice and long-term complications. J Urol 1997; **157**:28–32.

9 Singal RK, Razvi HA, Denstedt JD. Secondary ureteroscopy: results and management strategy at a referral center. J Urol 1998; **159**:52–5.

Percutaneous nephrolithotomy

Indications

Percutaneous nephrolithotomy (PCNL) is generally recommended for:

- Stones >2 cm in diameter (Fig. 6.12): stone-free rates for flexible ureterorenoscopy and laser lithotripsy are of the order of 50–60% in the hands of experts.[1] The 'average' surgeon may not be able to achieve such results, and therefore many surgeons will opt for PCNL for stones >2 cm in diameter and certainly for those >3 cm.
- Staghorn calculi[2] where it is the first line option (with ESWL and/or repeat PCNL or flexible ureterorenoscopy and laser lithotripsy being used for residual stone fragments).
- Stones <3 cm in diameter that have failed ESWL or one or more attempts at flexible ureterorenoscopy and laser fragmentation, and where watchful waiting is undesirable either because of symptoms (pain) or the relative risk of increase in stone size or stone migration into the ureter.
- Stones 1–2 cm in diameter represent a 'grey area': a number of factors determine the relative merits of PCNL versus flexible ureterorenoscopy or ESWL.
  - Stone composition (stone hardness): cystine stones are very hard. If they are >15 mm in diameter, many surgeons will opt for PCNL because of relatively low stone-free rates and the need for multiple procedures with the other options of ureterorenoscopy and ESWL.[3]
  - Stone density assessed by determination of the HU value. Stone fragmentation rates with ESWL are 80–100% for <500 HU, 70% for 500–1000 HU, and 25% for >1000 HU.[4] Many radiologists do not routinely report stone HU values and so the practical value of HU assessment is limited.
  - Lower pole stones >1 cm: ESWL and flexible ureterorenoscopy are less efficient. In a randomized trial of PCNL versus ESWL, PCNL achieved superior stone clearance (95% versus 21% stone-free rate).[5]
  - Lower pole anatomy: infundibulopelvic (IP) angle and infundibular (IF) length. The impact of so-called 'less favourable anatomy' (very acute IP angle (<40°) and long IF length (>3cm)) on outcomes of ESWL and flexible ureterorenoscopy is debatable.[6,7]
  - Presence of hydronephrosis: the success rate of ESWL in the presence of marked hydronephrosis is relatively poor when compared with absence of hydronephrosis (50% versus 70–80% stone clearance).[8] This may be because a proportion of patients with hydronephrosis have impaired peristalsis (hence the hydronephrosis) which prevents stone clearance after fragmentation with ESWL.

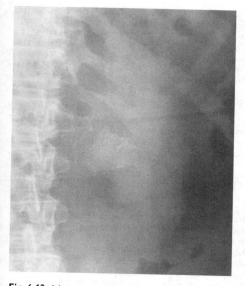

Fig. 6.12 A large stone occupying the renal pelvis. This is best treated by PCNL.

Contraindications

- Absolute:
  - Uncorrected bleeding disorders.
- Relative:
  - Pregnancy.
  - Severe respiratory disease.
  - Abnormal body configuration such that access to the stone will be technically very difficult or impossible.
  - Untreated infection (but with staghorn calculi it is not possible to render urine sterile until the stone has been removed; pre-operative loading with antibiotics may reduce sepsis rates).

Renal imaging prior to PCNL

Assess differential function of the kidney by MAG3 renography or a DMSA scan. Traditional teaching is that there is little benefit to be derived from operating on a kidney which has <10% function.

The traditional radiological method for determining the angle of approach and the most appropriate calyx for PCNL is IVU. However, IVU cannot detect whether a calyx is anterior or posterior in position and it provides only very limited information about the relationship of stones to each other within the collecting system. Clearly, it is not possible to remove a stone without knowing its precise location within the pelvi-calyceal system. CT urography (CTU) allows more accurate determination of stone location, size, and number. It also demonstrates the relationship of the planned track to adjacent organs such as the bowel. CTU sometimes demonstrates that stones thought to lie within the 'range' of a single track actually lie within geographically isolated calyces such that stone clearance may only be possible via multiple access tracks. It is sometimes apparent from the information provided by CTU that PCNL is simply not technically feasible. Increasingly we are moving towards the use of CTU as the imaging modality of choice in determining the feasibility, safety, and approach to PCNL.

Pre-operative preparation for PCNL

Culture the urine so that appropriate antibiotic prophylaxis can be given at the time of surgery. There are no hard and fast rules regarding length of antibiotic therapy prior to PCNL in those with confirmed positive urine culture. Prolonged courses run the risk of inducing resistant organisms and of causing antibiotic-associated infections such as *Clostridium difficile* induced diarrhea. Clearly, without removing the stone, eradication of infection is impossible. If no specific organism has been grown on pre-operative urine culture, we give patients 24 hr of intravenous cefuroxime prior to PCNL and intravenous gentamicin at induction of anaesthesia. This regimen is based on our local bacterial flora (yours may be different).

Group and save a serum sample in case heavy bleeding is encountered and blood transfusion is required. Most patients will require a general anaesthetic. However, patients with spinal cord injuries, absent sensation and limited respiratory function (e.g. tetraplegics) can undergo PCNL without anaesthesia, assuming they do not suffer from autonomic dysreflexia or spasms induced by manipulation of the urinary tract.

Operative technique

PCNL is the removal of a kidney stone via a 'track' developed between the surface of the skin and the collecting system of the kidney. The first step requires 'inflation' of the renal collecting system (pelvis and calyces) with fluid or air instilled via a ureteric catheter which is inserted cystoscopically (Fig. 6.13). Some surgeons also use diluted methylene blue mixed with the contrast agent, using the appearance of blue fluid from the end of the puncture needle as an indication of successful puncture of the calyceal system. Air has the advantage that it is lighter than contrast material and therefore will float up into the posterior calyces when the patient is in the prone position.

Prevent the ureteric catheter from falling out of the ureter by securing it to a urethral catheter. Aliquots of contrast media can then be injected into the collecting system of the kidney during attempts to perform needle nephrostomy puncture. Insertion of the ureteric catheter is done with the patient in a supine position. The patient is then repositioned prone to allow access to the flank for subsequent nephrostomy insertion. Pressure points are padded (e.g. feet and knees). The skin is cleansed with cleansing solution and an endo-urology drape with a plastic side pouch for the collection of irrigant fluid is positioned over the patient. A sterile drape is placed over the C-arm.

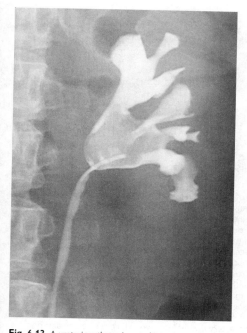

Fig. 6.13 A ureteric catheter inserted into the renal pelvis to dilate it with air or a radiocontrast agent.

The nephrostomy must be sited in such a way as to (a) allow a straight pathway into the renal calyx which contains the stone or allow access into the renal pelvis for staghorn stones and (b) minimize the risk of transecting a major renal vessel.

(a) The calyx of choice will be determined partly by the location of the stone as established by the pre-operative imaging (IVU or CTU), but also by the ease of access given the patient's morphology and position on the operating table (the kidneys will move anteriorly when the patient is moved from the supine to the prone position, and so the relationships to other structures as determined by the CT or IVU may have changed; the CT or IVU will have been done with the patient supine). Remember that the kidneys are rotated in three planes: coronally (the upper poles are more medial than the lower poles), transversely (the pelvis of the kidney lies 30° more anterior than the outer convex border), and in the sagittal plane (the kidney is angled ~10° posteriorly) (Fig. 6.14).

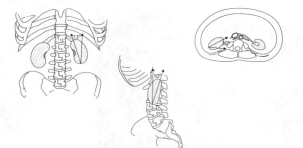

Fig. 6.14 Orientation of the kidneys in various planes. Reproduced with permission from Hinman, *Atlas of Urosurgical Anatomy*. WB Saunders, 1993.

- Knowledge of the structures surrounding the kidney helps avoid damage during the procedure. 'Overshooting' during puncture of the right kidney can lead to perforation of the right colon or duodenum, or damage to the liver or IVC. 'Overshooting' during puncture of the left kidney can lead to perforation of the splenic flexure, descending colon, or jejunum. Damage to the pancreas is rare.[9] An approach below the 12th rib is preferred to avoid the pleura (hydrothorax, haemothorax, pleural effusions, and atelectasis can occur with a supra-12th rib approach). However, access to the upper pole may only be possible by a supra-12th rib approach. Avoid hugging the lower surface of the rib which can damage the intercostal nerve and vessels (bleeding can be heavy).

(b) The main renal artery divides into two main branches: an anterior and posterior branch. The anterior division subdivides into the four anterior segmental arteries, which supply the anterior part of the kidney and the upper and lower poles (typically representing about 75% of renal blood flow). The posterior segmental artery supplies the rest of the posterior area of the kidney (typically representing about 25% of renal blood flow). However, many different arrangements on this theme occur. The segmental arteries divide into the interlobar arteries after crossing the renal sinus and become the arcuate arteries at the corticomedullary junction. Inter-*lobular* arteries branch off the arcuate arteries at right angles.

- A longitudinal depression is seen on the convex outer border of the kidney which marks the division between the distribution of the anterior and posterior branches of the renal artery. This depression is known as the white line of Brödel. It has been thought of as representing an avascular plane, but in fact Brödel himself warned against incisions in this region because he found that it would divide large branches of the anterior system. A plane posterior to the white line and just anterior to the posterior calyces represents the area of minimal vascularity between the anterior and posterior divisions of the renal artery.[10]

- In practice, it can be difficult positioning the track with such precision that it lies posterior to the white line of Brödel and just anterior to the posterior calyces, and generally a posterolateral path aimed end on to a posterior calyx is the safest way of avoiding damage to a division of the anterior and posterior branches.[11] A direct posterior puncture that is too medial risks injury to the posterior segmental artery—the artery most commonly injured in endo-urological procedures. If stones are present in an anterior calyx, puncture of anterior calyces may be required, but a posterior calyceal approach is preferred if at all possible. Avoid direct puncture of the renal pelvis because (i) a posterior branch of the renal artery may be damaged (in general terms, the more medial the puncture, the greater the risk of injuring larger branches of the renal artery) and (ii) the track will be unstable and therefore the nephroscope may easily slip out of the kidney (a transparenchymal puncture stabilizes the nephrostomy tube within the kidney).

With X-ray control and a haemostat to hold the needle (to avoid irradiating the surgeon's hand), an 18-gauge translumbar angiography needle is advanced towards the chosen calyx (Fig. 6.15). Confirmation that the needle is within the calyx is obtained by aspiration of air or fluid (whichever has been used to inflate the collecting system). Once the nephrostomy needle is in the calyx a guidewire is inserted into the renal pelvis to act as a guide over which the 'track' is dilated (Fig. 6.16). A 1 cm skin incision is made. The needle is removed, leaving the guidewire in place.

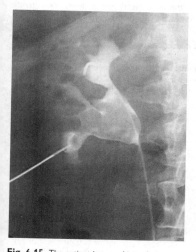

Fig. 6.15 The patient is turned into the prone position and a nephrostomy needle is inserted into a lower pole calyx.

Track dilatation can be achieved using fascial or balloon dilatation. Fascial dilators such as the Amplatz system consist of an 8Fr Polytef catheter (Cook Urological) tapered to fit over a 0.038 inch guidewire, over which a series of progressively larger polyurethane catheters are passed. An alternative system is the Alken coaxial dilator system which consists of stainless steel dilators of progressively larger size. Balloon dilatation is said to be faster, and therefore to involve less radiation, since it dilates the track to 30Ch in a single step rather than sequentially (a high-pressure balloon is used capable of developing 15 atm of pressure). However, the difference in radiation dose in the hands of an experienced surgeon or radiologist using his or her preferred technique of dilatation is probably fairly small. There is no good evidence to suggest that one technique is any better than the other in terms of minimizing haemorrhage, so use the technique you feel most comfortable with. An access sheath is passed over the dilator, down the track, and into the calyx, and a nephroscope can be advanced through this into the kidney. Use saline for irrigation to avoid causing hyponatremia from absorption of hypotonic irrigant fluids.

Use a Calcuson probe, inserted down the instrument channel of the nephroscope, to fragment the stone (Figs. 6.17–6.18, 📖 Fig. 6.6). Activate it in short bursts (~5 sec) to stop it from overheating. From time to time tighten the bolt that holds the probe onto the transducer; this tends to be loosened by the very-high-frequency vibration generated by the ultrasound transducer.

Large staghorn calculi may make placement of a guidewire in the collecting system difficult since, by occupying so much of the collecting system, they prevent passage of the wire into the renal pelvis. Very gentle dilatation is required to prevent displacement of the guidewire from within the collecting system.

Change in renal function as a consequence of track formation

Functional studies in both animals and humans have demonstrated that the reduction in renal function as a consequence of damage to functioning renal tissue during track formation is minimal.[12,13]

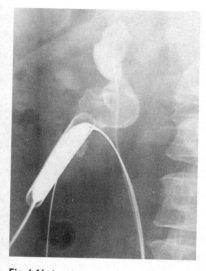

Fig. 6.16 A guidewire is inserted into the renal pelvis and down the ureter. The track is dilated over this guidewire using, in this case, a fascial balloon dilator.

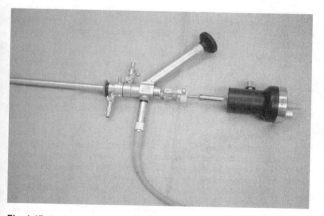

Fig. 6.17 The Calcuson probe in the instrument channel of the nephroscope.

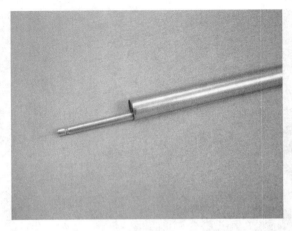

Fig. 6.18 The Calcuson probe extending from the end of the nephroscope.

Stone fragmentation techniques used during PCNL

A variety of instruments are used to fragment the stone and evacuate or remove the fragments.

- Ultrasonic probes fragment stones by shaking them to pieces at very high frequencies, and the fragmented stone is simultaneously sucked out through the centre of the probe. Provides 'industrial' stone removal, i.e. very efficient.
- Electrohydraulic lithotripsy; the advent of ultrasonic lithotripsy has made this a historical technique.
- Holmium laser lithotripsy: since this is a contact laser and the fibre diameter is small, this is a very inefficient form of lithotripsy for large renal stones.
- Pneumatic lithotripsy: very effective form of fragmentation. Fragments must be removed piecemeal, and therefore it is rather laborious compared with ultrasonic lithotripsy. Stone grabbers are used to remove large fragments.

Optimizing stone-free rates

Single-track puncture does not always allow access to every stone. Flexible nephroscopes can be used to negotiate a path around corners to otherwise inaccessible stones. Alternatively, flexible ureterorenoscopy can be carried out simultaneously, the aim being to limit the need for multiple punctures and thereby the associated morbidity (principally bleeding).[14] Following placement of a guidewire into the ureter and renal pelvis, an access sheath is placed to allow easy passage of the flexible ureteroscope. Stones in calyces that are likely to be inaccessible via the planned access track can either be fragmented with a holmium laser or moved, using a stone basket, to a site where they will be accessible. The patient can then be positioned prone to allow the percutaneous track to be made.

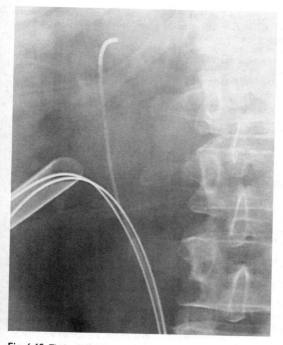

Fig. 6.19 The stone has been completely removed.

Post-operative nephrostomy drainage

The majority of surgeons place a nephrostomy tube post-PCNL, and these are designed for placement over a guidewire. This provides drainage of urine, can tamponade bleeding from the track, and, by keeping the track open, allows the possibility of 're-entry' into the collecting system if post-operative imaging shows incomplete stone clearance. A number of different types are available: locking pigtail catheters, Malecot catheters (Fig. 6.20), catheters with retaining balloons, Cope loop catheters, and circle loop catheters.

Nephrostomy tubes come in various sizes. Many surgeons prefer large-bore tubes (24–30Ch) to allow continued drainage of urine in the presence of heavy haematuria. Some use smaller-calibre tubes, but these can become blocked by clots and stone debris. The nephrostomy tube is usually removed on the second or third post-operative day.

There are two types of Malecot catheters—with and without a tail. An introducer is inserted through the catheter to straighten out the flanges and is locked into the Luer-Lok at the end of the tube. The Malecot catheter allows re-entry to the collecting system (hence Malecot catheters are known as re-entry nephrostomy tubes) to allow a 'second look' if residual stones require removal.

We leave the nephrostomy tube for approximately 24–48 hr post-PCNL and obtain a nephrostogram to check that there is free antegrade flow of contrast down the ureter (to exclude fragments of stone that have migrated into the ureter).

Tube-free PCNL

Tubeless or tube-free PCNL is feasible in selected patients. The aim is to avoid the discomfort associated with large bore nephrostomy tubes. A reduction in post-operative pain has been reported, but this approach prevents the facility for second-look PCNL if post-operative imaging after the first PCNL demonstrates residual stone fragments. Of course, such stone fragments can be managed by other techniques (ESWL or flexible ureterorenoscopy) if they are small, but if they are large, re-look PCNL may be the only sensible option.

Pain associated with the post-operative nephrostomy can be minimized by avoiding an intercostal tube location (avoid supra-12th rib puncture if possible).

Tube-free PCNL should be avoided if:
- There is a large volume of residual stone, such that a second PCNL is likely to be needed.
- There has been a pyonephrosis.
- Two or more access tracks have been required.
- There is evidence of bleeding.

Outcomes and complications of PCNL

Outcomes
- Small stones: the stone-free rate after PCNL is of the order of 90–95%.
- Staghorn stones: the stone-free rate after PCNL, combined with post-operative ESWL for residual stone fragments, is of the order of 80–85%.

Complications

Iatrogenic renal injury: renal haemorrhage after PCNL

PCNL is the surgical equivalent of a stab wound and serious haemorrhage (necessitating some form of intervention) occurs in approximately 1% of patients.[15,16]

Bleeding during or after PCNL can occur from vessels in the nephrostomy track itself, from an arteriovenous fistula, from an arteriocalyceal fistula, or from a pseudo-aneurysm which has ruptured. Track bleeding will usually tamponade around a large-bore nephrostomy tube, but this does not always control the bleeding.

Requirement for blood transfusion post-PCNL

There is a wide reported range of the percentage of patients requiring transfusion (3–23%).[17,18] Transfusion is more likely to be required for large complex stones (approximately 10%) and where an aggressive approach to stone clearance is undertaken. Not surprisingly, bleeding is

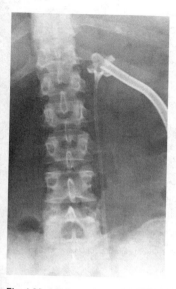

Fig. 6.20 A Malecot catheter used for drainage of the renal pelvis post-PCNL. Note the long tail extending into the ureter. Reproduced with permission from Reynard et al, 2006, *Oxford Handbook of Urology*, Oxford University Press.

likely to be more severe, and therefore the need for transfusion greater, with increasing number of punctures. Martin et al.[16] reported that when one or two punctures were required blood transfusion was necessary in 20% of cases, whereas when more than two punctures were required 40% of patients needed blood transfusion.

Traditional advice for control of persistent bleeding through the nephrostomy tube is to clamp the nephrostomy tube and wait for the clot to tamponade the bleeding. While this may control bleeding in some cases, in others a rising or persistently elevated pulse rate (with later hypotension) indicates the possibility of persistent bleeding and is an indication for renal arteriography and embolization of the arteriovenous fistula or pseudoaneurysm if found. Continued bleeding into the retroperitoneum can occur despite clamping the nephrostomy tube, and this may lead to haemodynamic compromise (Figs 6.21 and 6.22). Failure to stop the bleeding by embolization is an indication for renal exploration and control of the bleeding by the techniques described in 📖 Chapter 8.

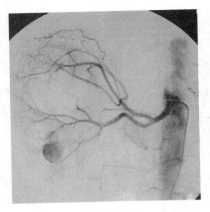

Fig. 6.21 Renal arteriography after PCNL where severe bleeding was encountered. An arteriovenous fistula has been found and is about to be embolized. Reproduced with permission from Reynard et al, 2006, *Oxford Handbook of Urology*, Oxford University Press.

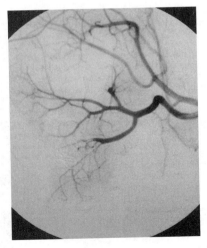

Fig. 6.22 Post-embolization of arteriovenous fistula (post-PCNL). Note the embolization coils in the lower pole. Reproduced with permission from Reynard et al, 2006, *Oxford Handbook of Urology*, Oxford University Press.

Arteriovenous or arteriocalyceal fistulae can sometimes occur following open renal surgery for stones or tumours, and again arteriography with embolization can be used to stop the bleeding in these cases. The bleeding usually occurs over a longer time course (days or even weeks), rather than as acute haemorrhage causing shock.

Sepsis
Septic shock occurs in 0.25–1.5% of patients undergoing percutaneous stone removal.[17,19,20] Probable infective organisms include *Proteus*, *Klebsiella*, *Enterobacter*, *Serratia*, and *Pseudomonas*, as well as *Escherichia coli*.

Pleural injury (pneumothorax), haemothorax, and pleural effusion
More likely with a supra-12th rib approach. Pleural effusion is said to occur in 10% of cases with a supra-12th rib approach.[21] Placement of a chest drain may be required.

Perforation of the renal pelvis
Consider placing an antegrade ureteral stent as well as leaving a nephrostomy tube, removing them when a contrast study shows no leak.[21,22]

Colonic perforation
Rare. It is more likely to occur in patients with a retrorenal colon. It is said to occur in ~0.5% of cases.[23] Perforation may be apparent at the time of operation or it may present in the post-operative period with sepsis, peritonitis (with intraperitoneal perforation), and drainage of faeces or gas either around or through the nephrostomy tube, or from the nephrostomy site following tube removal. There may be no symptoms, with the perforation being diagnosed only on the post-operative nephrostogram when contrast is seen within the colon.

Perforation of the duodenum
The diagnosis is made on the post-operative nephrostogram, which demonstrates a nephroduodenal fistula. Management is conservative: placement of a nephrostomy tube and a nasogastric tube to divert gastric secretions. A contrast study is repeated ~2 weeks post-operatively.[24]

Injury to the spleen and liver
Splenic injury is rare, although higher in patients with splenomegaly. Haemorrhage will usually be great and emergency laparotomy with splenectomy is usually required. Injuries to the liver are less common than those to the spleen (although more common with hepatomegaly). Conservative management (transfusion, bed rest) is usually successful, although open surgical exploration may be required.

Ureteric colic due to fragments of stones or blood clots in the ureter
This can usually be managed conservatively. Failure of stones to pass spontaneously can be managed using conventional techniques such as ESWL or ureteroscopic stone fragmentation.

Pancreatitis
Rare.[9]

Nephrocutaneous fistula
Rare. It can occur in the context of distal obstruction from a ureteric stone or blood clot. If drainage of urine from the site of the nephrostomy track is persistent, place a JJ stent or perform ureteroscopy to remove a ureteric stone if present.

Further reading

1 Thiruchelvam N, Mostafid H, Ubhayakar G. Planning percutaneous nephrolithotomy using multidetector computed tomography urography, multiplanar reconstruction and three-dimensional reformatting. *BJU Int* 2005; **95**:1280–4.

References

1 Grasso M, Conlin M, Bagley D. Retrograde ureteropyeloscopic treatment of 2 cm or greater upper urinary tract and minor staghorn calculi. *J Urol* 1998; **160**:346–51.

2 Segura JW, Preminger GM, Assimos DG et al. Nephrolithiasis clinical guidelines panel summary report on the management of staghorn calculi. *J Urol* 1994; **151**:1648–51.

3 Rudnick DM, Bennett PM, Dretler SP. Retrograde renoscopic fragmentation of moderate-size (1.5–3.0cm) renal cystine stones. *J Endourol* 1999; **13**:483–5.

4 Joseph P, Mandal AK, Singh SK et al. Computerized tomography attenuation value of renal calculus: can it predict successful fragmentation of the calculus by extracorporeal shock wave lithotripsy? A preliminary study. *J Urol* 2002; **167**:1968–71.

5 Albala DM, Assimos DG, Clayman RV et al. Lower pole I: a prospective randomized trial of extracorporeal shock wave lithotripsy and percutaneous nephrostolithotomy for lower pole nephrolithiasis—initial results. *J Urol* 2001; **166**:2072–2080.

6 Moody JA, Williams JC, Lingeman JE. Lower pole renal anatomy: effects on stone clearance after shock wave lithotripsy in a randomized population. *J Urol* 1999; **161**:378.

7 Madbouly K, Sheir KZ, Elsobky E. Impact of lower pole anatomy on stone clearance after shock wave lithotripsy: fact or fiction. *J Urol* 2001; **165**:1415–18.

8 Poulakis V, Dahm P, Witzsch U et al. Prediction of lower pole stone clearance after shock wave lithotripsy using an artificial neural network. *J Urol* 2003; **169**:1250–6.

9 Zagoria RJ, Dyer RB. Do's and don't's of percutaneous nephrostomy. *Acad Radiol* 1999; **6**:370–7.

10 Brödel M. The intrinsic blood vessels of the kidney and their significance in nephrotomy. Johns Hopkins Hosp Bull 1901; **12**:10–13.

11 Sampaio FJ. The dilemma of the crossing vessel of the uretopelvic junction: precise anatomic study. *J. Endourol* 1996; **10**:411–5.

12 Webb DR, Fitzpatrick JM. Percutaneous nephrolithotripsy: a functional and morphological study. *J Urol* 1985; **134**:587–91.

13 Chatham JR, Dykes TE, Kennon WG et al. Effect of percutaneous nephrolithotomy on differential renal function as measured by mercaptoacetyl triglycine nuclear renography. Urology 2002; **59**:522–5.

14 Marguet CG, Springhart WP, Tan YH et al. Simultaneous combined use of flexible ureteroscopy and percutaneous nephrolithotomy to reduce the number of access tracts in the management of complex renal calculi. *BJU Int* 2005; **96**:1097–1100.

15 Kessaris DN, Bellman GC, Pardalidis NP, Smith AG. Management of hemorrhage after percutaneous renal surgery. *J Urol* 1995; **153**:604–8.

16 Martin X, Murat FJ, Feitosa LC et al. Severe bleeding after nephrolithotomy: results of hyperselective embolization. *Eur Urol* 2000; **37**:136–9.

17 Segura JW, Patterson DE, LeRoy AJ et al. Percutaneous removal of kidney stones: review of 1000 cases. *J Urol* 1985; **134**:1077.

18 Stoller ML, Wolf JS, Jr, St Lezin MA. Estimated blood loss and transfusion rates associated with percutaneous nephrolithotomy. *J Urol* 1994; **152**:1977.

19 Rao PN, Dube DA, Weightman NC et al. Prediction of septicemia following endourological manipulation for stones in the upper urinary tract. *J Urol* 1991; **146**:955.

20 O'Keefe NK, Mortimer AJ, Sambrook PA et al. Severe sepsis following percutaneous or endoscopic procedures for urinary tract stones. *Br J Urol* 1993; **72**:277–83.

21 Pardalidis N, Smith AD Complications of stone treatment. In *Controversies in Endourology*, ed. Smith AD. Philadelphia, PA: WB Saunders, 1995, pp 179–85.

22 Dyer RB, Assimos DG, Regan JD Update on interventional uroradiology. *Urol Clin North Am* 1997; **24**:623.

23 Hadar H, Gadoth N. Positional relations of colon and kidney determined by perirenal fat. *Am J Roentgenol* 1984; **143**:773–6.

24 Culkin DJ, Wheeler JS, Jr, Canning JR. Nephro-duodenal fistula: a complication of percutaneous nephrolithotomy. *J Urol* 1985; **134**:528.

Stones at the pelvi-ureteric junction

It can be difficult to determine if stones which sit directly within the PUJ and are causing presumed obstruction (suggested by the presence of hydronephrosis) or confirmed obstruction (confirmed by MAG3 renography) are caused by a primary PUJO (through urinary stasis) or are themselves the cause of obstruction (a secondary cause of PUJO). Our policy and that of others is to treat the stone first, by PCNL if large and by ureteroscopy if small (ESWL is contraindicated in the presence of PUJO), allow a period of several weeks for any oedema caused by the presence of the stone to resolve, and then arrange a MAG3 renogram. The disadvantage of this approach is the need for a second procedure (e.g. antegrade endopyelotomy or laparoscopic pyeloplasty) at a later date. An alternative is to perform a combined PCNL and antegrade endopyelotomy. However, a proportion of such cases (the precise proportion being poorly defined) will have no primary PUJO and will therefore undergo an unnecessary procedure which is not without risk. As with so many problems in surgery, there is no correct answer, given the current evidence base.

Where a PCNL alone is performed and the post-operative nephrostogram shows no free flow of contrast past the PUJ (assuming that there is no residual fragment of obstructing stone), consider placement of a J stent before removing the nephrostomy. The J stent encourages antegrade flow of urine through the PUJ, allowing the PCNL track to heal and thereby discouraging the development of a nephrocutaneous fistula. Remove the stent after 2 weeks and then arrange a MAG3 renogram to determine if there is indeed a PUJO. If there is, and the patient develops loin pain characteristic of a PUJO, consider pyeloplasty. If the patient remains symptom free (no loin pain), the options include watchful waiting with serial MAG3 renograms to identify any decline in function (which would be an indication for pyeloplasty) or a pyeloplasty to reduce the subsequent risk of recurrent stone formation.

Open stone surgery

Indications

- Complex stone burden (projection of stone into multiple calyces, such that multiple PCNL tracks would be required to gain access to all the stone) (Fig. 6.23).
- Failure of endoscopic treatment (technical difficulty gaining access to the collecting system of the kidney, either ureterorenoscopically or percutaneously).
- Anatomical abnormality that precludes endoscopic surgery, e.g. retro-renal colon.
- Body habitus that precludes endoscopic surgery, e.g. gross obesity, kyphoscoliosis (open stone surgery can be difficult).
- Patient request for a single procedure where multiple PCNLs might be required for stone clearance.
- Non-functioning kidney.

Non-functioning kidney

Where the kidney is not working, the stone may, if relatively small, be left *in situ* if it is not causing symptoms (e.g. pain, recurrent urinary infection, haematuria). However, staghorn calculi should be removed, unless the patient has comorbidity that would preclude safe surgery, because there is a substantial risk of developing serious infective complications if the stone is left *in situ* (📖 p. 379). If the kidney is non-functioning the simplest way of removing the stone is to remove the kidney.

Functioning kidneys: options for stone removal

Small to medium sized stones

- Pyelolithotomy.
- Radical nephrolithotomy.

Staghorn calculi

- Anatrophic (avascular) nephrolithotomy.
- Extended pyelolithotomy with radial nephrotomies (small incisions over individual stones).
- Excision of the kidney, 'bench' surgery to remove the stones, and autotransplantation.

Operative technique

Pre-operative preparation

Culture the urine and, if organisms are grown, start an appropriate antibiotic 24–48 hr in advance of surgery.

Pyelolithotomy

Flank (supra-12th) or anterior subcostal extraperitoneal incision (a subcostal incision is usually too low). Divide the skin immediately above and parallel to the 12th rib. Extend it for 5–6 cm anterior to the tip of the rib (further if you think greater access will be required). Divide the subcutaneous fat down onto latissimus dorsi (overlying the rib) and external oblique. Divide latissimus dorsi as it lies over the rib, again keeping the

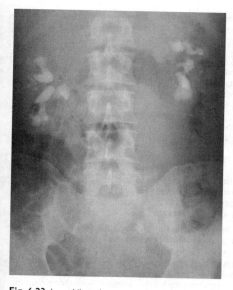

Fig. 6.23 Large bilateral stones involving multiple calyces. Several PCNL tracks would be required to gain access to all the stone.

line of the incision parallel with the top surface of the rib, and deep to latissimus dorsi divide serratus posterior. Just anterior to the tip of the 12th rib divide external oblique and beneath it internal oblique and transverses abdominis. Insert your index and middle finger and sweep them anteriorly to push the peritoneum out of harm's way. Beneath the divided latissimus dorsi will lie the intercostal muscles, which are divided from anterior to posterior (heading towards the vertebral column) along the top of the rib, taking care not to damage the underlying pleura. Divide the diaphragm as it inserts into the abdominal wall. For additional access, divide the costovertebral ligament so that the 12th rib can be swung downwards.

If you make a hole in the pleura a sudden escape of air during expiration will be heard. Divide fibres of attached diaphragm to reduce tension of the pleura and close the hole with a 4–0 absorbable suture, asking the anaesthetist to forcibly expand the lungs as you tie your last stitch so that residual air is forced out. Fill the wound with saline and ask the anaesthetist to expand the lung to check that no bubbles of air are escaping. Get a chest X-ray post-operatively.

The goal now is to expose an adequate area of the renal pelvis such that the stone can be removed through a renal pelvis incision. This incision avoids damaging any of the renal parenchyma. Start by opening

Gerota's fascia. Dissect the fat off the kidney until the kidney can be grasped by your assistant, who should then swing it towards the midline, in so doing exposing the posterior aspect of the kidney and thus the renal pelvis (the renal vein and artery lie anteriorly). Identify the ureter and encircle it with a sling. Using the ureter as a guide, work up towards the renal pelvis. Carefully dissect the fat off the posterior aspect of the renal pelvis. Insert stay sutures on either side of your intended incision line in the renal pelvis. Incise the pelvis transversely (roughly at a right angle to the line of the ureter) starting with a blade and using Pott's scissors to continue the incision, extending this as necessary in a U-shape, but keeping away from the PUJ (Figs 6.24 and 6.25). If there are small stones, pass a small catheter (8Ch) through the PUJ and down the ureter, to prevent migration of stones into the ureter. Use stone forceps to remove the stones. Stones that cannot be seen can be found using a flexible cystoscope inserted into the calyces.

Ask the anaesthetist to inflate the lung to check that there has been no inadvertent pleural injury. Close the incision with a 4–0 absorbable suture. Place a tube drain down to the closure line. Cover the pelvis in fat and close Gerota's fascia. Close the wound.

Extended pyelolithotomy (intra-sinusal pyeloinfundibulotomy) with radial nephrotomies (small incisions over individual stones)

This is done where stone extends into the calyces and, because of its size, cannot be pulled through the neck of the calyx without opening the latter. The approach is the same as for simple pyelolithotomy, but the plane between the kidney and each calyx involved with stone must be developed.

A thin film of fascia extending between the capsule of the kidney overlying the renal cortex and the renal pelvis is divided. Develop this plane by inserting a pair of curved scissors and gently spread them apart. Keep close to the wall of the renal pelvis. In so doing, the renal vessels will lift off with the perihilar fat. Use Gil-Vernet retractors to help exposure of this plane. Exposure of the renal artery and temporary clamping with a bulldog clamp can help by reducing the turgor of the renal parenchyma. Make an incision in the renal pelvis and extend this towards the neck of each involved calyx. For stones which cannot be removed through a tight calyceal neck, make radial nephrotomies over the stone and remove them through the renal parenchyma using a stone forceps to grasp it. The interlobar arteries, which are second-order branches from the renal artery, bifurcate at the base of each major calyx and follow a radial course towards the renal cortex where they form the arcuate arteries from which the afferent arterioles are derived. As a consequence, a radial nephrotomy, which extends from the cortex inwards towards the papilla, will avoid injury to arteries. Each nephrotomy need only be 1–2 cm in length.

If you cannot feel the stone through the parenchyma, grasp it with a stone forceps and push this towards the cortex. If you still cannot feel it, gently probe with a needle to 'sound' for the stone.

Close any nephrotomies you have made using absorbable sutures over bolsters of fat or Surgicel.® Close as for pyelolithotomy.

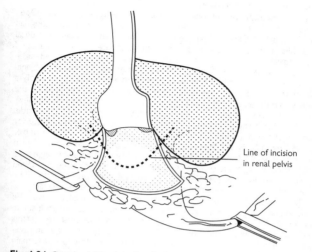

Fig. 6.24 Open pyelolithotomy: the incision in the renal pelvis. Reproduced from Blandy and Fowler, *Urology*, 2nd edn, 1996, Blackwell. Permission sought.

Line of incision in renal pelvis

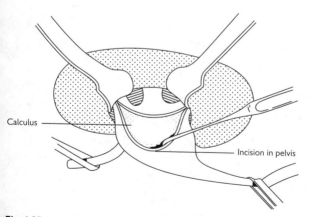

Calculus

Incision in pelvis

Fig. 6.25 The renal pelvis has been opened and the incision extended with Pott's scissors to expose the stone. Reproduced from Blandy and Fowler, *Urology*, 2nd edn, 1996, Blackwell. Permission sought.

Anatrophic nephrolithotomy
Flank (supra-12th) or anterior subcostal extraperitoneal incision. Open
Gerota's fascia. Expose the parenchyma of the kidney by dissecting off
the attached fat. Carefully expose the renal artery and its main segmental
branches (anterior and posterior). Place slings of different colours around
the arterial branches so that individual arteries can be clamped independently of each other (Fig. 6.26). There is no need to expose the renal
pelvis. Ask the anaesthetist to administer intravenous mannitol. Apply a
clamp to the posterior segmental artery and observe the area of the
kidney that blanches (this will be on the posterior surface of the kidney).
Mark the border of this area with light touches of the diathermy blade.
This is Brödel's line—the intersegmental (between anterior and posterior
segments) avascular (relatively) plane (Fig. 6.27). This line can be better
defined by intravenous injection of 10–20 mL of methylene blue, which
then diffuses into the kidney through the unclamped anterior segmental
arteries, colouring these regions blue, while the avascular segment supplied
by the posterior segmental artery is blanched. This procedure can be
repeated with other segmental arteries as required. Release the clamp.

Now cut a hole in a bowel bag to allow the bag to be placed over the
kidney. Place large dry swabs around the outside of the bag to insulate
the kidney from the surrounding body wall. Get the ice slush ready (this
will have been prepared previously). Ask the anaesthetist to give intravenous mannitol. Wait for this to circulate. Then apply a clamp to the main
renal artery. Place the ice slush around the kidney and leave it in place
for about 10 min to allow the kidney to cool. Incise the parenchyma of

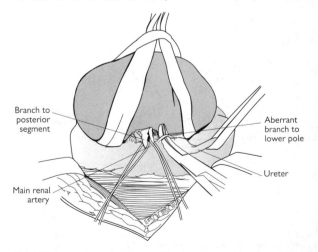

Branch to
posterior
segment

Aberrant
branch to
lower pole

Ureter

Main renal
artery

Fig. 6.26 Anatrophic nephrolithotomy. Slings have been positioned around the
renal vessels.

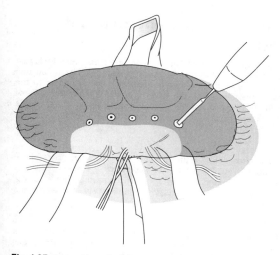

Fig. 6.27 Anatrophic nephrolithotomy. Brödel's line—the inter segmental avascular plane.

the kidney, if possible over the previously marked avascular line. Cut down onto the stone and extend the incision with Pott's scissors. Free the stone with forceps and remove it. Repair each opened calyx with a 5–0 absorbable suture. Avoid narrowing calyceal necks. Release the arterial clamp, and identify and suture ligate bleeding arteries and veins using figure-of-eight suture placement. Close the capsule with a continuous 4–0 absorbable suture. Place a drain. Close the wound.

Another option for open stone removal, depending on stone size and location, is lower pole partial nephrectomy.

Specific complications of open stone surgery

- Wound infection (the stones operated on are often infection stones).
- Flank hernia.
- Wound pain.
- Pneumothorax from pleural damage.
- Stricture of the PUJ if the pyelotomy incision has extended through the PUJ.

With PCNL these problems do not occur (apart from an occasional pneumothorax), blood transfusion rate is lower, analgesic requirement less, mobilization more rapid, and discharge earlier, all of which account for PCNL having replaced open surgery as the mainstay of treatment of large stones. There is a significant chance of stone recurrence after open stone surgery (as for any other treatment modality), and the scar tissue that develops around the kidney will make subsequent open stone surgery technically more difficult.

Ureteric stones: presentation and diagnosis

Ureteric stones usually present with sudden onset of severe flank pain which is colicky (waves of increasing severity are followed by a reduction in severity, but it seldom goes away completely). It may radiate to the groin as the stone passes into the lower ureter. Approximately 50% of patients with classic symptoms for a ureteric stone do not have a stone confirmed on subsequent imaging studies, nor do they physically ever pass a stone.[1]

Examination

Spend a few seconds looking at the patient. Ureteric stone pain is colicky—the patient moves around, trying to find a comfortable position. They may be doubled up with pain. Patients with conditions causing peritonitis (e.g. appendicitis, a ruptured ectopic pregnancy) lie very still. Movement and abdominal palpation are very painful.

Pregnancy test

Arrange a pregnancy test in pre-menopausal women (this is mandatory in any pre-menopausal woman who is going to undergo imaging using ionizing radiation). If positive, suggesting rupture of an ectopic pregnancy, refer to the gynaecologists; if negative, arrange imaging to determine whether they have a ureteric stone.

Dipstick or microscopic haematuria

Many patients with ureteric stones have dipstick or microscopic haematuria (and, more rarely, macroscopic haematuria), but 10–30% have no blood in their urine.[2,3]

The sensitivity of dipstick haematuria for detecting ureteric stones presenting acutely[3] is shown below:

- 95% on the first day of pain.
- 85% on the second day.
- 65% on the third and fourth days.

Thus, patients with a ureteric stone whose pain started 3–4 days ago may not have blood detectable in their urine. Dipstick testing is slightly more sensitive than urine microscopy for detecting stones (80% versus 70%) because blood cells lyse, and therefore disappear, if the urine specimen is not examined under the microscope within a few hours. Both ways of detecting haematuria have roughly the same specificity for diagnosing ureteric stones—about 60%. This means that the presence of blood in the urine in a patient with loin pain certainly does not mean a ureteric stone is present—the false positive rate for stones is high.

Remember, blood in the urine on dipstick testing or microscopy may be a coincidental finding, because of non-stone urological disease (e.g. neoplasm, infection) or a false-positive test (no abnormality is found in approximately 70% of patients with microscopic haematuria, despite full urological investigation).

Temperature

The most important aspect of examination in a patient with a ureteric stone confirmed on imaging is to measure their temperature. If the patient has a ureteric stone and a fever, they may have infection proximal to the stone. A fever in the presence of an obstructing stone is an indication for urine and blood culture, intravenous fluids and antibiotics, and nephrostomy drainage if the fever does not resolve within a matter of hours.

References

1 Smith RC, Verga M, McCarthy S, Rosenfield AT. Diagnosis of acute flank pain: value of unen-hanced helical CT. *Am J Roentgenol* 1996; **166**:97–101.

2 Luchs JS, Katz DS, Lane DS *et al.* Utility of hematuria testing in patients with suspected renal colic: correlation with unenhanced helical CT results. *Urology* 2002; **59**:839.

3 Kobayashi T, Nishizawa K, Mitsumori K, Ogura K. Impact of date of onset on the absence of hematuria in patients with acute renal colic. *J Urol* 2003; **1770**:1093–6.

Ureteric stones: diagnostic radiological imaging

The intravenous urogram (IVU), for many years the mainstay of imaging in patients with flank pain, has been replaced by CT urography (CTU) (Fig. 6.28). Compared with IVU, CTU:

- Has greater specificity (95%) and sensitivity (97%) for diagnosing ureteric stones[1]—it can identify other, non-stone, causes of flank pain (Fig. 6.29).
- Requires no contrast administration so avoiding the chance of a contrast reaction (risk of fatal anaphylaxis following the administration of low-osmolality contrast media for IVU is in the order of 1 in 100000[2]).
- Is faster, taking just a few minutes to image the kidneys and ureters. An IVU, particularly where delayed films are required to identify a stone causing high-grade obstruction, may take hours to identify the precise location of the obstructing stone.
- Is equivalent in cost to IVU in hospitals where high volumes of CT scans are done.[3]

If you only have access to IVU, remember that it is contraindicated in patients with a history of previous contrast reactions and should be avoided in those with hay fever, a strong history of allergies or asthma who have not been pre-treated with high-dose steroids 24 hr before the IVU. Patients taking metformin for diabetes should stop this for 48 hr prior to an IVU. Clearly, being able to perform an alternative test such as CTU in such patients is very useful.

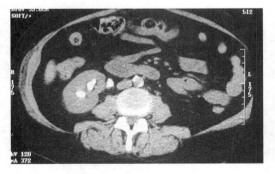

Fig. 6.28 A CT urogram. Reproduced with permission from Reynard *et al*, 2006, *Oxford Handbook of Urology*, Oxford University Press.

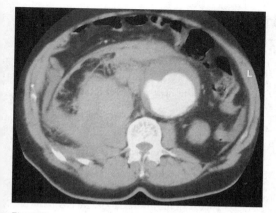

Fig. 6.29 A leaking aortic aneurysm identified on a CTU in a patient with loin pain. Reproduced with permission from Reynard et al, 2006, *Oxford Handbook of Urology*, Oxford University Press.

Where 24-hr CTU access is not available, admit patients with suspected ureteric colic for pain relief and arrange a CTU the following morning. When CT urography is not immediately available (between the hours of midnight and 8 am) we arrange urgent abdominal ultrasonography in all patients aged >50 years who present with flank pain suggestive of a possible stone to exclude serious pathology such as a leaking abdominal aortic aneurysm and to demonstrate any other gross abnormalities due to non-stone-associated flank pain.

Plain abdominal X-ray and renal ultrasound are not sufficiently sensitive or specific for routine use for diagnosing stones.

MR urography

This is an accurate way of determining whether a stone is present in the ureter or not[4]. However, at the present time, cost and restricted availability limit its usefulness as a routine diagnostic method of imaging in cases of acute flank pain. This may change as MR scanners become more widely available.

References

1 Smith RC, Verga M, McCarthy S, Rosenfield AT. Diagnosis of acute flank pain: value of unenhanced helical CT. *Am J Roentgenol* 1996; **166**:97–101.
2 Caro JJ, Trindale E, McGregor M. The risks of death and severe non-fatal reactions with high vs low osmolality contrast media. *Am J Roentgenol* 1991; **156**:825–32.
3 Thomson JM, Glocer J, Abbott C *et al.* Computed tomography versus intravenous urography in diagnosis of acute flank pain from urolithiasis: a randomized study comparing imaging costs and radiation dose. *Australas Radiol* 2001; **45**:291–7.
4 Louca G, Liberopoulos K, Fidas A *et al.* MR urography in the diagnosis of urinary tract obstruction. *Eur Urol* 1999; **35**:14.

Ureteric stones: acute management

While appropriate imaging studies are being organized, give pain relief.

- An NSAID, e.g. diclofenac (Voltarol) by intramuscular or intravenous injection, by mouth or per rectum provides rapid and effective pain control. The analgesic effect is partly anti-inflammatory and partly by reducing ureteric peristalsis.
- Where NSAIDS are inadequate, opiate analgesics such as pethidine or morphine are added.
- Calcium channel antagonists, e.g. nifedipine, may reduce the pain of ureteric colic by reducing the frequency of ureteric contractions.[1,2]

There is no need to encourage the patient to drink copious amounts of fluids or to give them large volumes of fluids intravenously in the hope that this will 'flush' the stone out. Renal blood flow and urine output from the affected kidney falls during an episode of acute, partial obstruction due to a stone. Excess urine output will tend to cause a greater degree of hydronephrosis in the affected kidney which will make ureteric peristalsis even less efficient than it already is (peristalsis, the forward propulsion of a bolus of urine down the ureter, can only occur if the walls of the ureter above the bolus of urine can coapt, i.e. close firmly together. If they cannot, as occurs in a ureter distended with urine, the bolus of urine cannot move distally).

Watchful waiting

In many instances, small ureteric stones will pass spontaneously within days or a few weeks, with analgesic supplements for exacerbations of pain.

Data on the rate of spontaneous stone passage are surprisingly limited.[3] Chances of spontaneous stone passage depend principally on stone size. Of stones 5 mm or less, 68% will pass spontaneously (95% CI 46–85%; meta-analysis of 224 patients); 47% of stones 6–10 mm in diameter will pass spontaneously (95% CI 36–59%; meta-analysis of 104 patients)[3]. The average time for spontaneous stone passage for stones 4–6 mm in diameter is 3 weeks.[4] Stones that have not passed in 2 months are unlikely to do so. Of those stones that do eventually pass, those 2 mm or less do so within 30 days, and those 2–6 mm in size do so within 40 days (but not all stones do pass and we cannot predict the chance of spontaneous passage in the *individual* patient). Therefore, accurate determination of stone size (on plain abdominal X-ray or by CTU) helps predict chances of spontaneous stone passage.

Medical expulsive therapy (MET)

There is growing evidence for the efficacy of MET,[3,5] the preferred agents being the smooth muscle-relaxing alpha-1 adrenergic adrenoceptor blockers. These increase spontaneous stone passage rates, reduce stone passage time, and reduce frequency of ureteric colic. The EAU/AUA Nephrolithiasis Guideline Panel meta-analysis showed that 29% more patients (CI 20–37%) taking tamsulosin passed their stones compared to controls.[3] Tamsulosin has been most studied in this setting, but terazosin and doxazosin seem to be equally effective. Whether stones in all segments of the ureter are equally responsive to alpha blockers remains to be determined.

In the same meta-analysis there was no significant difference in stone passage rates between those taking the calcium channel blocker nifedipine and control patients.

Glyceryl trinitrate patches do not aid stone passage or reduce frequency of pain episodes[6] and corticosteroids are of minimal, if any, benefit.[1-3]

A trial of MET is a very reasonable approach for many patients, but individual circumstances may dictate 'up-front' ESWL or ureteroscopy, e.g. the possible disruption to work and daily living activities from episodes of pain occurring while a stone is progressing towards eventual spontaneous passage may prompt the patient to request ESWL or ureteroscopy (e.g. commercial airline pilots cannot fly until stone-free, nor can those who fly for leisure).

MET is contraindicated where there is clinical evidence of sepsis (essentially fever) or deteriorating renal function. If you use a trial of MET, warn patients of the risks (drug side-effects, possible need for intervention in the form of ESWL, ureteroscopy or J stenting) and mention it is an 'off-label' (i.e. non-licenced) therapy. Arrange periodic follow-up imaging (usually a plain X-ray) to monitor stone position.

References

1 Borghi L et al. Nifedipine and methylprednisolone in facilitating ureteral stone passage: a randomised, double-blind, placebo controlled study. J Urol 1994; **152**:1095-8.

2 Porpiglia F et al. Effectiveness of nifedipine and deflazacort in the management of distal ureteric stones. Urology 2000; **56**:579-82.

3 Preminger GM et al. 2007 Guideline for the management of ureteral calculi (Joint EAU/AUA Nephrolithiasis Guideline Panel). J Urol 2007; **178**:2418-34.

4 Miller OF et al. Time to stone passage for observed ureteral calculi. J Urol 1999; **162**:688-91.

5 Hollingsworth JM et al. Medical therapy to facilitate urinary stone passage: a meta-analysis. Lancet 2006; **368**:1171-9.

6 Hussain Z et al. Use of glyceryl trinitrate patches in patients with ureteral stones: a randomized, double-blind, placebo-controlled study. Urology 2001; **58**:521-5.

Ureteric stones: indications for intervention to relieve obstruction and/or remove the stone

- Pain which fails to respond to analgesics or recurs and cannot be controlled with additional pain relief.
- Fever—have a low threshold for draining the kidney (usually done by percutaneous nephrostomy).
- Impaired renal function (solitary kidney obstructed by a stone, bilateral ureteric stones, or pre-existing renal impairment which worsens as a consequence of a ureteric stone). Threshold for intervention is lower.
- Prolonged unrelieved obstruction—this can result in long-term loss of renal function.[1] How long it takes for this loss of renal function to occur is uncertain but, generally speaking, the period of watchful waiting for spontaneous stone passage tends to be limited to 4–6 weeks.
- Social reasons—young, active patients may be very keen to opt for surgical treatment because they need to get back to work or their childcare duties, whereas some patients will be happy to sit things out. Airline pilots and some other professions are unable to work until they are stone-free.

Reference

1 Holm-Nielsen A, Jorgensen T, Mogensen P, Fogh J. The prognostic value of probe renography in ureteric stone obstruction. *Br J Urol* 1981; **53**:504–7.

Ureteric stones: emergency temporizing treatment ureteric stones

Where the pain of a ureteric stone fails to respond to analgesics or where renal function is impaired because of the stone, then temporary relief of the obstruction can be obtained by insertion of a JJ stent or percutaneous nephrostomy tube (a percutaneous nephrostomy tube can restore efficient peristalsis by restoring the ability of the ureteric wall to coapt).

The stone may pass down and out of the ureter with a stent or nephrostomy *in situ*, but in many instances it simply sits where it is and subsequent definitive treatment is required. While JJ stents can relieve stone pain, they can cause bothersome irritative bladder symptoms (pain in the bladder, frequency and urgency). JJ stents make subsequent stone treatment in the form of ureteroscopy technically easier by causing passive dilatation of the ureter.

The patient may elect to proceed to definitive stone treatment by immediate ureteroscopy (for stones at any location in the ureter) or ESWL (if the stone is in the upper and lower ureter—ESWL cannot be used for stones in the mid-ureter because this region is surrounded by bone, which prevents penetration of the shock waves) (Fig. 6.30). Local facilities and expertise will determine whether definitive treatment can be offered immediately. Not all hospitals have access to ESWL or endoscopic surgeons for 365 days a year.

Emergency treatment of an obstructed, infected kidney

Antibiotic delivery into an obstructed collecting system is impaired and so the septic patient with an obstructing stone should undergo urgent decompression of the collecting system, and definitive stone treatment (ESWL or ureteroscopy) should be delayed until the sepsis has resolved. The rationale for performing percutaneous nephrostomy rather than JJ stent insertion for an infected, obstructed kidney is to reduce the likelihood of

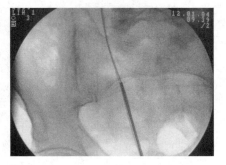

Fig. 6.30 Ureteroscopic stone fragmentation for a lower ureteric stone.
Reproduced with permission from Reynard *et al*, 2006, *Oxford Handbook of Urology*, Oxford University Press.

septicaemia occurring as a consequence of showering bacteria into the circulation. It has been theorized that this is more likely to occur with JJ stent insertion than with percutaneous nephrostomy insertion, that J stent insertion might damage the ureter (unlikely) and that monitoring of urine output and the facility for irrigation for a viscous pyonephrosis is possible with a nephrostomy but not a J stent. Nephrostomy insertion has the advantage that it avoids the need for a general anaesthetic, but J stent insertion can be performed with sedation and avoids the risk of bleeding from inadvertent puncture of a branch of the renal artery.[1]

The EAU/AUA Nephrolithiasis Guideline Panel[1] recommends that the system of drainage (J stent or percutaneous nephrostomy) is left to the discretion of the urologist, since both have been shown in a randomized trial of 42 patients with obstructing stones and a temperature of >38°C and/or white blood count of 17 000/mm^{3*} to be equally effective for the management of presumed obstructive pyelonephritis or pyonephrosis[2] in terms of time to normalization of temperature and white count (which takes approximately 2–3 days) and in-hospital stay. A 6- or 7-Ch J stent was used (with a Foley bladder catheter in 70%) or 8-Ch (occasionally larger) nephrostomy (plus a urethral catheter in 33%).

* An arbitrary definition of leucocytosis since patients with ureteric stones often have mildly elevated white blood count.

Table 6.6 Complications and problems associated with nephrostomy insertion and drainage (n=169)[1] and J stent[2,3] (none performed for relief of obstructed, infected kidney; n=226)

Complication	J stent (%)	Nephrostomy (%)
Failure of insertion	16	2
Sepsis in previously non-septic patient	—	3–4
Haemorrhage requiring transfusion	—	2
Stent occlusion	1–7	—
Tube displacement (tube falling out or for J stent migrating up or down)	0.1–7	5
Pleural effusion	—	1
Pneumonia/atelectasis	—	2
Ureteric perforation	6	—
Stent symptoms	Flank pain 15–20%; suprapubic pain 20%; urinary frequency 40%; haematuria 40%	—

1 Lee WJ et al. Emergency percutaneous nephrostomy: results and complications. *J Vasc Intervent Rad* 1994; **5**:135.
2 Pocock RD et al. Double J stents. A review of 100 patients. *Br J Urol* 1986; **58**:629.
3 Smedlev FH et al. J (pigtail) ureteric catheter insertions: a retrospective review. *Ann R Coll Surg (Engl)* 1988; **70**:377.

References

1 Preminger GM et al. 2007 Guideline for the management of ureteral calculi (Joint EAU/AUA Nephrolithiasis Guideline Panel). *J Urol* 2007; **178**:2418–34.
2 Pearle MS et al. Optimal method of urgent decompression of the collecting system for obstruction and infection due to ureteral calculi. *J Urol* 1998; **160**:1260.

Ureteric stones—indications for treatment

Almost 70% of stones 5 mm or less and almost 50% of stones 6–10 mm in diameter will pass spontaneously over a period of 3–6 weeks or there-abouts.[1] Stones that have not passed in 2 months are unlikely to do so although, much to the patient's and surgeon's surprise, large stones do sometimes drop out of the ureter at the last moment.

Indications for stone removal

- Pain which fails to respond to analgesics or recurs and cannot be controlled with additional pain relief.
- Impaired renal function (solitary kidney obstructed by a stone, bilateral ureteric stones, or pre-existing renal impairment which gets worsens as a consequence of a ureteric stone).
- Prolonged unrelieved obstruction (generally speaking ~4–6 weeks).
- Social reasons—young, active patients may be very keen to opt for surgical treatment because they need to return to work or childcare duties, whereas some patients will be happy to sit things out. Airline pilots and some other professions are unable to work until they are stone-free.

These indications need to be related to the individual patient—their stone size, their renal function, presence of a normal contralateral kidney, their tolerance of exacerbations of pain, their job and social situation, and local facilities (the availability of surgeons with appropriate skill and equipment to perform endoscopic stone treatment).

Twenty years ago, when the only options were watchful waiting or open surgical removal of a stone (open ureterolithotomy), surgeons and patients were inclined to 'sit it out' for a considerable time in the hope that the stone would pass spontaneously. Nowadays, the advent of ESWL and of smaller ureteroscopes with efficient stone fragmentation devices (e.g. the holmium laser) has made stone treatment and removal a far less morbid procedure, with a far smoother and faster post-treatment recovery. It is easier for both the patient and the surgeon to opt for intervention, in the form of ESWL or surgery, as a quicker way to relieve pain and to avoid unpredictable and unpleasant exacerbations of pain.

It is clearly important for the surgeon to inform the patient of the out-comes and potential complications of intervention, particularly given the fact that many stones would pass spontaneously if left a little longer, particularly now there is evidence for MET (medical expulsive therapy).

Reference

1 Preminger GM *et al.* 2007 Guideline for the management of ureteral calculi (Joint EAU/AUA Nephrolithiasis Guideline Panel. *J Urol* 2007; **178**:2418–34.

Ureteric stones: definitive treatment options

Definitive treatment options include the following.

- ESWL *in situ*, ESWL after 'push-back' into the kidney (i.e. into the renal pelvis or calyces), or after J stent insertion. There is now little call for 'push-back' ESWL in the era of small calibre semi-rigid ureteroscopes which have improved our ability to access the ureter and treat ureteric stones *in situ*.
- Ureteroscopy.
- PCNL.
- Open ureterolithotomy.
- Laparoscopic ureterolithotomy.

Basketing of stones (blind or under radiographic 'control') is a historical treatment (the potential for serious ureteric injury is significant).

The majority of urologists will nowadays opt for either ESWL or ureteroscopy. Stone clearance rates are higher after ureteroscopy, but those after ESWL fall not far behind and thus both are very reasonable treatment options (stone-free rates for ureteric stones after ESWL are in the order of 70–75%). Some hospitals do not, however, have ready access to ESWL or to staff with expertise in ureteroscopy and therefore the decision as to whether to proceed with one or other treatment will, to a very considerable degree, be influenced by local availability as well as by patient preference.

The ureter can be divided into two halves (proximal and distal to the iliac vessels) or into thirds (upper third from the PUJ to the upper edge of the sacrum; middle third from the upper to the lower edge of the sacrum; lower third from the lower edge of the sacrum to the VUJ).

EAU/AUA Nephrolithiasis Guideline Panel recommendations 2007[1]

These should be interpreted in the light of local facilities and expertise. Some hospitals have access to and expertise in the whole range of treatment options. Others may have limited access to a lithotripter or may not have surgeons skilled in the use of the ureteroscope.

Smaller ureteroscopes with improved optics and larger instrument channels and the advent of holmium laser lithotripsy have improved the efficacy of ureteroscopic stone fragmentation (to ~95% stone clearance) and reduced its morbidity. As a consequence, many surgeons and patients will opt for ureteroscopy, with its potential for a 'one-off' treatment, over ESWL where more than one treatment will be required and post-treatment imaging is required to confirm stone clearance (with ureteroscopy you can see that the stone has gone).

Many urology departments do not have unlimited access to ESWL and patients may therefore opt for ureteroscopic stone extraction.

The stone clearance rates for ESWL are dependent upon stone size. ESWL is more efficient for stones <1 cm in diameter compared with those >1 cm in size. Conversely, the outcome of ureteroscopy is somewhat less dependent on stone size.

Table 6.7 Efficacy outcomes (i.e. stone-free rates) of EAU/AUA Nephrolithiasis Guidelines Panel 2007. Median stone-free rates of ESWL and ureteroscopy (figures in brackets are 95% CI)

Stone position and size	ESWL (%)	Ureteroscopy (%)
Distal ureter <10 mm	86 (73–75)	97 (96–98)
Distal ureter >10 mm	74 (80–90)	93 (88–96)
Mid-ureter <10 mm	84 (65–95)	91 (81–96)
Mid-ureter >10 mm	76 (36–97)	78 (61–90)
Proximal ureter <10 mm	90 (85–93)	80 (73–85)
Proximal ureter >10 mm	68 (55–79)	79 (71–87)

Randomized controlled trials comparing ESWL and ureteroscopy are generally lacking. The EAU/AUA Nephrolithiasis Guidelines Panel 2007 meta-analysis suggests that:

- Proximal ureter <10 mm: ESWL leads to a marginally higher stone-free rate than ureteroscopy.
- Proximal ureter >10 mm: ureteroscopy results in a marginally higher stone-free rate than ESWL.
- For all mid-ureteric stones: ureteroscopy has a marginally higher stone-free rate than ESWL (but small patient numbers make comparison difficult).
- For all distal stones, ureteroscopy has a higher stone free rate than ESWL.

Thus, there are no great differences in stone-free rates between ESWL and ureteroscopy. Precisely which technique one uses will depend to a considerable degree on local resources (e.g. ready access to ESWL) and local expertise at performing ureteroscopy, particularly for upper tract stones.

Open ureterolithotomy and laparoscopic ureterolithotomy (less invasive than open ureterolithotomy) are used in the rare cases (e.g. very impacted stones) where ESWL or ureteroscopy have been tried and failed, or were not feasible.[1] Laparoscopic ureterolithotomy for large, impacted stones has a stone-free rate averaging almost 90%.

Reference

1 Preminger GM *et al.* 2007 Guideline for the management of ureteral calculi (Joint EAU/AUA Nephrolithiasis Guideline Panel. *J Urol* 2007; **178**:2418–34.

Ureteric stones: ureteroscopy for ureteric calculi

The instruments

Semi-rigid ureteroscopes have high density fibre-optic bundles for light ('non-coherently' arranged) and image transmission ('coherently' arranged to maintain image quality). For equivalent light and image transmission using glass rod lenses, thicker lenses are required than with fibre-optic bundles. As a consequence, semi-rigid ureteroscopes can be made smaller, while maintaining the size of the instrument channel. In addition, the instrument can be bent by several degrees without the image being distorted.

The working tip of most current models is in the order of 7 to 8 Ch, with the proximal end of the scope being in the order of 9 to 10 Ch. There is usually at least one working channel of at least 3.6 Ch.

Some surgeons advocate the use of flexible ureteroscopes for stones above the iliac vessels, whereas others use semi-rigid scopes for stones at all levels. There is no evidence that semi-rigid scopes are associated with a higher complication rate for treating proximal ureteric stones when compared with flexible scopes.[1] There is the distinct advantage of superior irrigant flow and illumination when using a semi-rigid ureteroscope rather than a flexible one.

Patient position

Position the patient as flat as possible on the operating table to 'iron out' the natural curves of the ureter (Fig. 6.31).

Placing the first guidewire

Perform a cystoscopy with either a flexible or rigid instrument. Negotiate a guidewire past the obstructing ureteric stone and into the renal pelvis. We use a Sensor® guidewire (Microvasive, Boston Scientific) which has a 3-cm long floppy, hydrophilic tip which is helpful in negotiating a way past the ureteric stone. The remaining length of the wire is rigid and covered in a smooth PTFE. Both properties aid passage of the ureteroscope.

To assist access of the ureteroscope into the ureter and up to the ureteric stone, place a safety guidewire, a dual lumen catheter for ureteric dilatation and a second guidewire, over which the semi-rigid ureteroscope will be passed. To pass the first guidewire, use one with a floppy end to facilitate passage of the wire past the obstructing ureteric stone and into the kidney. We find a Starter® guidewire has a tip which is a little too rigid to pass the stone safely without perforating the ureter

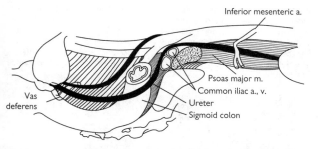

Fig. 6.31 Lateral view of the ureter. The lithotomy position will tend to exaggerate the curve of the ureter within the pelvis, so ureteroscope the patient with the legs in a neutral position. Reproduced with permission from Hinman, *Atlas of Urosurgical Anatomy*, WB Saunders, 1993.

(particularly when the stone is very impacted in the ureter) and we therefore prefer a Sensor® guidewire. This combines a very floppy end with a rigid shaft which makes manipulation of the wire easier than the very slippery hydrophilic Terumo Glidewire which, although very useful for negotiating a way past an impacted ureteric stone, is very difficult to hold. If the Sensor® guidewire will not pass the stone, switch to a straight or angled Terumo Glidewire. If this wire will not pass beyond the stone, pass a 4-Ch ureteric catheter over the wire, to a point just below the stone and use this to stabilize the Terumo Glidewire within the ureter as you attempt to negotiate the wire past the stone. Alternatively, advance the Terumo up to the stone—as it makes contact with an impacted stone it will tend to coil back on itself, but with continued pressure on the wire it may suddenly flick past the stone, into the proximal ureter. Failing this, attempt direct visual negotiation of the wire past the stone by advancing a semi-rigid ureteroscope over a guidewire positioned up to the stone. In the rare cases where it is not possible to reach the stone and where guidewire placement and J stenting fail, a nephrostomy followed by antegrade J stenting will be required (either under the same anaesthetic if a radiologist is available or as a later procedure). Following a period of J stenting, during which passive ureteric dilatation will occur, a second attempt at ureteroscopic stone removal will usually be successful.

Ureteric dilatation

Some surgeons do, others don't. Those who don't argue that dilatation is unnecessary in the era of modern, small calibre ureteroscopes. Those who do cite a higher chance of being able to advance the ureteroscope all the way up to the PUJ. Ureteric dilatation may be helpful where multiple passes of the ureteroscope up and down the ureter are going to be required for stone removal (alternatively, use a ureteric access sheath). Some surgeons prefer to place two guidewires into the ureter, one to pass the ureteroscope over ('railroading') and the other to act as a safety wire, so that access to the kidney is always possible if difficulties are encountered. This is the author's preference. The second guidewire is most easily placed via a dual-lumen catheter which has a second channel, through which the second guidewire can be easily passed into the ureter without requiring repeat cystoscopy (Fig. 6.32). This dual-lumen catheter has the added function of gently dilating the ureteric orifice to about 10-Ch. There is probably no long-term harm done to the ureter as a consequence of dilatation.[2]

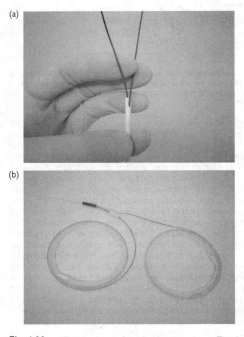

Fig. 6.32 (a) The distal end of the dual-lumen catheter. The dual-lumen catheter has a second channel, through which the second guidewire can be easily passed into the ureter. (b) The two guidewires in the proximal end of the dual-lumen catheter demonstrate the two channels.

Placing two guidewires using the dual lumen catheter

Position the first guidewire. The central channel of the dual-lumen catheter (the eye hole is at the end of the catheter) is fed over the first guidewire. Instil plenty of lubrication down the urethra. Then, with X-ray imaging over the bladder to allow imaging of the VUJ, pass the dual-lumen catheter down the urethra and into the lower ureter. There is no need to pass the dual lumen all the way up the ureter—the aim is to dilate the VUJ, the narrowest part of the ureter, to allow access for the ureteroscope, and to place a second guidewire into the ureter (we prefer to use an Amplatz Superstiff guidewire as the second wire because it is more rigid than the Sensor® guidewire, and, if used as the 'safety' wire, it holds the ureter in a straighter line, effectively 'ironing out' some of the curves of the ureter). Furthermore, the dual lumen may cause migration of a ureteric stone, if present, back into the kidney, necessitating a search for the migrated stone within the kidney. What would have been a straight-forward semi-rigid ureteroscopy suddenly becomes a more complex ureterorenoscopy.

Ureteroscopic irrigation systems

Use normal saline (high pressure irrigation with glycine or water would lead to fluid absorption from pyelolymphatic or venous backflow). Irrigation by gravity pressurization alone (the fluid bag suspended above the patient without any applied pressure) often provides a flow rate of irrigant fluid that is inadequate for visualization because the long, fine bore irrigation channels of modern ureteroscopes are inherently high resistance. Several methods are available for enhancing irrigant flow—hand-inflated pressure bags, foot pumps, and hand-operated syringe pumps. The author prefers a pressurized bag of saline, finding it difficult to use a hand-operated pump while holding both the ureteroscope and laser fibre, and having difficulty coordinating the action of his left foot with that of his right hand! No doubt other surgeons are able to do so with ease. Whatever system is used, use the minimal flow required to allow a safe view to avoid flushing the stone out of the ureter and into the kidney, from where you may not be able to retrieve it.

Ureteric stones: technique of semi-rigid ureteroscopy for treatment of ureteric calculi

Negotiating the curves of the urethra, and in particular finding your way from the bladder neck, across the bladder and into the ureteric orifice, is made considerably easier by the use of the second guidewire. If difficulty is encountered in passing the 'scope through the ureteric orifice, rotate it through 180° and try again.

Access sheaths are seldom helpful for the management of ureteric stones and indeed they can make ureteroscopic stone fragmentation more difficult.[1,4] For the ureterorenoscopic treatment of renal stones they can be very helpful.

Remember, only advance the 'scope under direct vision—you must be able to see the lumen of the ureter as you pass the 'scope. As you pass the 'scope up towards the stone, keep your finger on the valve on the irrigation channel so that you can control the rate of flow of irrigant, and thereby avoid flushing the stone back into the kidney, where it is less accessible. Clearly there is a compromise between trying to avoid proximal stone migration and yet having adequate vision to enable safe passage of the 'scope. Passing the ureteroscope over the guidewire helps to minimize pressure transmission to the stone. Once the stone is seen, close off the irrigation, remove the guidewire (retaining the safety wire) and pass the laser fibre or pneumatic lithotripter through the instrument channel of the 'scope. Make sure the end of the laser fibre is some distance from the lens of the 'scope since discharge of the laser too close to the lens will fracture the lens. Try to keep irrigant flow and pressure to a minimum. Fragment the stone using the laser or a pneumatic lithotripter.

Techniques for stone fragmentation: laser lithotripsy versus pneumatic lithotripsy

The main drawbacks of laser lithotripsy are:
- The dust cloud effect that occurs as the stone is fragmented. This temporarily obscures the view, and must be washed away before the laser can safely be re-applied.
- The potential for damage to the lens of the 'scope if the laser is discharged too close.
- It is all too easy when using the laser to fragment the stone into multiple large pieces which then have a tendency to move.

Targeting the laser on these mobile fragments can be difficult. Thus, you should try to maintain the stone in one piece, slowly painting the surface of the stone to vaporize it rather than creating large fragments.

The main drawback of pneumatic lithotripsy is a tendency to cause proximal stone migration. The laser generates small shock waves, but they are far less marked than those generated by pneumatic lithotriptors and proximal stone migration when using the laser is usually minimal (although of course high irrigant flow and pressure will cause proximal stone migration).

To stent or not to stent after ureteroscopy

The suggestion that a stent should be placed following 'complicated' ureteroscopy is all well and good, until one appreciates that 'complicated' has not been defined. The term means different things to different surgeons. Give serious consideration to stent placement if[5,6]:
- there has been ureteric injury (e.g. perforation—indicated by extravasation of contrast)
- there is mucosal trauma
- there are residual stones that might obstruct the ureter
- the patient has had a ureteric stricture that required dilatation
- the patient has a solitary kidney
- bilateral ureteroscopies have been performed.

Some authors suggest that, in cases where stone fragmentation takes longer than 45 minutes, a stent should be placed, because ureteric oedema and temporary post-operative obstruction may be more likely to occur than with shorter procedures.[1] This concept has not been rigorously tested.

Routine stenting after ureteroscopy for distal ureteric calculi is unnecessary.[7] Many urologists will place a stent after ureteroscopy for proximal ureteric stones.

An alternative to a J stent is the placement of a 4- or 6-Ch ureteric catheter which is secured in place by taping it to an indwelling urethral catheter. The two catheters can be removed the morning after ureteroscopy. Patients randomized to this form of drainage versus no drainage[9] had significantly less pain and required less analgesia, but urethral irritation is greater.

Management of steinstrasse

If there are signs of infection, commence antibiotics and arrange nephrostomy insertion. By decompressing the distended ureter, this may enhance peristalsis and assist spontaneous passage of the stones in the steinstrasse. ESWL to the lead fragment can be used for a steinstrasse in the proximal, mid-ureter and distal ureter. Ureteroscopy and stone fragmentation is an option, particularly for a steinstrasse in the distal ureter.

Complications of ureteroscopy

- Septicaemia.
- Ureteric perforation (2%) requiring either a JJ stent or, very occasionally, a nephrostomy tube where JJ stent placement is not possible.[11]
- New onset ureteric stricture (0.5–1.5%[8]).
- Ureteric avulsion (0–0.3% of 6178 patients).[12,13]

References

1 Knoll T, Alken P, Michel MS. Progress in management of ureteric stones. *Eur Urol Update Series* 2005; **3**:44–50.

2 Garvin TJ, Clayman RV. Balloon dilation of the ureter for ureteroscopy. *J Urol* 1991; **146**:742–5.

3 Harmon WJ et al. Ureteroscopy: current practice and long-term complications. *J Urol* 1997; **157**:28–32.

4 De Sio M, Autorino R, Damiano R et al. Expanding applications of the access sheath for ureterolithotripsy of distal ureteral stones. A frustrating experience. *Urol Int* 2004; **72**(Suppl.):55–7.

5 Jeong H, Kwak C, Lee SE. Ureteric stenting after ureteroscopy for ureteric stones: a prospective randomized study assessing symptoms and complications. *Br J Urol* 2004; **93**:1032–4.

6 Hollenbeck BK, Schuster TG, Seifman BD et al. Identifying patients who are suitable for stentless ureteroscopy following treatment of urolithiasis. *J Urol* 2003; **170**:103–6.

7 Srivastava A et al. Routine stenting after ureteroscopy for distal ureteral calculi is unnecessary: results of a randomized controlled trial. *J Endourol* 2003; **17**:871–77.

8 Sofer M, Watterson JD, Wollin et al. Holmium:YAG laser lithotripsy for upper urinary tract calculi in 598 patients. *J Urol* 2002; **167**:31–4.

9 Djaladat H et al. Ureteral catheterization in uncomplicated ureterolithotomy: a randomized, controlled trial. *Eur Urol* 2007; **52**:836–41.

10 Delvecchio FC et al. Assessment of stricture formation with the ureteral access sheath. *Urology* 2003; **61**:518–22.

11 Brooke Johnson D, Pearle MS. Complications of ureteroscopy. *Urol Clin NA* 2004; **31**:157–71.

12 Stoller ML, Wolf JS. Endoscopic ureteral injuries. In: JW McAninch (ed.) *Traumatic and Reconstructive Urology*. Philadelphia: WB Saunders; 1996, pp. 199–211.

13 Grasso M. Complications of ureteropyloscopy. In: SS Taneja, RB Smith, RM Ehrlich (eds) *Complications of Urologic Surgery*, 3rd edn. Philadelphia: WB Saunders; 2001, pp. 268–76.

Open ureterolithotomy

Indications

Open ureterolithotomy is essentially indicated for failed ureteroscopy, which can be due to failed access and/or failure of fragmentation.

Incision

- Upper third stones: supracostal or subcostal.
- Middle third stones: midline extraperitoneal. Push the peritoneum medially to expose the iliac vessels. Identify the ureter as it crosses anterior to the iliac vessels at the iliac bifurcation.
- Lower third stones: midline extraperitoneal, transperitoneal or a Gibson incision (an oblique muscle-splitting incision in the left or right iliac fossa).

Technique

Very gently mobilize the ureter above and below the stone so that you can place a sling above and then below the stone (alternatively use Babcock's forceps), thereby preventing proximal or distal migration of the stone. Palpate the stone. Make a vertical incision over the stone using a knife and extend it with Potts scissors (Fig. 6.33). Remove the stone. Close the ureter with interrupted 4-0 absorbable sutures passed through the adventitia to avoid narrowing its lumen (to preserve its vascularity).

For very low stones, approach the ureter transvesically by making a vertical incision in the bladder. Place a stay suture approximately 1 cm medial and distal to the ureteric orifice. Apply traction to the suture and make a transverse incision in the urothelium overlying the ureter approximately 3 cm proximal to the ureteric orifice. Locate the stone by palpation. Cut down onto it and remove it. Place a JJ stent. Close the bladder and leave a catheter in place for 10 days.

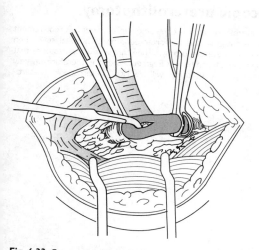

Fig. 6.33 Open ureterolithotomy. A vertical incision is made in the ureter, with Babcock's forceps placed above and below the stone to prevent proximal and distal migration.

Laparoscopic ureterolithotomy

Laparoscopic ureterolithotomy has comparable efficacy but less requirement for post-operative analgesia and a shorter duration of hospital stay when compared with open ureterolithotomy.[1] There are few ureteric stones that the ureteroscope cannot completely fragment, and it is therefore unlikely that laparoscopic ureterolithotomy will replace ureteroscopic ureterolithotomy.

Reference

1 Skrepetis K, Doumas K, Siafakas I, Lykourinas M. Laparoscopic versus open ureterolithotomy. A comparative study. *Eur Urol* 2001; **40**:32–6.

Management of ureteric stones in pregnancy

While hypercalciuria and uric acid excretion increase in pregnancy (predisposing to stone formation), so too do urinary citrate and magnesium levels (protecting against stone formation). The net effect is that the incidence of ureteric colic is the same as in non-pregnant women.[1] Ureteric stones occur in 1 in 1500–2500 pregnancies, mostly during the second and third trimesters. They are associated with a significant risk of pre-term labour (Hendricks 1991) and the pain caused by ureteric stones can be difficult to distinguish from other causes.

The hydronephrosis of pregnancy

Ninety per cent of pregnant women have bilateral hydronephrosis from weeks 6–10 of gestation and up to 2 months after birth (owing to the smooth muscle relaxant effect of progesterone and mechanical obstruction of the ureter from the enlarging fetus and uterus). Hydronephrosis is taken as surrogate evidence of ureteric obstruction in non-pregnant individuals but, because it is a normal finding in the majority of pregnancies, its presence *cannot* be taken as a sign of a possible ureteric stone. Ultrasound is unreliable for diagnosing the presence of stones in pregnant (and in non-pregnant) women (sensitivity 34%, i.e. it misses 66% of stones; specificity 86%, i.e. false-positive rate of 14%).[2]

Differential diagnosis of flank pain in pregnancy

Ureteric stone, placental abruption, appendicitis, pyelonephritis and all the other (many) causes of flank pain in non-pregnant women.

References
1 Coe FL, Parks JH, Lindhermer MD. Nephrolithiasis during pregnancy. *N Engl J Med* 1978; **298**:324–6.
2 Stothers L, Lee LM. Renal colic in pregnancy. *J Urol* 1992; **148**:1383–7.

Diagnostic imaging studies in pregnancy

Exposure of the fetus to ionizing radiation can cause fetal malformations, malignancies in later life (leukaemia) and mutagenic effects (damage to genes causing inherited disease in the offspring of the fetus). Fetal radiation doses during various procedures are shown in Table 6.8. While the recommended maximum radiation levels shown in the table are well above those occurring during even CT scanning, and a dose of 50 mGy or less is regarded as 'safe', every effort should be made to limit exposure of the fetus to radiation. Pregnant women may be reassured that the risk to the unborn child as a consequence of radiation exposure is likely to be minimal.

Plain radiography and IVU

These techniques have limited usefulness (the fetal skeleton and the enlarged uterus obscure ureteric stones; delayed excretion of contrast limits opacification of ureter; theoretical risk of fetal toxicity from the contrast material).

CTU

CTU is a very accurate method for detecting ureteric stones, but most radiologists and urologists are unhappy to recommend this form of imaging in pregnant women.

MRU

The American College of Obstetricians and Gynecologists and the US National Council on Radiation Protection state that, 'Although there is no evidence to suggest that the embryo is sensitive to magnetic and radiofrequency at the intensities encountered in MRI, it might be prudent to exclude pregnant women during the first trimester'.[1,2] MRU can therefore potentially be used during the second and third trimesters, but not during the first trimester. It involves no ionizing radiation and is very accurate (100% sensitivity for detecting ureteric stones), but is expensive and not readily available in most hospitals, particularly out of hours.

References

1 National Council on Radiation Protection and Measurement. *Medical Radiation Exposure of Pregnant and Potentially Pregnant Women.* NCRP Report no. 54, Bethesda, MD: NCRPM 1997.
2 American College of Obstetricians and Gynecologists Committee on Obstetric Practice. *Guidelines for Diagnostic Imaging During Pregnancy.* ACOG Committee Opinion no.158, Washington DC: ACOG, 1995.

Management of ureteric stones in pregnant women

Most (70–80%) will pass spontaneously.[1] Pain relief is provided by opiate-based analgesics; avoid NSAIDs as these can cause premature closure of the ductus arteriosus by blocking prostaglandin synthesis.

Indications for intervention are the same as in non-pregnant patients (pain refractory to analgesics, suspected urinary sepsis (high fever, high white count), high grade obstruction and obstruction in a solitary kidney).

Options for intervention

Options depend on the stage of pregnancy and on local facilities and expertise:

- JJ stent urinary diversion.[2]
- Nephrostomy urinary diversion.
- Ureteroscopic stone removal.

Aim to minimize radiation exposure to the fetus, and to minimize the risk of miscarriage and pre-term labour. General anaesthesia can precipitate pre-term labour and many urologists and obstetricians will err on the side of temporizing options such as nephrostomy tube drainage or JJ stent placement, rather than on operative treatment in the form of ureteroscopic stone removal.

Radiation doses of <100 mGy are very unlikely to have an adverse effect on the fetus.[2] In the United States the National Council on Radiation Protection has stated that, 'Fetal risk is considered to be negligible at <50 mGy when compared to the other risks of pregnancy, and the risk of malformations is significantly increased above control levels at doses >150 mGy'.[3] The American College of Obstetricians and Gynecologists has stated that, 'X-ray exposure to <50 mGy has not been associated with an increase in fetal anomalies or pregnancy loss'.[4]

References

1 Stothers L, Lee LM. Renal colic in pregnancy. *J Urol* 1992; **148**:1383–7.
2 Hellawell GO, Cowan NC, Holt SJ, Mutch SJ. A radiation perspective for treating loin pain in pregnancy by double-pigtail stents. *Br J Urol Int* 2002; **90**:801–8.
3 National Council on Radiation Protection and Measurement. *Medical Radiation Exposure of Pregnant and Potentially Pregnant Women.* NCRP Report no. 54, Bethesda, MD: NCRPM 1997.
4 American College of Obstetricians and Gynecologists Committee on Obstetric Practice. *Guidelines for Diagnostic Imaging During Pregnancy.* ACOG Committee Opinion no.158, Washington DC: ACOG, 1995.

Additional reading

Doyle LA, Cronan JJ, Breslaw BH, Ridlen MS. New techniques of ultrasound and color doppler in the prospective evaluation of acute renal obstruction: do they replace the intravenous urogram? *Abdom Imaging* 1995; **20**:58–63.

Table 6.8 Fetal radiation dose after various radiological investigations

Procedure	Mean fetal dose (mGy)	Risk of inducing fetal cancer (up to age 15 years)
KUB X-ray	1.4	–
IVU 6 shot	1.7	1 in 10 000
IVU 3 shot		
CT—abdominal	8	
CT—pelvic	25	
Fluoroscopy for JJ stent insertion	0.4	1 in 42 000

Bladder stones

Bladder stones are composed of struvite (i.e. they are infection stones) or uric acid (in non-infected urine).

In adults, bladder stones are predominantly a disease of men aged >50 years with bladder outlet obstruction due to BPE (benign prostatic enlargement). They also occur in the chronically catheterized patient, representing a manifestation of chronic urinary infection. In chronically catheterized spinal cord injury patients the chance of developing a bladder stone is 25% over 5 years (similar risk whether urethral or suprapubic location).[1]

In children, bladder stones are still endemic in Thailand, Indonesia, North Africa, the Middle East, and Burma, where they are usually composed of a combination of ammonium urate and calcium oxalate. A low-phosphate diet in these areas (a diet of breast milk and polished rice or millet) results in high peaks of ammonia excretion in the urine.

Diagnosis

May be symptomless (incidental finding on KUB X-ray or bladder ultrasound or at cystoscopy, the common 'presentation' in spinal patients who have limited or no bladder sensation). In the neurologically intact patient there is suprapubic or perineal pain, haematuria, urgency and/or urge incontinence, recurrent UTI, and LUTS (hesitancy, poor flow). Bladder stones are visible on KUB X-ray or ultrasound.

Treatment

Most stones are small enough to be removed cystoscopically (endoscopic cystolitholapaxy), using stone-fragmenting forceps for those that can be engaged by the jaws of the forceps, and EHL or pneumatic lithotripsy for those that cannot. Large stones are removed by open surgery (open cystolitholapaxy) (Fig. 6.34, ☐ p. 476).

Endoscopic cystolitholapaxy

Small stones can be engaged in a stone punch such as the Mauermayer punch (Fig. 6.35). Manipulate the stone into the jaws of the instrument while ensuring that the irrigant is flowing (this pushes the mucosa of the bladder away from the jaws of the stone punch). Before crushing it, gently move the entrapped stone from side to side to ensure that the bladder mucosa is not trapped in the jaws.

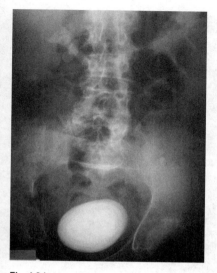

Fig. 6.34 A large bladder stone. The sensible option is open cystolithotomy.

(a)

(b)

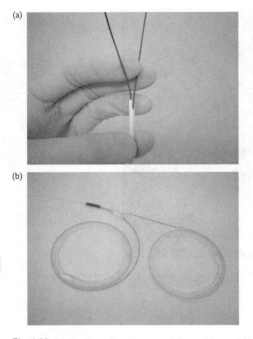

Fig. 6.35 (a) The Mauermayer stone punch for crushing small bladder stones.
(b) The open jaws of the Mauermayer stone punch.

For stones that are too large to fit within the jaws of the stone punch, but are not large enough to warrant open stone surgery, use an EHL probe (Fig. 6.36) or pneumatic lithotripter to fragment the stone into pieces of a suitable size for further fragmentation with the stone punch. When using EHL, ensure that the bladder contains enough fluid to ensure that the wall is pushed away from the EHL probe, and therefore out of harm's way from the powerful electrical discharge. Discharging the device too close to the wall of the bladder risks either bladder perforation or damage to bowel adjacent to the bladder. As with laser lithotripsy, avoid discharging the EHL probe too close (within 5 mm) to the lens of the cystoscope, since this can fracture. Get into the habit of moving your foot off the control pedal when not fragmenting the stone, and switch the EHL machine off whenever you withdraw the EHL probe from the cystoscope, since inadvertent discharge of the device could harm the patient, your cystoscope, or you! Evacuate fragments of stone with an Ellik evacuator.

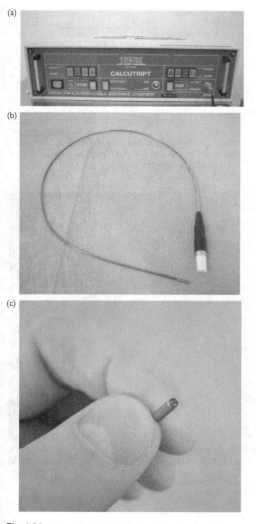

Fig. 6.36 (a) An EHL generator (b) The EHL probe for bladder stone fragmentation. (c) End view of the EHL probe showing the electrode.

Open cystolitholapaxy

Insert a urethral catheter and attach it to a giving set connected to a bag of glycine (to allow use of the diathermy probe to make the cystotomy). This can be used to inflate the bladder and thereby push the peritoneal contents (small bowel) out of the way, thus avoiding inadvertent bowel injury. A Pfannenstiel incision provides good access. Separate the rectus muscles in the midline, and then inflate the bladder with glycine. Place two stay sutures on either side of your intended incision line. Your assistant should be ready with the sucker, to evacuate the glycine from the opened bladder. Make a midline incision in the bladder using diathermy (Fig. 6.37). This should be extended sufficiently to allow removal of the stones. Close the bladder in one or two layers using an absorbable suture. Place a tube drain down to the closure line. Close the rectus fascia and superficial fascia. Use clips for the skin or interrupted sutures (the urine is often infected and wound infection can occur).

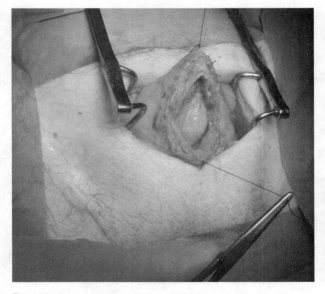

Fig. 6.37 Open cystolithotomy. The bladder has been opened between stay sutures to allow the removal of the contained stones.

Chapter 7

Surgery for upper tract obstruction and other ureteric surgery

Pelvi-ureteric junction obstruction in adults

History

Numerous treatment options for pelvi-ureteric junction (PUJ) obstruction have been developed over the last century.

- 1886 Trendelenburg: first description of open repair.
- 1903 Albarran: ureterotome externe—first attempt at endosurgical repair.[1]
- 1943 Davis et al.: intubated ureterotomy.[2]
- 1983 Wickham and Kellett: endoscopic pyelolysis.[3]
- 1984 Ramsay et al.: antegrade endopyelotomy.[4]

Retrograde endopyelotomy

This procedure has evolved over the last decade with the development of ureteroscopic and fluoroscopic techniques. It has clear advantages over the antegrade approach as percutaneous access is not required. Retrograde endopyelotomy can be performed in one of three ways:

- Using a rigid ureteroscope and a cold/hot/laser incision.
- Flexible ureteroscope with hot/laser incision.
- Using the Acucise device (a balloon catheter with an overlying fine cutting wire) which was introduced in 1993.[5]

Some surgeons place an indwelling ureteral stent (4.8–7Fr) 1–2 weeks prior to surgery to drain the obstructed kidney.[6,7] This prevents further episodes of renal colic and facilitates passage of the ureteroscope at the time of endopyelotomy. The disadvantage is that it may bring significant stent symptoms in some patients.

Indications

- Symptomatic PUJ obstruction.
- Urinary tract infections.
- Progressive renal deterioration.

Absolute contraindications[8–10]

- Strictures >2 cm.
- Poor renal function (≤ 20%).
- Untreated bleeding diathesis.
- Active urinary tract infection.

Relative contraindications[11,12]

- Massive hydronephrosis.
- High insertion of ureter at PUJ.
- Renal anomalies.
- Crossing vessels (controversial).

Immediate pre-operative preparation

- Informed consent: this should include the surgeon's results.
- Pre-operative urine cultures checked.
- Pre-operative clotting screen checked.
- Patient's side marked and signed by surgeon.
- Patient imaging on screen in theatre.

- Prophylactic intravenous antibiotics: gentamicin 240 mg plus cefuroxime 1.5 g at induction plus three post-operative doses of cefuroxime 750 mg.
- Prophylactic heparinization: unfractionated heparin 5000 IU twice daily or fractionated heparin once daily until discharge.
- C-arm in theatre with radiation protection gowns for use.

Patient positioning
Dorsal lithotomy with legs in supports.

Operative technique[7]
Place a stiff guidewire into the kidney under fluoroscopic guidance and place an open-ended ureteral catheter (5Fr) over the wire. This allows irrigation and protection of the ureter from the electrocautery or laser. Advance the rigid or flexible ureteroscope up the ureter over a separate second guidewire under fluoroscopic control. Once at the PUJ, inspect for pulsations visually. Make a lateral incision with electrocautery or a holmium laser (1–1.5 J setting). The incision needs to be full thickness down to peri-ureteral fat and along the whole length of the stricture. Balloon dilate the PUJ to 24Fr, place a stent of your choice over the guidewire and leave *in situ* for 4 weeks.

Acucise endopyelotomy also requires initial placement of a stiff guidewire (0.035 inch). Railroad a ureteral catheter over the wire and drain residual urine in the renal pelvis.

Replace the guidewire. Prealign the Acucise device for a lateral incision and then place over the guidewire and advance to a position just distal to the stricture. Attach the Sureseal II (Applied Medical Resources, Rancho, Santa Margarita, CA) over the guidewire to the centre port of the Acucise catheter and perform a retrograde pyelogram with dilute contrast. Do not use normal saline as the irrigation fluid and dilute the contrast with sterile water or glycine.

Advance the Acucise catheter slowly until the radio-opaque markers straddle the PUJ. This can be checked by rotating the C-arm laterally. Inflate the balloon partially to confirm correct placement and keep the cautery on standby mode at this point. When the position is correct, inflate the balloon to 2.2 cc and apply 75 W (pure cut) of cautery for 3–5 sec. Inflate the Acucise balloon to maximum and leave for 10 min to tamponade. Full-thickness incision can be monitored by observing the disappearance of the balloon waist or extravasation of contrast. Place a 7Fr stent or 10Fr endopyelotomy stent over the guidewire and leave for 4–6 weeks. Place a Foley catheter initially to monitor active bleeding. The patient can usually be discharged the same day or the following morning.

Signs of bleeding after endopyelotomy include haemodynamic instability, a flank mass, ecchymosis, haematuria and decreased haematocrit.

Remove the stent after 4–6 weeks.

Outcomes and complications[5,10,13-22]

Success rates of 73–90% for ureteroscopic endopyelotomy (UE)[13-16] and 66–84% for Acucise[5,10,17-22] have been reported. Operative duration is 33–100 min with UE and 90.2–180 min with Acucise. Hospital stay is 0.38–6 days with UE and 0.52–5 days with Acucise. Both procedures are associated with lower opiate use, shorter hospital stay, and shorter convalescence compared with antegrade endopyelotomy and open and laparoscopic pyeloplasty.

Complications occur in 2.5–21% of UE and 0–13.6% of Acucise patients. Average drops in haemaglobin are 1.8 mg for both. However, transfusions are reported in 1–9%, with transcatheter embolization performed in 4%. UTIs occur in 2% and stent symptoms in 3–5%.

Follow-up is probably required for 2 years. Most failures are reported within 7 months of surgery, although 13% of failures have been reported in the second year of follow-up. Succesful outcomes ideally require the patient to be completely asymptomatic with normal MAG3 renograms or IVPs post-operatively. Pre-operative imaging is required.

No clear difference between UE and Acucise outcomes has been demonstrated, and the decision should rest with the surgeon's preference and experience.

Percutaneous endopyelotomy

Percutaneous management of PUJ obstruction was first described by Wickham and colleagues in 1983.[4] The term 'endopyelotomy' was first coined by Smith and colleagues in 1986.[23] It is specifically indicated for patients for whom an open approach has failed, and is also suitable for patients with pyelocalyceal stones that can be managed at the same time.

Indications

• Symptomatic PUJ obstruction.
• Urinary tract infections/stones.
• Progressive renal deterioration.
• Causal hypertension (rarely).

Absolute contraindications[8-10]

• Strictures >2 cm.
• Poor renal function (≤ 20%).
• Untreated bleeding diathesis.
• Active urinary tract infection.

Relative contraindications[11-12]

• Massive hydronephrosis.
• High insertion of ureter at PUJ.
• Renal anomalies.
• Crossing vessels (controversial).

Immediate pre-operative preparation

• Informed consent: this should include the surgeon's results.
• Check pre-operative urine cultures.
• Patient's side marked and signed by surgeon.
• Patient imaging on screen in theatre.

- Prophylactic intravenous antibiotics: gentamicin 240 mg plus cefuroxime 1.5 g at induction plus three post-operative doses of cefuroxime 750 mg.
- Prophylactic heparinization: unfractionated heparin 5000 IU twice daily or fractionated heparin once daily until discharge.
- C-arm in theatre with radiation protection gowns for use.

Patient positioning
Prone position.

Operative technique[24]
Access is needed across the PUJ obstruction initially to allow for a safe endopyelotomy. Place an initial hydrophilic guidewire into the kidney under fluoroscopic guidance and then place an open-ended ureteral catheter (5Fr) over the wire. Remove the wire and then use the catheter for contrast injection to guide percutaneous access. Percutaneous access follows the description under PCNL (📖 p. 416).

The original description[4] of the technique of endopyelotomy involved a cold knife under direct vision. With two guidewires in place across the PUJ, a direct vision 'endopyelotome' is used. This is a hook-shaped cold knife which can completely incise the full thickness of the PUJ from lumen out to peri-ureteral and peri-pelvic fat. Extend the incision several millimeters into the normal ureter.

Although a lateral incision is recommended, the ureter does sometimes insert into the renal pelvis on the anterior or posterior wall. In these cases an anterior or posterior incision may be required, marsupializing the proximal ureter into the renal pelvis. Direct vision allows the crossing vessels to be seen and avoided.

Following complete incision, place a 14/7Fr endopyelotomy stent over the guidewire in an antegrade fashion. Position the large-diameter end of the stent across the PUJ. If this stent is difficult to place, use a standard 8Fr internal stent. Some authors recommend placing a nephrostomy tube for 24–48 hr, though tubeless percutaneous endopyelotomies have been reported.[25] Place a Foley catheter initially to monitor active bleeding.

Variations of this technique have been described. These include a stent first–hot knife technique.[24] This involves placing the stent in position first with the potential advantages of obviating concern about avulsing the PUJ during stent placement after the endopyelotomy and better definition of the PUJ allowing more precise incision.

Use a Bugbee electrode or Collins knife on a 24Fr resectoscope to marsupialize the proximal ureter into the renal pelvis. In high insertion PUJ, extend the incision all the way to the dependent renal pelvis under vision. If stones are present they should be removed prior to the endopyelotomy so that fragments do not migrate into the peri-ureteral and peri-pelvic tissues.

Leave the stent for 4–6 weeks. Avoid strenuous exercise for 8–10 days. The use of prophylactic antibiotics for the period of stenting is controversial.

Follow-up involves repeat imaging (IVP and MAG3) a month after stent removal and then after 6, 12, and 24 months. The duration and timing of imaging follow-up is controversial, but 2 years is a common period.

Outcomes and complications

Success rates range from 57% to 100% (mean 73.5%) with follow-up between 2 and 96 months.[26] Other series report 85–90% success rates for both primary and secondary PUJ obstruction.[27–29]

Complications are the same as those reported for PCNL (📖 p. 426). Haemorrhage is slightly less than with PCNL, possibly because of the thinner renal cortex experienced in PUJ obstruction.

Open dismembered pyeloplasty

Kuster[30] described the first pyeloplasty in 1891. Fenger[31] then applied the Heineke–Mickulicz principle to reconstruction of the PUJ. Schwyzer[32] introduced flap techniques in 1923, and these were successfully modified by Foley.[33] Culp and DeWeerd[34] reported their spiral flap in 1951, and this was followed by the vertical flap of Scardino and Prince[35] in 1953. In 1949, Anderson and Hynes[36] described the dismembered pyeloplasty.

The dismembered pyeloplasty is generally accepted as the treatment of choice. It can be universally applicable for repair of PUJ obstruction. It has the advantage of being applicable to high as well as dependent ureteral insertions, reduction of the redundant pelvis, or straightening of a lengthy or tortuous ureter. It also allows transposition of the PUJ when crossing vessels are present.

It has become clear with time that whichever technique is used, the anastomosis needs to be widely patent and watertight without tension, and the reconstructed PUJ should allow a funnel-shaped transition between pelvis and ureter with dependent drainage.

Indications

- Symptomatic PUJ obstruction.
- Urinary tract infections/stones.
- Progressive renal deterioration.
- Causal hypertension (rarely).
- Impaired renal function in a solitary kidney or bilateral disease.

Contraindications

- Lengthy or multiple proximal ureteral strictures.
- PUJ obstruction in a small inaccessible intra-renal pelvis.

Immediate pre-operative preparation

- Informed consent: ideally this should include the surgeon's results and success rates.
- Patient's side marked and signed by surgeon.
- Patient imaging on screen in theatre.
- Prophylactic antibiotics: gentamicin 240 mg plus cefuroxime 1.5 g at induction plus three post-operative doses of cefuroxime 750 mg.
- Prophylactic heparinization: unfractionated heparin 5000 IU twice daily or fractionated heparin once daily until discharge. There is some controversy with regard to this approach as compressions boots may provide a similar level of protection against thrombosis with fewer haemorrhagic events.
- Shave in theatre.

- Initial cystoscopy, retrograde pyelogram, and JJ stent insertion (6Fr, 28 cm) on affected side. We prefer to do this as a final check for stones and stricture as this can alter the surgery required. The stent can be placed antegrade during the pyeloplasty, but we do it at cystoscopy to be certain of its position and aid in ureteric identification in difficult cases during the pyeloplasty. The stent is 28Fr as this allows the J at the renal end to lie well above the anastomosis and not potentially cantilever on it, leading to urine leak and loosening of sutures. A JJ stent is placed for dismembered pyeloplasty and all the flap techniques described below.
- Catheterize patient: 12–14Ch catheter.

Patient positioning

Retroperitoneal approach. Flank (lateral decubitus position) with the affected side upwards. Flank position with table broken so that lumbar support is raised to maximum height. It is vital to pad soft tissues and bony sites carefully to minimize the risk of neuropraxia. In particular, the downside shoulder (axillary roll and posterior back support), hip, knee, and ankle should be padded (we prefer a pillow between the legs, buttock support posteriorly, and gel ankle supports). Body-warming devices and compression boots are also recommended.

Operative technique

Various incisions have been described including an anterior extraperitoneal and posterior lumbotomy. An anterior transperitoneal approach may also be of value when there have been previous flank incisions or when bilateral PUJ obstructions exist. The retroperitoneal approach allows direct exposure to the PUJ with minimal mobilization of the renal pelvis and proximal ureter and is our preferred route.

Make a subcostal or supra-12th rib incision. Cut the various muscles down to the retroperitoneum. Identify the proximal ureter lying on the psoas muscle and dissect it proximally to the renal pelvis. Care needs to be taken not to strip the peri-ureteral tissue as this may compromise the ureteric blood supply and a successful outcome. Place a stay suture in the ureter distal to the level of obstruction to aid with the anastomosis and orientation. Two stay sutures are then placed at the medial and lateral aspects of the dependent portions of the pelvis. Excise the PUJ; if the renal pelvis is particularly large, redundant pelvis can also be removed. Spatulate the lateral aspect of the ureter with Pott's scissors. Bring the apex of the spatulated ureter to the inferior border of the lateral renal pelvis and bring the medial portion of the ureter to the superior edge of the pelvis. Perform the anastomosis with a fine interrupted or running suture such as 4–0 Vicryl. Place the suture full thickness in a watertight fashion (Fig. 7.1).

If a crossing vessel is present at the PUJ, the dismembered pyeloplasty can be transposed to the other side of the vessel.

Place a 20Fr Robinson drain in the renal bed.

Post-operatively, remove the urinary catheter when the drain is dry and the drain 24 hr later if there has been no further drainage.

The JJ stent is removed via flexible cystoscopy 4 weeks post-operatively and the first MAG3 renogram is performed at 3 months.

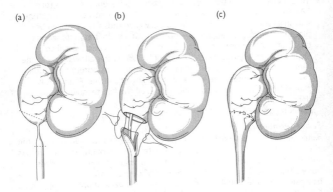

Fig. 7.1 Andersson Huynor dismembered pyecoplasty. Redrawn with permission from Walsh et al., *Campbell's Urology*, 8th edn., 2002, WB Saunders.

Other flap techniques

Foley Y–Vplasty

This was originally designed for PUJ obstruction with high ureteric insertion. It is contraindicated when transposition is required and pelvic reduction is needed.

Tissue mark a wide-based triangular or V-shaped flap. Position the base of the V on the dependent medial aspect of the renal pelvis and the apex at the PUJ. Carry the incision from the apex of the flap onto the lateral aspect of the ureter and extend distally beyond the stenosis and several millimetres onto normal calibre ureter. The initial incision is with a scalpel and is then developed with Pott's scissors. Bring the apex of the pelvic flap to the apex of ureteric incision distally and suture with 4–0 Vicryl. Close the posterior and anterior walls with 4–0 Vicryl interrupted sutures (Fig. 7.2).

Culp–DeWeerd spiral flap

This technique is best suited to a large extra-renal pelvis with the ureter inserted in the dependent position. It is best suited to a long segment of proximal ureteric narrowing/stricture.

Outline the flap with a broad base situated obliquely on the dependent renal pelvis. The base needs to be lateral to the PUJ (between ureteric insertion and renal parenchyma) to preserve blood supply to the flap. The flap can be spiralled posterior to anterior or vice versa. The length of the flap is determined by the length of ureter needed to be bridged, but the ratio of flap length to width should not exceed 3:1 to preserve vascular integrity. It is wise to outline the flap longer than what is perceived to be needed as flap shrinkage tends to occur when the pelvis is

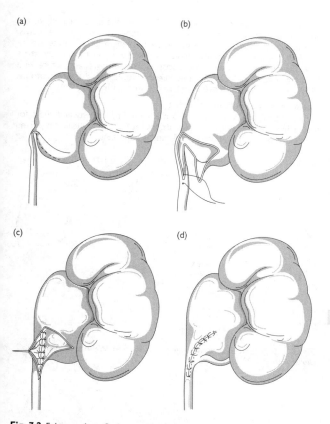

Fig. 7.2 Foley y-r plasty. Redrawn with permission from Walsh *et al.*, *Campbell's Urology*, 8th edn., 2002, WB Saunders.

incised. Any excess can be removed. Continue the medial aspect of the flap incision down the ureter beyond the obstructed segment. Rotate the apex of the flap down to the apex of the ureterotomy and close the posterior and anterior walls with 4–0 Vicryl interrupted sutures (Fig. 7.3).

Scardino–Prince vertical flap
This has a limited use today for relatively long areas of proximal ureteral narrowing when the ureter is situated at the medial margin of a large box-shaped extra-renal pelvis. It cannot bridge the same gap as a spiral flap. The flap is similar to the spiral flap except that the base is situated more horizontally on the dependent aspect of the renal pelvis. Form the

flap from straight incisions which converge from the base vertically to the apex superiorly on the posterior or anterior aspect of the pelvis. The length of the flap is determined by the length of the ureter to be bridged. Continue the medial incision down the ureter beyond the stricture. Develop the flap with Pott's scissors, rotate down, and suture with a interrupted 4–0 Vicryl to the inferior aspect of the ureterotomy. Then close the flap with 4–0 Vicryl interrupted sutures (Fig. 7.4).

Outcomes and complications[37–41]

Mean success rates are 92.6% for dismembered pyeloplasty and 80.5% for flap techniques. Complication rates are low at 6%. Urinary leak is reported in 5–12.5% of cases, infection in 1.5%, and ileus in 4.6%.

(a)   (b)   (c)

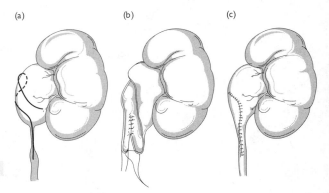

Fig. 7.3 Culp de weera. Redrawn with permission from Walsh et al., *Campbell's Urology*, 8th edn., 2002, Elsevier.

(a)   (b)   (c)

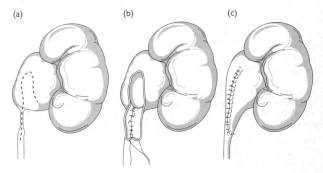

Fig. 7.4 Scordino price vertical flap. Redrawn with permission from Walsh et al., *Campbell's Urology*, 8th edn., 2002, Elsevier.

Laparoscopic pyeloplasty
See ☐ Chapter 5, p. 340.

JJ stenting for PUJO

A JJ stent may be an acceptable alternative treatment in the elderly, with or without significant comorbidity, who are experiencing significant complications from their PUJ obstruction. This can be done under local anaesthetic, although six-monthly changes are required.

Poorly functioning renal units (probably <15%) will be best served with nephrectomy.

References

1 Albarran J. Operations plastiques et anastomoses dans la traitment des retentions de veim. Thesis Paris, 1903.
2 Davis DM, Strong GH, Drake WM. Intubated ureterotomy: a new operation for ureteral and ureteral pelvic strictures. *Surg Gynaecol Obstet* 1943; **76**:513–23.
3 Wickham JEA, Kellet MJ. Percutaneous pyelolysis. *Eur Urol* 1983; **9**:122–4.
4 Ramsay JWA, Miller RA, Kellett MJ *et al.* Percutaneous pyelolysis: indications, complications, and results. *Br J Urol* 1983; **56**:586–8.
5 Chandoke PS, Clayman RV, Stone AM *et al.* Endopyelotomy and endoureterotomy with the Acucise ureteral cutting balloon device: preliminary experience. *J Endourol* 1993; **7**:45–51.
6 Thomas R, Monga M, Klein EW. Ureteroscopic retrograde endopyelotomy for management of ureteropelvic junction obstruction. *J Endourol* 1996; **10**:141–5.
7 Nakada SY, Johnson M. Ureteropelvic junction obstruction: retrograde endopyelotomy. *Urol Clin North Am* 2000; **27**:677–84.
8 Badlani GH, Karlin G, Smith AD. Complications of endopyelotomy: analysis in series of 64 patients. *J Urol* 1988; **140**:473–5.
9 Kim FJ, Herrell SD, Johoda AE *et al.* Complications of Acucise endopyelotomy. *J Endourol* 1998; **12**:433–6.

10 Preminger GM, Clayman RV, Nakada SY et al. A multicentre clinical trial investigating the use of a fluoroscopically controlled cutting balloon catheter for the management of ureteral and ureteropelvic junction obstruction. *J Urol* 1997; **157**:1625–9.

11 Shalhav AL, Giusti G, Elbahnasy AM et al. Endopyelotomy for high-insertion ureteropelvic junction obstruction. *J Endourol* 1998, **12**:127–30.

12 Van Cangh PH, Wilmart JF, Opsomer RJ et al. Long-term results and late recurrence after endoureteropyelotomy: a critical analysis of prognostic factors. *J Urol* 1994; **151**:934–7.

13 Clayman RV, Basler JO, Kavoussi LR et al. Ureteronephroscopic endopyelotomy. *J Urol* 1990; **144**:246–52.

14 Conlin MJ, Bagley DH. Ureteroscopic endopyelotomy at a single setting. *J Urol* 1998; **159**:727–31.

15 Meretyk I, Meretyk S, Clayman RV. Endopyelotomy: comparison of ureteroscopic retrograde and antegrade percutaneous techniques. *J Urol* 1992; **148**:775–83.

16 Thomas R, Monga M, Klein EW. Ureteroscopic retrograde endopyelotomy for management of ureteropelvic junction obstruction. *J Endourol* 1996; **10**:141–5.

17 Nadler RB, Rao GS, Pearle MS et al. Acucise endopyelotomy: evolution of a less-invasive technology. *J Urol* 1996; **156**:1094–7.

18 Faerber GJ, Richardson TD, Farah N et al. Retrograde treatment of ureteropelvic junction obstruction using the ureteral cutting balloon catheter. *J Urol* 1997; **157**:454–8.

19 Gelet A, Combe M, Ramackers JM et al. Endopyelotomy with the Acucise cutting balloon device. *Eur Urol* 1997; **31**:389–93.

20 Kim FJ, Herrell SD, Johoda AE et al. Complications of Acucise endopyelotomy. *J Endourol* 1998; **12**:433–6.

21 Gill HS, Liao JC. Pelvi-ureteric junction obstruction treated with Acucise retrograde endopyelotomy. *Br J Urol* 1998; **82**:8–11.

22 Cohen TD, Gross MB, Preminger GM. Long-term follow up of Acucise incision of ureteropelvic junction obstruction and ureteral strictures. *Urology* 1996; **47**:317–23.

23 Badlani G, Karlin G, Smith AD. Percutaneous surgery for ureteropelvic junction obstruction (endopyelotomy): technique and early results. *J Urol* 1986; **135**:26–8.

24 Streem SB. Percutaneous endopyelotomy. *Urol Clin N Am* 2000; **27**:685–93.

25 Bellman GC, Davidoff R, Candela J et al. Tubeless percutaneous renal surgery. *J Urol* 1997; **157**:1578–82.

26 Gerber GS, Lyon ES. Endopyelotomy: patient selection, results and complications. *Urology* 1994; **43**:2–10.

27 Kletscher BA, Segura JW, LeRoy AJ et al. Percutaneous antegrade endoscopic pyelotomy: review of 50 consecutive cases. *J Urol* 1995; **155**:701–3.

28 Motola JA, Badlani GH, Smith AD. Results of 212 consecutive endopyelotomies: an 8 year follow up. *J Urol* 1993; **149**:453–6.

29 Shalhav AL, Giusti G, Elbahnasy AM et al. Adult endopyelotomy: impact of aetiology and antegrade versus retrograde approach on outcome. *J Urol* 1998; **160**:685–9.

30 Kuster. Ein fall von resection des ureter. *Arch Klin Chir* 1892; **44**:850.

31 Fenger C. Operation for the relief of valve formation and stricture of the ureter in hydro or pyonephrosis. *JAMA* 1894; **22**:335–43.

32 Schwyzer A. New pyeloureteric plastic operation for hydronephrosis. *Surg Clin North Am* 1923; **3**:1441.

33 Foley FEB. New plastic operation for stricture at the ureteropelvic junction. *J Urol* 1937; **38**:643–5.

34 Culp OS, DeWeerd JH. A pelvic flap operation for certain types of uretero-pelvic obstruction. Preliminary report. *Mayo Clin Proc* 1951; **26**:483–8.

35 Scardino PL, Prince CL. Vertical flap ureteropelviplasty: preliminary report. *South Med J* 1953; **46**:325–31.

36 Anderson JC, Hynes W. Retrocaval ureter: a case diagnosed preoperatively and treated successfully by a plastic operation. *Br J Urol* 1949; **21**:209–14.

37 Graversen HP, Tofte T, Genster HG. Uretero-pelvic stenosis. *Int Urol Nephrol* 1987; **19**:245–51.

38 Guys JM, Borella F, Montfort G. Ureteropelvic junction obstructions: prenatal diagnosis and neonatal surgery in 47 cases. *J Paediatr Surg* 1988; **23**:156–8.

39 Mikkelson SS, Rasmussen BS, Jensen TM et al. Long-term follow up of patients with hydronephrosis treated by Anderson-Hynes pyeloplasty. *Br J Urol* 1992; **79**:121–4.

40 Nguyen DH, Aliabadi H, Ercole CJ et al. Non-intubated Anderson–Hynes repair of ureteropelvic junction obstruction in 60 patients. *J Urol* 1989; **142**:704–6.

41 Eden CG. Treatment options for pelvi-ureteric junction obstruction: implications for practice and training. *Br J Urol* 1997; **80**:365–72.

Management of ureteric strictures

Ureteral strictures are relatively rare and occur in a number of benign and malignant conditions:

- Congenital.
- Infection (e.g. tuberculosis, schistosomiasis).
- Iatrogenic (e.g. ureteroscopy, gynaecological, or other pelvic surgery).
- Radiation.
- Malignancy.
- Stones.

Not all ureteric strictures require surgical intervention. In dealing with ureteral strictures it is helpful to divide the ureter into proximal, middle, and distal parts. Most strictures occur in the distal ureter from iatrogenic, malignant, and infective causes, (during endoscopic or pelvic surgery) these are the iatrogenic causes.

Nephrostomies or JJ stents can be used both palliatively, i.e. to relieve symptoms and restore renal function, and therapeutically. Therapeutically, JJ stents can be used to intubate ureters that have been ligated during other pelvic surgery. The injury is not recognized during the pelvic surgery and only becomes evident post-operatively. JJ stenting will be therapeutically successful in 50% of cases.

Nephrostomy tracts can be used therapeutically as part of an antegrade approach to a ureteral stricture. Three endoscopic techniques exist to treat ureteral strictures: catheter dilatation, balloon dilatation, and endo-incision. These techniques are the same as for the retrograde approach described earlier for PUJ obstruction.

The first end-to-end anastomosis of a divided ureter was described by Tauffer in 1885. Boree reported cutting the ureteric ends obliquely to reduce the chance of stenosis. Transuretero-ureterostomy was also performed in this time period. Boari[1] described his bladder flap operation in 1894, and Sir John Simon performed uretero-intestinal anastomosis in 1852. The psoas hitch was popularized by Turner-Warwick and Worth[2] in 1969. Endoscopic procedures to treat or palliate ureteric strictures have been a very recent development and are still undergoing scrutiny.

Ureteric strictures are an uncommon cause of obstructive uropathy. Other than those caused by accidental suture ligation, they tend to develop slowly, producing chronic obstructive uropathy.

Conservative management

Specific mention needs to be made of infective causes of ureteric strictures (tuberculosis and schistosomiasis). In both these cases chemotherapy may suffice. The disease needs to be treated when inflammation and oedema, rather than fibrosis, are present.

With tuberculosis, the lower third of the ureter is most commonly affected. Anti-tuberculous treatment is initiated and weekly full-shot IVUs are performed. If there is no improvement after 4 weeks, prednisolone is added to the regimen. If no further improvement is seen in the subsequent 4 weeks, surgical intervention is required. An alternative approach is to place a JJ stent in combination with the chemotherapy. This may improve outcome in terms of both initial success and subsequent surgery if chemotherapy fails.[3]

Ureteric strictures occur in 25% of cases of urinary schistosomiasis; 80% of these strictures are in the lower third of the ureter. Medical treatment is the initial approach with or without a JJ stent, and if this fails surgical intervention.

Endoscopic techniques

There are four general endosurgical techniques for treating ureteral strictures:[4–8]

- JJ stent insertion.
- Catheter dilatation.
- Balloon dilatation.
- Endo-incision.

Indications[6,8–9]

- Benign ureteric strictures <1 cm.
- Palliation of malignant ureteric strictures <1 cm.

Contraindications[6,8–9]

- Stricture length >1 cm.

Relative contraindications[5,6,10–11]

- Ischaemic or radiation-induced strictures.
- Mid-ureteric location.

Immediate pre-operative preparation
- Informed consent: this should include the surgeon's results and possible need to do an open surgical repair.
- Check pre-operative urine cultures.
- Patient's side marked and signed by surgeon.
- Patient imaging on screen in theatre.
- Prophylactic intravenous gentamicin 240 mg plus cefuroxime 1.5 g.
- Prophylactic TED stockings and compression boots.
- C-arm in theatre with radiation protection gowns for use.

Patient positioning
Dorsal lithotomy with legs in supports.

Operative technique
The first step is to pass a guidewire beyond the stricture with the tip placed into the kidney under fluoroscopic guidance. A Terumo (0.035 inch) guidewire is usually the easiest to place as its hydrophilic coating facilitates passage through the stricture. Then place an open-ended ureteral catheter (5Fr) over the wire and exchange the Terumo for a stiffer guidewire such as a Bentson or Amplatz Superstiff.

In cases where a suture has been tied around the ureter, if a ureteric stent can be placed this can be definitive treatment and should be left for 3 months. Following removal an IVU should be performed 4 weeks later and, if normal, after a further 3 months.[12]

In all other cases, catheter or balloon dilatation or retrograde incision via a ureteroscopic or fluoroscopic approach can be performed. Retrogradely, these techniques are similar for those described for PUJ obstruction.

Similarly, a percutaneous approach to upper or midureteric strictures can be performed following the same description of an antegrade endopyelotomy. The incision in the mid-ureter is made laterally, except over the iliac vessels where it is placed anteromedially.

An endo-incision also uses the same modalities as endopyelotomy, i.e. cold knife, endosurgical probe, or laser (Nd:YAG, KTP, or Ho:YAG). The incision needs to be full thickness. Retroperitoneal fat will usually be seen in the upper, middle, and proximal distal ureter. Retroperitoneal fat may not be seen in marked fibrosis; if the peri-ureteric fat has been seen, no further incision should be made because of the risk of haemorrhage.

Place a stent (14Fr Nephrostent, 7 or 8Fr double pigtail, or 10Fr nephrostomy (for antegrade approach)). Leave a urethral catheter *in situ* for 24–36 hr. If a nephrostomy is in place, perform a nephrostogram after 48 hr and cap the Nephrostent. Remove the Nephrostent or internal JJ stents after 4–6 weeks.

If the stricture has caused complete obstruction, it will not be possible to perform a retrograde approach as neither a guidewire nor contrast will pass.[13,14] The limits of the stricture need to be ascertained from a combined nephrostogram and retrograde ureterogram. If the occlusion is <1 cm an endosurgical approach can be tried, but if it is >1 cm open surgery is recommended.[14]

If the complete obstruction is in the proximal or middle ureter, the technique described for approaching the completely obstructed PUJ is followed. The indwelling stent should be left for 12 weeks.[14]

If the complete obstruction is in the distal ureter, place a nephrostomy tube. A purely fluoroscopic or combined fluoroscopy and endoscopic incision can then be followed.

In the fluoroscopic approach, introduce a stiff guidewire via the nephrostomy antegrade to the proximal level of the stricture. Fill the bladder with contrast. Use the C-arm to position the guidewire tip, pointing directly at the bladder in both anteroposterior and lateral views. Introduce a cystoscope and forcibly advanced the guidewire into the bladder. Once the guidewire enters the bladder grasp it and bring it out through the urethral meatus. Pass a 4–8 mm balloon dilator antegrade into the stricture and dilate for 10 min. Then place either a Nephrostent or an indwelling ureteric stent with a nephrostomy. If a nephrostomy is placed a nephrostogram is performed on the third post-operative day and removed if no extravasation is seen. The stents are left for 6–12 weeks.

The second option is to place an antegrade guidewire to the proximal level of the stricture, followed by a flexible ureteroscope over the wire. Introduce a resectoscope with a Collings knife attached or an optical urethrotome per urethra. Position the cystoscope with the C-arm so that it lies next to the flexible ureteroscope. Turn off the cystoscope light and the theatre lights and make the incision to the bright light coming from the ureteroscope. Once the ureteroscope is uncovered, retrieve the guidewire and place a Nephrostent or indwelling stent plus nephrostomy and a urethral catheter left *in situ*. If a nephrostomy is placed, a nephrostogram is performed on the third post-operative and removed if there is no extravasation.

If peri-vesical fat is seen at the time of incision, a cystogram is performed at 7–10 days and the catheter is removed if no leak is seen. Otherwise, the urethral catheter is removed on the second post-operative day. The stent remains in place for 4–6 weeks.[15]

An alternative for totally obstructed ureters if the above procedure fails is a nephrovesical stent.[15] This involves inserting one end of the stent into the renal pelvis via a percutaneous nephrostomy puncture. The body of the stent is tunnelled subcutaneously towards the bladder. The distal end of the stent is then placed into the bladder via a percutaneous puncture. The stent needs to be changed every 4 months using a combined cystoscopic and percutaneous cut-down technique.

Outcomes and complications[3–16]

- Ureteric stent insertion for ligatures will succeed in 50% of cases.
- Balloon dilatation is successful in 55% (range 45–80%) of cases.
- Endoureterotomy has been reported to achieve patency in 70% (range 55–80%) of cases.

The wide variability is due to differences in technique, data collection, and type of stricture. However, the length of stricture is the most important determinant with those >1 cm rarely responding to an endo-surgical approach. Ischaemic strictures (40% success) do less well than non-ischaemic strictures (58% success).

Strictures in the upper and lower ureter that can be marsupialized at their upper border into the renal pelvis or bladder respectively do better than middle ureteric strictures and those bounded by normal ureter on each end (80% versus 25%). The duration of the stricture has not been shown to clearly influence the outcome.

Metallic stents have also been used to treat unfavourable ureteric strictures. Numerous stents have been described: Wallstents, Palmer–Schatz, Accuflex, Memokath. The first three are meshed stents which allow urothelial ingrowth and are incorporated into the ureter. If complications occur, their removal is often impossible.

References

1 Boari A. *La uretero-cisto-neostomia*. Rome: Societa Editrice Dante Aligghieri, 1894.

2 Turner-Warwick RT, Worth PHL. The psoas bladder-hitch procedure for the replacement of the lower third of the ureter. *Br J Urol* 1969; **41**:701–9.

3 Shin KY, Park HJ, Lee JJ et al. Role of early endourologic management of tuberculous ureteral strictures. *J Endourol* 2002; **16**:755–8.

4 Glanz S, Gordon PH, Butt K et al. Percutaneous balloon dilatation of the ureter. *Radiology* 1983; **143**:795–801.

5 Smith AD. Management of iatrogenic ureteral strictures after urological procedures. *J Urol* 1988; **140**:1372–4.

6 Meretyk S, Albala DM, Clayman RV et al. Endoureterotomy for treatment of ureteral strictures. *J Urol* 1992; **147**:1502–6.

7 Preminger GM, Clayman RV, Nakada SY et al. A multicentre clinical trial investigating the use of a fluoroscopically controlled cutting balloon catheter for the management of ureteral and ureteropelvic junction obstruction. *J Urol* 1997; **157**:1625–9.

8 Netto NR, Jr, Ferreira U, Lemos GC et al. Endourological management of ureteral strictures. *J Urol* 1990; **144**:631–4.

9 Chang R, Marshall FF, Mitchell S. Percutaneous management of benign ureteral strictures and fistulas. *J Urol* 1987; **137**:1126–31.

10 Lang EK. Antegrade ureteral stenting for dehiscence, strictures and fistulae. *Am J Roentgenol* 1984; **143**:795–801.

11 O'Brien WM, Maxted WC, Pahira JJ. Ureteral stricture: experience with 31 cases. *J Urol* 1988; **140**:737–40.

12 Cormio L, Battaglia M, Traficante A, Selvaggi FP. Endourological treatment of ureteric injuries. *Br J Urol* 1993; **72**:165–8.

13 Bagley DH, Huffmann J, Lyon E et al. Endoscopic ureteropyelotomy: opening the obliterated ureteropelvic junction with nephroscopy and flexible ureteropyeloscopy. *J Urol* 1985; **133**:462–4.

14 Bagley DH. Endoscopic ureteroureterostomy. *J Urol* 1990; **143**:235a.

15 Cubelli V, Smith AD. Transurethral ureteral surgery guided by fluoroscopy. *Endourology* 1987; **2**:8.

16 Desgrandchamps F, Cussenot O, Bassi S et al. Percutaneous extra-anatomic nephrovesical diversion: preliminary report. *J Endourol* 1993; **7**:323–6.

The omental wrap involves four steps.[2] First, liberate the hepatic and splenic flexures by dividing the hepatocolic and splenocolic ligaments and fully mobilize the ascending and descending colons medially. In the second step, detach the greater omentum from the transverse colon along its bloodless line of adhesion. Thirdly, divide the omentum in the midline and free each half from the greater curvature of the stomach by dividing some of the short gastric vessels on each side of the midline. The right half of the omentum receives its arterial blood supply from the gastro-epiploic branch of the pancreaticoduodenal artery and the left side by the middle colic artery. Wrap the omental flaps completely around each ureter, extending from the hilum of the kidney to the point where the ureter crosses the common iliac artery.

The fibrosis can invade the ureter, although usually only a short segment is involved. Resection of the ureter and uretero-ureterostomy is necessary. If extensive ureteral invasion is present an ileal ureter may be required.

Outcomes[3–6]

Recurrent obstruction is reported in 10–50% of cases.[3–6] Development of obstruction in the apparently uninvolved kidney occurs in 20–40% cases of unilateral obstruction.[3–4] Mortality is 5–28% in some series; however, many of these deaths occur years after surgery and appear to be related to age, the degree of renal impairment pre-operatively, and comorbidity.[3] Ureteric leak is seen in 14–17%,[4,5] intestinal obstruction in up to 14%,[4] ileus in 6%,[5] recurrent UTI in 17%,[5] aortic thrombosis in 6%,[5] wound infection in 11%,[5] and deep vein thrombosis in 10–11%.[4–5]

References

1 Albarran J. Retention renale par perl externe de l'uretere. *Proc Verb Fr Urol* 1905; **9**:511–17.
2 Tresidder GC, Blandy JP, Singh M. Omental sleeve to prevent recurrent retroperitoneal fibrosis the ureter. *Urol Int* 1972; **27**:144–8.
3 Baker LRI, Mallinson WJW, Gregory MC *et al.* Idiopathic retroperitoneal fibrosis: a retrospective analysis of 60 cases. *Br J Urol* 1987; **60**:497–503.
4 Tiptaft RC, Costello AJ, Paris AMI *et al.* The long-term follow-up of idiopathic retroperitoneal fibrosis. *Br J Urol* 1982; **54**:620–4.
5 Cooksey G, Powell PH, Singh M *et al.* Idiopathic retroperitoneal fibrosis: a long-term review after surgical treatment. *Br J Urol* 1982; **54**:628–31.
6 Osborn DE, Rao PR, Barnard RJ *et al.* Surgical management of idiopathic retroperitoneal fibrosis. *Br J Urol* 1981; **53**:292–6.

Ureteric re-implantation

Various open surgical techniques to treat ureteral strictures have been adopted. Which one is adopted depends on the position and length of ureteric defect to be bridged, but intra-operative flexibility is required. Ureteric re-implantation can also be used for distal ureteric injuries occurring either intra-operatively or secondary to trauma or for distal ureteric tumours following local excision.

Uretero-ureterostomy

This technique can only be used for short defects as tension on the anastomosis will nearly always lead to an anastomotic stricture. The determination of whether adequate mobility can be achieved is often only possible intra-operatively.

Indications[1,2]
- Ureteric stricture ≤ 2–3 cm in upper/mid ureter.

Contraindications[1,2]
- Ureteric strictures >3 cm.
- Lower-third ureteric strictures.

Immediate pre-operative preparation
- Informed consent.
- Patient's side marked and signed by surgeon.
- Patient imaging on screen in theatre.
- Prophylactic intravenous antibiotics: cefuroxime 1.5 g plus gentamicin 240 mg at induction.
- Prophylactic heparinization: unfractionated heparin 5000 IU twice daily or fractionated heparin once daily until discharge plus TED stockings plus compression boots intra-operatively.
- Abdominal shave in theatre.
- Catheterize patient: 12–14Ch catheter.

Patient positioning
- Lateral: loin incision, upper ureter.
- Supine: Gibson incision, middle ureter.

Operative technique
A subcostal incision is made. Skin, connective tissue, and muscle layers are opened as previously discussed. Develop the retroperitoneal space with the peritoneum mobilized and retracted medially. The ureter is attached to the posterior peritoneum and is usually most easily identified as it crosses the common iliac vessels. Mobilize the ureter using a right angle. Care needs to be taken to preserve the adventitia which loosely attaches the blood supply to the ureter. The ureter is mobilized as the clinical setting dictates and this equates to avoiding tension on the anastomosis once the strictured area has been excised. Minimal handling of the ureter with non-toothed forceps is recommended. Correctly orientate the ureter and then spatulate the two ends for 5–6 mm. Perform the spatulation at both ureteral ends at 180° to each other. Place a 4–0 Vicryl suture in the corner of one ureteral segment and the apex of the other.

Suture the opposite corner and apex similarly. Run interrupted sutures up each side of the anastomosis. Place a JJ stent before completion of closure (methylene blue is put into the bladder via the catheter and visualization of the refluxing methylene blue at the anastomotic site indicates correct positioning of the stent in the bladder). Mobilize retroperitoneal fat or omentum to surround the anastomosis. Place a 20Fr Robinson drain close to but not over the anastomosis.

The Foley catheter can usually be removed after 1–2 days. The drain can be removed when there has been 24–48 hr of minimal drainage (<50 mL) following catheter removal. If drainage persists the fluid, should be sent for creatinine assessment which will determine if it is urine or serous fluid.

Endoscopically remove the JJ stent via a flexible cystoscope at 4 weeks.

Outcomes
Success rates are 90%.[3] Fistulae have been reported in up to 4%.

Uretero-neocystostomy
Indications[1,2]
- Ureteric stricture ≤4–5 cm in lower ureter.
- Lower-third ureteric injuries <5 cm from bladder due to intra-operative injury or trauma.

Contraindications[1,2]
- Lower ureteric strictures >5 cm.

Immediate pre-operative preparation
- Informed consent.
- Patient's side marked and signed by surgeon.
- Patient imaging on screen in theatre.
- Prophylactic intravenous antibiotics: cefuroxime 1.5 g plus gentamicin 240 mg at induction.
- Prophylactic heparinization: unfractionated heparin 5000 IU twice daily or fractionated heparin once daily until discharge plus TED stockings plus compression boots intra-operatively.
- Abdominal shave in theatre.
- Catheterize patient: 12–14Ch catheter.

Patient positioning
- Supine.

Operative technique
This involves an extra-vesical Lich—Gregoire re-implantation[3,4] via a lower midline or Pfannensteil incision. Ideally, an extra-peritoneal approach is adopted. Identify the ureter as it crosses the common iliac arteries and proximally mobilize. Take care not to skeletonize the ureter and thereby preserve its adventitia and blood supply. Excise the affected length of ureter. Perfom a direct uretero-neocystostomy if a tension-free anastomosis is possible. Fill the bladder with saline via the catheter until it is moderately full. Dissect the peritoneum off the posterior aspect of the bladder where implantation is intended. Preserve major blood vessels (e.g. superior vesical artery) during peri-vesical dissection. Open the

serosal and muscular layers of the detrusor along a straight course cephalad to the ureterovesical junction with the opening continued through the bladder mucosa. Placement in the more mobile lateral bladder wall is discouraged as this may result in ureteral kinking. It is not necessary to tunnel the ureter, which is placed intraluminally. JJ stents are controversial, but Foley catheters are placed urethrally. The detrusor is then closed over the ureter with 3–0 PDS or Vicryl sutures.

A 20Fr Robinson drain is placed in the peri-vesical space. The Foley catheter is removed at 7–10 days and, if placed, the JJ stent at 6–8 weeks.

Outcomes

Incidence of complications after the repair of iatrogenically injured ureter is not reported. Complication rates after repair of traumatic injuries is 25%.[5–7] Prolonged leakage at the anastomosis is the most common genito-urinary complication, presenting as urinoma, abscess, or peritonitis. Drain placement at the time of surgery minimizes this risk and allows its earlier identification. Delayed complications include ureteral stricture and retained ureteral stent leading to stone formation.

Uretero-neocystotomy plus psoas hitch

This procedure was first described by Zimmerman et al.[8] in 1960. It has the advantage of maintaining urothelial continuity. It also avoids compromising the function of a normal contralateral ureter and the risks of chronic urinary tract infections and electrolyte abnormalities, problems associated with transuretero-ureterostomy and ileal substitution, respectively.

Indications[1,2]
- Ureteric stricture ≤6–10 cm in lower ureter[1,2] (generally up to pelvic brim).
- Lower-third ureteric injuries <10 cm from bladder caused by intra-operative injury or trauma.
- Distal ureteral fistulae.
- Distal ureteric tumours.
- Failed uretero-neocystotomy.

Contraindications[1–2]
- Lower ureteric strictures >10 cm.
- Small contracted bladder.

Operative technique

The initial operative preparation and patient position are the same as for a neocystotomy. Make a lower midline or Pfannensteil incision. Develop the space of Retzius and mobilize the bladder, dividing the contralateral obliterated umbilical artery, freeing the peritoneal attachments, and dividing the vas deferens or round ligaments. This will usually provide adequate bladder mobility to bridge the ureteral defect, but if not, the urachus, ipsilateral obliterated umbilical artery, and superior vesical artery can also be divided.

Identify the affected ureter is as it crosses the iliac vessels and mobilize it down to the diseased segment. Divide the ureter just proximal to the diseased segment. Place a fine stay suture on the normal proximal ureter. Fill the bladder with 200 mL of normal saline and then enter the bladder via an anterior or oblique anterior cystotomy. Place a finger directly into the bladder, advancing the ipsilateral bladder to the psoas muscle. Fix the bladder to the psoas tendon using two to four 0–PDS sutures. The sutures are placed vertically to avoid injury to the genitofemoral nerve, and not too deep to avoid branches of the femoral nerve. The bladder is fixed prior to the re-implantation to avoid kinks in the distal ureter. Then re-implant the ureter using either a non-refluxing submucosal tunnel or a refluxing-type direct reanastomosis. Place a JJ stent and close the bladder with full-thickness running 20 Vicryl sutures.

A 20Fr Robinson drain is placed in the perivesical space. Remove the JJ stent at 7–14 days.

Outcomes

Success rates are >95%. The most common complications are urinary fistulae and ureteral obstruction. A direct refluxing anastomosis does not appear to carry greater complications when compared with a non-refluxing anastomosis.

Uretero-neocystotomy plus Boari flap

This technique, first described by Boari in 1894, is required for lower ureteric strictures 12–15 cm long[1,2] or to bridge lower ureteric defects 10–15 cm long. A spiralled Boari flap can reach the renal pelvis in some circumstances. Ideally, bladder outlet obstruction and neurogenic dysfunction should be addressed pre-operatively.

Indications[1,2]

- Ureteric stricture ≤15 cm in lower ± middle ureter.[1,2]
- Lower-third ureteric injuries <15 cm from bladder caused by intra-operative injury or trauma.
- Distal ureteral fistulae.
- Distal ureteric tumours.

Contraindications[1,2]

- Lower ± middle ureteric strictures >15 cm.
- Small contracted bladder.

Operative technique

The initial operative preparation and patient position is the same as for a neocystostomy. Make a lower midline or Pfannensteil incision. A midline incision allows easier access to the upper ureter. Develop the space of Retzius and mobilize the bladder, dividing the umbilical ligaments, freeing the peritoneal attachments, and dividing the vas deferens or round ligaments and contralateral superior vesical artery. Mobilize the upper ureter down to the diseased or injured portion, taking care to preserve the adventitia.

Identify the ipsilateral superior vesical artery or one of its branches as the posterolateral bladder flap is outlined based on this vessel. Fill the bladder with 200 mL normal saline. Mark out the base of the flap at least 4 cm in width. Continue the flap obliquely across the anterior bladder wall with the tip of the flap being at least 3 cm wide. The flap length should equal the estimated ureteral defect plus 3–4 cm if a non-refluxing anastomosis is desired. An open-ended ureteric catheter can be placed in the contralateral ureter at this point to protect it during the surgery and removed prior to closing the bladder.

Secure the distal end of the flap to the psoas minor tendon or psoas major muscle with two to four 2–0 Vicryl sutures. Deliver the ureter through the posterior flap and spatulate anteriorly. Perform a standard mucosa to mucosa anastomosis with interrupted 4–0 Vicryl making sure there is no tension. Some authors propose routine placement of a JJ stent in the affected ureter, although this remains controversial.[6] The flap is then rolled anteriorly and closed using a continuous 2–0 Vicryl suture. The ureteral adventitia can be secured to the distal aspect of the flap with 4–0 Vicryl and the base of the flap secured to the psoas with 3–0 Vicryl. Close the bladder in one or two layers with 2–0 Vicryl. The bladder is drained with a urethral catheter. A Robinson or similar drain is placed in the pelvis adjacent to the Boari flap.

A cystogram is performed 2 weeks post-operatively. If the bladder is healed, the urethral catheter is removed.

Outcomes[9–11]

Successful outcomes are seen in 85% of patients. Recurrent stricture formation is the most common complication (A tunnel-and-cuff anastomosis rather than an end-to-end anastomosis reduces this complication significantly). Early complications of wound and urinary sepsis occur in 20% and 10%, respectively.

References

1 Hinman F. Ureter. In *Reconstruction Atlas of Urologic Surgery.*, ed. Hinman F. Philadelphia, PA: WB Saunders, 1989, pp 636–93.
2 Galal H, Lazica A, Lampel A et al. Management of ureteral strictures by different modalities and effect of stents on upper tract drainage. *J Endourol* 1993; **7**:411–17.
3 Gregoir W, Van Regemorter GV. Le reflux vesico-ureteral congenital. *Urol Int* 1964; **18**:122.
4 Lich R, Howerton LW, Goode LS et al. The ureterovesical junction of the newborn. *J Urol* 1964; **92**:436–8.
5 Elliott SP, McAninch JW. Ureteral injuries from external violence: the 25-year experience at San Francisco General Hospital. *J Urol* 2003; **170**:1213–16.
6 Bright TC 3rd, Peters PC. Ureteral injuries due to external violence: 10 years experience with 59 cases. *J Trauma* 1977; **17**:616–20.
7 Ghali AM, El Malik EM, Ibrahim AI et al. Ureteric injuries: diagnosis, management, and outcome. *J Trauma* 1999; **46**:150–8.
8 Zimmerman IJ, Precourt WE, Thompson CC. Direct uretero-cysto-neostomy with the short ureter in the cure of ureterovaginal fistula. *J Urol* 1960; **83**:113–15.
9 Motiwala HG, Shah SA, Patel SM. Ureteric substitution with Boari bladder flap. *Br J Urol* 1990; **66**:369–71.
10 Cukier J. L'operation de Boari. *Acta Urol Belg* 1966; **34**:15–28.
11 Bowsher WG, Shah PJR, Costello AJ et al. A critical appraisal of the boari flap. *Br J Urol* 1982; **54**:682–5.

Repair of ureterocoele

Ureterocoele is cystic dilatation of the terminal ureter. They occur more frequently in females (4:1), and almost exclusively in whites. Ten per cent are bilateral and 80% arise from upper poles of duplicated systems. Single-system ureterocoeles (often referred to as simple ureterocoeles) are usually seen in adults and tend not to have the severe obstructive and dysplastic problems associated with duplex systems. However, they can be complicated by stones and infection. Under these circumstances surgery may be required, and this can be achieved endoscopically for single-system intra-vesical ureterocoeles.

Indications[1]

- Single-system intra-vesical ureterocoeles.

Relative contraindications[1]

There is continuing controversy with regard to these:
- Ectopic ureterocoeles.
- Duplex collecting systems.

Operative technique

The initial operative preparation and patient position are the same as for cystoscopy (☐ Chapter 2, p. 14). The bladder is assessed cystoscopically. The ureterocoele is either incised[2] or punctured.[3] Keep the bladder relatively empty.
- *Incision* Make a transverse full-thickness incision distally on the ureterocoele as close to the bladder as possible without rupturing it. A Collins knife, cold knife, or the metal stylet of a ureteral catheter can be used. If a Collins knife is used, set the cautery to cutting at 150 W.
- *Puncture* Perform the puncture with a 3Fr Bugbee electrode. Set the cutting current to 150 watts. Place the Bugbee electrode low on the front ureterocoele wall and puncture. Apply flank pressure to visualize urine efflux after puncture, confirming adequate drainage.

Successful decompression of the upper tract can be documented by a KUB ultrasound 1 month post-operatively.

Outcomes[1–3]

No data are available from adult endoscopic incision. Data from paediatric series show re-operation rates of 0–100% for all cases of endoscopic incision/puncture. The rates for intra-vesical single systems are lower (7–50%) than those for ectopic ureterocoeles. Successful decompression is common (94%) and the incidence of recurrent urinary tract infections appears to be reduced.

References

1 Byun E, Merguerian PA. A meta-analysis of surgical practice patterns in the endoscopic management of ureterocoeles. *J Urol* 2006; **176**:1871–7.

2 Monfort G, Morisson-Lacombe G, Guys JM *et al.* Simplified treatment of ureterocoeles. *Chir Pediatr* 1985; **26**:26–30.

3 Hagg MJ, Mourachov PV, Snyder HM *et al.* The modern endoscopic approach to ureterocoele. *J Urol* 2000; **163**:940–3.

Chapter 8

Trauma to the genitourinary tract and other urological emergencies

Essentials in the initial evaluation of the trauma patient

Mechanics of trauma

Penetrating trauma

Need for tissue debridement and potential for reconstruction is determined by type and extent of tissue damage. Type and extent of tissue damage in penetrating injuries is determined by:

- Kinetic energy.
- Cavitation.
- Secondary missiles.

Kinetic energy

$$\text{Kinetic energy} = \text{missile mass} \times (\text{missile velocity})^1$$

The amount of tissue damage is directly proportional to the kinetic energy transferred to tissues in the path of the missile. Increases in velocity exponentially increase energy transfer and hence the likelihood of multiple organ injuries. Based on the energy exchanged, penetrating injuries are classified as low, medium, and high energy (Table 8.1). Shotguns have unique wounding characteristics because pellets disperse on contact. At close range they can cause massive tissue destruction. At longer range they inflict insignificant wounds.

Cavitation

Tissue is pushed aside producing a path of destruction:

$$\text{higher energy} = \text{larger cavity}$$

Part of the cavity produced is permanent (visible to the examiner) and part is temporary (occurs momentarily after impact and quickly disappears). Tissues with low tensile strength (e.g. parenchymal organs (liver, kidney, spleen)) develop larger cavitations than tissues with greater tensile strength (e.g. bone, muscle, tendon).

Secondary missiles

Created when a bullet or its fragments impart sufficient kinetic energy to dense tissue such as bone and, occasionally, metal objects (e.g. buttons, buckles). Secondary missiles created in this way can be unpredictable and highly destructive.

Blunt trauma

Unlike penetrating trauma, where a large force and energy is applied to a relatively small area, the forces applied in blunt trauma and the transfer of energy are more complex. For example, in motor vehicle accidents, biomechanical interactions are intricate and difficult to assess. Head-on collisions usually result in large energy transfer to victims and are associated with highest mortality, followed by side impacts, roll-overs, and rear-end collisions.

Table 8.1 Penetrating injury classification according to missile energy

Kinetic energy of missile	Typical weapon type
Low	'Hand-driven' weapons, e.g. knives; some handguns
Medium	Handguns with projectile modifications e.g. hollow-point or expanding bullets
High	Assault and hunting rifles

Initial resuscitation of the traumatized patient

The resuscitation of the traumatized patient is usually initiated in the field by the paramedic team, and is continued systematically once the patient reaches the emergency department by a rapid, multidisciplinary priority-based approach. The goals of resuscitation are:

- Restoration of cardiac, pulmonary, and neurological function.
- Diagnosis of immediate life-threatening conditions.
- Prevention of complications from multisystem injuries.

The initial resuscitation process can be divided into three phases.

Primary survey

ABC

Assess the patient's **A**irway, **B**reathing, and **C**irculation.

- Airway and breathing:
  - Establish a secure airway.
  - Ventilate by oxygen mask or endotracheal intubation and mechanical ventilation.
  - Immobilize the cervical spine.
- Circulation: assess circulatory function by pulse rate and blood pressure. The most common cause of hypotension in the polytraumatized patient is hypovolaemia secondary to haemorrhage. With hypovolaemic shock an immediate bolus of intravenous isotonic crystalloid solution should be given and the patient's response (PR, BP) assessed.

Radiological imaging

Determined by local facilities. Increasingly, in the severely traumatized patient, CT of chest, abdomen, and pelvis is used to identify significant chest, abdominal, and pelvic injuries. If CT is not available, arrange supine chest, abdomen, and pelvic X-rays to identify the presence of rib and pelvic fractures and to identify the presence of significant quantities of blood in chest, abdomen, and pelvis. In patients with persistent hypotension from presumed bleeding, search for occult haemorrhage using a diagnostic peritoneal lavage or focused abdominal ultrasound.

Hypovolaemic shock is not always associated with hypotension. In young patients compensatory mechanisms (e.g. rapid vasoconstriction) can compensate for as much as a 35% volume loss without significant decreases in blood pressure.

Remember non-hypovolaemic causes of hypotension:
- Tension pneumothorax.
- Cardiac tamponade.
- Myocardial infarction.
- Neurogenic (spinal cord injury).

Urinalysis
Routinely performed in every trauma patient because it provides valuable information regarding the likelihood of injuries to the upper and lower urinary tract. However, the absence of haematuria does not exclude a urinary tract injury (e.g. haematuria may be absent in acceleration/deceleration renal injuries.

As life-threatening injuries are found during the primary survey, resuscitation efforts are initiated concurrently (e.g. chest drain for pneumothorax). The decision to transfer a patient from the emergency room to either the operating room or the angiography suite is made during the primary survey.

Secondary survey
Performed after completion of the primary survey:
- Perform a complete history and physical examination from head to toe.
- Arrange selective skeletal X-rays, according to physical findings.

Definitive survey
During this phase, focus attention on identifying specific organ injuries using clinical and radiographic means. Genitourinary injuries are usually recognized during the definitive survey.

During all phases of the initial resuscitation, assess vital signs (blood pressure, respiratory rate, blood gases, urinary output, and body temperature) continually. Vascular pressure monitoring, using central venous and pulmonary arterial catheters, can be performed selectively. Frequent re-evaluation should be performed to detect changes in the patient's condition and the appropriate actions should be taken.

Arrange radiographic renal imaging in the haemodynamically stable patient with:[1-3]

- Any *penetrating* injury to the abdomen, flanks, back, or lower chest.
- Any *blunt* injury presenting with any of the following:
  - Gross haematuria.
  - Microscopic haematuria and an initial blood pressure <90 mmHg.
  - Any clinical indicator of renal injury.

In patients who sustain blunt trauma and are haemodynamically stable with only microscopic haematuria, a clinical diagnosis of a low-grade renal injury can be made accurately without the need for radiographic renal assessment.

The haemodynamically unstable patient

Surgical staging (as opposed to radiological staging) is required in patients who are too unstable to undergo the appropriate clinical and radiographic evaluation. In these cases, a one-shot IVP is performed 10 min after intravenous infusion of 2 mL/kg contrast material.[4] The primary purpose of this limited study is to assess the presence and function of the contralateral kidney, since emergency nephrectomy of the injured kidney may be required to save the patient's life.

Pediatric renal injuries

Paediatric renal injuries are evaluated similarly, except that a further distinction is made regarding the degree of microhaematuria with blunt trauma. Specifically, a finding of >50 erythrocytes per high-power field warrants radiographic imaging.

Renal injury classification

On the basis of the radiographic and/or clinical information obtained, renal injuries are classified into five grades according to severity (Fig. 8.2).

- Grade I   Contusion or subcapsular haematoma.
- Grade II   <1 cm parenchymal laceration.
- Grade III >1 cm parenchymal laceration *without* urinary extravasation.
- Grade IV   Deep parenchymal laceration *with* urinary extravasation or a contained vascular injury.
- Grade V   Shattered kidney or avulsion of the renal pedicle.

Management of renal injuries (Fig. 8.1)

Low-grade renal injuries (grades I, II) can be observed.[5,6] High-grade renal injuries (grades III–V), with associated intra-abdominal organ injuries requiring laparotomy, and most renovascular injuries should be explored and reconstructed.[7] Overall, ~95% of blunt and >50% of penetrating renal injuries can be safely managed non-operatively.[8] Bed rest is recommended (usually until the urine is visibly clear), with antibiotics if there is urinary extravasation.

Percutaneous angiographic techniques are becoming increasingly important in managing renal injuries. They can be particularly useful in the case of iatrogenic renal injury at the time of PCNL.[9] Arterial embolization can be used to control both acute and delayed renal bleeding, as an adjunct to non-operative management.

Although most renal injuries do not require intervention, when surgery is indicated, it should be performed expeditiously and carefully. Indications for renal exploration are shown in Table 8.2. The aims of renal exploration are to achieve renal preservation, except in cases of renal pedicle avulsion where a nephrectomy is performed as a life-saving measure.

Explore the traumatized kidney through a midline transperitoneal incision extending from the xiphoid process to the pubic symphysis (this allows an exploratory laparotomy to determine the presence of associated injuries and allows control of the great vessels). Control bleeding by direct pressure with swab-sticks and abdominal packs until the anaesthetist has stabilized the patient.

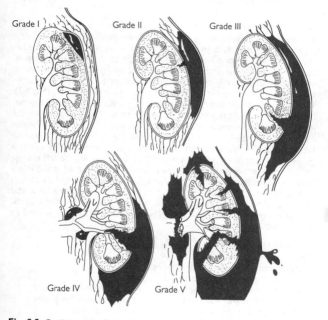

Fig. 8.2 Grading system for renal injuries: American Association for the Surgery of Trauma Organ Injury Severity Scale. Reproduced from McAninch, *Traumatic and reconstructive urology*. Philadelphia, PA. WB Saunders, 1996. Permission sought.

Table 8.2 Indications for renal exploration

Absolute
- Haemodynamic instability from renal haemorrhage suggested by an expanding or pulsatile retroperitoneal haematoma

Relative
- Urinary extravasation
- >25% non-viable renal parenchyma
- Renovascular injury
- Persistent bleeding (>2 units transfused per 24 hr)
- Incomplete radiographic staging
- Laparotomy for associated injuries

Getting renal vascular control

It is preferable to achieve renal vascular control before attempting renal repair. The renal vessels are accessed by retracting the transverse colon and small bowel superiorly and placing them on the patient's chest, exposing the root of the mesentery and the ligament of Treitz. A retroperitoneal incision is made directly over the aorta (superior to the inferior mesenteric artery) and extented superiorly to the ligament of Treitz (Fig. 8.3). With a large retroperitoneal hematoma, palpation of the aorta may not be possible. In this case, the inferior mesenteric vein, which lies to the left of the aorta, serves as a visible guide allowing for the retroperitoneal incision to be made just medial to this vessel. The retroperitoneal incision first exposes the left renal vein which should be looped as it serves as a guide to the remaining renal vessels. If the injury involves the left kidney, the left renal artery is then identified posteriorly and looped. If the injury is to the right kidney, after looping the left renal vein the right renal vein is identified medially followed by the right renal artery posteriorly, and both are looped (Fig. 8.4). The vessels are left unoccluded unless significant bleeding is encountered. Warm ischemia time should be limited to approximately 30 min.

Renal reconstruction

General principles:
- Obtain broad exposure of the entire kidney.
- Debride non-viable parenchyma.
- Achieve meticulous haemostasis of renal parenchymal vessles with 4–0, monofilament (slides easily through tissue) absorbable sutures.
- Close the collecting system with 4–0 absorbable sutures.
- Re-approximate the parenchymal edges (renorrhaphy).
- Isolate the repair from surrounding organs.

Upper and lower pole renal injuries can be managed with partial nephrectomy, whereas a renorrhaphy suffices for most mid-renal injuries (Figs. 8.5 and 8.6). In either case, the collecting system should be closed and the parenchymal defect approximated. An absorbable gelatin sponge bolster alone or in conjunction with an omental flap can be used to cover the defect. Injuries to the main renal vessels can be repaired with 5–0 vascular sutures; segmental vessels usually can be safely ligated (Fig. 8.7). Vascular occlusion is necessary when repairing renovascular injuries.

Outcome

Aggressive accurate staging of renal trauma is important in avoiding renal loss. Although most renal injuries are managed non-operatively, renal salvage can be achieved in the majority of cases requiring exploration when adequate expertise is readily available.

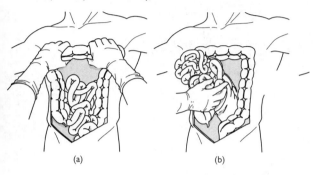

(a)   (b)

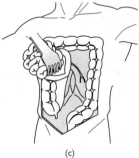

(c)

Fig. 8.3 (a) Transverse colon retracted. (b) Small bowel retracted. (c) Exposure of the retroperitoneum over the abdominal aorta.

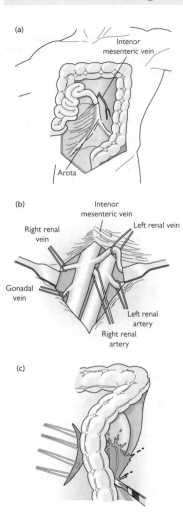

Fig. 8.4 (a) Incision made over the abdominal aorta or medial to the inferior mesenteric vein. (b) Exposed renal vessels. (c) Gerota's fascia opened.

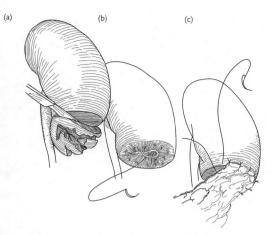

Fig. 8.5 Technique for partial nephrectomy following renal trauma. (a) Partial (polar) nephrectomy. (b) Closure of collecting system. (c) Omental advancement flap. Reproduced from McAninch, *Traumatic and reconstructive urology*. Philadelphia, PA. WB Saunders, 1996. Permission sought.

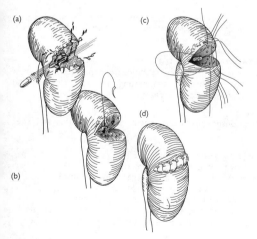

Fig. 8.6 Technique of renal repair. (a) Deep renal laceration. (b) Closure of pelvis and ligation of parenchymal vessels. (c) Renal Defect closure. (d) Completed renorrhaphy over a gelatin sponge. Reproduced from McAninch, *Traumatic and reconstructive urology*. Philadelphia, PA. WB Saunders, 1996. Permission sought.

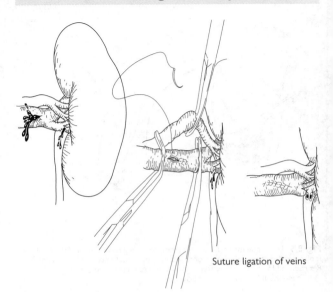

Suture ligation of veins

Fig. 8.7 Technique of segmental vessels ligation. Reproduced from McAninch, *Traumatic and reconstructive urology*. Philadelphia, PA. WB Saunders, 1996. Permission sought.

Early complications of renal trauma

The precise frequencies of these complications depend on a number of factors including the proportion of penetrating versus blunt injuries and the proportion of paediatric to adult cases.

Delayed bleeding

Can occur after conservative management of renal injuries and after surgical repair.
- Incidence:
  - 1.5% of surgically treated patients.[10]
  - 4% of surgically treated penetrating injuries.[11]
  - 1–6% of paediatric blunt injuries managed non-operatively.[12]
  - 20% of conservatively managed stab injuries.[12]
- 75% require surgery, and 60% of these require nephrectomy (the impact of modern angiographic embolization techniques on the need for surgical exploration and nephrectomy rates remains to be established).

Urinary extravasation and urinoma formation

- Due to injury to collecting system.
- Frequency: blunt injury 2–20%; penetrating injury 10–25%.[11,12] May be considerably more likely to occur in children.[13] CT has a higher sensitivity compared with IVU for detecting extravasation.
- Low-volume non-infected urinary extravasation often heals spontaneously and serial CT imaging to detect resolution is often all that is necessary. For large-volume extravasation consider a trial of JJ stenting. Renal repair for persistent prolonged extravasation is rarely necessary.
- Urinoma: a chronic urine collection in the retroperitoneum surrounded by a pseudocapsule (a pseudocyst: no true epithelial lining).
  - May present as an abdominal mass, ileus, vague abdominal pain.
  - Diagnosed by ultrasound or CT.
  - Management: percutaneous drainage with or without JJ stenting (often successful); open drainage and collecting system repair.

Abscess formation

- Follows infection of peri-renal haematoma and/or extravasated urine and/or devitalized kidney. May also occur as a consequence of associated injury to large or small bowel. Incidence after renal injury is low.
- Presentation: flank pain, fever, ileus.
- CT or ultrasound is diagnostic.
- Treat by percutaneous drainage.

Renal arteriovenous fistulae

- Can occur with blunt and penetrating injuries and post-surgical repair of renal injury. Most common cause is percutaneous renal biopsy, i.e. iatrogenic. Often small and heal spontaneously. Incidence reported to be as high as 15% (if looked for with renal arteriography).[14]
- Many remain undiagnosed now that renal arteriography is not used in renal trauma staging.
- Presentation and signs: retroperitoneal bleeding, collecting system bleeding (heavy haematuria), microscopic haematuria, abdominal bruit, hypertension, tachycardia, high output heart failure.
- Diagnosis is confirmed by selective renal arteriography (look for early opacification of renal vein and IVC).
- Indications for treatment: cardiac compromise (heart failure, hypertension), persistent haematuria, progressive enlargement of fistula.
- Small fistulae (e.g. post renal biopsy; most post blunt trauma) resolve spontaneously on arteriographic follow-up. Those occurring after stab wounds are said to be more likely to persist than those after blunt trauma or low-velocity gunshot wounds.
- Treatment: arterial embolization (treatment of choice), partial nephrectomy, complete nephrectomy.

Ureteral injuries

Aetiology

Internal trauma

Most commonest cause of ureteral trauma is iatrogenic following uretero-scopy, hysterectomy, oophorectomy, low anterior colon resection, laser ablation of endometriosis (burns to ureter), abdominal aneurysm repair, spinal surgery, and total hip replacement.

External trauma

Three per cent of all genitourinary injuries from external trauma involve the ureter. Most external ureteral injuries occur from gunshot wounds and are almost always associated with multiple organ injuries, most commonly to the small intestine, colon, liver, and iliac vessels. Ureteral injuries from blunt trauma are rare; they usually occur in children during rapid deceleration and are most commonly associated with injuries to the liver, spleen, and skeletal system.[1]

Diagnosis

Prompt diagnosis is the first step towards a successful outcome.

External ureteral trauma

Diagnosis is complicated by the presence of multiple organ injuries and the absence of early clinical and laboratory findings specific for ureteral trauma. Early clinical indicators of ureteral trauma are vague or non-existent. Delayed signs or symptoms of a ureteral injury include prolonged ileus, urinary obstruction, urinary leakage, azootemia, fever, persistent flank pain, fistula formation, and eventually sepsis. Haematuria is absent in approximately 30% of ureteral injuries from an external mechanism. Overall, >90% of ureteral injuries from external trauma are identified immediately.

Arrange radiographic investigations in any patient with penetrating or blunt abdominal trauma to the flank or abdomen, or in those who after abdominal or pelvic surgery present with signs or symptoms suggestive of a possible ureteral injury.

Internal (iatrogenic) trauma

Although ureteric injury is a well-recognized complication of pelvic surgery and flank pain is not a 'normal' post-operative symptom of pelvic surgery, fewer than half of iatrogenic ureteral injuries are recognized promptly. Symptoms and signs include flank pain, per vaginal fluid leak, unexplained fever, and flank tenderness.[2]

Making the diagnosis (Fig. 8.8)

External trauma

In the context of external trauma arrange a CT scan with delayed films post contrast administration to give adequate time for excretion of contrast into the collecting system and ureter, thereby allowing visualization of the ureter. In the stable patient where a diagnosis of ureteric injury is suspected, but the CT scan has not confirmed such an injury, perform retrograde ureterography (easier said than done in the poly-traumatized patient).

Internal (iatrogenic) trauma

When you are called to the operating theatre because of a suspected ureteric injury, while still on the telephone tell the operating surgeon to control any bleeding, pack the wound, and cover it, and instruct them to do *nothing more*. Advise them *not* to attempt repair or mobilization of the ureter until you have arrived. Ask the surgeon to call the radiographer and arrange for transfer of a C-arm into theatre so that you can carry out a retrograde ureterogram if necessary.

If the surgeon has already 'repaired' the ureter and simply asked you to be present to endorse his repair, you are in a tricky situation. Once you, as a urologist, have been asked to be involved in the case, should any untoward complications occur as a consequence of the repair to the ureter, you will be held at least partly responsible. The safest option in such cases is to take the repair down and start again. 'Starting again' means starting from the point of diagnosis, which involves checking that the rest of that ureter has not been injured (double ligation or division of one ureter has been reported) and checking (by inspection or retrograde ureterography) that the contralateral ureter has not been injured.

When you arrive, the atmosphere in the operating theatre may be tense. Remain calm and approach the case in a methodical way. Optimize exposure of the suspected injury site by packing bowel out of the way, controlling bleeding, and ensuring that the theatre lights are appropriately positioned. Ensure that the retractor you like using is available. Remember that you must examine *both* ureters.

In the context of a suspected intra-operative ureteric injury (e.g. during hysterectomy), your options for diagnosis/exclusion of a ureteric injury are as follows.

- *Direct inspection of the ureter* A good way of inspecting the ureter for injury, but requires exposure of a considerable length of ureter to establish that it has not been injured. The process of exposure can itself damage the ureter. Lower ureteric exposure is more difficult than upper ureteric exposure. If you are in any doubt about the integrity of the ureter, perform retrograde ureterography. The mechanism of trauma is helpful in assessing the level of ureteral injury.
- *Extravasation after injection of methylene blue into the ureter* Look for leakage of dye from a more distant section of ureter (will miss a ligation injury).
- *On-table IVU* Technically difficult, and does not always demonstrate the presence or site of injury.

- *On-table retrograde ureterography*. Do this either cystoscopically or via an incision made in the bladder. Contrast extravasation is the radiographic *sine qua non* of ureteral injury. It is a very accurate method of establishing the presence or absence of a ureteric injury. Both ureters should be examined, since bilateral injuries can occur (Fig. 8.9).

Where no contrast extravasation is seen at retrograde ureterography, but where there has been extensive use of diathermy or the laser around the ureter (e.g. in the context of laparoscopic endometrial laser ablation), assume that the ureter may have been injured and insert a JJ stent. The ureteric wall may remain intact for several days after a burn and therefore may not leak contrast at retrograde ureterography. Assuming that an injury has occurred, stenting the ureter is the safe option. Remove the stent 6 weeks later and repeat a retrograde study at the time of stent removal to confirm that there is no contrast leak.

Classification of ureteric injuries

Ureteral injuries are classified on the basis of radiographic or intra-operative findings.

- Grade I   Contusion or haematoma without devascularization.
- Grade II   <50% transection.
- Grade III >50% transection.
- Grade IV   Complete transection with >2 cm devascularization.
- Grade V   Avulsion with >2 cm devascularization.

Management of ureteral injuries (Fig. 8.8)

Selection of the appropriate management depends on the patient's condition, the delay between injury and its recognition, and the grade and nature of the injury.

External ureteral injuries

Most patients with external ureteral injuries require prompt operative exploration for management of their associated abdominal injuries. Repair the ureter using one of the options described below.

Internal (intra-operative) injuries identified intra-operatively
Stable patient

Repair the injured ureter immediately using one of the options described below.

Unstable patient

Place a percutaneous nephrostomy or ureteric stent and drain the site of injury. Subsequent reconstruction can be scheduled electively. In the shocked patient you may consider tying the ureter off at the site of the leakage with a long non-absorbable suture. This allows dilatation of the ureter so that your interventional radiologist can subsequently place a nephrostomy tube under X-ray control a day or so later. The non-absorbable suture allows easier identification of the ureter when you come back later for definitive repair.

Diagnosis and management of ureteral injuries
(Abdominal or rapid deceleration injury)

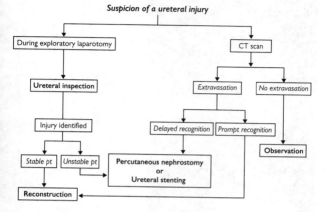

Fig. 8.8 Diagnosis and management of ureteral injuries.

Iatrogenic ureteric injuries diagnosed days or weeks post-operatively

In general terms, the best time to repair the ureter is intraoperatively.

However, the diagnosis of most iatrogenic ureteral injuries is delayed. Management should be tailored to the particular circumstances of the injury and the patients overall condition. Up to 50% of iatrogenic ureteral injuries with heal with renal drainage alone (using a JJ stent of percutaneous nephrostomy).[3,4] The appropriate imaging studies should be performed to characterize the injury and surgical repair usually deferred for at least 6 weeks to allow for resolution of postoperative inflammation and edema. However, favourable outcomes have been reported after early repair (after 7 days), and the time of the original injury is nowadays seen as a less important determinant of time of definitive repair. Blandy et al.[5] reported favourable results of repair (by Boari flap) of iatrogenic ureteric injuries in 43 patients, 28 (65%) of whom underwent definitive repair within 6 weeks of injury.

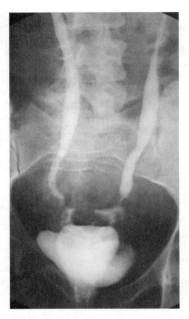

Fig. 8.9 Retrograde ureterography demonstrating bilateral ureteric injuries.

Options for definitive treatment of ureteric injuries

Specific reconstructive techniques depend on the location and extent of injury and range from simple JJ stenting to an anterior bladder wall flap or ileal interposition (Fig. 8.10).

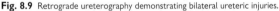

Summary of techniques for ureteric injury dependent on level of injury

- JJ stenting: for contusions, crush injuries (recognized within a few days of injury), ligation injuries (recognized within a few days of injury), partial transactions.
- Grade II–IV transections involving the middle or upper third of the ureter are usually best managed by primary uretero-ureterostomy (Fig. 8.11). The middle and upper third of the ureter can usually be mobilized enough to allow a tension-free anastomosis. The distal ureter usually cannot be mobilized enough to bridge such defects.
- The distal lower third of the ureter is best managed by submucosal bladder re-implantation (Fig. 8.12) rather than primary uretero-ureterostomy (because of the relatively tenuous blood supply of the lower third of ureter below the take-off of the internal iliac artery). If the ureter cannot be tunnelled into the bladder without tension, re-implant into a psoas hitch.

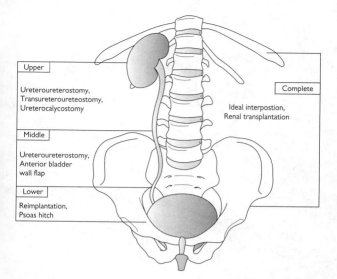

Fig. 8.10 Options for management of ureteric injury depending on level of injury.

- The entire lower third of the ureter is best managed by a psoas hitch in conjunction with ureteral re-implantation (Fig. 8.13).
- The entire lower two-thirds of the ureter is best managed with an anterior bladder wall flap (Boari flap), in conjunction with a psoas hitch (Fig. 8.14). This procedure should not be used in patients with prior pelvic irradiation or neurogenic bladder disease.
- Alternatively, injuries involving the distal half of the ureter with insufficient bladder capacity or severe pelvic scarring can be managed by trans-uretero-ureterostomy (Fig. 8.15).
- Ureterocalycostomy is used for extensive injuries to the ureteropelvic junction and proximal ureter (Fig. 8.16). The lower pole of the involved kidney is amputated, exposing the infundibulum of the inferior calyx. The ureter is generously spatulated, allowing for a direct end-to-end ureterocalyceal anastomosis.
- Complete ureteral avulsion: a segment of ileum can be interposed as a ureteral substitute. A modification of the standard technique is the Monti procedure (Fig. 8.17).
- Solitary kidney or compromised renal function or complete ureteral avulsions can be managed by renal autotransplantation nephrectomy, in the context of a vascular graft procedure (e.g. an aortobifemoral graft).
- Permanent cutaneous ureterostomy.

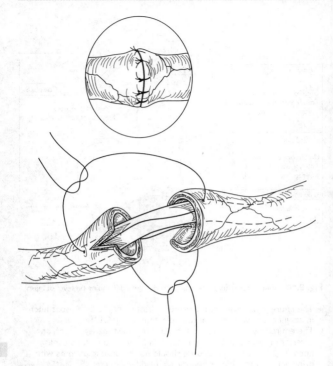

Fig. 8.11 Primary ureteroureterostomy with spatulation of both ends.
Reproduced from McAninch, *Traumatic and reconstructive urology*. Philadelphia, PA.
WB Saunders, 1996. Permission sought.

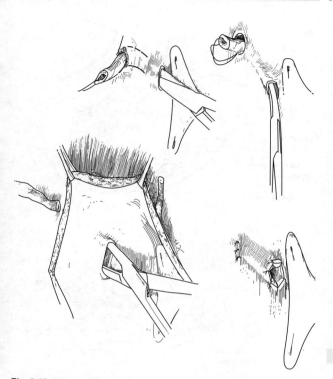

Fig. 8.12 Submucosal reimplantation of the ureter into bladder using an intra- and extravesical approach. Reproduced from McAninch, *Traumatic and reconstructive urology*. Philadelphia, PA. WB Saunders, 1996. Permission sought.

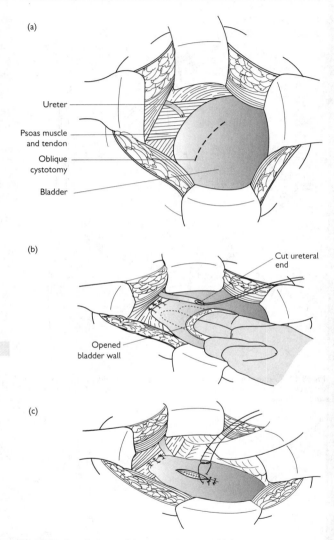

(a)

Ureter

Psoas muscle
and tendon

Oblique
cystotomy

Bladder

(b)

Cut ureteral
end

Opened
bladder wall

(c)

Fig. 8.13 Reimplantation of the ureter using a psoas hitch.

(a)

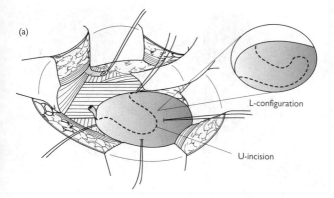

L-configuration

U-incision

(b)

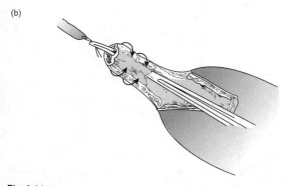

Fig. 8.14 Reimplantation of the ureter using a Boari flap.

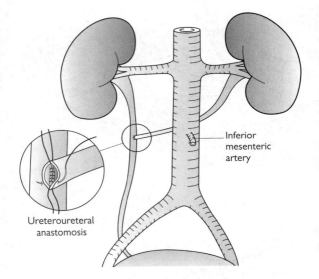

Fig. 8.15 A transureteroureterostomy.

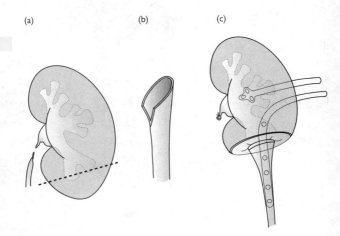

Fig. 8.16 A ureterocalycostomy. (a) Amputated inferior pole. (b) Spatulated proximal ureter. (c) Completed anastomosis with appropriate drainage tubes.

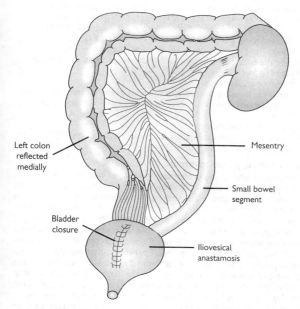

Fig. 8.17 Ileal interposition.

JJ stenting

JJ stenting may be adequate for definitive treatment of some injuries, particularly where the injury does not involve the entire circumference of the ureter and therefore continuity is maintained across the region of the ureteric injury. In situations where a ligature has been applied around the ureter, and this has been immediately recognized such that viability of the ureter has probably not been compromised, remove the ligature and place a JJ stent (cystoscopically if this is feasible or, if not, by opening the bladder).[2] Generally speaking the stent is maintained in position for 3–6 weeks. At the time of stent removal perform a retrograde ureterogram to confirm that there is no persistent leakage of contrast from the original site of injury, and to see if there is evidence of ureteric stricturing.

Factors other than the level of injury are important in determining the type of repair. Gunshot wounds characteristically cause considerable 'collateral damage' to the ureter and surrounding tissues, and this may not be apparent at the time of surgery. Delayed necrosis can occur in such apparently normal-looking ureters. If such an injury is suspected, a JJ stent should be placed.

General principles of ureteric repair

- In intra-operatively diagnosed injuries, the ureter has already been exposed. In elective ureteric reconstruction, use a midline abdominal incision to allow wide access to the ureter. Alternatively, the incision can be tailored to the specific procedure, e.g. a subcostal incision can be used for upper and mid-ureteral injuries and a Gibson (muscle-splitting) incision for lower ureteral injuries.
- Debride the ends of the ureter so that the edges to be anastomosed are bleeding freely.
- Tension-free anastomosis.
- For complete transaction spatulate the ends of the ureter to allow a wide anastomosis (the circumference of the repair will tend to shrink by ~20%).
- Place a stent across the repair.
- Perform a mucosa-to-mucosa anastomosis to achieve a watertight closure.
- Place a drain down to the site of the anastomosis.

Primary closure of partial transection of the ureter

A partial transaction of the ureter can be repaired over a JJ stent as long as the injury has not been caused by a gunshot wound, in which case there may well be a blast effect causing more extensive necrosis than is immediately apparent at the time of surgery. Such injuries are better managed by excising the affected segment of ureter and performing a primary uretero-ureterostomy. Mobilize the ends of the ureter to allow a tension-free anastomosis to be done. After completing 2/3 of the anastomosis, pass a guidewire into the renal pelvis and pass the stent up into the renal pelvis. To introduce the stent into the lower ureter, remove the guidewire and place it in a side hole of the stent, so as to straighten the end of the stent so that it can be introduced into the distal end of the ureter (Fig. 8.18). It is easier to place the guidewire through a side hole in the *middle* of the stent, because this makes it easier to disengage the wire from the stent. The stent can be pulled out of the bladder as the guidewire is withdrawn if the latter has been placed through a side hole near the *end* of the stent). Thread the stent and guidewire down the ureter and into the bladder. Instil some diluted methylene blue into the bladder via the catheter and fill the bladder with saline, clamping the catheter so that the bladder can be distended. When the JJ stent reaches the bladder and the guidewire is withdrawn, blue fluid refluxes up the stent, confirming that the distal end of the stent is in the bladder. We use 4–0 Vicryl (i.e. absorbable suture material) to close the hole in the ureter. Place a drain down to the site of the repair.

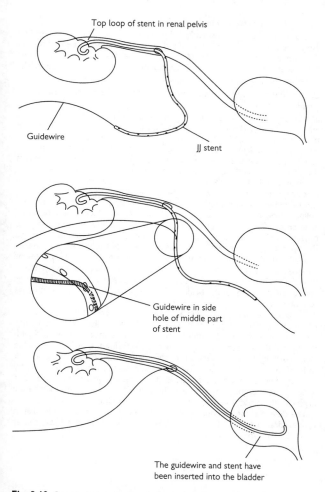

Top loop of stent in renal pelvis

Guidewire

JJ stent

Guidewire in side
hole of middle part
of stent

The guidewire and stent have
been inserted into the bladder

Fig. 8.18 Open technique for introducing a ureteral stent through a
ureterotomy. Reproduced from Hashim *et al. Urological emergencies in clinical
practice.* Springer-Verlag. London, 2005. Permission sought.

Primary uretero-ureterostomy (Fig 8.11)

This is anastomosis of one end of the ureter to the other end. Debride the ureteric ends, spatulate them, and perform a tension free end-to-end anastomosis over a stent using 4–0 Vicryl. If the defect between the ends of the ureter is of a length where a tension-free anastomosis is not possible, consider interposing a segment of ileum.

Uretero-neocystostomy: re-implantation of the ureter directly into the bladder (Fig. 8.12)

Identify the end of the proximal ureter. If the injury has been recognized intra-operatively, the end will usually be easily identifiable. However, if there has been a delay in recognizing the injury, the end of the ureter may be encased in a mass of fibrous and oedematous tissue. In such cases, trace the ureter down as far as you can, and transect it as it enters the area of fibrosis. Place a stay suture through the end of the ureter.

Open the bladder between stay sutures. Create a hole or tunnel through which the ureter will be anastomosed to the bladder. The ureter can be either anastomosed to the bladder in a refluxing fashion or tunnelled through the muscle of the bladder to produce a non-refluxing anastomosis. In the former situation, place a right-angled forceps on the outside of the bladder at the site of intended re-implantation, cut onto the tip of the forceps, and simply draw the end of the ureter (by the stay suture) into the bladder. Spatulate the end of the ureter on its anterior surface using Pott's scissors. Perform the anastomosis over a JJ stent. Place the first suture through all layers of the posterior wall of the ureter and take a deep bite of the bladder. The remaining sutures can be mucosa to mucosa only.

For a non-refluxing anastomosis, create a submucosal tunnel in the wall of the bladder. Use a pair of McIndoe or Addson scissors. Make a small cut in the mucosa of the bladder, and then tunnel under the mucosa with the tips of the scissors, rapidly opening and closing the tips to create the tunnel. After ~2 cm (allowing a ratio of tunnel length to ureteric diameter ratio of ~3:1), turn the scissors over and cut onto their ends with diathermy so that they can exit the bladder. Exchange them for a Robert's forceps, which is used to grasp the suture in the end of the ureter. Anastomose the ureter to the bladder in the same way as for the refluxing anastomosis.

The defect in the bladder is then closed, in the same axis as the ureter. Place a drain down to the site of bladder closure and leave the catheter in the bladder for 2 weeks.

Psoas hitch[5] (Figs 8.13 and 8.19)

A psoas hitch is fashioned by making an incision in the bladder which lies at right angles to the long axis of the ureter. This essentially lengthens the bladder, allowing it to reach the ureter, which can be anastomosed to the bladder without tension.

Inflate the bladder with a few hundred millilitres of water (saline would short-circuit the diathermy). Use a sterile giving set attached to a 1 L bag of water. Control the inflow and outflow yourself. Mark out the site of the incision in the distended bladder, using a marker pen if you find this easier, and apply stay sutures around the edges of the incision; these make it easier to manipulate the tissues and also create less tissue damage than using forceps.

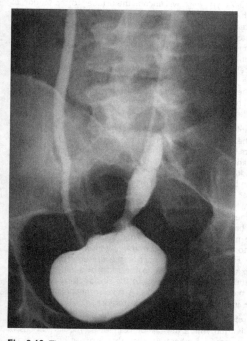

Fig. 8.19 The appearance of a psoas hitch on a post-operative cystogram.

Place two stay sutures on each side of the planned incision. As the incision is made, pull the stay suture apart until you have produced an incision that is long enough to breach the defect. Alternatively, place two fingers inside the bladder and elevate the bladder towards the cut ureter. Divide the contralateral superior vesical vessels to achieve an adequate length of bladder. The psoas hitch should reach well above the iliac vessels so that it can be anchored to the psoas minor tendon (psoas major tendon if the former is absent). To achieve this length the incision in the bladder may have to comprise as much as 50% of the circumference of the bladder.

Hitch stitches are used to anchor the bladder to the psoas minor tendon. They take tension off of the uretero-vesical anastomosis and also prevent tension at this site developing as the bladder fills and empties. Place the hitch stitches (2–0 Vicryl) which will anchor the bladder to the tendon of psoas minor at this time, first to ensure that an adequate length of bladder is taken for tension-free ureter-to-bladder anastomosis, and secondly so that the anastomosis can be performed in a position that will avoid kinking the ureter. Clip the stitches, but do not tie them yet: 'Having sited the position of the hitch-sutures, it is often easier to create the ureteric tunnel before actually anchoring the bladder.'[4] When placing the hitch stitches, be careful not to place your sutures too deeply as it is possible to hit the genitofemoral nerve (which lies on psoas major) and even the femoral nerve (which lies deep to the psoas major).

Boari flap (8.14)
A Boari flap is able to bridge a greater defect than a psoas hitch. Place stay sutures in the inflated bladder around the edges of the flap. The flap will receive all its blood supply from its base and should therefore be at least 4 cm wide and have a length-to-width ratio of no more than 3:1.

Inflate the bladder as for a psoas hitch. Measure the defect and make sure that you can bridge it with your Boari flap with a few centimetres to spare. Remember that if you prefer to re-implant the ureter in a non-refluxing fashion, you will need an extra ~3 cm of length to allow the ureter to be tunnelled into the bladder.

Fold the flap backwards. If more length is required, small transverse incisions can be made in the side of the flap. Pulling these lengthways enables the flap to be lengthened. Perform the re-implantation as described above and then close the bladder. Start at the ureter end, folding the sides of the flap towards each other in the form of a tube. Complete the bladder closure, place a drain down to the site of closure, and leave the catheter in the bladder for 2 weeks. A reverse nephropexy can be used to alleviate any mild tension of the anastomosis.

Trans-uretero-ureterostomy (Fig. 8.15)
This procedure is used where the bladder cannot be mobilized or is of small volume (e.g. post-radiotherapy), such that a psoas hitch or Boari flap cannot be made without tension at the uretero-vesical anastomosis. The damaged ureter is swung over to the normal ureter and the two are anastomosed in an end-to-end fashion.

First, check that the 'recipient' ureter has not been injured. Perform an on-table retrograde ureterogram. There must be an adequate length of ureter to swing over to the opposite ureter. Remember that just above the pelvic brim the ureters are the closest together of any point throughout their course (6–7 cm apart), and therefore the least amount of mobilization will be required at this point.

Ideally, the caecum should be mobilized to avoid having to tunnel the ureter through the retroperitoneum, which runs the risk of angulating or constricting the ureter. The 'donor' ureter (the cut ureter) should be brought over to the opposite ureter above the inferior mesenteric artery. Make a longitudinal incision in the recipient ureter that is slightly longer than the diameter of the donor ureter. By cutting the end of the donor ureter obliquely, you can increase its length slightly and this may help reduce the chances of post-operative obstruction.

Place a 4–0 Vicryl suture from outside to inside at the top end of the recipient ureter and then pass it from inside to outside of the donor ureter. Do the same at the bottom end. Complete the back wall of the anastomosis from inside the ureter, and the front wall from the outside. Before completing the anastomosis, place a JJ stent into the recipient ureter, and complete the anastomosis. Place a drain down to the site of the anastomosis.

Ureterocalycostomy (Fig. 8.16)

Ureterocalycostomy can be used for extensive injuries to the ureteropelvic junction and proximal ureter. The lower pole of the involved kidney is amputated, exposing the infundibulum of the inferior calyx. The ureter is generously spatulated, allowing for a direct end-to-end ureterocalyceal anastomosis. This procedure involves excessive renal dissection and is fraught with a high incidence of anastomotic stricture.

Alternative procedures for managing ureteric injuries

Alternative procedures, where the segment of damaged ureter is very long, include autotransplantation of the kidney into the pelvis and replacement of the ureter with ileum (Fig. 8.17). Specialized surgical texts can be consulted for details on how to perform such procedures. Very occasionally, where the patient's life expectancy is very limited, ureteric injuries can be managed by a permanent cutaneous ureterostomy.

When a ureter has been injured in a patient who has undergone a vascular graft procedure (e.g. an aortobifemoral graft), traditional teaching advocated nephrectomy because of the potential for graft infection as a consequence of infection of urine which might leak from the site of a ureteric anastomosis. However, renal failure is a significant cause of death after aneurysm repair, particularly in the context of emergency (ruptured) aneurysm repair. Therefore preservation of as much functioning renal tissue as possible is clearly desirable in such patients, and this would tend to sway one away from nephrectomy. Such injuries can be safely repaired. Isolation of the repair with an omental flap and adequate intra- and peri-ureteral drainage limits the liklihood of graft infection.

Outcome

A delay in diagnosis is the most important contributory factor in morbidity related to ureteral injury. Maintain a high index of suspicion in the poly-traumatized patient or the patient who has undergone pelvic surgery.

Complications of ureteral injuries

- Prolonged urinary extravasation.
- Infection.
- Urinoma.
- Fistula.
- Ureteric stricture.

References

1 Elliott SP, McAninch JW. Ureteral injuries from external violence: the 25 year experience at San Francisco General Hospital. *J Urol* 2003; **170**:1213–16.

2 Assimos DG, Patterson LC, Taylor CL. Changing incidence and aetiology of iatrogenic ureteral injuries. *J Urol* 1994; **152**:2240–6.

3 Ku JH, Kim ME, Jeon YS, Lee NK, Park YH. Minimally invasive management of ureteral injuries recognized late after obstetric and gynaecologic surgery. *Int J Care Injured* 2003; **34**:480.

4 Blandy JP, Badenoch DF, Fowler CG *et al.* Early repair of iatrogenic injury to the ureter and bladder after gynecological surgery. *J Urol* 1991; **146**:761.

5 Turner-Warwick R, Worth PHL. The psoas bladder hitch procedure for the replacement of the lower third of the ureter. *Br J Urol* 1969; **41**:701.

Bladder injuries

Aetiology

The bladder is second to the kidneys in frequency of injury, accounting for approximately 25% of all genitourinary injuries.

External bladder injuries

External bladder injuries are caused by either blunt or penetrating trauma to the lower abdomen, pelvis, or perineum.

- *Blunt trauma* leading to pelvic fracture is the more common mechanism of bladder injury (95% of blunt bladder ruptures occur in association with a pelvic fracture and in this situation associated injuries such as long-bone fractures, central nervous system, and chest injuries are common). The bladder may also rupture following a sudden deceleration, such as in a high-speed motor vehicle accident or fall, or an external blow to the lower abdomen, particularly if the bladder is full.
- *Penetrating injuries* account for approximately 25% of external bladder injuries in North America and are most commonly the result of gunshot wounds.

Internal bladder injuries

The bladder is the most frequently injured organ during pelvic surgery. Iatrogenic bladder injuries can occur during:

- Transurethral surgery:
  - Transurethral resection of bladder tumour (TURBT).
  - Cystoscopic bladder biopsy.
  - Transurethral resection of prostate (TURP) (0.25% of TURP in the UK National Prostatectomy Audit.[1]
  - Cystolitholapaxy.
- Gynaecological procedures:
  - Abdominal hysterectomy.
  - Caesarean section, especially as an emergency.
  - Pelvic mass excision.
- Colon resection.
- Total hip replacement (very rare).

Predisposing factors include scarring from prior surgery or radiation, inflammation, and extensive tumor burden.

Diagnosis (Fig. 8.20)

Suspect a bladder injury after any external lower abdominal or pelvic trauma. Abdominal pain and distention are usual (Fig. 8.21). The patient may be unable to urinate. The hallmark of a bladder injury is haematuria. Gross haematuria occurs in at least 95% of bladder ruptures from blunt injury, and the remainder have microscopic haematuria. In contrast, approximately half of patients with penetrating bladder injuries present with gross haematuria.[2]

In pelvic fracture haemodynamic instability is common because of extensive pelvic haemorrhage. Perform pelvic and rectal examinations (look for blood on the finger indicating a rectal and/or vaginal tear).

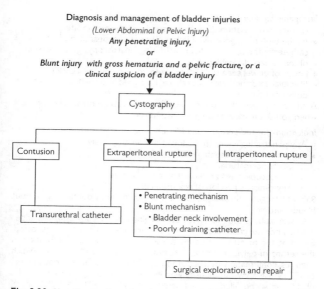

Diagnosis and management of bladder injuries
(Lower Abdominal or Pelvic Injury)
Any penetrating injury,
or
**Blunt injury with gross hematuria and a pelvic fracture, or a
clinical suspicion of a bladder injury**

↓

Cystography

Contusion — Extraperitoneal rupture — Intraperitoneal rupture

Transurethral catheter

• Penetrating mechanism
• Blunt mechanism
  • Bladder neck involvement
  • Poorly draining catheter

Surgical exploration and repair

Fig. 8.20 Algorithm for diagnosis and management of bladder injuries.

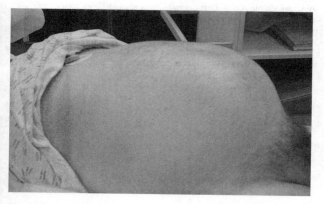

Fig. 8.21 Gross distension of the abdomen following bladder perforation during a TURBT.

Iatrogenic bladder injuries
- Urinary extravasation through a wound, drain, or drain site.
- At the time of surgery a visible laceration, the appearance of a Foley catheter in the operative field, or (during laparoscopy) gas distension of the urinary drainage bag.
- Loops of bowel seen through the resectoscope during TURBT.
- Ellik evacuator not sucking back, i.e. fluid goes into the bladder but does not come back out.

A bladder perforation during TURBT is usually immediately apparent when you see marked abdominal distension.

Indications for radiographic bladder imaging
- Any penetrating injury to the lower abdomen or pelvis.
- Any blunt injury presenting with:
  - Gross haematuria.
  - Microscopic haematuria and a pelvic fracture.
  - Any clinical suspicion of bladder injury.

95% of iatrogenic bladder injuries are diagnosed intra-operatively without bladder imaging.

Cystography is the most accurate imaging test for diagnosing a bladder injury. Prior to catheterization the urethral meatus must be inspected. Blood at the meatus is a contraindication to urethral catheterization in the setting of pelvic trauma as it strongly suggests a urethral injury which requires confirmation by retrograde urethrography. Either conventional or CT cystography can be used with equivalent accuracy. In each case the bladder must be filled in a *retrograde* manner with at least 350 mL of contrast (in children use 60 mL of contrast plus 30 mL per year of age up to a maximum of 400 mL. With CT cystography the contrast should be further diluted (approximately 5:1) to avoid a white out effect which can obscure visualization). Post-drainage films should be obtained only with conventional cystography since a posterior leak may be obscured by the mass of contrast filling the bladder (on post-drainage films a 'wisp' of extra-vesical contrast will be seen in such cases). The cystogram phase of an IVU or CT with IV contrast alone are not adequate for diagnosis of a bladder rupture since the diluted contrast is not sufficient in adequately imaging the bladder.[3]

Classification

Bladder injuries are classified based on the extent of injury seen radiographically.

- Grade I — Contusion, intramural haematoma, or partial-thickness laceration (haematuria, normal urethrogram, no contrast leak on cystogram).
- Grade II — Extra-peritoneal bladder wall laceration <2 cm.
- Grade III — Extra-peritoneal bladder wall laceration >2 cm or intra-peritoneal bladder wall laceration <2 cm.
- Grade IV — Intra-peritoneal bladder wall laceration >2 cm.
- Grade V — Intra- or extra-peritoneal bladder wall laceration extending into bladder neck or ureteral orifice (trigone).

Management of bladder injuries (Fig. 8.20)

Management depends on the overall status of the patient, the grade of the injury, and the extent of any associated injuries.

- Bladder contusions and haematomas: treat by transurethral catheter drainage alone until the haematuria completely resolves.
- Extra-peritoneal bladder lacerations (Fig. 8.22) can usually be managed non-operatively, provided that there is good catheter drainage and no infection.
- Indications for repair of extra-peritoneal bladder lacerations:
  - Involvement of bladder neck.
  - Concomitant vaginal or rectal injury (high risk of severe pelvic sepsis if not surgically repaired).
  - Intra-vesical bone fragments from pelvic fracture (if demonstrated on pelvic CT).
  - Where conservative management of an extra-peritoneal bladder rupture with catheter drainage is started, but there is persistent urinary bleeding impeding adequate catheter drainage.
- Intra-peritoneal bladder lacerations all require surgical exploration (Fig. 8.23). Expose the bladder through a midline infraumbilical incision. In the case of a bladder perforation due to a pelvic fracture, avoid dissection of the pelvic haematoma associated with the pelvic fracture (Fig. 8.24). Make a peritoneotomy and inspect the abdominal viscera. In the context of TURBT, inspect the bowel for diathermy damage and bowel perforates.

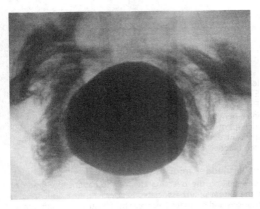

Fig. 8.22 An extra-peritoneal bladder perforation. The ill-defined extravasation of contrast is limited to the tissues around the bladder.

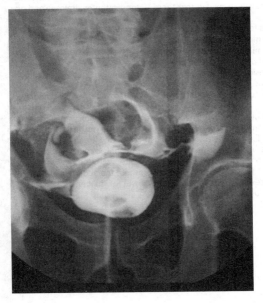

Fig. 8.23 An intra-peritoneal bladder perforation. Loops of bowel are outlined by the contrast that has leaked through the perforation into the peritoneal cavity.

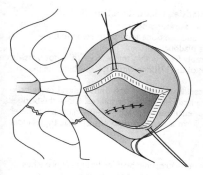

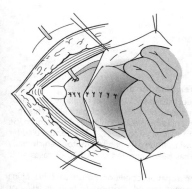

Fig. 8.24 For bladder perforations due to pelvic fracture, explore the bladder through an anterior midline incision and avoid dissection of the pelvic haematoma associated with the pelvic fracture.

General principles of bladder reconstruction
- Inspect the bladder neck and ureteric orifices.
- Debride non-viable tissue and use bone forceps to remove bone fragments poking into the bladder.
- Suture lacerations, preferably from within the bladder (it is not possible to get round the back of the bladder without disturbing the pelvic haematoma.

Prior to bladder closure insert a suprapubic and transurethral catheter in males;[3] in females, a transurethral Foley catheter suffices. Close the bladder in two layers using absorbable sutures (e.g. Vicryl 3–0). Maintain catheter drainage for 7–10 days. Perform a cystogram to ensure that the bladder has healed.

Outcome
- Mortality in patients with non-iatrogenic bladder trauma approaches 20%, usually as a consequence of the associated injuries rather than the bladder laceration.
- Early complications of bladder injury:
  - Bleeding.
  - Urinary extravasation.
  - Infection.
- Long-term complications (rare):
  - Fistula formation.
  - Urinary incontinence.
  - Bladder instability.

Spontaneous rupture after bladder augmentation
An augmented bladder (ileocystoplasty, gastrocystoplasty, detrusor myectomy) can rupture spontaneously in ~5–10% of patients.[4] This may occur many years after augmentation. Ileocystoplasties are said to be more likely to rupture than are gastrocystoplasties.[4,5] Augmented bladder rupture may also occur following trauma (e.g. after motor vehicle accidents). Spontaneous rupture has been reported in 1 of 50 of cases after detrusor myectomy.[6]

Patients with underlying neuropathic conditions, such as spina bifida and spinal cord injury, usually have limited awarness of bladder filling or of pelvic pain, and diagnosis of perforation of an augmented bladder in such patients may be delayed because the pain, although usually present, is not usually severe enough to make one think that a serious event has occurred. Have a high index of suspicion in such patients who may present with abdominal pain, vague in onset and nature, combined with fever or sepsis. Arrange a cystogram. A normal cystogram or CT does not necessarily exclude a diagnosis of perforation. Where there are clinical signs such as persistent or progressive abdominal distension, consider exploratory laparotomy even though imaging studies may be normal. Management usually consists of immediate laparotomy and repair of the perforation, but in cases where there is severe sepsis, this should be managed prior to exploration.

Further reading

1 Cass AS, Gleich P, Smith C. Simultaneous bladder and prostatomembranous urethral rupture from external trauma. *J Urol* 1984; **132**:907–8.

References

1 Neal DE. The National Prostatectomy Audit. *Br J Urol* 1997; **79**(Suppl 2):69–75.
2 Cass AS, Luxenberg M. Features of 164 bladder ruptures. *J Urol* 1987; **138**:743–5.
3 Volpe MA, Pachter EM, Scalea TM *et al.* Is there a difference in outcome when treating traumatic intraperitoneal bladder rupture with or without a suprapubic tube? *J Urol* 1999; **161**:1103–5.
4 DeFoor W, Tackett L, Minevich E *et al.* Risk factors for spontaneous bladder perforation after augmentation cystoplasty. *Urology* 2003; **62**:737–41.
5 Shekarriz B, Upadhyay J, Demirbilrk S *et al.* Surgical complications of bladder augmentation: comparison between various enterocystoplasties in 133 patients. *Urology* 2000; **55**:123–8.
6 Stohrer M. *Spinal Cord* 1997; **35**:456–62.

Testicular injuries

Aetiology
- Most testicular injuries result from blunt trauma (80%) and are usually unilateral. The most common causes are sports-related injuries, motor vehicle accidents, and assaults.
- Penetrating testicular injuries most frequently result from gunshots with one-third involving both testes. Most are associated with multiple injuries including to the thigh, penis, perineum, pelvis, urethra and femoral vessels.

Diagnosis
Based on history and physical examination.

History
- Typically scrotal pain and swelling after a direct blow to the scrotum.
- Any penetrating injury to the scrotum suggests the likelihood of testicular involvement.

Examination
- Scrotal discoloration.
- A tender firm scrotal mass that fails to transilluminate, suggesting a haematocoele.
- Often examiantion is limited by patient discomfort, making it difficult to assess the extent of a testicular injury accurately by clinical means alone.
- Degree of injury may be out of proportion to the physical findings.
  For these reasons, the diagnosis of a blunt testicular injury should be confirmed by scrotal ultrasound.

Ultrasound findings
A heterogeneous intra-testicular echo pattern with loss of contour definition is the most common ultrasonographic finding of a testicular rupture. Extruded testicular tissue or disruption of the tunica albuginea can be seen on occasion, but is not a required sonographic criterion to confirm a rupture.

Classification
Testicular injuries are classified based on clinical and imaging information.
- Grade I   Contusion or haematoma.
- Grade II   Subclinical laceration of tunica albuginea.
- Grade III Laceration of tunica albuginea with <50% parenchymal loss.
- Grade IV   Major laceration of tunica albuginea with >50% parenchymal loss.
- Grade V   Total testicular destruction or avulsion.

Management

- All penetrating testicular injuries and any blunt testicular injury suggestive of a tunical laceration should be surgically explored and repaired.
- Use a transverse scrotal skin incision to expose the testis.
- Having completely exposed the testis, epidydimis and spermatic cord drain the haematocoele, judiciously debride extruded seminiferous tubules, and reapproximate the tunica albuginea.
- For complete testicular destruction (usually a consequence of gunshot injuries), orchidectomy may be the only option.

Outcome

Prompt diagnosis and exploration are critical in limiting complications of testicular injuries, including infection, chronic pain, atrophy, and delayed orchidectomy. With preservation of testicular parenchyma, normal endocrine function is usually maintained.

Further reading

1 Cass AS. Testicular trauma. *J Urol* 1983; **129**:299.
2 Gomez RG, Castanheira ACC, McAninch JW. Gunshot wounds to the male external genitalia. *J Urol* 1993; **150**:1147.
3 Kratzik CH, Hainz A, Kuber W et al. Has scrotal ultrasound influenced the therapy of blunt scrotal trauma. *J Urol* 1989; **142**:1243.
4 McDermot JP, Gray BK. Bilateral testicular atrophy following blunt trauma. *Br J Urol* 1989; **63**:215.
5 chuster G. Traumatic rupture of the testicle and a review of the literature. *J Urol* 1982; **127**:1194.

Anatomy of degloving incision for repair of penile fracture (Fig. 8.26)

The skin of the penis is very mobile (to allow expansion during erection). Beneath it lies the dartos fascia (also known as the superficial fascia of the penis) which is continuous with the superficial fascia of the groin and perineum (Colles' fascia). Within the dartos fascia run superficial penile arteries and the superficial dorsal vein. The dartos fascia is only loosely attached to Buck's fascia and therefore, along with the skin, can be mobilized off Buck's fascia.

Buck's fascia (the deep fascia of the penis) is a dense elastic fascial layer which is firmly attached to the underlying tunica albuginea of the corpora cavernosa and corpus spongiosum, which it encloses. It also encloses the deep dorsal vein, the dorsal arteries, and the dorsal nerves.

General principles of penile reconstruction include:

- Identification of the all injuries (penile shaft, urethra, and neurovascular bundle).
- Maximal preservation of penile tissue.
- Watertight closure of the tunica albuginea.

The goal of surgery is preservation of genitourinary function and maintenance of cosmesis.

Foreign bodies in the urethra or bladder and foreign bodies attached to the penis

Patients may present either acutely or months or even years after the object was inserted.

Symptoms

- Pain on voiding.
- Suprapubic pain.
- Haematuria.
- Urinary retention.
- Volunteered history that they have inserted something into the urethra (sometimes no such history is forthcoming).

Examination and investigations

The object may be protruding from the urethral meatus or you may be able to feel it within the urethra. Arrange a plain X-ray of the pelvis and genitalia to locate the foreign body if it is radio-opaque or alternatively an ultrasound scan. If no foreign body is seen, ascending urethrography or flexible cystoscopy can be used to identify its presence and location.

Treatment

Removing the foreign body can be a challenge. Occasionally it may be voided spontaneously, but more often than not you have to go in after it. Use a flexible cystoscope if the object is smooth and small enough to be grasped in a stone basket or grabbed with forceps. It may be possible to retrieve the object using a rigid cystoscope or wide-bore resectoscope under general anaesthetic. If this fails, remove the bladder via an open cystostomy. If the object is made of glass, such as a thermometer, it may be safer to avoid attempting to remove it per urethra because of the danger that it might break and damage the urethra or even become lodged within it. A formal open cystostomy is the safest way of retrieving glass objects.

Outcome

- Penile injuries can be diagnosed easily and should be managed promptly, usually surgically.
- Complications include soft tissue necrosis, erectile dysfunction, urethral stricture and urethrocutaneous fistule.

Further reading

1 Aboseif S, Gomez R, McAninch JW. Genital self-mutilation. *J Urol* 1993; **150**:1143–6.
2 Agrawal SK, Morgan BE, Shafique M, Shazely M. Experience with penile fractures in Saudi Arabia. *Br J Urol* 1991; **67**:644–6.
3 Asgari MA, Hosseini SY, Safarinejad MR *et al.* Penile fractures: evaluation, therapeutic approaches and long-term results. *J Urol* 1996; **155**:148–9.
4 Bertini JE, Corriere JN. The aetiology and management of genital injuries. *J Trauma* 1988; **28**:1278–81.
5 Gomez RG, Castanheira AC, McAninch JW. Gunshot wounds to the male external genitalia. *J Urol* 1993; **150**:1147–9.
6 Johnin K, Kushima M, Koizumi S, *et al.* Percutaneous transvesical retrieval of foreign bodies penetrating the urethra. *J Urol*. 1999; **161**:915–16.
7 Osca JM, Broseta E, Server G, *et al.* Unusual foreign bodies in the urethra and bladder. *Br J Urol.* 1991; **68**:510–12.
8 Romilly CS, Issac MT. Male genital self-mutilation. *Br J Hosp Med* 1996; **55**:427–31.
9 van Ophoven A, deKernion JB. Clinical management of foreign bodies of the genitourinary tract. *J Urol* 2000; **164**:274–87.

Scrotal injuries

Aetiology

- Necrotizing infections (Fournier's gangrene).
- Avulsion injuries to scrotum.
- Penetrating scrotal injuries from gunshot or stab wounds (infrequent).

Fournier's gangrene

A necrotizing fasciitis affecting the genitalia and perineum. Primarily affects males, particularly the elderly, although serious infection can occur in young men. Necrosis and subsequent gangrene of infected tissue occurs. A source of infection can be identified in 75% of cases, most commonly from the colorectum, urinary tract, or skin. The most common colorectal sources include peri-anal, peri-rectal, and ischio-rectal abscesses, rectal instrumentation, and colonic perforation. Urethral strictures and indwelling catheters are the most common urological sources of sepsis. Skin sources include abscesses or pressure sores; they can also occur as complications of surgery, including vasectomy, insertion of a penile prosthesis, and diathermy for genital warts.

Conditions which predispose to the development of Fournier's gangrene include diabetes and local trauma to the genitalia and perineum.

Risk factors

- Alcohol abuse.
- Diabetes mellitus.
- Immunosuppressive states (e.g. transplant patients, chemotherapy, HIV/AIDS).
- Prolonged bed rest.
- Local trauma (including surgery) to genitalia or perineum. The 'trauma' may be trivial (e.g. zipper injuries to the foreskin, circumcision).

Diagnosis

Presentation of necrotizing scrotal infections is often dramatic (over a very short time course—just a few hours), with pain often out of proportion to the initial physical signs. Findings include swelling, tenderness of the affected area, crepitus, and fever, often following a seemingly trivial injury to the external genitalia, although there is not always a history of trauma or surgery. The clinical course is rapidly progressive. Blisters (bullae) may appear in the skin and within a matter of hours areas of skin necrosis may develop. Septic shock is common. The condition advances rapidly; hence its alternative name of spontaneous fulminant gangrene of the genitalia.

Both aerobic and anaerobic pathogens are responsible, with *E.coli*, *Bacteroides*, *Streptococcus*, *Klebsiella*, *Staphylococcus*, and *Clostridium* cultured most commonly. Scrotal, urethral, and abdominal imaging (using sonography, retrograde urethrography, and CT, respectively) can be selectively employed to identify the source of infection.

Although blood tests may be abnormal (e.g. elevated white count), the diagnosis is clinical, and is based on awareness of the condition and a high index of suspicion.

Management

Necrotizing infections

Principles of management:
- Prompt resuscitation.
- Antibiotics.
- Immediate surgical debridement.
- Reconstruction at a later date.

Initiate fluid resuscitation and correction of electrolyte abnormalities simultaneously with intravenous broad-spectrum antibiotic therapy to cover Gram-positive, Gram-negative, and anaerobic bacteria. Immediate surgical debridement remains the mainstay of treatment. This is performed in the operating room under general anesthesia. Urinary and faecal diversion may be required to limit wound contamination. Percutaneous cystostomy drainage is used in most cases to divert urine; additionally, a colostomy is necessary in ~30% of patients.

Start parenteral hyper-alimentation early to enhance healing. Perform further surgical debridement (usually required within 24–48 hr), and repeat as often as necessary to ensure removal of all infected tissue. Where facilities allow, consider treatment with hyperbaric oxygen therapy. There is some evidence that this may be beneficial.[1]

Scrotal reconstruction is performed only after the infection has been adequately controlled.

Avulsion injuries to the scrotum

Usually a consequence of heavy machinery or motor vehicle accidents. Diagnosis is easy and is based on physical examination. Scrotal ultrasonography can be used to evaluate the testes if there is a suspicion of their involvement.

Penetrating scrotal injuries

Explore penetrating scrotal injuries promptly. Diagnosis is easy and is based on physical examination. Principles of management include lavage, debridement, haemostasis, and reconstruction. Usually these injuries can be closed primarily. Most scrotal injuries do not directly involve the testes, as they are protected by their mobility, the cremasteric reflex, and the strength of the tunica albuginea. Consequently, testicular coverage rather than repair is usually the concern with extensive scrotal injuries.

Outcome

Aggressive resuscitation and wound care with control of infection and careful reconstruction are necessary for the successful management of scrotal injuries. In this way, mortality, which can approach 30% for necrotizing scrotal infections, can be minimized.

References

1 Pizzorno R, Bonini F, Donelli A et al. Hyperbaric oxygen therapy in the treatment of Fournier's gangrene in 100 male patients. J Urol 1997; **158**:837–40.

Tissue transfer techniques in genital reconstructive surgery

Genital skin defects can be managed by:
- Primary approximation.
- Tissue transfer techniques:
  - Grafts.
  - Flaps.

Primary approximation is the preferred method of wound closure where possible. It is limited by the size of the defect and the need to create a tension-free closure.

A **graft** is a portion of integument, completely detached from its donor site and transferred to a host bed where it acquires a new blood supply.

A skin **flap** consists of a portion of skin and subcutaneous tissue attached to the surrounding skin by a vascular pedicle. The vascular supply, maintained through the pedicle, ensures the viability of the flap until it acquires a new blood supply from the host bed. The graft is either excised and transferred to its new site with the blood supply intact, or the blood supply is re-established at the recipient site.

Graft or flap?

Consider:
- Recipient site requirements.
- Donor site morbidity.
- Operative complexity.
- Patient factors.

In general, grafts are simpler and should be considered initially. They are predominantly autografts (derived from the patient's own tissues), with allografts (derived from another human subject) and xenografts (animal derived) limited to use as biological dressings.

Skin grafts

Classification

Skin grafts are classified according to their constituents (Fig. 8.27).

Split-thickness grafts

These are skin autografts, cut at the split-thickness level, which contain the epidermis and a portion of the dermis (superficial dermis). Split-thickness skin grafts can be subdivided by the amount of dermis they contain:
- Thin (0.02–0.03 cm).
- Intermediate (0.03–0.04 cm).
- Thick (0.04–0.05 cm).

The thinner the graft, the greater the interface of fibrous tissue between the dermis and the recipient site, resulting in greater contraction. However, a thin split-thickness skin graft has a higher likelihood of survival because it is more stable during the phase of plasmatic absorption and can wait longer for vascularization. Moreover, a thin split-thickness graft does not contain hair follicles and consequently will not permit hair growth (useful for non-hair-bearing genital areas, e.g. penis).

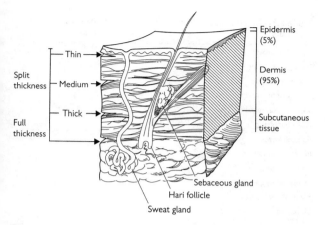

Fig. 8.27 Composition of skin grafts. Reproduced from McAninch, *Traumatic and reconstructive urology*. Philadelphia, PA. WB Saunders, 1996. Permission sought.

Full-thickness grafts

These contain the epidermis and the entire thickness of the dermis (superficial and deep dermis). The fat must be trimmed from the under-surface of the dermis to facilitate graft vascularization. Because of their thickness, these grafts have less tendency to contract, but they are revascularized more slowly, requiring optimal host conditions for survival. Their size is limited by the need to close the donor site primarily or with a split-thickness skin graft. After tissue transplantation, full-thickness grafts will resemble normal skin more closely in colour and texture. In addition, full-thickness grafts achieve better sensation than split-thickness grafts (Table 8.3).

Dermal grafts

These are a variant of full-thickness skin grafts in which the epidermis has been excluded. They are primarily used for elevation of soft tissue contour defects. The advantage of removing both the superficial and deep surfaces of the dermis is the enhanced graft survival from improved vascularization by means of the superior dermal surface. In genital reconstruction, these grafts are commonly used for replacement of the tunica albuginea in cases of Peyronie's disease.

Table 8.3 Characteristics of split-thickness and full-thickness skin grafts

Split thickness
Enhanced survival
Non-hair-bearing
Rapid donor site epithelialization
Variable contracture
Easily harvested
Full thickness
Improved colour match
Hair growth
Increased sensation
Minimal contracture
Donor site closure required

Techniques

Selection of donor site depends on the size and colour match of the defect. If possible, select an area that can be hidden readily by either anatomical structures or clothing. For genital reconstruction, split-thickness skin grafts can be obtained from the abdomen, thighs, and buttocks (Fig. 8.28). Cover the donor site with antibiotic fine mesh gauze. Full-thickness skin and dermal grafts can be harvested from the groin, retro-auricular area or antecubital flexor crease. Undermine the wound edges to mobilize the skin so that it can be re-approximated without tension. A split-thickness graft may be needed for closure in larger defects.

Split-thickness skin grafts can be harvested using either a knife or dermatome (drum-type or electric) (Fig. 8.29). Full-thickness skin and dermal grafts are cut freehand with a scalpel.

Before applying a graft to the host bed, excise all necrotic tissue, exposing a clean non-infected bleeding base. Place the skin graft on the recipient bed with the dermal undersurface in contact with the wound. Dermal grafts can be applied with their superior surface towards the wound, facilitating graft vascularization by eliminating any remaining adherent subcutaneous fat between host and graft. Secure the graft with fine non-absorbable sutures or staples placed in an interrupted fashion. Once the graft is in position, immobilization is essential for revascularization; this is best provided by a tie-over dressing. For penile grafting, a splint may be also applied to fix the penis in an upright position limiting the amount of post-operative edema and preventing graft shifting.

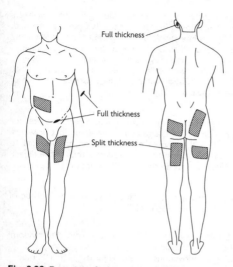

Fig. 8.28 Donor sites for harvesting split-thickness and full-thickness grafts.
Reproduced from McAninch, *Traumatic and reconstructive urology*. Philadelphia, PA.
WB Saunders, 1996. Permission sought.

(a) (a)

(c)

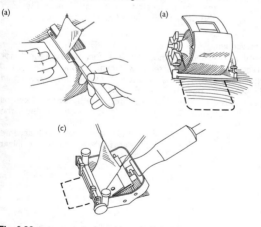

Fig. 8.29 Instruments for harvesting split-thickness skin grafts: (a) knife for harvesting
a split-thickness skin graft; (b) drum-type dermatome; (c) electric dermatome.
Reproduced from McAninch, *Traumatic and reconstructive urology*. Philadelphia, PA.
WB Saunders, 1996. Permission sought.

There are two distinct phases in graft survival. During the first, *imbibition*, the graft vessels fill with fibrinogen-free fluid and cells from the host bed. The graft is nurtured by this interstitial fluid and plasma for approximately 48 hr until circulation is established. During the second phase, *inosculation*, there is an ingrowth of new capillaries from the host's vessels, allowing revascularization of the graft's own capillary plexus. This process is gradual, resulting in adequate graft circulation within 4–5 days. Common causes of graft failure are shown in Table 8.4.

Flaps

Flaps are used to resurface wounds that are unsuitable recipient sites for skin grafting. These include areas of large composite tissue loss or where excess bulk is required. A flap should be selected on its potential to provide coverage. It should conform to the desired contour of the defect, preserve donor function, and provide an aesthetically acceptable result.

Classification

Flaps can be classified according to their vascular supply, their method of movement, or their composition (Table 8.5).

Blood supply

Random flaps (Fig. 8.30) receive their blood supply from the 'random' intradermal and subdermal vascular plexus. Consequently, they lack an anatomically identifiable arteriovenous system. Their use in genital reconstruction is limited; they are more frequently used in urethral reconstruction and, occasionally, in closing perineal defects.

Axial flaps (Fig. 8.31) incorporate at least one artery and vein in the pedicle. Because of their larger length-to-width ratio, these flaps can reach more positions through a greater arc of mobility and are preferable to random flaps.

Method of movement

Advancement flaps (Fig. 8.32) are moved directly forward from the donor site to the recipient site without lateral movement or rotation.

Rotational flaps (Fig. 8.33) are semicircular flaps that are moved in an arc around a fixed pivot point to fill a defect.

Interpolation flaps (Fig. 8.34) are taken from nearby donor sites and transposed to the recipient site. The pedicle must pass over or under the tissue to reach the recipient area.

Free flaps (Fig. 8.35) have a defined axial vascular supply that is severed at the donor site and microsurgically reanastomosed to the recipient vessels.

Table 8.4 Common causes of graft failure

Poor contact between the graft and host, usually from haematoma or seroma
Graft displacement from improper immobilization
Poor donor site vascularity
Infection (usually group A beta-haemolytic streptococci and *Pseudomonas aeruginosa*)
Technical errors
Poor graft storage

Table 8.5 Classification of flaps

Based on vascular supply
Random
Axial
Based on method of movement
Local
Advancement
Rotational
Interpolation
Distant
Free (microvascular)
Based on composition
Simple
Cutaneous
Muscle
Compound
Myocutaneous
Fasciocutaneous

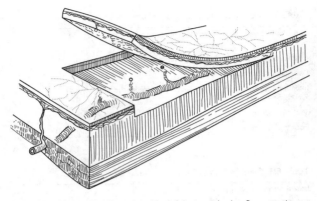

Fig. 8.30 A random flap. Reproduced from Schreiter & Jordan, *Reconstructive urethral surgery*; Springer, 2005. Permission sought.

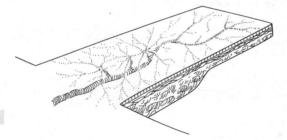

Fig. 8.31 An axial flap. Reproduced from Schreiter & Jordan, *Reconstructive urethral surgery*; Springer, 2005. Permission sought.

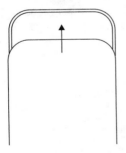

Fig. 8.32 An advancement flap.

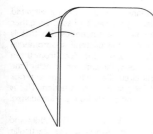

Fig. 8.33 A rotational flap.

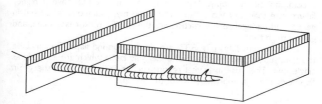

Fig. 8.34 An interpolation flap.

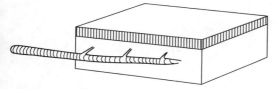

Fig. 8.35 A free flap.

Composition

Cutaneous flaps consist of skin and subcutaneous tissue which is elevated above the muscular fascia. Their vascular supply can be based on either a random or an axial pattern. An example of a cutaneous flap that is frequently used for genital reconstruction is the bilateral superomedial thigh flap. This is an axial flap whose blood supply is derived from three main sources: the deep external pudendal artery, the anterior branch of the obturator artery, and the medial femoral circumflex artery. The anterior scrotal cutaneous flap can also be used for genital reconstruction. This is a random rotational flap which receives its blood supply from the intradermal scrotal plexus.

Muscle flaps are comprised of a specific muscle alone. Their bulk and malleable characteristics permit them to conform to the particular wound characteristics and to fill large defects. Examples of muscle flaps include the rectus abdominis and gluteus maximus, both of which have very limited use in genital reconstruction.

Myocutaneous (musculocutaneous) flaps (Fig. 8.36) are compound flaps which consist of superficial muscles and their overlying skin, sharing a common blood supply. They are more complex and have a higher failure rate than cutaneous flaps. The three myocutaneous flaps used in genital and perineal reconstruction are the gracilis, tensor fascia lata, and gluteal thigh flaps.

Fasciocutaneous flaps (Fig. 8.37) are also compound flaps. They include the skin, subcutaneous tissue, and underlying fascia which are elevated as single unit. Their use in genital reconstruction is limited, with the groin flap being the only representative of this group.

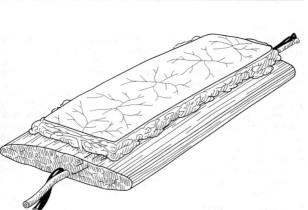

Fig. 8.36 A myocutaneous flap. Reproduced from McAninch, *Traumatic and reconstructive urology*. Philadelphia, PA. WB Saunders, 1996. Permission sought.

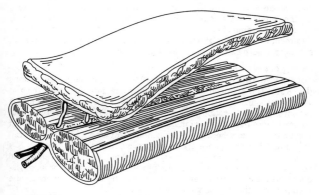

Fig. 8.37 A fasciocutaneous flap. Reproduced from McAninch, *Traumatic and reconstructive urology*. Philadelphia, PA. WB Saunders, 1996. Permission sought.

Techniques

Skin flaps grow with the patient. They maintain their original colour and texture with little change. Hair growth will continue as all the skin appendages are included in the flap. Sensation is re-established by the ingrowths of nerve fibres from the surrounding skin, as well as from the recipient bed, but it can take up to 3 years.

Pre-operative decision-making is the critical factor affecting the fate of any flap. Often the size of the defect is under-estimated; donor site restrictions, such as compromised vasculature by previous abdominal surgery or radiation, must also be considered. Intra-operatively, careful attention to detail in the design and execution of the flap is critical. With an axial flap, vascular isolation should be meticulous. Another important consideration is avoiding functional loss at the donor site. With myocutaneous flaps, errors in tunnelling are the most common cause of flap failure. Tension or kinking of the pedicle can similarly result in flap necrosis from decreased perfusion.

Penile reconstruction

Extensive loss of penile skin occurs infrequently. There may also be loss of skin in the scrotum, perineum, or abdomen. The objective of penile reconstruction should be to maintain the functional properties of the penis as a conduit of urine and semen, and its erectile capabilities, while providing an acceptable cosmetic appearance.

With extensive penile tissue loss, as with burns, necrotizing infections, and over-zealous circumcision, various techniques can be used depending on the extent of the defect and the experience of the surgeon. It is important to remember that in all infected cases, the initial mainstay of treatment is thorough debridement. All necrotic tissue must be removed, providing a clean base for tissue transplantation.

Penile grafts

Total penile skin loss is best managed by split-thickness skin grafting (Fig. 8.38). The graft can be harvested from the anterior lateral thigh at various thicknesses, depending on the local wound conditions and the patient's erectile function. Thinner grafts have improved survival but contract more than thicker grafts, and consequently may limit subsequent erections. In cases where erectile function is not a concern, the graft can be meshed, facilitating coverage and improving survival.

Full-thickness skin grafts are rarely used in complete penile denudation because of the size of the donor site required and the need for its subsequent closure. For partial penile skin loss, full-thickness skin grafts can be used provided that the donor site is hairless.

Penile flaps

Skin flaps have limited use for penile skin replacement. Their cumbersome nature, hair-bearing characteristics, and torsional effect on the erect penis make them cosmetically inferior to skin grafts. In certain cases, an anterior scrotal cutaneous flap can be rotated to cover a limited proximal penile skin defect. Alternatively, in a sexually inactive patient, a bipedicle scrotal flap has been described for covering the entire penile shaft.

Scrotal reconstruction

The viscoelastic properties of the scrotum allow unique extensibility, permitting even large scrotal skin defects to be closed primarily without tension. When skin is insufficient for primary closure, as with extensive avulsions, necrotizing infections, or burns, scrotal replacement is needed. As with penile reconstruction, careful timing and planning are necessary to ensure a successful result. In cases of severe infection, initial management consists of aggressive debridement with frequent dressing changes. Faecal and urinary diversion may often be necessary to avoid wound soilage.

Testicular thigh pouches

Thigh pouches offer the simplest temporary coverage for the exposed testicles. Any infection must first be adequately controlled to avoid dissemination. Thigh pouches can be fashioned by dissecting the subcutaneous tissue from the thigh fascia, followed by creation of a separate pocket for implantation of each testicle. In severely debilitated patients, thigh pouches can be used as a permanent solution for testicular coverage.

Scrotal grafts

The entire scrotum can be reconstructed with a continuous single meshed split-thickness skin graft (Fig. 8.38a). Before grafting, the testicles should be sutured together in the midline to prevent inferior migration. Full-thickness skin grafts are not used in scrotal reconstruction because of the large surface area needed for coverage.

Scrotal flaps

When additional tissue bulk is preferred, or with large concomitant perineal defects, flaps should be used for scrotal reconstruction. The most versatile flap for scrotal reconstruction is the bilateral superomedial thigh flap (Fig. 8.38b). It is raised off the underlying fat distally and, more proximally, off the fascia lata covering the origin of the gracilis and adductor longus muscles. After the thigh flaps are elevated, they can be transferred to create a saccular neoscrotum by suturing both distal margins together in the midline. A drain should be used to prevent accumulation of serosanguinous fluid. The donor sites are closed primarily, avoiding skin grafts. Alternatively, a gracilis myocutaneous flap can be used to reconstruct the scrotum. This is technically more difficult and may lead to an inferior cosmetic result.

Tissue expanders

Tissue expanders have been used to reconstruct a two-compartment system. Provided that adjacent perineal or inguinal skin is uninvolved, tissue expanders can be placed on each side of the midline with gradual expansion over a 2–3 month period. The primary disadvantage is the time it takes to complete the reconstruction and the multiple procedures involved. Alternatively, rapid intraoperative tissue expansion can be used, selectively, limiting the long-term process involved with standard tissue expansion.[1]

Reference

1 Kwon E, Pareek G, Fracchia JA, Armenakas NA. Scrotal reconstruction using rapid intraoperative tissue expansion: A preliminary report. *J Urol* 2008; **179**:207.

Anterior urethral injuries (Fig. 8.39, 8.40)

Aetiology
- The most frequent urethral injuries are iatrogenic, e.g. inadvertent Foley catheter balloon inflation in the urethra, traumatic lower urinary tract endoscopy (cystoscopy, transurethral surgery). They are often minor and under-reported.
- External trauma
  • Usually caused by a blow to the perineum (Fig. 8.41) or motor vehicle accident. Usually straddle injuries, with forceful contact of the perineum with a blunt object such as bicycle cross-bar or the top of a fence. They usually involve the relatively immobile bulbar urethral segment rather than the mobile penile urethra.
  • Penetrating anterior urethral injuries result predominantly from gunshot wounds. Often these occur in conjunction with penile or testicular trauma. Stab wounds are an uncommon cause of anterior urethral trauma.
  • Penile amputations and penile ruptures (penile fracture).

Diagnosis
Suspect an anterior urethral injury with the above history combined with pain on urination or complete inability to void, and haematuria.

Signs are blood at the meatus and a perineal swelling or haematoma (which may extend superiorly to the abdomen and chest and inferiorly to the scrotum, perineum and medial thighs) (Fig. 8.42).

Any patient with a history suggestive of a urethral injury or any clinical indicator of urethral trauma should undergo dynamic retrograde urethrography before any attempt is made at transurethral catheterization. Instil ~20–30 mL of undiluted water-soluble contrast material into the urethra under fluoroscopic guidance. Extravasation of contrast material is diagnostic of a urethral injury. The presence of haematuria in the context of a straddle injury, but where there is no urethral contrast extravasation, suggests an anterior urethral contusion.

Classification
Urethral injuries, both anterior or posterior, are classified as follows.

- Grade I   Contusion: blood at the urethral meatus, normal urethrogram
- Grade II   Stretch injury: elongation of the urethra without extravasation on urethrography
- Grade III Partial disruption: extravasation of contrast at injury site with contrast visualized in the bladder
- Grade IV   Complete disruption: extravasation of contrast at injury site without bladder visualization; <2 cm urethral separation
- Grade V   Complete disruption: complete transection with >2 cm urethral separation or extension in the prostate or vagina

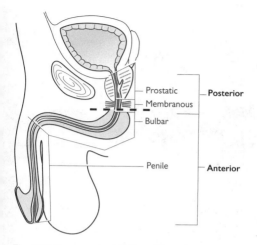

Fig. 8.39 The anatomic subdivisions of the urethra.

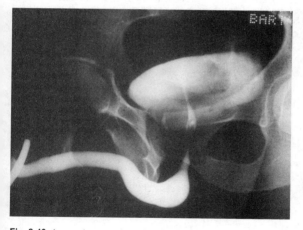

Fig. 8.40 A normal retrograde urethrogram demonstrating the subdivisions of the anterior and posterior urethra.

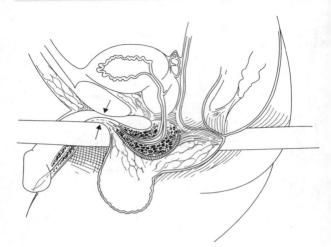

Fig. 8.41 A common mechanism of external blunt trauma to the anterior urethra. Reproduced from McAninch, *Traumatic and reconstructive urology*. Philadelphia, PA. WB Saunders, 1996. Permission sought.

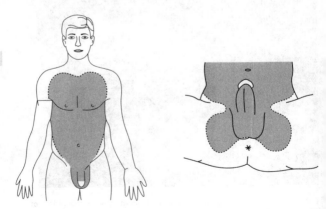

Fig. 8.42 Butterfly bruising following rupture of Buck's fascia. Reproduced from Reynard *et al.* 2006, *Oxford Handbook of Urology*, Oxford University Press.

Management of anterior urethral injuries (Fig. 8.43)
The goal of initial treatment for any trauma to the urethra is avoidance of any manoeuvre that can potentiate the injury combined with urine diversion.

Urethral contusions and stretch injuries: transurethral catheterization maintained for 7–10 days.

Urethral disruption: blind passage of a transurethral catheter is strongly contraindicated.

- Urinary diversion by means of a percutaneous suprapubic cystostomy is the easiest and safest option, and is indicated for:
  - All *blunt* anterior urethral disruptions except in association with penile ruptures.
  - Haemodynamic instability.
  - Multiple associated injuries of non-genital organs.
  - Penetrating injury with a large urethral defect requiring extensive reconstruction (grade IV or V).
- Keep the cystostomy tube in place for at least 6 weeks (obviously longer if repair of other injuries is ongoing) at which time retrograde and voiding cysto-urethrograms are performed to identify the extent of injury. The appropriate reconstructive procedure can be scheduled, as needed, usually 8–12 weeks after the initial injury.
- Select *partial* anterior urethral disruptions can be bridged using a flexible cystoscope to pass a guidewire followed by a council-tip catheter into the bladder. When attempted, this procedure should be done gently and aborted promptly if resistance or poor visualization is encountered.
- Immediate anterior urethral repair. Attempt only for:
  - Penetrating urethral disruption, provided that the patient is haemodynamically stable, without multiple injuries.
  - Any urethral injury associated with a penile rupture.

Technique of repair of anterior urethral disruptions
Small mucosal tears
Use interrupted fine absorbable sutures placed in a watertight fashion without compromising the urethral luminal size. Use a 16Fr Foley catheter to stent the repair. More extensive partial disruptions and select complete disruptions are managed by primary excision and re-anastomosis (Fig. 8.44). The corpus spongiosum is mobilized distally, obtaining sufficient length for tension-free anastomosis. The urethral ends are spatulated and the anastomoses performed over an 18Fr Foley catheter using interrupted 5–0 absorbable sutures and ensuring a tension-free watertight repair. Remove the urethral catheter 2 weeks after surgery and arrange a voiding cysto-urethrogram.

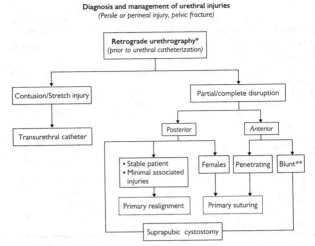

Diagnosis and management of urethral injuries
(Penile or perineal injury, pelvic fracture)

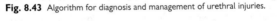

* In females only, proceed to urethroscopy
** Except in association with penile fractures

Fig. 8.43 Algorithm for diagnosis and management of urethral injuries.

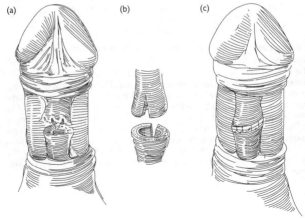

Fig. 8.44 Technique of repair of anterior urethral disruption (a) debride, (b) spatulate, (c) anastomose. Reproduced from McAninch, *Traumatic and reconstructive urology*. Philadelphia, PA. WB Saunders, 1996. Permission sought.

If, at the time of initial exploration, the urethra is found to be so extensively disrupted that primary anastomosis is not feasible, either urethral marsupialization or suprapubic urinary diversion should be performed. Urethral replacement with grafts or flaps should be avoided in the acute trauma setting, as contamination or decreased blood supply can compromise such a repair.

Outcomes

Potential complications of anterior urethral injuries include stricture, infection, sacculation, fistula, erectile dysfunction, chordee, and incontinence. Early diagnosis, prompt urinary diversion coupled with judicious use of antibiotics, and the appropriate urethral reconstruction can decrease their incidence.

Further reading

1 Cass AS, Godec CJ. Urethral injury due to external trauma. *Urology* 1978; **11**:607.
2 Husmann DA, Boone TB, Wilson WT. Management of low velocity gunshot wounds to the anterior urethra: the role of primary repair versus urinary diversion alone. *J Urol* 1993; **150**:70–2.
3 Marsh HP, King Q, Kourambas J, Reynard JM. Penile fracture with complete rupture of the urethra. *BJU Int* 2000; **85**:169.
4 Pierce JM. Disruptions of the anterior urethra. *Urol Clin North Am* 1989; **16**:329–34.
5 Sellett T. Iatrogenic urethral injury due to preinflation of a Foley catheter. *JAMA* 1971; **217**:1548.

Posterior urethral injuries

Aetiology

Injuries to the posterior urethra occur almost exclusively with pelvic fractures. Specifically, with a crush or deceleration-impact injury, the severe shearing forces necessary to fracture the pelvis are transmitted to the prostato-membranous junction, the weakest portion of the urethra, resulting in its disruption. Overall, the posterior urethra is injured in up to 10% of male pelvic fractures and up to 4% of female pelvic fractures.

Diagnosis

Suspect a posterior urethral injury in any patient with a pelvic fracture and blood at the meatus or vaginal introitus. Other signs and symptoms include haematuria, pain on urination, and inability to void.

A high-riding prostate is an unreliable finding. Rectal examination in pelvic fracture is done not to assess prostate location, but rather to determine the possible presence of a concomitant rectal injury in both men and women (blood on the gloved finger). In addition, a complete pelvic examination should be performed on female patients to exclude a coexisting vaginal injury.

Any patient suspected of having a urethral injury should undergo dynamic retrograde urethrography before transurethral catheterization.

Classification

See anterior urethral injuries (📖 p. 576).

Management of posterior urethral injuries (Fig. 8.43)

Initial management

The initial approach to the management of posterior urethral injuries depends on the patient's overall condition. Most patients with pelvic fracture have significant coexisting trauma (abdomen, chest, head, long bones) and therefore immediate consideration should be given to resuscitative measures and treatment of these associated injuries.

Associated bladder injuries

Approximately 15% of male and 70% of female patients with posterior urethral disruptions have an associated bladder rupture. The diagnosis of bladder rupture in the context of a posterior urethral disruption is made visually during placement of an open suprepubic cystotomy or radiographically, by performing a cystogram, after first placing a large bore suprepubic tube (16Fr) using image-guidance (sonography or CT scan).

Placement of an open suprapubic cystostomy

The bladder is exposed via a midline incision allowing:

• Accurate and safe placement of a suprapubic catheter.
• Inspection of the posterior wall of the bladder for injuries and penetrating bone fragments.
• Bladder repair and removal of any bone fragments.
• Opening the peritoneal cavity so that the intra-abdominal contents can be inspected.

Avoid extending the lower end of your midline incision (and the incision in the bladder) too close to the pelvic haematoma—aim to avoid disturbing the latter. If you are having difficulty identifying the bladder, do not hesitate to open the peritoneum and locate the bladder from above downwards. Once you have found the bladder, place two 2–0 stay sutures of Vicryl on either side of the midline and incise between them to open the bladder. Look inside for bladder tears and repair these with 3–0 Vicryl. Remove any bone fragments within the bladder. Flush the wound with a gentamicin solution and repair the bladder. Place a suprapubic catheter close to the midline cystotomy incision. Close the bladder in two layers.

Injury specific management options

As with anterior urethral injuries, posterior urethral contusions and stretch injuries can be managed with transurethral catheterization alone (Fig. 8.43).

The easiest, safest, and most readily available initial management option for any posterior urethral disruption is the placement of a suprapubic cystostomy, preferably using an open approach to identify and repair coexisting bladder injuries as described above (Fig. 8.45). After the patient has adequately recovered from the associated injuries and the urethral injury has stabilized, the urethra can be evaluated radiographically and the appropriate reconstructive procedure planned.

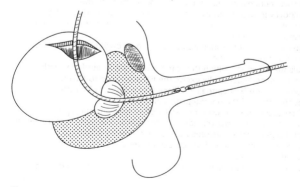

Fig. 8.45 A catheter is placed through a cystotomy and advanced to the urethral meatus, and a second catheter is tied to it. The second catheter is then withdrawn into the bladder.

In rare instances, a transpubic approach is additionally used in order to improve visualization of the prostato-membranous regions (e.g. with severe posterior urethral displacement or multiple fistulous tracts). Through a separate lower abdominal incision extending to the base of the penis, remove a wedge of pubis with a Gigli saw. Orthopaedic sequelae of pubic resection are negligible because the anterior two-thirds of the pelvic ring is non-weight bearing.

Disruption of the female urethra requires immediate surgical repair. This is because any tear involving the short female urethra will probably extend to the bladder neck and disrupt the sphincteric mechanism. Prompt urethral and bladder neck reconstruction is necessary to avoid post-traumatic incontinence.

Outcome

Posterior urethral injures can result in devastating long-term consequences. For a young person, the potential complications of impotence, stricture and incontinence often create life-long morbidity. Management of these injuries can be complex and depends on the individual case and the surgeon's expertise. As a general rule, initial suprapubic cystostomy is the simplest option. Alternatively, primary realignment can be attempted. The advantage of this latter procedure is its lower subsequent stricture rate (~50% vs. 95%). Contemporary series suggest similar erectile dysfunction and incontinence rates of 40% and 10%, respectively, for both procedures.

Further reading

1 Jackson DH, Williams JL. Urethral injury: a retrospective study. *Br J Urol* 1974; **46**:665–76.

2 Koraitim MM, Marzouk ME, Atta MA, Orabi SS. Risk factors and mechansim of urethral injury in pelvic fracture. *Br J Urol* 1996; **77**:876–80.

3 Kotkin L, Koch MO. Impotence and incontinence after immediate realignment of posterior urethral trauma: result of injury or management? *J Urol* 1996; **155**:1600–3.

4 Lowe MA, Mason JT, Luna GK *et al*. Risk factors for urethral injuries in men with traumatic pelvic fractures. *J Urol* 1988; **140**:506.

5 Cass AS, Gleich P, Smith C. Simultaneous bladder and prostatomembranous urethral rupture from external trauma. *J Urol* 1984; **132**:907–8.

6 Elliott DS, Barrett DM. Long-term follow-up and evaluation of primary realignment of posterior urethral disruptions. *J Urol* 1997; **157**:814–16.

7 Zingg EJ, Casanova GA, Isler B *et al*. Pelvic fractures and traumatic lesions of the posterior urethra. *Eur Urol* 1990; **18**:27.

Pelvic fractures

Aetiology

Pelvic trauma can be divided by mechanism into low-energy and high-energy groups based on the energy exchanged in the impact.

- Low-energy mechanisms (approximately one-third of all pelvic fractures) usually result in isolated fractures of the pelvic ring without damaging the integrity of the pelvic structures:
  - domestic falls.
  - sports injuries.
  - low-velocity vehicular accidents.
- High-energy mechanisms (approximately two-thirds of all pelvic fractures) often result in multiple fractures of the pelvic ring:
  - most commonly occur from motor vehicle and motorcycle accidents (both drivers and pedestrian injuries)—classically from 'run-over' injuries.
  - falls from heights >4 m.

Associated injuries with high-energy pelvic trauma are common and include extremity fractures (tibia and femur) and injuries to the central nervous system, chest, and abdomen. Intra-abdominal injuries occur in ~20% of high-energy pelvic trauma, most commonly to the liver, lower urinary tract, spleen, diaphragm, and bowel. Two-thirds of the lower urinary tract injuries involve the bladder and one-third involve the urethra.

Diagnosis

With pelvic fractures, accurate injury assessment depends not only on the traditional history, physical, laboratory, and radiographic examinations but also on the details of the mechanism of injury (including the type, direction, and magnitude of the force involved).

The initial evaluation of any patient suspected of having a pelvic fracture should include a manual examination of the pelvic ring for rotational instability. Examination of the abdomen often demonstrates voluntary guarding with suprapubic dullness to percussion. A digital rectal examination should be performed on all patients and a vaginal examination on all females to identify concomitant injuries. A complete blood count will suggest the degree of blood loss. Radiographs of the cervical spine, chest, abdomen, anteroposterior pelvis and extremities should be performed on all high-energy pelvic fractures; imaging of low-energy fractures can be confined to the pelvis.

In haemodynamically *unstable* patients, first identify and control bleeding. The pelvis should be stabilized using either a proprietary device or simply a bed sheet as a binder. This manoeuver decreases pelvic volume, stabilizes the fracture, and potentially limits venous bleeding. Military antishock trousers (MAST) can also be used to limit further blood loss by increasing blood return from the lower extremities to the central circulation. Initially, thoracic and abdominal sources of bleeding must be excluded. Chest radiographs suffice for excluding significant thoracic bleeding. Once this is ruled out, the next diagnostic step should be peritoneal lavage. This is preferably performed using a supra-umbilical open technique. False-positive results can occur because the pelvic haematoma can contaminate the findings. In order to limit false readings, a positive aspiration is considered when gross rather than microscopic blood is obtained. A negative lavage is accurate in ruling out an intra-peritoneal injury but can miss a retroperitoneal injury. Alternatively, focused abdominal ultrasonography can be used for the initial evaluation of the intra-abdominal organs. The results of these tests are essential in triaging unstable patients between the operating room and the angiography suite.

A patient who is haemodynamically unstable should not be taken for CT imaging.

In haemodynamically stable patients, additional radiographs should be obtained to identify and classify all injuries; this is preferably accomplished using CT of the pelvis and abdomen.

Classification

Although several classifications of pelvic fractures have been proposed, the most comprehensive is the Young system which is based on the type and direction of the injurious force applied to the pelvic ring.

Young classification system

- Lateral compression injuries: transverse fractures of pubic rami, either ipsilateral or contralateral to posterior injury
  - Type I   Sacral compression on side of impact
  - Type II   Crescent (iliac wing) fracture on side of impact
  - Type III Type I or II injuries on side of impact; contralateral open-book (anteroposterior compression) injury
- Anterio-posterior compression injures: symphyseal diastasis and/or longitudinal rami fracture
  - Type I   Slight widening of pubic symphysis and/or anterior sacro-iliac (SI) joint; stretched but intact anterior SI, sacrotuberous and sacrospinous ligaments; intact posterior SI ligaments
  - Type II   Widened anterior SI joint; disrupted anterior SI, sacrotuberous and sacrospinous ligaments; intact posterior SI ligaments
  - Type III Complete SI joint disruption with lateral displacement; disrupted anterior SI, sacrotuberous and sacrospinous ligaments; disrupted posterior SI ligaments
- Vertical shear injuries: symphyseal diastasis or vertical displacement anteriorly and posteriorly, usually through the SI joint, but occasionally through the iliac wing and/or sacrum.
- Combined mechanical injuries: Combination of other injury patterns (most commonly lateral compression and vertical shear injuries):
  - Lateral compression injuries occur from a laterally applied force and result in stretching not tearing of the pelvic ligaments; they are not usually associated with significant haemorrhage.
  - Anteroposterior compression injuries result from forces applied to the anterior or posterior superior iliac spine areas either directly or indirectly via the lower extremities or ischial tuberosities. They result in pelvic ligament tears, open symphysis and SI joints, and significant bleeding.

- Vertical shear injuries occur when the pelvis is stressed vertically or longitudinally. The classic mechanism is a fall from a height, landing on an extended lower extremity. In addition these injuries can occur when a victim is struck from above (by a falling object) or by forces applied to the pelvis from an extended lower extremity during a motor vehicle accident (by extending the leg against the floorboard just prior to impact). Such injuries result in significant trauma to the pelvic ligaments.

Management of pelvic fractures

Low-energy pelvic fractures can usually can be managed non-operatively with gentle mobilization and protected weight bearing. Prolonged bed rest, pelvic suspension, and body casts are not advised.

Treatment of high-energy pelvic fractures depends on the patient's overall condition, associated injuries, and the specifics of the pelvic disruption (Fig. 8.47). Pelvic stabilization should be performed promptly. This can be accomplished immediately with a temporary device or within the first 4 hr after the injury (once the patient is haemodynamically stable) with an external fixator. The external fixator can easily be applied in the resuscitation suite and may be all that is required to stabilize the fracture. Its limitation is that it allows reduction of only anterior and not posterior pelvic ring disruptions.

If, despite these manoeuvres, haemodynamic instability persists, those patients with a positive peritoneal lavage should undergo exploratory laparotomy and those with a negative lavage should be taken for pelvic angiography with attempt at embolization.

Once the patient has been effectively haemodynamically stabilized and all associated injuries addressed, definitive management of the pelvic fracture can be accomplished using internal fixation. Internal fixation is usually deferred for several days to allow resolution of the retroperitoneal bleeding. This is performed in the operating room using a variety of techniques depending on the pelvic fracture pattern.

Outcome

Potential complications of pelvic fractures include:
- long-term pain and disability.
- infection.
- thrombo-embolism.

Most importantly, prompt identification and control of pelvic haemorrhage is pivotal in decreasing mortality related to pelvic fracture.

Acute diagnosis and management of high-energy pelvic fractures

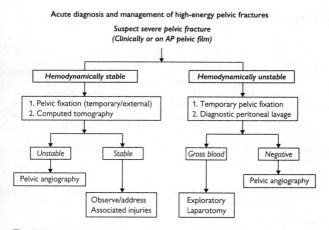

Fig. 8.47 Algorithm for diagnosis and management of high-energy pelvic fractures.

Further reading

1 Latenser BA, Gentilello LM, Tarver AA et al. Improved outcome with early fixation of skeletally unstable pelvic fractures. *J Trauma* 1991; **31**:28.
2 Leung KS, Chien P, Shen WY et al. Operative treatment of unstable pelvic fractures. *Injury* 1992; **23**:31.
3 Tile M. *Fractures of the pelvis and acetabulum*. Baltimore, MD: Williams & Wilkins, 1984.
4 Tile M. Pelvic ring fractures. Should they be fixed? *J Bone Joint Surg* 1988; **70B**:1.

Paraphimosis

Definition

The foreskin is retracted from over the glans of the penis, and cannot then be pulled back over the glans into its normal anatomical position (the foreskin becomes trapped behind the glans). Paraphimosis affects males at any age, but is most common in teenagers or young men. It also occurs in elderly men who have had the foreskin retracted during catheterization, but not been returned to its normal position. It can occur in an otherwise normal foreskin, which if left in the retracted position may become oedematous to the point where it cannot be reduced. Occasionally a phimotic foreskin (a tight foreskin which is difficult to retract off the glans) is retracted, and it is then impossible for it to be put back in its normal position.

History

Ask the patient if he is normally able to retract the foreskin (suggesting an otherwise normal foreskin if he can, and a phimotic one if he cannot).

Examination

Usually painful, oedematous foreskin. It may become so engorged with oedema fluid that the appearance can be very confusing for those who have never seen it. Occasionally a small area of ulceration of the foreskin may develop in a paraphimosis that has been present for several days, which those unfamiliar with the condition may misinterpret as a malignant or infective process.

Treatment

The patient will usually have applied pressure to the oedematous foreskin in an attempt to reduce it, and usually the attending doctor does the same, sometimes successfully reducing the foreskin, but more often than not failing to do so (depending on the duration of the paraphimosis).

Options

- 'Iced-glove' method:[1] apply topical lidocaine gel to the glans and foreskin. Wait for 5 min until anaesthesia of the area is achieved. Place ice and water in a rubber glove and tie a knot in the cuff of the glove to prevent the contents from pouring out. Also tie-off the four fingers of the glove. Place the thumb of the glove over the penis so that the penis lies within it and in contact with the ice and water. This may reduce the swelling and allow reduction of the foreskin.
- Granulated sugar has been used to reduce the oedema (by an osmotic effect).[2] The sugar can be placed in a condom or glove applied over the end of the penis. The process of reduction may take several hours.
- Hyaluronidase (1 mL; 150 U/cc) has been injected via a 25G hypodermic needle into the prepuce.[3] This breaks down hyaluronic acid and decreases the oedema.
- The Dundee technique.[4]
- Dorsal slit.

The Dundee technique (Fig. 8.48)

Give the patient a broad-spectrum antibiotic such as ciprofloxacin 500 mg by mouth. Apply a ring block to the base of the penis using a 26G needle. Use 10 mL of 1% plain lidocaine or 10–20 mL of 0.5% plain bupivicaine (Marcaine) to the skin at the base of the penis. Wait for 5 min. Touch the skin of the prepuce to check that the penis has been anaesthetised. Try pricking the skin of the penis with a sterile needle and ask the patient if he can feel it to make sure that it is well anaesthetised. Occasionally inadequate anaesthesia is achieved and the patient will require a general anaesthetic. In children, a general anaesthetic is usually required.

Clean the skin of the foreskin and the glans with an antiseptic. Using a 25G needle make approximately 20 punctures into the oedematous fore-skin. Firmly squeeze the foreskin to force the oedema fluid out (Fig. 8.48). Small 'jets' of oedema fluid will be seen. Once the foreskin has been decompressed, it can usually be returned to its normal position. Discharge the patient on a 7 day course of ciprofloxacin as a prophylactic measure and recommend daily baths with careful cleaning of the glans and skin with soap and water. The patient should be advised to dry the foreskin carefully and always return it to its normal position afterwards.

Dorsal slit

Tis is usually performed under general anaesthetic or ring block. Make an incision in the tight band of constricting tissue. Pull the foreskin back over the glans, checking that it can move easily. If you make a longitudinal incision, this can be closed transversely, thus essentially lengthening the circumference of the foreskin and hopefully preventing further recurrence of the paraphimosis (Fig. 8.49).

If, having had a dorsal slit, the patient is concerned about the cosmetic appearance, or if the underlying cause of the paraphimosis was a phimo-sis, then he can undergo circumcision at a later date. We have avoided immediate circumcision in such cases, because the gross distortion of the normal anatomy of the foreskin can make circumcision difficult and lead to a less than perfect cosmetic result.

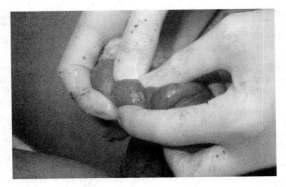

Fig. 8.48 Reduction of paraphimosis using the Dundee technique. Reproduced with permission from Reynard and Barua, Reduction of paraphimosis the simple way. *British Journal Urology International*; **83**: 859–60, Blackwells © 1999.

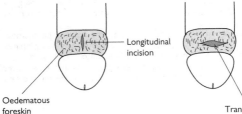

Fig. 8.49 A dorsal slit with the longitudinal incision closed transversely. Reproduced from Hashim et *al. Urological emergencies in clinical practice.* Springer-Verlag. London, 2005. Permission sought.

References

1 Houghton GR. The 'iced-glove' method of treatment of paraphimosis. *Br J Surg* 1973; **60**:876–7.
2 Kerwat R, Shandall A, Stephenson B. Reduction of paraphimosis with granulated sugar. *Br J Urol* 1998; **82**:755.
3 DeVries CR, Miller AK, Packer MG. Reduction of paraphimosis with hyaluronidase. *Urology* 1996; **48**:464–5.
4 Reynard JM, Barua JM. Reduction of paraphimosis the simple: the Dundee technique. *BJU Int* 1999; **83**:859–860.

Priapism

Definition

A pathological condition of penile erection which persists beyond or is unrelated to sexual stimulation.

Classification

- Ischaemic (veno-occlusive) priapism is the most common. It is a low-flow state resulting from an imbalance of the vasoconstrictive and vasorelaxatory mechanisms. It leads to penile compartment syndrome, characterized by hypoxia, hypercapnia, and acidosis. With prolonged ischemia, the cavernosal tissue is irreversibly damaged.
- Non-ischaemic (arterial) priapism is a high-flow state resulting from acute trauma. The ensuing unregulated cavernous arterial flow leads to the formation of an arterial-lacunar fistula and release of nitrous oxide which inhibits vasoconstriction and coagulation.

Aetiology

Approximately 30% of cases are idiopathic. Drugs are responsible for approximately four-fifths of the remaining 70% of cases, most commonly as a consequence of intracavernosal injections of vasoactive agents for management of erectile dysfunction. Other factors are listed in Table 8.6.

Diagnosis (Fig. 8.50)

Take an in-depth history and carry out a physical examination focusing on predisposing factors, as the aetiology will determine appropriate management. Pertinent historical findings include current medications or recreational drugs, and known hypercoagulable states or haematological disorders. In addition, the characteristics of the erection, including duration, and quality and presence of pain, should be elicited. In ischaemic priapism the erection is painful, while in the non-ischaemic type it is painless.

Helpful laboratory tests include full blood and platelet count, sickle test, and urine screening for metabolites of cocaine or psychoactive drugs. However, do not delay treatment by waiting for test results.

Aspiration of corporal blood is helpful in distinguishing ischaemic from non-ischaemic priapism. Blood gas values of pH <7.25, PO_2 <30 mmHg, and PCO_2 >60 mmHg suggest ischaemic priapism, whereas values similar to arterial blood suggest non-ischaemic priapism. Alternatively, penile duplex Doppler ultrasonography can be used to assess cavernosal blood flow and distinguish the two types of priapism.

Treatment (Fig. 8.50)

Therapy is directed by the type of priapism. Specifically, in ischaemic priapism treatment is aimed at increasing venous drainage, while in non-ischaemic priapism, it is aimed at decreasing arterial inflow. Ischaemic priapism requires immediate intervention, whereas non-ischaemic priapism does not; this is because the penis is well perfused in the latter type. Contributory underlying disease should be treated simultaneously.

Table 8.6 Aetiological factors in priapism

Drugs

Antihypertensives (labetalol, prazosin, phenoxybenzamine)

Intra-cavernosal vasoactive agents (papaverine, phentolamine, alprostadil)

Antidepressants (trazodone)

Antipsychotics (chlorpromazine)

Hormones (gonodotropin-releasing hormone)

Heparin

Alcohol

Cocaine

Total parenteral nutrition (high lipid content)

Haematological disorders

Sickle-cell disease

Leukaemia

Polycythemia

Neurological disorders

CNS and spinal cord disorders

Diabetic autonomic neuropathy

Metabolic disorders

Amyloidosis

Fabry's disease

Malignancies

Genitourinary cancers (renal, bladder, prostate, penile, urethral)

Colorectal cancer

Multiple myeloma

Trauma

Blunt or penetrating penile, pelvic, or perineal injuries

Non-ischaemic priapism

Treatment options for non-ischaemic priapism range from observation to embolization. These patients can be safely followed to allow for spontaneous closure of the fistula. Usually, this does not occur and intervention is required. Selective internal pudendal arteriography and superselective embolization with autologous clot injection is the procedure of choice; alternate embolization materials should be a last resort as they are associated with permanent arterial occlusion which leads to erectile dysfunction.

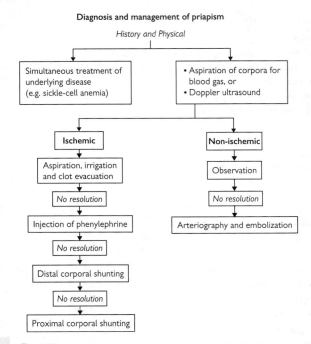

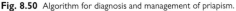

Fig. 8.50 Algorithm for diagnosis and management of priapism.

Ischaemic priapism

Ischaemic priapism is initially treated by corpora cavernosal aspiration, saline irrigation. and clot evacuation (using a 19 or 21G butterfly needle). If this is unsuccessful, a dilute alpha-agonist solution is injected intracorporally. Phenylephrine is preferred because of its low beta-adrenergic activity. The recommended dose is 500 mcg injected intracavernosally every 5–10 min up to a maximum dose of 1.5 mg. Patients should be closely monitored during injection, because hypertension, bradycardia, palpitations, arrhythmia, and cardiac arrest can occur.

An oral alternative beta-agonist is terbutaline (5 mg initially, followed by a further 5 mg if no response after 15 min).

For ischaemic priapism from sickle cell anaemia, use phenylephrine combined with analgesics, hydration, oxygen, tranquillizers, and (usually) blood transfusion (exchange transfusion to lower HbS concentrations).

If conservative measures fail, surgical intervention is necessary. The goal of surgery is to shunt blood away from the engorged corpora caversona. This is accomplished by a variety of techniques. Explain to the patient, and document your explanation carefully, that there is a high likelihood of post-operative impotence.

- Glans-cavernosal shunts: fast and least invasive. Try these first before resorting to the other techniques. Examples include the Winter procedure (Tru-Cut needle through the glans) (Fig. 8.51) or direct incision of the glans (Ebbehoj and Al-Ghorab procedures). Local or general anaesthetic can be used. For local anaesthetic apply a penile base ring block. Clean the skin of the penis. Insert a Tru-Cut biopsy needle through the glans in the midline, well dorsal of the meatus (to avoid entering the urethra), and head towards the right corpus cavernosum. 'Biopsy' the right corpus cavernosum and then repeat the procedure on the left side. Compression or suture closure may be required for the puncture site.
- Where detumescence is not achieved consider a larger proximal shunt. This can be performed by creating a caverноso-spongiosal shunt (Quackels procedure) (Fig. 8.52), a caverноso-saphenous shunt (Grayhack procedure) (Fig. 8.53), or a caverноso-dorsal vein shunt (Barry procedure) (Fig. 8.54). Intra-corporal pressure monitoring is helpful in ensuring satisfactory detumescence, as this can be difficult to evaluate clinically because of persistent penile edema. A successful outcome is achieved with an intra-corporal pressure <40 cmH_2O.

Quackels cavernoso-spongiosal shunt procedure (Fig. 8.52)

Pass a urethral catheter (to allow easy identification and therefore protection of the urethra). Incise the penile skin longitudinally just distal to the penoscrotal junction (the corpus spongiosum is thicker here than distally), overlying the junction between the corpus spongiosum and the corpus cavernosum of one side. Incise Buck's fascia and expose the corpus spongiosum and corpus cavernosum over a distance of ~3 cm. Suture the walls of the corpus spongiosum and corpus cavernosum together with 5–0 prolene. Now make a longitudinal incision in the corpus spongiosum (not too deep to avoid the urethra) and corpus cavernosum.

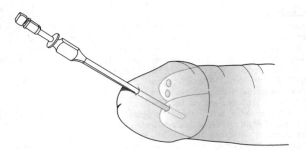

Fig. 8.51 The Winter glans-cavernosal shunt procedure.

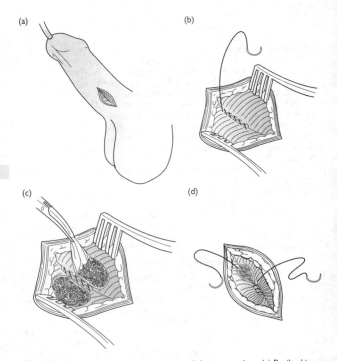

Fig. 8.52 The Quackels cavernoso-spongiosal shunt procedure. (a) Penile skin incision. (b) Exposure of corporus cavernosum and spongiosum. (c) Incised corpora. (d) Creation of the cavernoso-spongiosal anastomosis.

Suture the edges of the corpus spongiosum and corpus cavernosum together with prolene. Close the fascia and skin. Repeat on the opposite side if detumescence is not achieved.

Grayhack cavernoso-saphenous shunt procedure (Fig. 8.53)

Incise the penile skin longitudinally just distal to the penoscrotal junction and expose the tunica albuginea over one corpus cavernosum. Make a skin crease incision in the groin (as for high ligation of the sapheno-femoral junction in varicose vein surgery). Expose the long saphenous vein and dissect it over a length that will allow it to reach the corpus cavernosum. Ligate and divide the vein distally (it should remain connected proximally to the femoral vein). Create a subcutaneous tunnel between the groin incision and the penis. Excise an ellipse of tunica from the corpus cavernosum. Gently pass the saphenous vein through the subcutaneous tunnel to the penile incision and suture the vein to the corpus cavernosum using 5–0 prolene. Close the fascia and skin.

Barry cavernoso-dorsal vein shunt procedure (Fig. 8.54)

Deglove the penis. Incise the dartos fascia and deep to this Buck's fascia. Dissect the dorsal penile vein from its bed (beware the dorsal artery and nerves). Tie the distal end of the vein with an absorbable suture. Incise the tunica of one corpus cavernosum at a point where the dorsal vein will easily reach. Anastomose the vein to the corpus with 7–0 prolene. Replace the skin. Post-operatively, compression dressings should be avoided. Intra-corporal pressure determinations or penile duplex Doppler ultrasonography are helpful adjuncts for monitoring results.

Stuttering priapism

Stuttering or intermittent priapism is a recurrent form of ischaemic priapism which usually occurs in patients with sickle cell anaemia. The goal is prevention of subsequent episodes. To this end, oral phenylephrene hydrochloride twice daily or intra-cavernosal self-administration of phenylephrine 500 mcg can be used. Alternatively, in patients where erectile dysfunction is not a concern, anti-androgens or gonadotrophin-releasing hormone agonists can be tried.

Outcome

Following priapism, erectile dysfunction occurs in approximately 50% of patients and is due to corporal fibrosis. The most important determining factor for subsequent erectile function is the duration of priapism. Consequently, rapid intervention is important in minimizing this untoward consequence.

Further reading

1 Montague DK, Jarow J, Broderick GA *et al.* American Urological Association guideline on the management of priapism. *J Urol.* 2003; **170**:1318–24.

2 Keoghane SR, Sullivan ME, Miller MA. The aetiology, pathogenesis and management of priapism. *BJU Int* 2002; **90**:149–54.

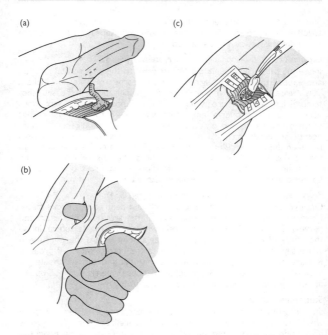

Fig. 8.53 The Grayhack cavernoso-saphenous shunt procedure. (a) Dissection of the superficial septenous vein. (b) Creation of a subcutaneous tunnel. (c) Creation of a cavernoso-saphenous anastomosis.

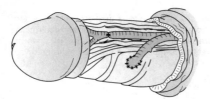

Fig. 8.54 A Barry cavernoso-dorsal vein shunt procedure.

Testicular torsion

Definition and aetiology

A twist of the spermatic cord resulting in strangulation of the blood supply to the testis and epididymis.

During descent of the testis into the scrotum, the parietal layer of tunica vaginalis does not immediately fuse with the fascial layers of the scrotum. Therefore it is possible for the testis, with its covering visceral and parietal layers of tunica, to twist within the scrotum i.e. the twist occurs outside the two layers of the tunica. This is called an extra-vaginal torsion and is the type that occurs in the neonatal or prenatal period.

Intra-vaginal torsion, in which the testis with its covering layer of visceral tunica twists within the parietal layer of the tunica vaginalis, is more common in young boys, adolescents, and adults. The essential anatomical reason for torsion is that the entire surface of the testis and the spermatic cord are covered in visceral tunica vaginalis, such that the testis has the configuration of a bell-clapper lying within the scrotum (Figs 8.55 and 8.56).

Testicular torsion can occur at any age but is most common during adolescence (peak at age 13–15 years). The left side is said to be affected more often, and 2% are said to present with torsion of both testes.

Predisposing factors and mechanism

Presence of a narrow mesenteric attachment from the spermatic cord onto the testis and epididymis (Fig. 8.56). The entire surface of the testis, together with a length of spermatic cord, is covered with the visceral layer of tunica vaginalis such that the testis can twist on the spermatic cord. This permits additional testicular mobility and freedom of the testicle to rotate within the tunica vaginalis. The reason why this occurs more commonly during puberty is because of the significant testicular growth that occurs at this age.

Testicular torsion occurs less frequently during the neonatal period. The mechanism is distinct from torsion occurring after this period in that the newly descended testis is incompletely attached to the gubernaculum, resulting in extra-vaginal torsion, i.e. the entire testis, epididymis, and tunica vaginalis are twisted together in a vertical axis. In contrast, pubertal torsion is intra-vaginal, i.e. the testicle and spermatic cord twist within the parietal tunica vaginalis.

Diagnosis

The classic presentation of testicular torsion is sudden onset of severe unilateral scrotal pain and swelling (except in the 2% with bilateral torsion!). There may be a history of a blow to the testis in the hours before the acute onset of pain. Some patients report similar episodes occurring in the past, with spontaneous resolution of the pain, suggesting an episode of torsion with spontaneous detorsion.

They may have a slight fever. Often the physical examination is difficult because of severe pain and tenderness. The testicle may have a horizontal lie and be situated higher in the scrotum. The cremasteric reflex is usually, but not always, absent (positive Rabinowitz's sign).[1] The cremasteric reflex, which can normally be elicited by stroking the finger along inside of the thigh resulting in upwards movement of the ipsilateral testis, is absent with torsion. Elevation of the involved testicle does not ameliorate the symptoms (negative Prehn's sign). There may be scrotal wall erythema. In the neonate, pain may be absent, and the only finding may be a hard enlarged hemiscrotal mass.

A urinalysis should be performed in all patients presenting with acute hemiscrotal pain. With testicular torsion, the urinalysis is usually clear. The presence of pyuria and bacteriuria is more indicative of an infectious process.

The imaging modality of choice for diagnosing testicular torsion is colour duplex Doppler ultrasonography.[2] Colour Doppler ultrasound will show reduced arterial blood flow to the involved testicle. Alternatively, radionuclide scintigraphy can be used and shows decreased uptake of the radio-isotope in the affected testis, an indication of absent blood flow to that testis.[3] Useful though these tests may be, they are not readily available in many hospitals.

If testicular imaging is not available or the findings are equivocal, surgical exploration should be performed immediately.

Differential diagnosis

The differential diagnosis encompasses all potential causes of an acute scrotum, including torsion of the appendix testis or appendix epididymis, acute epididymitis, strangulated inguinal hernia, haematocoele, trauma, tumor, Henoch–Schönlein purpura, and viral inflammation. Rarely a ureteric stone, with radiation of pain to the ipsilateral testis, can masquerade as a torsion. Usually the history and physical and laboratory examinations will assist in making the correct diagnosis. For example, in acute epididymitis, fever and pyuria are common and Doppler ultrasonography shows epididymotesticular hypervascularity. A history of trauma may suggest a haematocoele.

Treatment

Testicular torsion is a urologic emergency.

The treatment of testicular torsion is immediate surgical exploration with attempts at reduction and bilateral orchidopexy. Undertake this as a matter of urgency. Delay in relieving the twisted testis can result in permanent ischaemic damage to the testis with subsequent atrophy and loss of hormone and sperm production. Furthermore, as the testis undergoes necrosis, the blood–testis barrier breaks down and an autoimmune reaction has been shown to develop (sympathetic orchidopathia) in animal models.[4,5] Whether this occurs in humans to the extent that spermatogenesis is impaired is uncertain.[6] The autoantibodies so produced can then damage the contralateral testis, thereby impairing hormone production and spermatogenesis of this side as well. A delay of >6 hr in relieving the torsion increases the risk that ischaemic necrosis will take place.

Surgical approach to orchidopexy for testicular torsion

Explore the involved testis through a midline incision (allows easy access to both testes, rather than making two incisions). Incise the tunica vaginalis and deliver the testis (Fig. 8.55). Manually reduce the spermatic cord and observe the testicle for return of its normal color. Wrap it in saline gauze while the contralateral testis is pexed through a small scrotal incision. Re-examine the twisted testis for viability. If it appears viable, fix it to the dartos or parietal layer of tunica vaginalis. If the testis is felt to be necrotic, remove it to avoid infection and development of anti-testicular antibodies that can affect fertility. In cases where orchidectomy is necessary, a testicular prosthesis can be placed at the same time.

Technique of testicular fixation

Suture fixation

There is some controversy surrounding the best technique for fixation. Some surgeons fix the testis within the scrotum with suture material, inserted at two or three points, arguing that this reduces the risk of re-torsion.[7,8] Some use absorbable sutures and others use non-absorbable sutures. Absorbable sutures may disappear, exposing the patient to the risk of subsequent re-torsion (15 of 16 patients with recurrent torsion had undergone previous orchidopexy using absorbable suture material[9]). Those who use absorbable sutures argue that the fibrous reaction around the absorbable sutures used to fix the testis will prevent re-torsion and that the patient may be able to feel non-absorbable sutures, which can be uncomfortable (although this should not occur if the sutures are placed medially, i.e. into the septum between the two testes).

If you use suture fixation, pass the sutures through the visceral layer of the tunica vaginalis covering the testis, through the tough tunica albuginea of the testis, and then through the parietal layer of the tunica vaginalis, which lines the inner surface of the scrotum (Fig. 8.56). Clip the ends of each suture as it is placed, and tie them only once all three have been placed. (Tying each one after it has been placed can make it difficult to insert the next suture).

Dartos pouch fixation

Other surgeons have argued that the testis should be fixed within a dartos pouch[10] to avoid breaching the blood–testis barrier which could, in theory, expose both testes to the risk of sympathetic orchidopathia. In a review of 387 patients who had undergone unilateral or bilateral orchidopexy, Coughlin[11] reported that the use of testicular suture material was strongly associated with infertility. Concerns have also been expressed about a possible increased cancer risk in testes that have been suture fixed.[10]

If you use dartos pouch fixation, open the tunica vaginalis, bring the testis out, and untwist it. Develop a dartos pouch in the scrotum by holding the skin with forceps and dissecting with scissors between the skin and the underlying dartos muscle. Once you have started to develop this space, it can be enlarged by inserting your two index fingers and pulling them apart. Place the testis in this pouch. A few absorbable sutures can be used to attach the cord near the testis to the inside of the dartos pouch. This can help to prevent re-torsion of the testes (which can occur in testes that have been placed in a dartos pouch). The dartos can then be closed over the testis and the skin approximated in a separate layer.

Many surgeons continue to use suture fixation and, indeed, operative surgery textbooks describe this technique for use in testicular fixation for torsion.[12] Whatever technique you use, remember to fix **both** testes because the bell-clapper abnormality which predisposes to torsion can occur bilaterally.

If you find an appendix testis or appendix epididymis at the time of scrotal exploration, whether there is a testicular torsion or not, remove it (with diathermy or by ligating it with a small suture) so that it cannot twist in the future, which may result in an unnecessary repeat scrotal exploration. If we find that the testis is not twisted, we assume that it had undergone torsion, but had untwisted once the patient had been anaesthetized, or that the diagnosis could be epididymo-orchitis. If there is free fluid surrounding the testis, we take a swab and send this for culture. We fix the testis and the contralateral testis as a prophylactic measure.

Complications

Complications of torsion include infection (with a missed torsion), haematoma, and recurrent torsion. Orchidopexy decreases the likelihood but does not exclude the possibility of re-torsion, and the patient or parents should be aware of this.

References

1 Nelson CP, Williams JF, Bloom DA. The cremasteric reflex: a useful but imperfect sign in testicular torsion. *J Pediatr Surg* 2003; **38**:1248–9.

2 Al Mufti RA, Ogedegbe AK, Lafferty K. The use of Doppler ultrasound in the clinical management of acute testicular pain. *Br J Urol* 1995; **76**:625–7.

3 Melloul M, Paz A, Lask D et al. The value of radionuclide scrotal imaging in the diagnosis of acute testicular torsion. *Br J Urol* 1995; **76**: 628–31.

4 Cerasaro TG, Nachtscheim DA, Otero F, Parsons L. The effect of testicular torsion on contralateral testis and the production of antisperm antibodies in rabbits. *J Urol* 1984; **135**:577–9.

5 Wallace DMA, Gunter PA, London GV et al. Sympathetic orchidopathia, an experimental and clinical study. *Br J Urol* 1982; **54**:765–8.

6 Anderson JB, Williamson RCN. The fate of the human testis following unilateral torsion of the spermatic cord. *Br J Urol* 1986; **58**:698–704.

7 Thurston A, Whitaker R Torsion of testis after previous testicular surgery. *Br J Surg* 1983; **70**:217.

8 Phipps JH. Torsion of testis following orchidopexy. *Br J Urol* 1987; **59**:596.

9 Kuntze JR, Lowe P, Ahlering TE. Testicular torsion after orchidopexy. *J Urol* 1985; **134**:1209–10.

10 Frank JD, O'Brien M. Related articles: fixation of the testis. *BJU Int* 2002; **89**:331–3.

11 Coughlin HT, Bellinger MF, La Porte RE, Lee PA. Testicular suture: a significant risk factor for infertility among formerly cryptorchid men. *J Pediatr Surg* 1998; **33**:1790–3.

12 Hinman F, Jr. *Atlas of Urologic Surgery*. Philadelphia, PA: WB Saunders, 1998.

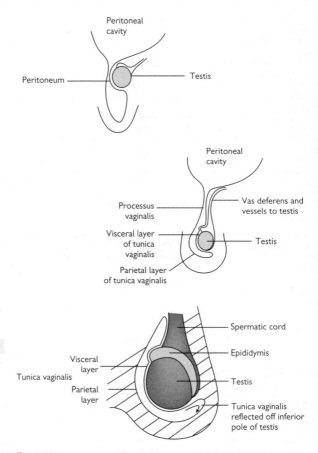

Fig. 8.55 The posterior surface of the testis is fused to the posterior scrotum. Reproduced from Hashim et al. *Urological emergencies in clinical practice.* Springer-Verlag. London, 2005. Permission sought.

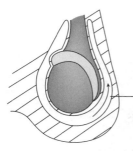

Visceral layer of tunica vaginalis covering the entire testis and spermatic cord

Fig. 8.56 The entire surface of the testis, together with a length of spermatic cord, is covered with the visceral layer of tunica vaginalis such that the testis can twist on the spermatic cord. Reproduced from Hashim et al. *Urological emergencies in clinical practice*. Springer-Verlag. London, 2005. Permission sought.

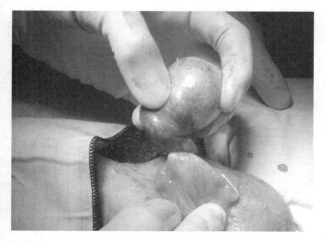

Fig. 8.57 Testicular torsion at scrotal exploration.

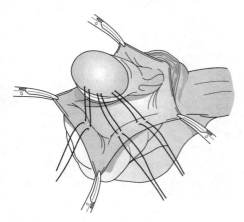

Fig. 8.58 Suture fixation of the testis to the parietal layer of the tunica vaginalis.

Scrotal and penile surgery

Circumcision

The difficulty of circumcision is underestimated. A poor circumcision has lifelong cosmetic and functional consequences for your patient.

Indications

- Non-retractile foreskin at the age of sexual activity.
- Recurrent balanoposthitis: a superficial inflammation of the glans (balano) and prepuce (posthitis). In neonates and infants due to ammoniacal dermatitis.
- Reduction of risk of UTI in neonatal boys (710-fold risk reduction up to age of 3 months).
- Lichen sclerosus et atrophicus (LSA) (balanitis xerotica obliterans (BXO)).
- Neoplasia of prepuce.
- To prevent penile cancer in the context of a non-retractile foreskin (but estimated that 900 circumcisions are required to prevent one case of penile cancer).
- Phimosis: a narrowed preutial opening which prevents withdrawal of the prepuce over the glans (usually in the context of a prepuce scarred by recurrent balanoposthitis).
- Voiding obstruction (pinhole prepuce).
- Reduction of risk of HIV transmission.
- Cultural or religious reasons.

Contraindications

- Hypospadias.
- Epispadias.

Development of the foreskin

The newborn boy's foreskin is adherent to the glans (such that in approximately 50% of newborns even the external urethral meatus cannot be visualized) and remains so in 80% at 3 months and in 10% at 3 years. By the early teens the foreskin has completely separated from the glans.

Alternatives to circumcision

Phimosis may respond to topical steroids (0.05% betamethasone ointment) applied to the area of phimosis twice daily for 2 months, combined with gentle daily retraction of the foreskin to encourage separation of the glans and foreskin.

Technique

Prepare the skin of the penis, prepuce, and glans. If the prepuce is too tight to retract, keep some skin prep on the trolley and clean the glans once the prepuce has been excised. Hold the flaccid penis without tension and mark the coronal sulcus with a pen. On the ventral surface mark a V-shape with the apex towards the meatus. This extension of the ventral skin flap aids in reconstructing the frenulum. Cut through the skin where marked with a 15 blade. Coagulate any obvious vessels at this stage with bipolar diathermy, or tie and divide vessels with 3–0 absorbable ties. Apply two straight artery forceps to the foreskin dorsally either side of the midline.

Cut the full thickness of the foreskin between these forceps with dissecting scissors over a distance of ~5 mm to create a short dorsal slit. Insert the closed blades of the scissors into this incision between the two layers of foreskin and gently develop the plane between the skin layers to the level of the circumferential cut in the coronal sulcus. Withdraw the scissors and extend the incision through the outer layer of skin to meet the circumferential incision. If the circumferential incision has not gone through the full thickness of the outer skin layer then complete this incision now with the scissors. Extend the dorsal slit through the inner layer of skin. It is important that you visualize the corona as you do this and do not take this incision closer than 5 mm to the corona. Using knife or scissors cut circumferentially around the corona keeping a margin of 5 mm of skin on the corona. Cut through the frenulum last; this minimizes bleeding from the frenular artery before you are able to control it. The freed prepuce should be sent for histology. Control bleeding vessels with bipolar diathermy or 3–0 ties. Be meticulous about haemostasis. Close the wound with 4–0 absorbable sutures. Try to pick up some of the subcutaneous tissue but take small bites through the skin edges. Starting at the frenulum, bring the apex of the V on the shaft skin up to the frenulum using a horizontal mattress suture. Use this stitch as a ventral stay suture. Place a second stay stitch dorsally. With the two stays on gentle stretch, close each side of the wound. Use either a running suture or interrupted sutures 5 mm apart. Wrap the wound with paraffin gauze and then with a single piece of dressing gauze. Secure with tape.

Alternative techniques

The dorsal slit can be made through both outer and inner skin layers at the same time. This technique is more rapid but it is more difficult to ensure that each layer is cut to the correct distance.

In the sleeve technique[1] the two circumferential incisions are made first. With the foreskin fully retracted (and both circumferential incisions and the intervening sleeve of foreskin exposed) join the two incisions with a dorsal incision (Fig. 9.1) Lift one edge and free the skin from the underlying dartos layer (Fig. 9.2).

Anaesthesia for circumcision

Circumcision is usually performed under general or spinal anaesthesia, although it can be performed under a local anaesthetic penile ring block alone (this block is also useful for post-operative analgesia when circumcision is performed under general anaesthesia and for reducing the discomfort associated with reduction of paraphimosis or priapism). The sensory innervation of the penis is by the dorsal nerves of the penis which arise as the first branches of the pudendal nerves in Alcock's canal. These nerves are best blocked by injecting local anaesthetic into the triangular space defined by the inferior border of the symphysis above, the corpora inferiorly, and Buck's fascia anteriorly. Having cleaned the skin, insert a 23G needle just under the symphysis to one side of the midline and pass it through the tough Buck's fascia. Aspirate and then inject 9 mL of a mixture made from 15 mL 0.5% bupivacaine and 5 mL 2% lidocaine *without adrenaline*. Inject a further 9 mL on the opposite side. Use the remaining 2 mL of local anaesthetic to raise a bleb of skin at the penoscrotal junction to block branches of the perineal nerve. Local anaesthetic containing adrenaline causes vasoconstriction and may result in penile ischaemia. If this occurs, it may be possible to salvage the situation with a caudal block (causes sympathetic blockade) or by iloprost infusion.[2,3]

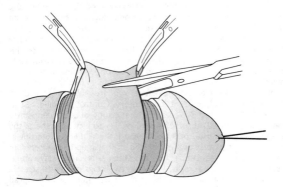

Fig. 9.1 Make the two circumferential incisions.

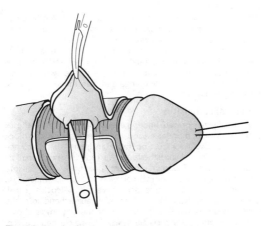

Fig. 9.2 Free the skin from the underlying dartos layer.

Post-operative advice

Some degree of post-operative oedema and bruising is normal after circumcision. Warn the patient or parents that blood from the wound may turn black (because of reduction of haemoglobin) and this can give the erroneous impression of penile ischaemia. Reassurance is all that is needed.

Complications of circumcision

- Post-operative bleeding (frequently on the ventral aspect of the penis) is due to an inadequately controlled frenular artery. It often settles with firm pressure, but if not may require an additional stitch.
- Infections usually settle with antibiotics but occasionally a stitch or two may need to be removed.
- Removal of too much skin: if this occurs, it is probably best to dress the open wound and allow healing by secondary intention (use a Vaseline gauze dressing). Immediate closure will result in a buried penis.
- Removal of too little skin may not correct a phimosis. The excess residual skin may become oedematous since the lymphatics draining the prepuce have been divided during circumcision. Excision of the excess skin may be required.
- Skin bridges can appear some time after circumcision and should simply be divided.
- Hyper- or hypo-aesthesia of the glans: some men report loss of sensation in the glans (thought to be due to decreased sensitivity secondary to cornification of the epithelium of the glans), while others report heightened sensation.[4]
- Meatal stenosis.
- Urethrocutaneous fistula due to inadvertent division of the external meatus during circumcision.

References

1 Tucker SC, Cerqueiro J, Sterne GD, Bracka A. Circumcision: a refined technique and 5 year review. *Ann R Coll Surg Engl* 2001; **83**:121–5.
2 Burke D, Joypaul V, Thomson MF. Circumcision supplemented by dorsal penile nerve block with 0.75% ropivacaine: a complication. *Reg Anesth Pain Med* 2000; **25**:424–7.
3 Berens R, Pontus SP, Jr. A complication associated with dorsal penile nerve block. *Reg Anesth* 1990; **15**:309–10.
4 Fink KS, Carson CC, DeVillis RF. Adult circumcision outcome study: effect of circumcision on erectile function, penile sensitivity and sexual activity and satisfaction. *J Urol* 2002; **167**:2113–16.

Meatotomy

Indication

To overcome narrowing of the navicular fossa in adults (usually prior to urethral instrumentation).

Technique

Pass a no.10 scalpel blade 1–2 cm into the meatus, bevel up. Holding the penis firmly, withdraw the blade whilst applying gentle upward pressure. Repeat until the cystoscope/resectoscope will pass. (Fig. 9.3).

Complications

Bleeding is usually gentle and stops spontaneously. If not, gentle pressure against a catheter will tamponade it.

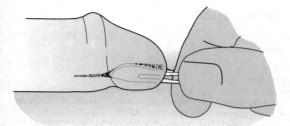

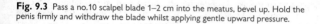

Fig. 9.3 Pass a no.10 scalpel blade 1–2 cm into the meatus, bevel up. Hold the penis firmly and withdraw the blade whilst applying gentle upward pressure.

Hydrocele repair

Indications

Symptomatic hydrocele.

Technique

Lord's procedure[1]

This procedure has the advantage that dissection in the scrotum is minimized, with a reduction in the risk of post-operative haematoma. Since the tunica sac is not excised, the scrotum can still be bulky after the repair of large hydroceles, which may be best managed by partial excision of the tunica.

Shave, prep, and drape the supine patient. Grasp the hydrocele sac firmly so that the skin is under tension. Incise transversely (about 4–5 cm), avoiding obvious vessels (Fig. 9.4). Continue the incision through the dartos layer until the tunical sac is exposed. Hold the skin edges apart with Allis forceps (Fig. 9.5). Bluntly dissect the tunica away from the dartos by sweeping the tip of your index finger under the edge of the incision. This creates a sub-dartos space to which the testis can be returned at the end of the procedure. Incise the tunical sac and collect the fluid in a receiver or with a sump sucker. Enlarge the incision in the tunica and deliver the testis away from the scrotum, allowing the inverted tunica sac to stretch out behind it (Fig. 9.6). Starting at the free edge of the tunica, pick up bites of tunica at 1 cm intervals from the free edge towards the testis using a 3–0 absorbable suture. Do not tie this suture. Put several similar sutures in place around the circumference of the testis (Fig. 9.7). Tie the sutures. As you do so, the tunica will gather up and concertina behind the testis. Check for haemostasis. Return the testis to the scrotum. To do this you may need to further enlarge the space within the dartos layer with a finger tip. Using two Allis forceps grasp the dartos layer at each end of the incision. Close the dartos, taking good bites with a running 3–0 absorbable suture. Close the skin with a running or interrupted 4–0 absorbable suture. Apply a scrotal support.

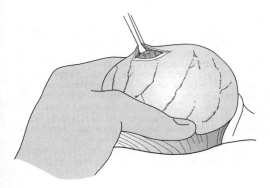

Fig. 9.4 Grasp the hydrocele firmly and make a skin incision.

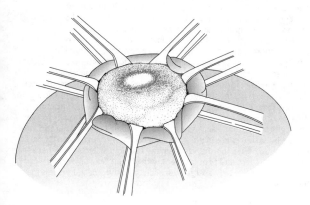

Fig. 9.5 Hold the skin edges apart with Allis forceps.

Jaboulay procedure

In this procedure the whole hydrocele sac is delivered from the scrotum. Since the sac can be excised there is less residual scrotal bulk, making this the procedure of choice for large or thick-walled hydroceles. Expose the hydrocele sac as in Lord's procedure. The incision may need to be larger. Gently free the hydrocele sac from the scrotum with finger-tip dissection and deliver the intact sac. Open the hydrocele sac anteriorly taking care not to damage the testis. Drain the fluid and enlarge the opening in the tunica. If the sac is large, excise the excess tunica, taking care not to damage the spermatic cord. Reflect the remaining sac behind the testis and epididymis and suture the edges of the sac to each other with a running 3–0 suture (Fig. 9.8). Ensure that the closure is not tight around the cord at the superior pole of the testis. Check for haemostasis, return the testis to the scrotum, and close as described above.

Complications

● Haematoma: the laxity of the scrotum means there is no natural tamponade after scrotal surgery. Haemostasis in the scrotum must be meticulous to prevent haematoma formation. Placement of a drain is rarely necessary at the time of surgery, but a drain should be placed if haemostasis is suboptimal. If a scrotal haematoma does form, most can be managed conservatively (give antibiotics to reduce the risk of secondary infection). Large, tense, or infected haematomas should be drained.
● Infection: most infections are superficial and should settle with antibiotics.
● Recurrence: hydroceles recur when the redundant tunica vaginalis adheres to itself, forming a closed space in which fluid re-accumulates. Recurrent hydroceles should be re-explored, but the patient should be warned that all the complications are more frequent when operating on a recurrence.
● Damage to the testicular vascular pedicle and to the vas deferens: care should be taken to identify the testicular vessels (damage can cause testicular atrophy) and the vas (damage may impair fertility). If necessary, isolate them and protect them with sloops. Scrotal anatomy can be grossly distorted by a large hydrocele, and the vas and vessels may be widely separated.

Aspiration and sclerotherapy

Aspiration of a hydrocele is an alternative to surgical repair in an unfit man. Place the scrotal skin on tension over the hydrocele sac and infiltrate a small bleb of local anaesthetic. Pass a large-bore cannula into the hydrocele, attach a syringe, and aspirate to dryness. A sclerosing agent (e.g. phenol, tetracycline, sodium tetradecylsulfate (STDS)) can then be instilled into the hydrocele sac. Some surgeons have found that sclerotherapy is as efficacious as surgery and has a lower morbidity, but multiple injections of sclerosant may be required.[2,3] However, others report high recurrence rates and morbidity with sclerotherapy, and advocate that it should be reserved for men where surgery carries an unacceptably high risk.[4,5]

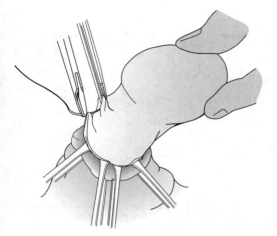

Fig. 9.6 Deliver the testis away from the scrotum, allowing the inverted tunica sac to stretch out behind it.

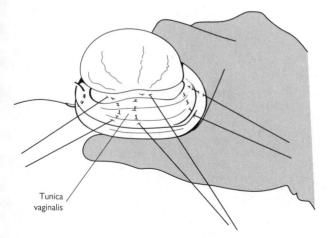

Tunica
vaginalis

Fig. 9.7 Pick up bites of tunica at 1 cm intervals from the free edge towards the testis using a 3–0 absorbable suture. When these are tied, the tunica will concertina behind the testis.

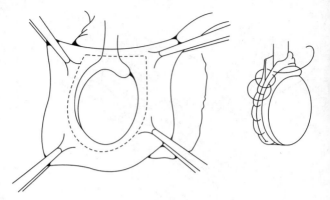

Fig. 9.8 Reflect the remaining sac behind the testis and epididymis and suture the edges of the sac to each other. Redrawn from Marshall, *Textbook of Operative Urology*, Philadelphia, PA: WB Saunders. Permission sought.

References

1 Lord PH. A bloodless operation for the radical cure of idiopathic hydrocele. *Br J Surg* 1964; **51**:914–16.

2 Shan CJ, Lucon AM, Arap S. Comparative study of sclerotherapy with phenol and surgical treatment for hydrocele. *J Urol* 2003; **169**:1056–9.

3 Beiko DT, Kim D, Morales A. Aspiration and sclerotherapy versus hydrocelectomy for treatment of hydroceles. *Urology* 2003; **61**:708–12.

4 Sigurdsson T, Johansson JE, Jahnson S, Helgesen F, Andersson SO. Polidocanol sclerotherapy for hydroceles and epididymal cysts. *J Urol* 1994; **151**:898–901.

5 Thomson H, Odell M. Sclerosant treatment for hydroceles and epididymal cysts. *BMJ* 1979; ii:704–5.

Vasectomy

Indication
- Unwanted fertility.
- Prevention of recurrent epididymo-orchitis.

Preparation
Warn the patient that other methods of contraception should be used until he has had a negative semen analysis, that vasectomy should be considered permanent and irreversible, that vasectomy has a recognized failure rate of 1:2000, and that failure means they may have been given the 'all clear' but subsequently become fertile again (because of spontaneous recanalization). Also discuss the complications listed below.

Techniques
'Scalpel' vasectomy
Arrange for the patient to shave the scrotum prior to surgery. Stand on the patient's right. Isolate the vas under the scrotal skin by placing the index and middle fingers of the left hand behind the vas and stretching the skin over it using the left thumb (Fig. 9.9). Aim to have just the vas under the skin and to have the skin taut over the vas. Inject 2 mL of 1% lidocaine with adrenaline 1:200 000 into the skin directly over the vas, and then a further 1–2 mL a little deeper along the line of the vas proximally. The aim of this manoeuvre is to infiltrate the perivasal sheath to achieve a vasal nerve block. Make a 1 cm incision with a 15 blade through the skin and subcutaneous tissue over the vas until the white shiny surface of the vas is exposed. Pick up the vas using Allis forceps, an artery forceps, or Li vas ring forceps (see below). Lift the vas away from the scrotum and free it further from its sheath over 1–2 cm using longitudinal incisions with the 15 blade. Reapply the forceps to the isolated vas. If the vas is freed from its sheath, it should be easy to lift a loop of several centimetres. Occasionally it is necessary to sweep adherent sheath and vessels from the under-surface of the vas with a swab. If vessels are damaged during this manoeuvre, control them with diathermy. Excise a 1–2 cm length of vas and occlude the vas using one of the techniques described below. Return the vasal ends to the scrotum and close the fascia and skin with absorbable sutures.

'No-scalpel' Li vasectomy[1]
This method was developed in China. It uses a tiny puncture hole and is associated with fewer complications. It requires special instruments and is harder to learn, but is quicker to do when proficient. The skin is anaesthetized over the midline raphe and a vasal nerve block administered to both vasa as described above. The vas is grasped through the anaesthetized skin using a small ring forcep such that the scrotal skin is as tight as possible over the vas. One blade of a specialized sharp curved clamp is used to puncture the skin and vas wall (Fig. 9.10). This blade is withdrawn and the closed instrument is re-introduced through the skin puncture. The blades are gently opened until the vas is seen. One blade is then

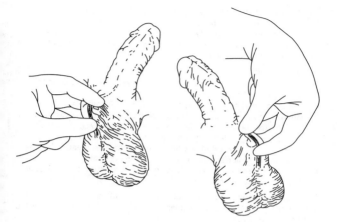

Fig. 9.9 Isolate the vas under the scrotal skin by placing the index and middle fingers of the left hand behind the vas and stretching the skin over the vas using the left thumb. Reproduced from Li et al., J. Urol. 1991; **145**: 341–4, Elsevier. Permission sought.

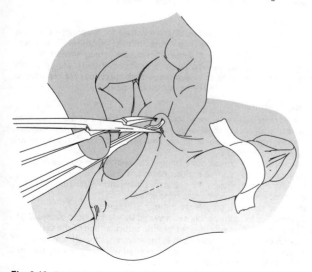

Fig. 9.10 One blade of a specialized sharp curved clamp is used to puncture the skin and vas wall.

used to puncture the vas, and the open clamp is rotated to deliver the vas (Fig. 9.11). At the same time the ring forceps is released from the scrotal skin and re-applied to the delivered vas. Excise and occlude the vas as described below. The second vas is manipulated to the same puncture site and the procedure repeated.

Occluding the vas

- Suture ligation, e.g. 3–0 absorbable. If the ends of the vas slough then recanalization may be more likely.
- Haemoclips: perhaps less likely to slough, may be palpable.
- Diathermy: pass a needle electrode down each end of the vas for 1 cm and cauterize sufficiently to destroy the mucosal surface but not to cause full-thickness desruction of the vas.
- Folding the vas over: fold the ends of the vas back to create a J-shape and secure the folded vas with a tie. May still necrose.
- Fascial interposition: separate the two vasal ends into different fascial planes and close the fascia with a suture.

The ideal technique should be effective, quick, and add no morbidity. It is the author's preference to use diathermy alone. This technique is supported by a very large UK series.[2]

Alternatives

The author prefers bilateral incision. By placing the incisions laterally it is easier to minimize the amount of tissue between skin and vas.

Useful aside

Should you send off the excised segments of vas for histological confirmation? It is the author's preference not to do this. Whatever the histology report, your management is determined by the semen analysis. If many motile sperm remain, re-exploration is indicated; if there are no motile sperm, there is no need to re-explore. If both specimens are reported as vas deferens they could still be from the same side.

Complications

Complications post-vasectomy are a potential source of litigation. Make sure that you discuss them with your patient pre-operatively, that you document that you have done so, and that your operative notes are detailed (and legible!).

- Haematoma: 2% overall but incidence depends on experience of the surgeon.[3] Warn your patient that occasionally there is extensive bruising after vasectomy. Like all scrotal haematomas, should only be explored if very tense, painful, or infected.
- Infection: about 3% on average but higher in some series.[4–6]
- Sperm granuloma (probably experienced by every patient eventually). These occur when sperm leak from the testicular end of the vas. They present as a palpable lump in the scrotum, although they are rarely troublesome. They may be associated with early re-canalization and may be the site of chronic scrotal pain.

- Primary failure of vasectomy (early failure) is where spermatozoa are still present in the post-operative semen analyses. This may be because of early re-uniting of the cut ends of the vas (spontaneous recanalization) or because one (or both!) vasa have been incorrectly identified and that it was not the vas that was cut. Either way, re-exploration is necessary with redo vasectomy. The risk of pregnancy resulting from spontaneous rejoining of the ends of the vas after previous negative semen analysis is 1 in 2000–3000.[2,7]
- Chronic testicular pain: the frequency of chronic testicular pain is hard to determine but it is certainly a common cause for complaint. In one series, 2% of men who had undergone vasectomy regretted the decision because of the testicular pain.[8]

Vasovasostomy[9]

Best results are obtained when this procedure is performed using an operating microscope. This is a highly complex procedure using micro-surgical skills. The technique is covered briefly here to allow a surgeon to assist at and understand the principles of vasovasostomy. Refer to the references for a detailed description.

Indications

- Vasectomy reversal.
- Obstructive azoospermia.

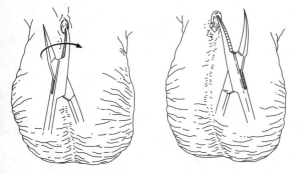

Fig. 9.11 One blade is used to puncture the vas and the open clamp is rotated to deliver the vas. Redrawn from Walsh et al. *Campbell's Urology* 8th edn. Philadelphia, PA, WB Saunders 2002. Permission sought.

Preparation

Obtain details of previous vasectomy. How much vas was excised? Which occlusion technique was employed? Take a fertility history from patient and partner. Examine the scrotum for testicular size and consistency, to assess the vasal gap, and to identify sperm granulomata.

Technique

If you can feel both ends of the vas, make scrotal incisions over the gap. If not, use 2–3 cm vertical incision just below the inguinal scrotal junction such that the incision can be extended in to the groin if necessary. Find and grasp the occluded vasal ends with Babcock clamps. Dissect the vas in both directions until the ends can be approximated without tension. Clear adventitia from the ends of the vas to expose the ends, but without disturbing the delicate perivasal vasculature. Cut the occluded ends of the vas until the lumen can be seen. Both ends of the vas should bleed. Pass a 2–0 monofilament suture along each end to ensure patency. Hold the two ends in apposition with a vas clamp.

Use an operating microscope. Mark the suture sites (six dots) with a fine marker on each end of the vas (Fig. 9.12) The dots lie midway between the mucosal and outer muscular layers and are equally spaced circumferentially. The anastamosis is performed in two layers. Using 10–0 double-ended nylon sutures, place three mucosal sutures anteriorly and tie. Place two 9–0 nylon sutures between the mucosal sutures, passing from the outside of the vas through the muscularis and emerging close to but not through the mucosa (Fig. 9.13). Rotate the anastamosis through 180° and place three further 10–0 sutures through the marked dots and tie. Place four 9–0 sutures between the mucosal sutures. Another layer of four to six 9–0 sutures is placed through the adventitia of the vas and a final (fourth) layer of 7–0 sutures is placed through the vasal sheath.

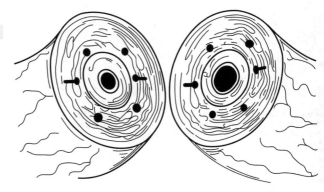

Fig. 9.12 Mark the suture sites (six dots) with a fine marker on each end of the vas. Redrawn from Walsh et al., *Campbell's Urology* 8th edn. Philadelphia, PA, WB Saunders 2002. Permission sought.

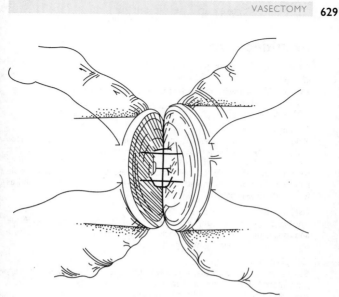

Fig. 9.13 The anastamosis is performed in two layers. Redrawn from Walsh *et al.*, *Campbell's Urology* 8th edn. Philadelphia, PA, WB Saunders 2002.

References

1 Li SQ, Goldstein M, Zhu J, Huber D. The no-scalpel vasectomy. *J Urol* 1991; **145**:341–4.
2 Haldar N, Cranston D, Turner E, MacKenzie I, Guillebaud J. How reliable is a vasectomy? Long-term follow-up of vasectomised men. *Lancet* 2000; **356**:43–4.
3 Kendrick JS, Gonzales B, Huber DH, Grubb GS, Rubin GL. Complications of vasectomies in the United States. *J Fam Pract* 1987; **25**:245–8.
4 Appell RA, Evans PR. Vasectomy: etiology of infectious complications. *Fertil Steril* 1980; **33**:52–3.
5 Randall PE, Ganguli L, Marcuson RW. Wound infection following vasectomy. *Br J Urol* 1983; **55**:564–7.
6 Randall PE, Ganguli LA, Keaney MG, Marcuson RW. Prevention of wound infection following vasectomy. *Br J Urol* 1985; **57**:227–9.
7 Philp T, Guillebaud J, Budd D. Late failure of vasectomy after two documented analyses showing azoospermic semen. *BMJ (Clin Res Ed)* 1984; **289**:77–90.
8 McMahon AJ, Buckley J, Taylor A, Lloyd SN, Deane RF, Kirk D. Chronic testicular pain following vasectomy. *Br J Urol* 1992; **69**:188–91.
9 Goldstein M, Li PS, Matthews GJ. Microsurgical vasovasostomy: the microdot technique of precision suture placement. *J Urol* 1998; **159**:188–90.

Orchidectomy

Simple orchidectomy

Indications
- Testicular pain: warn the patient the pain may remain unresolved.
- Testicular abscess.
- Missed torsion.

Technique
Make a midline or transverse scrotal incision. Cut through the dartos until the tunica vaginalis is seen. Incise the tunica to expose the testis. Deliver the testis, and clamp the vas and other cord structures either together or separately. Suture ligate the vessels with an 0 absorbable suture and tie off the vas with a 2–0 tie (Fig. 9.14). Close the wound as for a hydrocele repair.

Useful aside
The cord can retract a long way when you cut it. Finding it again is difficult and usually means extending the incision. Therefore do not cut your suture until you are sure that haemostasis has been secured.

Complications
Scrotal haematomas usually resolve, but should be drained if very uncomfortable or infected. Leave a drain if you are worried about haemostasis, but this should not be necessary.

Subcapsular orchidectomy

Indication
Androgen deprivation in prostate cancer. This operation removes the testicular tissue but leaves the tunica albuginea intact. There is more residual bulk than after a simple orchidectomy which may reduce the psychological impact of bilateral orchidectomy.

Procedure
Deliver the testis as described above. Incise the tunica albuginea along the full length of the testis. Evert the edged of the tunica (grasp with Allis or artery forceps if necessary) and sweep out the testicular tissue using a gauze swab held taut over the index finger (Fig. 9.15). Control bleeders with diathermy or clip and tie. Close the tunica albuginea with a running 3–0 absorbable suture (Fig. 9.16).

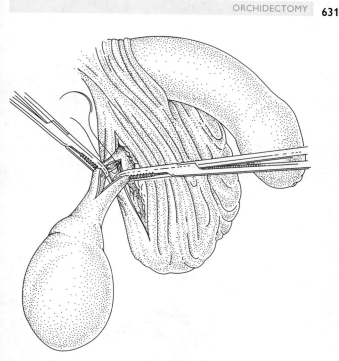

Fig. 9.14 The testis is delivered through a scrotal incision and the vessels are suture ligated. Reproduced from Whitfield, *Rob and Smith's operative surgery: Genitourinary surgery, Vol 2.* Butterworth Heinemann, Oxford, 1993. Permission sought.

Radical orchidectomy and insertion of testicular prosthesis

Indications

* Testicular tumour.
* Atrophic testis.
* Maldescent of testis.

Technique

Supine position. Prep and drape the lower abdomen from the umbilicus to the scrotum. Incise the skin 2 cm above and parallel to the inguinal ligament (as for inguinal herniorraphy). Divide the superficial fasciae (with diathermy) to expose the external oblique aponeurosis. Ensure that you visualize the external ring. Incise the external oblique from the ring in the line of its fibres to the approximate position of the internal ring (Fig. 9.17).

(a)

(b)

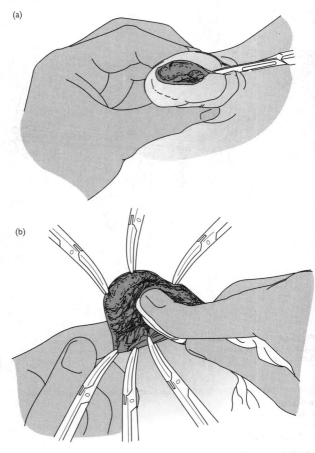

Fig. 9.15 (a) The testis is delivered through a scrotal incision. Incise the tunica albuginea. (b) Using a swab wrapped around your finger, sweep the contents of the testis off of the tunica albuginea.

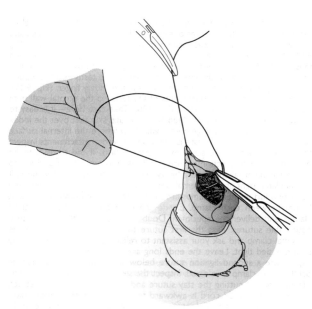

Fig. 9.16 Close the tunica albuginea with a running 3–0 absorbable suture.

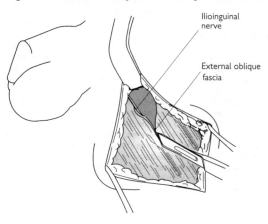

Ilioinguinal
nerve

External oblique
fascia

Fig. 9.17 Incise the external oblique from the ring in the line of its fibres to the approximate position of the internal ring.

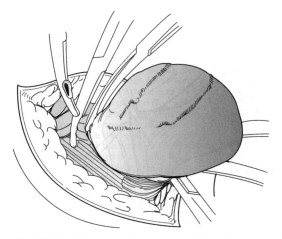

Fig. 9.20 Divide the gubernacular attachments of the testis to the scrotal wall.

Complications

Warn the patient to expect some swelling of the inguinal wound and bruising tracking down in to the scrotum. Large haematomas should be drained. If there is evidence of ongoing blood loss, suspect retroperitoneal bleeding from a retracted and inadequately controlled vascular pedicle. Explore the wound through the original incision, but be prepared to extend it and dissect retroperitoneally to find and control the vessels. Infected prostheses manifest with ongoing pain, sepsis, and purulent discharge. They are rarely salvageable with antibiotics and should be removed. Send the prosthesis for culture and irrigate the wound thoroughly. A prosthesis that has been in for a while but is uncomfortable or high-riding can be removed by enucleating it from its pseudo-capsule through a scrotal incision.

References

1 Adshead J, Khoubehi B, Wood J, Rustin G. Testicular implants and patient satisfaction: a questionnaire-based study of men after orchidectomy for testicular cancer. *BJU Int* 2001; **88**:559–62.

2 Simms MS, Huq S, Mellon JK. Testicular prostheses: a new technique for insertion. *BJU Int* 2004; **93**:179.

Epididymectomy

Indications

- Chronic epididymitis.
- Chronic epididymal pain.
- Tuberculous epididymitis.

Warn the patient about the possibility of testicular loss because of compromise to the testicular blood supply. This may occur acutely or by progressive atrophy of the testis after the procedure.

Procedure

Incise the scrotal skin either through the midline raphe or transversely. Cut through the layers of the scrotum with knife or diathermy to expose the tunica vaginalis. Carefully open the tunica and deliver the testis. Identify the junction between the straight and convoluted portions of the vas. Clamp and divide the vas here and tie the ends with 3–0 absorbable ties. Follow the convoluted vas to the tail of the epididymis. Hold the epididymis under tension away from the testis to make the attachments between epididymis and testis more obvious (Fig. 9.21). Sharply dissect the epididymis away from the testis. Take care not to damage the testicular vascular pedicle which enters the testis medial to the epididymis at the junction of the middle and upper thirds of the testis. Ligate the efferent ducts to the epididymis at the superior pole of the testis and remove the specimen. Close the edges of the tunica over the epididymal defect with 3–0 absorbable sutures (Fig. 9.22). Replace the testis and close the scrotum.

Complications

As in all scrotal surgery, be meticulous with haemostasis and leave a drain if bleeding has been problematic during the procedure. If a haematoma does occur, then re-exploration and drainage may be necessary. There is little you can do about damage to the testicular vascular pedicle. Atrophy is unpredictable and may be incomplete.

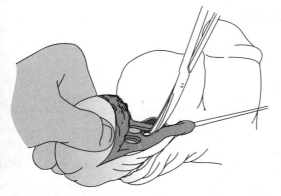

Fig. 9.21 Hold the epididymis under tension away from the testis to make the attachments between epididymis and testis more obvious and sharply dissect the epididymis away from the testis.

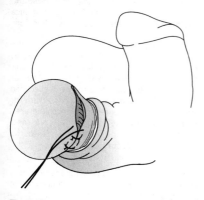

Fig. 9.22 Close the edges of the tunica over the epididymal defect.

Testicular biopsy

Indications
- For diagnosis of suspected carcinoma *in situ* in the at-risk testis (e.g. germ cell tumour of contralateral testis).
- Evaluation of male subfertility.

Preparation
If the biopsy is for evaluation of spermatogenesis, liaise with the IVF or andrology laboratory staff to ensure proper handling and rapid processing of the specimen, which needs to be examined fresh.

Techniques

Incision biopsy under local anaesthesia
Gently pull the testis inferiorly and grasp the cord just inferior to the external ring. Infiltrate a total of about 5 mL of plain lidocaine (1–2%) or bupivicaine (0.25–0.5%) into the cord medially and laterally. Avoid puncturing the vas. Grasp the testis firmly with the skin held taut over it. Infiltrate a further 2 mL of local anaesthetic into the skin and dartos over the upper pole of the testis. Incise the skin, dartos, and tunica vaginalis for about 1 cm transversely over the superior pole of the testis. Hold the edges of the tunica vaginalis apart with artery forceps. Expose the tunica albuginea of the medial or lateral aspects of the upper pole (these are the least vascular areas). Identify an avascular region of the tunica albuginea (some surgeons use loupes or a microscope for this). Incise the tunica albuginea over 3–4 mm with a 15 blade. Squeeze the testis to promote extrusion of a bead of tubules 4–5 mm in diameter. Excise this bead with fine sharp scissors (Fig. 9.23). Handle the specimen as little as possible to avoid distorting the architecture. Either pass the fresh specimen to the andrology technician or place the specimen in Bouin's medium for histological examination (formalin distorts the testicular architecture). Close the tunica albuginea with 4–0 absorbable sutures. Observe carefully for haemostasis and insert more sutures if necessary. Close the tunica vaginalis and the dartos/skin with 4–0 absorbable sutures.

Percutaneous needle biopsy
This technique is widely used in the evaluation of spermatogenesis. It is quicker to perform than an incision biopsy. Specimens obtained are smaller than with an incision biopsy and there is a greater risk of distorted architecture. There may also be a greater risk to testicular vessels/epididymes and this technique should not be used when previous surgery/biopsies may have distorted the scrotal anatomy.

Perform a local anaesthetic cord block as described above. Grasp the testis so that the skin is taut over the intended biopsy site (usually the upper pole). Prep the skin. Use a 20 g bevelled needle with a stylette (e.g. Testicular Biopsy Needle, Portland Surgical Products Pty Ltd, Portland, Australia). Push the needle in to the bulk of the testis. Remove the stylet and attach a 20 mL syringe to the needle. The syringe should have a small

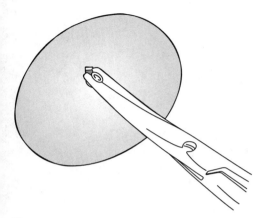

Fig. 9.23 Incise the testis and excise the testicular tubules with sharp scissors.

volume (about 0.5 mL) of heparinized saline within it to facilitate withdrawing the plunger under pressure and to aid evacuation of the specimen into a receptacle. Move the needle–syringe in and out a few times (the excursion is a few millimetres so that the needle tip remains in the testis) whilst applying negative pressure to the plunger of the syringe. Gently withdraw the needle. You may find that some tubules have not been drawn in to the needle but remain attached to the needle tip as it is withdrawn through the scrotal skin. Carefully snip these off flush with the skin using sterile scissors so that the needle can be fully withdrawn with these tubules still attached. Place the tip of the needle into a small receptacle (e.g. an Eppendorf tube) containing the appropriate solution (see above) and gently depress the plunger of the syringe to evacuate any tubules that have been aspirated in to the needle. Apply an occlusive dressing, and advise the patient to remain supine for a couple of hours and to avoid strenuous activity for a week.

Surgery for male factor infertility

Surgical management of male factor infertility

Testicular biopsy (📖 Chapter 9).

Vasography[3]

Vasography is indicated when there is azoospermia in combination with normal spermatogenesis on testicular biopsy. It is usually performed immediately prior to attempted surgical repair of an obstruction, which is presumed to be present on the basis of a normal FSH level (which implies that spermatogenesis is normal). Make a midline incision in the scrotum nearer the peno-scrotal junction, rather than placing the incision towards the lower pole of the testis. Deliver the testis. Dissect out the vas deferens to identify the junction between the straight and convoluted vas. Using operating loupes or a microscope for magnification, incise the vasal sheath longitudinally. Make a transverse incision into the vas to expose the lumen, without transecting the vas. If any fluid leaks out collect it on a slide and arrange microscopy—if there are no sperm in the vasal fluid the obstruction must be more proximal (i.e. on the testis side of the vasal incision). Cannulate the vas and instil some saline or Ringer's solution. Free flow rules out obstruction. Where there is doubt, instil 50% indigo carmine and catheterize the bladder. Blue staining of the urine confirms patency. If the vas is obstructed more distally it is usually dilated and fluid from the vasotomy contains large amounts of sperm. Before formal vasography the bladder should be catheterized. The catheter balloon is filled with 5 mL of air and pulled onto the bladder neck. The vas is cannulated and 0.5 mL of contrast is injected to determine the site of obstruction. If the obstruction is at the level of the ejaculatory ducts, injection of indigo carmine at this stage aids subsequent transurethral resection (see below). If the site of the obstruction is in the inguinal canal, inguinal vasovasostomy may be appropriate. Obstruction at other sites may not be reconstructable but collection of sperm from the vas may allow subsequent fertilization by IVF. If the vasa are patent but the vasal fluid contains no sperm, vaso-epididymostomy is appropriate.

Vaso-epididymostomy[3]

This is a demanding microsurgical technique best performed by a sub-specialist. The principles are described below.

Deliver the testis and expose the vas as described above. Prepare the vesicular end of the vas as for vasovasostomy (📖 p. 627). Incise the tunica vaginalis and expose the epididymis. The site of epididymal obstruction may be manifested by a noticeable transition from dilated to collapsed tubules. The tunica over the epididymis is incised and dilated loops of epididymal tubules are dissected free. The vas is drawn through the opening in the tunica and secured to it with 6–0 sutures. A dilated epididymal tubule is incised and aspirated fluid examined to confirm the presence of sperm. A mucosa to mucosa anastamosis is performed with 10–0 sutures, and then the muscular and adventitial layers of the vas are secured to the tunica with 9–0 sutures. In appropriately selected cases, vaso-epididymostomy will result in the appearance of sperm in about 70% of men,[4] but a significant proportion of initially patent anastamoses will subsequently close. Modifications of the surgical technique may result in enhanced outcomes.[3]

Transurethral resection of the ejaculatory ducts

Ejaculatory duct obstruction is usually congenital but may be a consequence of chronic prostatitis or extrinsic compression by cysts of ducts within the prostate or seminal vesicles. If initial investigations are suggestive of obstruction, trans-rectal ultrasound is often a helpful diagnostic tool. If the ejaculatory ducts or seminal vesicles are dilated, fluid can be aspirated and examined for the presence of spermatozoa. At the same time indigo carmine mixed with radio-opaque contrast can be introduced. X-ray screening will then allow localization of the probable point of obstruction. If these investigations demonstrate distal ejaculatory duct obstruction, proceed with trans-urethral resection. The veru montanum is resected with a loop. Avoid incising the bladder neck and the urethral sphincter distally. The dilated ejaculatory duct is usually rapidly exposed and the presence of indigo carmine confirms that the ducts have been entered.

After this procedure sperm are detectable in the ejaculate of about 50% of appropriately selected men.[5] Such men may still need to undergo IVF/ICSI if the semen quality is poor. Complications include reflux of urine into the ejaculatory ducts (which can result in epididymitis) and retrograde ejaculation.

Sperm retrieval techniques

Sperm retrieval techniques are used in men whose azoospermia is due to abnormalities of the vas deferens which cannot be reconstructed. Sperm are also retrieved in men undergoing an attempt at reconstruction (since success rates may be low and retrieved sperm can be stored for subsequent attempts at IVF).

Microsurgical epididymal sperm aspiration (MESA)

MESA is the oldest and most invasive of the sperm retrieval techniques. The testis is delivered, the tunica vaginalis is opened, and the epididymis is inspected. The tunica of the epididymis is opened over a dilated tubule. Effluxing fluid is examined for the presence of spermatozoa. If none are found, the epididymotomy is closed with bipolar diathermy and a different (usually more proximal) site selected. Once an appropriate site is found, a micropipette is positioned adjacent to the epididymotomy and effluxing fluid collected by capillary action. The quantity of collected fluid can be increased by gentle pressure on the epididymis. Multiple pipettes can be filled in this way. The fluid is passed to an IVF technician for subsequent handling. The epididymis is known to be important for sperm maturation, and in normal males the most motile sperm are found in the cauda epididymis. This does not appear to be the case in men with obstructive azoospermia, and the most motile sperm are often in the proximal epididymis.

Percutaneous epididymal sperm aspiration (PESA)

Ask your assistant to hold the testicle firmly by grasping the lower two-thirds. Stabilize the caput of the epididymis carefully between the thumb and index finger. Introduce a 27 gauge butterfly needle with a short length of plastic tubing attached to the caput in alignment with the rete testes. Gently aspirate using a 1 mL syringe filled with appropriate medium (check with your IVF laboratory). Examine the aspirated fluid for the presence of sperm. If sperm are present, gently massage the epididymis to propel fluid into the tubing. At the end of the procedure apply firm pressure to the aspiration site for 5 min.

Some surgeons doubt the adequacy of this technique and report that the quality of the sperm produced and the subsequent pregnancy rate are lower than with an open technique.[3] Others report that PESA is as successful as MESA but with fewer complications.[6,7]

Testicular sperm aspiration (TESA)

This technique is very similar to PESA. Grasp the testis firmly with the scrotal skin stretched taut. Pass a 19 gauge needle attached to a 20 mL syringe from the anterior surface of the inferior pole towards the superior pole. Move the needle rapidly in and out five or six times, with each pass of the needle in a slightly different direction. Then slowly withdraw the needle from the testis whilst maintaining negative pressure on the syringe. Carefully free any tubules attached to the tip of the needle using fine forceps and place them in a sterile tube containing culture medium. Disconnect the needle and flush it through with culture medium to wash any fluid within the needle into the sterile tube.

TESA is easy to perform and is comparable to open techniques in terms of sperm recovery.[8]

ICSI and the role of 'surgery' in the treatment of male infertility

ICSI (intra-cytoplasmic sperm injection) has revolutionized the treatment of male factor infertility. In ICSI, a sperm is injected directly into an oocyte; only one sperm is needed per oocyte retrieved. In theory any man from whom a single viable sperm can be obtained can become a biological father. The availability of ICSI and the relative ease with which sperm can be obtained by minimally invasive techniques (PESA and TESA) has led some to question the value of invasive techniques (vaso-epididymostomy) which have unpredictable success rates. Even after attempted reconstruction ICSI may still be necessary, but its success may have been compromised by the advancing age of the female partner whilst the results of surgery on the male partner are awaited. Although some take the view that everything possible should be done to allow 'natural' conception,[3] others recognize that going straight to ICSI may be a pragmatic first choice.[9]

Varicoceles

Varicoceles are found in 15% of all men, but in 35% of men with primary infertility. Whether treating a varicocele is effective in increasing pregnancy rates in subfertile couples is controversial, but the current consensus (including a Cochrane review) is that it is not,[10,11] although this remains a highly controversial question.[12] Varicoceles are also treated because they may be the cause of chronic scrotal discomfort or for cosmetic reasons. In adolescents, varicoceles are associated with ipsilateral reduction in testicular growth. The discrepancy in testicular size recovers in most boys after treatment of the varicocele.

Techniques for the treatment of varicoceles

Embolization (📖 p. 658)

In our practice embolization is the treatment of choice for previously untreated varicoceles.

Surgical approaches

The spermatic veins can be approached abdominally (retroperitoneally) after their exit through the deep ring, within the inguinal canal, or sub-inguinally before they enter the canal. Scrotal approaches have been used in the past but have fallen out of favour because of the risk to the testicular artery and difficulty in determining how much of the pampiniform plexus should be excised.

Complications

There are three principal complications: varicocele recurrence, hydrocele formation, and testicular atrophy secondary to inadvertent damage to the testicular artery. Recurrences occur when not all the draining veins are divided and collaterals are established. When non-microsurgical techniques are used, the incidence of recurrence is about 10–15%; with microsurgery the incidence is 1–2%.[13–15] The inguinal and subinguinal approaches allow access to external spermatic and gubernacular veins which do not drain into the cord and may be responsible for some cases of recurrence.[16] Delivery of the cord alone will allow access to most external spermatic collaterals, but to ensure control of all external spermatic veins and gubernacular veins the testis must be delivered (Fig. 10.1). If draining lymphatics are divided, development of hydroceles is more likely.[17] Damage to lymphatics (and to the testicular artery) is less likely if loupes or the operating microscope are used.[13–15]

Abdominal (retroperitoneal or Palomo) approach

This is a good approach if there has been prior inguinal surgery. The advantage of this approach is that the whole vascular pedicle (i.e. artery and vein) can be ligated. This is reported to reduce the risk of recurrence since there is little danger of leaving a draining vein behind. When the testicular artery is taken at this level, collateral supply (vasal and cremasteric) ensures the viability of the testis (although the effect on

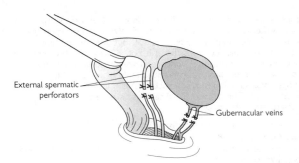

External spermatic perforators

Gubernacular veins

Fig. 10.1 Delivery of the testis allows access to most spermatic collaterals.

spermatogenesis is not known). There are also fewer veins at this level (usually no more than two). However, since lymphatics are disrupted in this approach, the incidence of post-operative hydrocele may be greater. Recurrence rates may be slightly higher (~15%) with this approach if the artery is not taken.[18,19] This may be because preserved fine peri-arterial veins may communicate with spermatic veins as several levels and can gradually dilate over time.

The supine patient is tilted a little head up to fill the veins. Make a short oblique incision over the internal ring (about 2 cm medial to the anterior superior iliac spine). Open the external oblique aponeurosis in the line of its fibres and split internal oblique and transversus abdominis. Sweep the peritoneum medially and identify the gonadal vessels as they run towards the vas (Fig. 10.2) Gentle traction on the testis may bring the cord structures in to relief. Place a right-angle clamp behind the vessels to lift them into the wound. Some surgeons put loupes on at this stage to facilitate identification of the vessels. Separate the veins from the artery and lymphatics. Papaverine solution dripped on the artery will make it dilate. It is does not matter if the artery is divided (see above) but most surgeons will leave it intact if the veins can be identified with confidence. Ligate each vein individually with 3–0 absorbable ties (Fig. 10.3). Close the wound in layers.

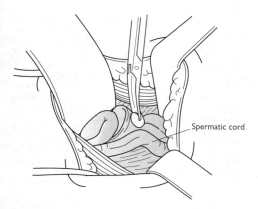

Fig. 10.2 Abdominal approach.

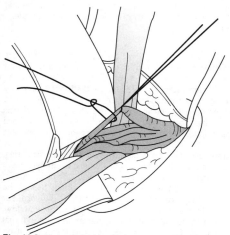

Fig. 10.3 Abdominal approach, Ligating each vein.

Spermatic cord

Inguinal varicocelectomy (Ivanissevich)

This approach is usually easier and quicker than the retroperitoneal approach, especially in the obese patient. The patient is positioned supine with 10° of head up. Make an incision beginning medially at the external ring (2 cm above and lateral to the pubic tubercle) following the line of the inguinal canal for 4 cm. Divide the superficial fascia and sweep the adventitia away to expose the ring and the external oblique aponeurosis. Open the aponeurosis from the superficial ring to just above the deep ring. Take care not to damage the ilioinguinal nerve just deep to external oblique. Mobilize the cord above, below, and behind using a peanut swab. There may be a cremasteric vein entering the posterior aspect of the cord (running from the external ring). If left, this can be a source of recurrence and it should be divided. Pass a vessel loop or tape behind the cord and elevate it out of the wound (Fig. 10.4). Consider delivery of the testis and control of gubernacular and external spermatic veins (see above). Open the internal spermatic fascia in the line of the cord. Clip the ends of the tape or vessel loop to your drapes to suspend the cord structures (Fig. 10.5). Using loupes or a microscope begin to separate out and identify the artery, lymphatics, and internal spermatic veins (usually three). The artery is often adherent to the undersurface of a large vein. Application of 1% papaverine may help to identify the artery; some surgeons use a fine Doppler probe. The artery must not be tied at this level. Tie off the veins with 4–0 absorbable ties and divide them. Close the wound in layers.

Subinguinal (Marmar) approach[15,20]

The advantage of this approach is that the spermatic vessels are approached at their most superficial and so there is no need to disrupt fascial planes. However, the technique is demanding; the veins are yet to unite and so are often multiple and the testicular artery may have already divided into several branches which may be more difficult to identify than the larger main testicular artery. The approach is perhaps best used when there has been prior inguinal surgery, when the cord is lax and the testis is low lying, and when the surgeon is a confident microsurgeon.

Make a 2–3 cm transverse incision is directly over the superficial ring. Open the superficial fascia and identify the cord where it emerges from the deep ring. Free its attachments with a peanut swab. Lift the cord out with a Babcock clamp and pass two tapes or Penrose drains behind the cord (Fig. 10.6). The distal tape can be held fairly taut to fix the cord, but the proximal tape should be fairly lax to avoid occluding the arterial flow. Consider delivery of the testis and control of gubernacular and external spermatic veins (see above). Open the external spermatic fascia. Put on loupes or bring in the operating microscope. The dissection of the cord is as described above.

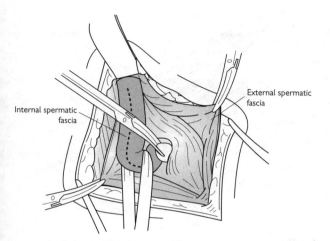

Fig. 10.4 Inguinal varicocelectomy, a vessel loop or tape is placed behind the cord to elevate it out of the wound.

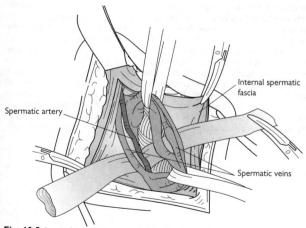

Fig. 10.5 Inguinal varicocelectomy, suspending the cord structures.

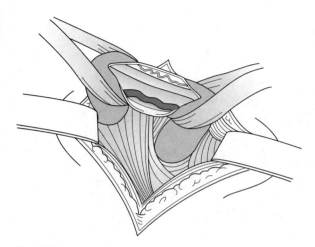

Fig. 10.6 Sub-inguinal approach, passing two tapes or Penrose drains behind the cord.

Laparoscopic treatment of varicoceles

In essence the laparoscopic approach to a varicocele is the same as the retroperitoneal approach and the advantages and disadvantages in terms of outcome are the same. As in the open retroperitoneal approach the surgeon has the choice whether to divide the whole vascular pedicle or to preserve the artery and lymphatics. Arguably the greater magnification of the laparoscope facilitates identification and preservation of the artery and lymph vessels. Critics of the laparoscopic approach state that it is time consuming, expensive in terms of equipment, and carries a risk of iatrogenic damage to other structures.[3,21] However, as more urologists become adept at laparoscopy, operating times and complications are likely to fall. In one recent study the laparoscopic approach was judged to be superior to a microsurgical subinguinal approach and took less time.[22]

References

1 WHO laboratory manual for the examination of human semen and semen-cervical mucus interaction, 3rd edn. Cambridge University Press, 1992.

2 Sigman M, Jarrow JP. Male infertility. In Campbell's Urology, 8th edn, ed. Walsh PC, Retik AB, Darracott Vaughan E, Wein AJ. Philadelphia, PA: WB Saunders, 200, pp 1475–531.

3 Goldstein M. Surgical management of male infertility and other scrotal disorders. In Campbell's Urology, 8th edn, ed. Walsh PC, Retik AB, Darracott Vaughan E, Wein AJ. Philadelphia, PA: WB Saunders, 200, pp 1532–87.

4 Schlegel PN, Goldstein M. Microsurgical vasoepididymostomy: refinements and results. J Urol 1993; 150:1165–8.

5 Schroeder-Printzen I, Ludwig M, Kohn F, Weidner W. Surgical therapy in infertile men with ejaculatory duct obstruction: technique and outcome of a standardized surgical approach. Hum Reprod 2000; 15:1364–8.

6 Madgar I, Seidman DS, Levran D et al. Micromanipulation improves in-vitro fertilization results after epididymal or testicular sperm aspiration in patients with congenital absence of the vas deferens. Hum Reprod 1996; 11:2151–4.

7 Tsirigotis M, Pelekanos M, Yazdani N, Boulos A, Foster C, Craft IL. Simplified sperm retrieval and intracytoplasmic sperm injection in patients with azoospermia. Br J Urol 1995; 76:765–8.

8 Tournaye H, Clasen K, Aytoz A, Nagy Z, Van Steirteghem A, Devroey P. Fine needle aspiration versus open biopsy for testicular sperm recovery: a controlled study in azoospermic patients with normal spermatogenesis. Hum Reprod 1998; 13:901–4.

9 Nicopoullos JD, Gilling-Smith C, Ramsay JW. Male-factor infertility: do we really need urologists? A gynaecological view. BJU Int 2004; 93:1188–90.

10 Kamischke A, Nieschlag E. Varicocele treatment in the light of evidence-based andrology. Hum Reprod Update 2001; 7:65–9.

11 Evers JL, Collins JA. Surgery or embolization for varicocele in subfertile men. Cochrane Database Syst Rev 2004: CD000479.

12 Ficarra V, Cerruto MA, Liguori G et al. Treatment of varicocele in subfertile men. The Cochrane review: a contrary opinion. Eur Urol 2006; 49:258–63.

13 Cayan S, Kadioglu TC, Tefekli A, Kadioglu A, Tellaloglu S. Comparison of results and complications of high ligation surgery and microsurgical high inguinal varicocelectomy in the treatment of varicocele. Urology 2000; 55:750–4.

14 Goldstein M, Gilbert BR, Dicker AP, Dwosh J, Gnecco C. Microsurgical inguinal varicocelectomy with delivery of the testis: an artery and lymphatic sparing technique. J Urol 1992; 148:1808–11.

15 Marmar JL, Kim Y. Subinguinal microsurgical varicocelectomy: a technical critique and statistical analysis of semen and pregnancy data. J Urol 1994; 152:1127–32.

16 Kaufman SL, Kadir S, Barth KH, Smyth JW, Walsh PC, White RI, Jr. Mechanisms of recurrent varicocele after balloon occlusion or surgical ligation of the internal spermatic vein. Radiology 1983; 147:435–40.

17 Szabo R, Kessler R. Hydrocele following internal spermatic vein ligation: a retrospective study and review of the literature. J Urol 1984; 132:924–5.

18 Homonnai ZT, Fainman N, Engelhard Y, Rudberg Z, David MP, Paz G. Varicocelectomy and male fertility: comparison of semen quality and recurrence of varicocele following varicocelectomy by two techniques. Int J Androl 1980; 3:447–58.

19 Rothman CM, Newmark H, 3rd, Karson RA. The recurrent varicocele: a poorly recognized problem. Fertil Steril 1981; 35:552–6.

20 Marmar JL, DeBenedictis TJ, Praiss D. The manament of varicoceles by microdissection of the spermatic cord at the external inguinal ring. Fertil Steril 1985; 43:583–8.

21 Hirsch IH, Abdel-Meguid TA, Gomella LG. Postsurgical outcomes assessment following varicocele ligation: laparoscopic versus subinguinal approach. Urology 1998; 51:810–5.

22 McManus MC, Barqawi A, Meacham RB, Furness PD, 3rd, Koyle MA. Laparoscopic varicocele ligation: are there advantages compared with the microscopic subinguinal approach? Urology 2004; 64:357–61.

Chapter 11

Uroradiological intervention

Percutaneous nephrostomy

Indications

Percutaneous nephrostomy (puncture of the collecting system by a percutaneous approach) is central to many urological procedures. It is used to relieve obstruction (e.g. an infected obstructed kidney caused by a ureteric calculus, malignant obstruction from pelvic cancer) and to provide access for intra-renal surgery (percutaneous nephrolithotomy, ablation of renal pelvis TCC) or diagnostic procedures (antegrade pyelography, Whittaker test for upper tract obstruction).

Preparation

Anticoagulation or impaired clotting is a contraindication. Prepare and drape as for open surgery. Local anaesthesia (± sedation) is sufficient for insertion of a nephrostomy tube up to 12Fr. Administer broad-spectrum IV antibiotics if puncturing an infected system. Wear radiation protection.

Technique

Depending on where you work, percutaneous renal access may be the preserve of the interventional radiologist, the urologist, or both. Ultrasound guidance alone may be sufficient for puncture (especially of dilated systems), but fluoroscopy may also be required and facilitates depth perception. The procedure can also be guided by CT or MRI. The patient is positioned prone. The puncture site is typically in the posterior axillary line approximately midway between the iliac crest and the 12th rib. Many factors may dictate the chosen site (body habitus, position and rotation of the kidney, position of other organs, location of stone/tumour, previous punctures). If the aim of the procedure is to gain access to the ureter, puncturing the collecting system superiorly allows more direct access into the ureter for a ureteroscope and other instruments. Aim to puncture through the parenchyma into a posterior calyx (less chance of damaging intra-renal vessels). The initial puncture is usually with a 16–18 gauge needle. A guidewire is inserted along the needle, the needle is removed, and dilatation of the tract performed to the required size.

Complications of percutaneous renal access

- Bleeding (rarely necessitating selective arterial embolization or even nephrectomy).
- Damage to another viscus (spleen, gall bladder, liver, colon).
- Pneumothorax.
- Injury to the renal pelvis.
- Septicaemia.

Renovascular procedures

Embolization

Embolization is used to stop bleeding, to ablate failed kidneys or prior to nephrectomy. Bleeding may be a consequence of trauma, iatrogenic, or from renal tumours (e.g. bleeding angiomyolipoma or renal cell carcinoma).

Various materials can be employed to achieve embolization, including metal coils, glue, foam particles, balloons, and alcohol.

Renovascular hypertension

Renal artery angioplasty or the placement of a renal artery stent may be valuable in cases where hypertension is shown to be due to a renovascular cause (renal artery stenosis, fibromuscular dysplasia).

Varicocele

Placement of metal coils or injection of sclerosant into the gonadal vein has become a common treatment for varicoceles, and in our unit is the initial treatment of choice. Percutaneous occlusion techniques have the advantage that the whole length of the gonadal vein can be occluded, as can feeding tributaries if necessary. There is also no risk to the testicular artery or of damage to lymphatics (which enhances the risk of hydrocele formation) (📖 Chapter 10). Embolization is always preceded by venography to demonstrate the size of the varicocele and the venous anatomy. Success rates are ~90%.[1]

Reference

1 Beddy P, Geoghegan T, Browne RF, Torreggiani WC. Testicular varicoceles. *Clin Radiol* 2005; **60**: 1248–55.

Chapter 12

Surgery for disorders of erectile function, ejaculation, and seminal vesicles

Physiology of erection

The relaxation of penile corporeal smooth muscle, an essential step for penile erection, is controlled locally by autonomic dilator nerves and the vascular endothelium. The pelvic nerves appear to mediate penile erection via two circulatory events. The first is a prompt dilatation of penile resistance vessels causing a greatly increased arterial inflow. The second is a rapid filling of the corpora cavernosa and an increase in cavernosal pressure.

This is attributed to sudden opening of low-resistance shunt vessels, the helicine arteries, diverting part of the increased arterial inflow into the cavernous bodies. The penile rigidity may also be enhanced by muscular compression of the blood-distended cavernous bodies through contraction of the ischiocavernosus muscles.

The blood vessels, intrinsic smooth muscles of the penis and surrounding striated muscles, are controlled by nerves arising from three different parts of the peripheral nervous system: the thoracolumbar sympathetic, the lumbosacral parasympathetic, and the lumbosacral sympathetic. Normal erection requires participation of all three of these systems. The sympathetic pre-ganglionic fibres arise from the lower thoracic (T10) and upper lumbar (L3) spinal cord segments. The sympathetic fibres probably have both erectile and anti-erectile properties. The parasympathetic pre-ganglionic neurons are located in the sixth lumbar to fourth sacral spinal cord segments. The sacral parasympathetics in the pelvic nerves are the primary efferent system for generating penile erection, inducing vasodilation in the penile blood vessels and increased blood flow to the cavernous tissue.

At a molecular level, penile smooth muscle relaxation follows a decrease in free calcium in the sarcoplasma. Calmodulin dissociates from myosin light-chain kinase and inactivates it. When myosin is dephosphorylated from myosin light-chain kinase and detaches from the actin filament, the muscle relaxes. A second or alternative mechanism involving the NO–cGMP pathway directly, causing relaxation by decreasing the rate of cross-bridge recruitment through phosphorylation, may also exist.

cAMP and cGMP are the second messengers involved in penile smooth muscle relaxation. They activate cAMP- and cGMP-dependent protein kinases, which in turn phosphorylate certain proteins and ion channels. This leads to opening of potassium channels and hyperpolarization, sequestration of intracellular calcium by the endoplasmic reticulum, and inhibition of voltage-dependent calcium channels, blocking calcium influx. Subsequently the cytosolic free calcium drops and the penile smooth muscle relaxes.[1]

Reference

1 Dean RC, Lue TF. Physiology of penile erection and pathophysiology of erectile dysfunction. *Urol Clin North Am* 2005; **32**:379–95.

Physiology of ejaculation

Ejaculation requires coordinated activity of seminal fluid deposition in the posterior urethra followed by antegrade expulsion. Three distinct phases have been described.

- Bladder neck contraction.
- Emission.
- Ejaculation.

These events occur in a systematic way. During emission, seminal fluid is deposited in the posterior urethra by contraction of the smooth muscles of the prostate, seminal vesicles, and vas deferens. This is initiated by reflex activity in the thoracolumbar sympathetic nerves. The bladder neck contracts simultaneously (pressures as high as 500 cmH$_2$O are generated) to prevent retrograde seminal flow into the bladder. Once the seminal fluid is in the posterior urethra, the peri-urethral skeletal and external sphincter muscles contract and relax rhythmically, expelling the semen in a pulsatile manner from the urethra. This phase is controlled via stimulation of the perineal branch of the pudendal nerve (S2–4). Although skeletal muscles under somatic control are involved, all the events of the ejaculatory process are involuntary once the reflex has been initiated.

Ejaculation usually involves genital sensory input coordinated with erotic imagery from the cerebral cortex. It can occur through activation of the cerebrum alone, as evidenced by nocturnal emissions.

The ejaculatory volume is normally 2–6 mL, of which 0.1–0.2 mL comes from sperm mixed with secretions from the glands of Littre and Cowper, 0.5 mL from prostatic secretions, and 2–2.5 mL from seminal vesicle fluid. Fructose is only present in the seminal vesicle portion. The pH of normal ejaculate is 7.2–8. Prostatic secretions are slightly acidic whilst seminal vesicle are alkaline.[1]

Reference

1 Master VA, Turek PJ. Ejaculatory physiology and dysfunction. *Urol Clin North Am* 2001, **28**:363–74.

Evaluation of impotence[1,2]

History and examination

- Clues to psychogenic origin: sudden onset, early collapse of erection, good-quality self-stimulated or early morning erections, premature ejaculation, relationship problems/changes, major life events, psychological problems.
- Clues to organic cause: gradual onset, lack of tumescence, normal ejaculation, normal libido, risk factors e.g. vascular, endocrine, neurological, pelvic operations, radiotherapy or trauma, medications, smoking, high alcohol, recreational or body-building drugs.
- Erectile dysfunction may be the first presenting feature of a depressive illness. Also beware of anxiety states, psychosis, body dysmorphic disorder, gender identity problems, and alcoholism.

Drug causes

- Antihypertensives: β-blockers/thiazides/hydralazine >α-blockers, ACE inhibitors, calcium-channel blockers.
- Diuretics: thiazides/potassium-sparing diuretics/carbonic anhydrase inhibitors >loop diuretics.
- Antidepressants: e.g. SSRIs, tricyclics, MAOIs.
- Antipsychotics: e.g. phenothiazines, carbamazepine, risperidone.
- Hormonal agents: e.g. CPA, LHRH analogues, oestrogens.
- Lipid regulators: gemfibrozil/clofibrate >statins.
- Anticonvulsants e.g. phenytoin, carbamazepine.
- Antiparkinsonian, e.g. levodopa.
- Ulcer healing: H_2 antagonists >proton pump inhibitors.
- Miscellaneous: allopurinol, indomethacin, disulfiram.

Examination

- Blood pressure, peripheral pulses.
- Genitalia: testicular size, penile fibrosis, retractable foreskin.
- Digital rectal examination in men >50 years with life expectancy ≥10 years.

Investigations

- Exclude diabetes: fasting venous plasma glucose.
- Lipid profile: if not done in previous 12 months.
- Testosterone: free and morning (7–11a.m.)
- LH/prolactin (if testosterone low).
- U&E (if renal impairment is suspected).
- LFTs (if liver impairment is suspected).
- Sickle cell (African Caribbean patients).

References

1 Montague DK, Jarow JP, Broderick GA *et al.* Chapter 1: The management of erectile dysfunction: An AUA update. *J Urol* 2006, **174**:230–9.
2 *European Association of Urology Guidelines*. Arnhem: European Association of Urology, 2006.

Surgery for impotence: vascular surgery

This covers two areas: penile revascularization and venous leak (veno-occlusive) surgery.

Penile revascularization surgery

Functional arterial disease needs to have been initially demonstrated on either penile Doppler (poor peak systolic velocities, i.e. <25 cm/sec) or dynamic infusion cavernosometry and cavernosography (DICC) (a gradient of >30 mmHg between penile occlusion pressure and mean brachial pressure). Pudendal arteriography should then be performed.[1] The arteriogram will also allow selection of the preferred recipient vessel[2] (Fig. 12.1). Ideally the inferior epigastric artery is anastomosed end to end or end to side to a branch of the dorsal penile artery as this allows the most efficient run-off. Failing this, a saphenous vein connected to the femoral artery can serve as the arterial input and an isolated segment of the deep dorsal vein with good communicators to the intracavernous tissue as the recipient vessel.[3]

Indications[1,4]
- Recently acquired erectile dysfunction due to discrete focal arterial lesions on pudendal arteriography in a healthy young patient (<40 years).
- Ideally post-traumatic.

Absolute contraindications[1,4]
- Insulin-dependent diabetes.
- Smoking.
- Neurological disease.
- Pre-existing systemic atherosclerosis or major veno-occlusive dysfunction.

Immediate pre-operative preparation
- Genital shave.
- Prophylactic IV antibiotics: cefuroxime 1.5 g at induction of anaesthesia.
- TED stockings.
- 14Fr Foley urethral catheterization.

Patient positioning
Supine with legs slightly abducted.

Operative technique
Make a lower midline or transverse abdominal incision (two-thirds of the way from pubic bone to umbilicus). Dissect out the inferior epigastric artery, usually at the lateral edge of the rectus muscle, with accompanying veins. Ligate any branches encountered during the dissection with 4–0 Vicryl. Dissect the inferior epigastric artery as far proximally as possible, usually close to the umbilicus. Tie any other small branches near its origin to maximize available arterial length. Harvesting the artery distally to the common femoral artery will usually provide adequate length. Papaverine should be applied topically to the artery throughout the dissection.

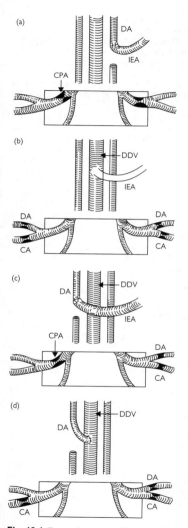

Fig. 12.1 Types of arteriographic patterns and the associated types of bypass procedures. DDV, Deep dorsal vein; DA, dorsal artery; IEA, inferior epigastric artery; CA, cavernosal artery; CPA, common penile artery. Reproduced from Hatzichristou and Goldstein, *Surgery Annual*, 1993, **25**(2): 207–29. Permission sought.

Make a curvilinear incision two fingerbreadths lateral to the shaft of the penis from the pubic tubercle to the median scrotal raphe. The side of this incision depends on the side of the best-quality inferior epigastric artery. Identify the ipsilateral tunica albuginea at the middle of the penile shaft and perform blunt finger dissection proximally to the ipsilateral crus to the level of the ischiopubic ramus. Then carry out blunt finger dissection distally, avoiding injury to the fundiform ligament and allowing inversion of the penis. Further distal dissection bluntly allows the plane between Buck's and Colles' fascias to be established.

Prepare the recipient vessel. If the deep dorsal vein is used, it is approached from the distal end of the penis near the glans. Vascular control is achieved here with care to avoid the posterior emissary branches and the dorsal nerve. Tie off the initial multiple branches near the glans penis with 4–0 Vicryl together with large trunks of the deep dorsal vein that anastomose to the spongiosum laterally along the shaft of the penis. This will prevent post-operative glans hyperaemia. Follow the vein proximally with liberal application of topical papaverine. Ligate the vein under the symphysis pubis. Assess retrograde flow in the deep dorsal vein to the corpora by placing a 19 gauge butterfly needle in one corpora, observing free flow of corporal blood in the butterfly and injecting diluted methylene blue into the isolated deep dorsal vein. If the methylene blue drains through the butterfly needle, a valveless system exists (60% of cases). If not, the valves in the deep dorsal vein are then destroyed using a 2 mm Fogarty balloon catheter or a 2 mm Lemaitre valve cutter.

The transfer route of the neo-arterial inflow is then prepared prior to distal transaction of the inferior epigastric artery. Identify the internal inguinal ring lateral to the origin of the inferior epigastric artery and, using blunt finger dissection along the inguinal canal, pass a finger to the defect between the fundiform and suspensory ligaments at the base of the penis. Preservation rather than division of these ligaments may be important in preventing injury to cutaneous nerves in the fundiform ligaments which supply the base of the penis and in preserving penile length. Then dissect the artery between ligaclips. Pass a fine right-angled instrument through the fenestration and up the inguinal canal to the internal inguinal ring. Grasp the surrounding veins ± the artery, avoiding crush injury to the artery, and slowly transfer. Undue tension or twisting must be avoided. Once the artery is transferred, check its pulsatility distally and observe its origin for twisting. Close the abdominal incision at this point.

Remove the adventitia from the vessels only at the site of anastomosis. This prevents the adventitia from being trapped in the lumen and causing thrombosis.

Flush the inferior epigastric artery with dilute heparin and clamp the vessels with vascular bulldog clips. Perform the anastomosis microscopically (10× magnification) using 8–0 to 10–0 prolene interrupted.

Release the bulldog clips and close the skin with 4–0 Vicryl. Apply a loose elastic dressing to the penis for 24 hr. Resumption of sexual activity should start 6 weeks post-operatively.[2]

Outcomes and complications[3,5-15]

- Success is reported in 20–78% of cases. However, the patient's perception of success does not clearly correlate with pre- and post-operative objective testing, making interpretation of these results difficult. Penile oedema is common, although it is minimized by the elastic dressing and resolves 2–3 weeks post-operatively.
- Penile numbness is quite common, but should recover in 12–18 months unless a major penile sensory nerve has been injured.
- Penile shortening from scar entrapment occurs in up to 20% of cases. This may require Z-plasty incisions to relax. Mechanical disruption has been reported, probably because sexual activity has been initiated too soon after surgery.
- Glans hyperaemia can occur with deep dorsal vein arterialization when a communicating vein is missed during the distal dissection.

Venous leak surgery

Significant controversy exists with regard to this surgery and the AUA and EAU no longer recommend its use.[1,4]

It is difficult to distinguish functional abnormalities from anatomical defects. It is also not known how to determine what percentage of erectile dysfunction is due to veno-occlusive erectile dysfunction independent of general arterial hypofunction, how to diagnose this condition accurately, how often arterial insufficiency coexists, and whether there is a subset of patients with veno-occlusive disorder who will benefit from this surgery.

Indications
- Uncertain.

Absolute contraindications
- Uncertain.

Immediate pre-operative preparation
- Genital shave.
- Prophylactic IV antibiotic: cefuroxime 1.5 g at induction of anaesthesia.
- TED stockings.
- 14Fr Foley urethral catheterization.

Patient positioning
Supine with legs slightly abducted.

Operative technique
Make a peri-penile anterior scrotal incision. This allows the penis to be inverted into the wound for access to the all important venous channels along the penile shaft. Identify the communicating veins between the superficial and deep penile veins, dissect them out, and ligate with 4–0 Vicryl. Dissect the penis more proximally and release the suspensory ligament in the infrapubic region. Isolate the communicating veins to the perineal side wall and infrapubic region and divided to expose the deep venous drainage system.

Make an incision in Buck's fascia to expose the deep dorsal penile vein. Divide the vein and tie with 4–0 Vicryl. Dissect the vein proximally and distally, ligating all the communicators and communicators from the circumflex vessels. Take care to stay in the midline to avoid potential injury to the more lateral dorsal penile arteries and penile sensory nerves. Take the dissection of the deep dorsal vein distally 1–1.5 cm from the glanular sulcus, where the truncal origins of the vein are dissected and ligated. Proximally the deep dorsal vein is ligated under the pubis with a 1–0 Vicryl tie. The cavernosal veins will be seen in this area and need to be dissected out and ligated. An intra-operative cavernosometry is then performed using a large butterfly needle placed in one of the corpora to assess the adequacy of veno-occlusion.

Reattach the suspensory ligament from pubis to midline tunica albuginea in the midline sulcus where the deep dorsal vein had been. Place a fenestrated drain in the infrapubic region, exiting via a separate stab wound and secured with a 0 silk tie.

Close the layers carefully with equal side-to-side approximation, otherwise dense fixation of the scrotal or infrapubic skin to the penile shaft will occur. Use bipolar diathermy throughout to minimize risk of injury to arteries and nerves. Apply a loose elastic dressing to the penile shaft.

Outcomes and complications[16–31]

- Success is reported in 12.5–61% of cases. However, patient's perception of success does not clearly correlate with pre- and post-operative objective testing, making interpretation of these results difficult. Penile oedema is common, although it is minimized by the elastic dressing and resolves 2–3 weeks post-operatively.
- Penile numbness is quite common, but should recover in 12–18 months unless a major penile sensory nerve has been injured.
- Penile shortening from scar entrapment occurs in up to 20% of cases. This may require Z-plasty incisions to relax.

References

1 Montague DK, Jarow JP, Broderick GA et al. Chapter 1: The management of erectile dysfunction: an AUA update. *J Urol* 2006; **174**:230–9.
2 Hatzichristou D, Goldstein I. Penile microvascular arterial bypass: Indications and surgical considerations. *Ann Surg* 1993; **25**:207–27.

3 Sharlip ID. The role of vascular surgery in arteriographic and combined arteriographic and venous impotence. *Semin Urol* 1990; **8**:129–37.

4 *European Association of Urology Guidelines*. Arnhem: European Association of Urology, 2006.

5 Belker, Bennett AH. Applications of microsurgery in urology. *Surg Clin North Am* 1988; **68**:1177–8.

6 Furlow WL, Fisher J, Knoll LD et al. Current status of penile revascularization with deep dorsal vein arterialization: experience with 95 patients. *Int J Impot Res* 1990; **2**(Suppl 2):348–9.

7 Sohn MH, Sikora RR, Bohndorf KK et al. Objective follow up after penile revascularization. *Int J Impot Res* 1992; **4**:73–84.

8 Bock D, Lewis RW. Treatment of vasculogenic impotence: penile revascularization. *Int J Impot Res* 1992; **4**:223–30.

9 Kawanishi Y, Kimura K, Nakanishi R, Kojima K, Numata A. Penile revascularization surgery for arteriogenic erectile dysfunction: the long-term efficacy rate calculated by survival analysis. *BJU Int* 2004; **94**:361–8.

10 Wespes E, Wildschutz T, Roumeguere T, Schulman CC. The place of surgery for vascular impotence in the third millennium. *J Urol* 2003; **170**:1284–6.

11 Rao DS, Donatucci CF. Vasculogenic impotence: arterial and venous surgery. *Urol Clin North Am* 2001; **28**:309–19.

12 Jarow JP, DeFranzo AJ. Long-term results of arterial bypass surgery for impotence secondary to segmental vascular disease. *J Urol* 1996; **156**:982–5.

13 Sarramon JP, Bertrand N, Malavaud B, Rischmann P. Microrevascularization of the penis in vascular impotence. *Int J Impot Res* 1997; **9**:127–33.

14 Kaufman JM, Kaufman JL, Fitch WP 3rd. Deep dorsal vein arterialization in arteriogenic impotence: use of the dorsal artery as a neoarterial source. *Int J Impot Res* 1995; **7**:157–64.

15 Lizza EF, Zorgniotti AW. Experience with the long-term effect of microsurgical penile revascularization. *Int J Impot Res* 1994; **6**:145–52.

16 Da Ros CT, Teloken C, Antonini CC, Sogari PR, Souto CA. Long-term results of penile vein ligation for erectile dysfunction due to cavernousal disease. *Tech Urol* 2000; **6**:172–4.

17 Popken G, Katzenwadel A, Wetterauer U. Long-term results of dorsal penile vein ligation for symptomatic treatment of erectile dysfunction. *Andrologia* 1999; **31**:77–82.

18 Schultheiss D, Truss MC, Becker AJ et al. Long-term results following dorsal penile vein ligation in 126 patients with veno-occlusive dysfunction. *Int J Impot Res* 1997; **9**:205–9.

19 Berardinucci D, Morales A, Heaton JP, Fenemore J, Bloom S. Surgical treatment of penile veno-occlusive dysfunction. Is it justified? *Urology* 1996; **47**:88–92.

20 Hassan AA, Hassouna MM, Elhilali MM. Long-term results of penile venous ligation for corporeal venous occlusion. *Can J Surg* 1995; **38**:537–41.

21 Vale JA, Feneley MR, Lees WR, Kirby RS. Venous leak surgery: long-term follow-up of patients undergoing excision and ligation of the deep dorsal vein of the penis. *Br J Urol* 1995; **76**:192–5.

22 Kim ED, McVary KT. Long-term results with penile vein ligation for venogenic impotence. *J Urol* 1995; **153**:655–8.

23 Stief CG, Djamilian M, Truss MC, Tan H, Thon WF, Jonas U. Prognostic factors for the postoperative outcome of penile venous surgery for venogenic erectile dysfunction. *J Urol* 1994; **151**:880–3.

24 Hwang TI, Yang CR. Penile vein ligation for venogenic impotence. *Eur Urol* 1994; **26**:46–51.

25 Freedman AL, Costa Neto F, Mehringer CM, Rajfer J. Long-term results of penile vein ligation for impotence from venous leakage. *J Urol* 1993; **149**:1301–3.

26 Montague DK, Angermeier KW, Lakin MM, Ignaut CA. Penile venous ligation in 18 patients with 1 to 3 years of followup. *J Urol* 1993; **149**:306–7.

27 Wespes E, Delcour C, Preserowitz L, Herbaut AG, Struyven J, Schulman C. Impotence due to corporeal veno-occlusive dysfunction: long-term follow-up of venous surgery. *Eur Urol* 1992; **21**:115–19.

28 Austoni E, Colombo F, Mantovani F, Trinchieri A. Venous surgery in erectile dysfunction: therapeutic strategy and results. *Urol Int* 1992; **49**:63–8.

29 Gilbert P, Sparwasser C, Beckert R, Treiber U, Pust R. Venous surgery in erectile dysfunction. The role of dorsal-penile-vein ligation and spongiosolysis for impotence. *Urol Int* 1992; **49**:40–7.

30 Knoll LD, Furlow WL, Benson RC. Penile venous ligation surgery for the management of cavernosal venous leakage. *Urol Int* 1992; **49**:33–9.

31 Lue TF. Penile venous surgery. *Urol Clin North Am* 1989; **16**:607–11.

Surgery for impotence: penile prosthesis

This operation is exclusively aimed at improving the patient's erectile function. Patients need to be aware they will probably experience penile shortening; restoration of the full natural erection length is not possible and the procedure is irreversible. In some countries it can be financially prohibitive because of lack of reimbursement.

Two major types of prosthesis exist: malleable (semi-rigid) or inflatable. Malleable prostheses are silicone elastomer rods which are placed in the corpora cavernosa and orientated by the patient according to needs (Fig. 12.2). Examples include AMS 600–650 and the Mentor Acuform.

Inflatable implants include two- and three-piece prostheses. The only two-piece implant is the Ambicor, where inflatable cylinders are implanted into the corpora cavernosa and a single pump placed in the scrotum (Fig. 12.3). Three-piece prostheses have an additional reservoir which is placed in the laterovesical space or intraperitoneally (Fig. 12.4). Examples are AMS 700CX, 700 Ultrex, and Mentor Titan. Three-piece implants coated with antibiotics (InhibiZone, AMS) or a hydrophilic substance (Resist, Mentor) have recently been introduced to attempt to reduce the infection risk.

Selection of the appropriate device for any one individual is based on the patient's preference, the cost of the device, and surgeon preference.

Indications[1,2]

- Patients with erectile dysfunction who fail to achieve a satisfactory response to non-surgical treatments.
- Need to have an irreversible organic cause of erectile dysfunction.
- Post-priapism with non-responsive erectile dysfunction.

Relative contraindications[1,2]

- Spinal cord injury (increased risk of infection and prosthetic erosion).
- Diabetes mellitus (controversial increased risk of infection).
- Pre-existing infection.
- Genital lesions, bleeding scars, dermatitis.

The last two can be treated and the prosthetic surgery re-dated following resolution.

Immediate pre-operative preparation

- Five days povidone iodine genital scrub preoperatively.
- Genital shave.
- Prophylactic IV antibiotics: gentamicin 240 mg plus cefuroxime 1.5 g or vancomycin 1 hr before and for 48 hr post-operatively followed by ciprofloxacin (500 mg twice daily) for 7–10 days.
- TED stockings.
- Minimize traffic in theatre (reduces infection risk).
- 14Fr Foley urethral catheterization (protects and helps identify urethra throughout procedure).

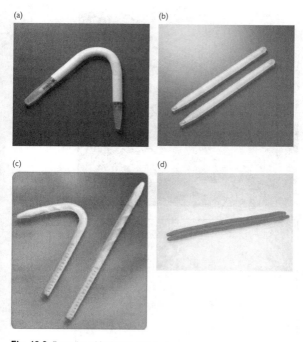

Fig. 12.2 Examples of four semi-rigid devices.

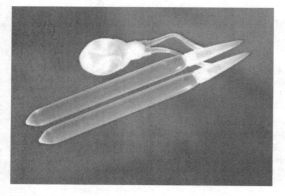

Fig. 12.3 Two-piece device (Ambicor).

(a)

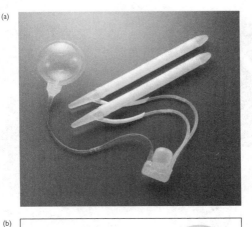

(b)

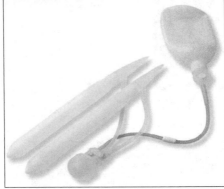

Fig. 12.4 Three-piece devices.

Patient positioning
Supine with arms by side.

Operative technique
Malleable prosthesis
A infrapubic, scrotal, or subcoronal approach can be used (with no clear advantage for any). Expose the tunica albuginea and incise laterally, extending for 2.5–4 cm with scissors. With a subcoronal incision the corporotomy is started distally 2–3 cm from the edge of the glans and extended proximally. With scrotal or infrapubic incisions, the most proximal aspect of the corporotomy is 6–7 cm from the crural end.

Dilate the corpus cavernosum cavity. Hegar or Rossello dilators can be used. In patients who have had priapism-induced fibrosis, fibrosis secondary to prosthesis infection, fibrosis secondary to Peyronie's disease, or fibrosis secondary to intracavernosal injections, it is sometimes necessary to use a smaller Hegar dilator, an optical urethrotome, or sharp dissection. Dilatation needs to be performed carefully. At the crural end, the dilator needs to abut on the ischial tuberosity as this is the most common site of intra-operative perforation. At the glans, the dilator tip needs to be advanced laterally, allowing proper placement of the cylinder and avoiding an SST deformity. Urethral perforation can occur with aggressive dilatation distally or in patients with distal corporal fibrosis. Dilatation is generally straightforward, and problems should alert the surgeon to incorrect plane, cross-over into the adjacent corpora, or perforation. Place corporeal closure sutures at this stage, although not tied as this allows easier and safer closure for inflatable devices. A Furlow cylinder inserter or other measuring cylinder is then used to measure the diameter and length of the corpus cavernosa. If the length falls between two prostheses, use the shorter one. Irrigate the corporeal spaces with antibiotic solution. Place a cylinder of appropriate length into the relevant corporeal space. Rear tip extenders are advised as these allow intracavernosal adjustment if required. Malleable devices are most easily placed by putting the crural tip in first. Close the corporotomies and skin with 4–0 Vicryl. Tape the penis to the lower abdomen for comfort.

Remove the urethral catheter several hours post-operatively. Attempts can be made at intercourse 4–6 weeks post-operatively if the wounds have healed adequately

Inflatable prosthesis

The same incision and approach is used as for the malleable prosthesis.

Inflatable devices have a placement tool incorporating a suture attached to a Keith needle (which is placed through the glans). This aids their insertion into the corpora. If the inflatable cylinder has attached tubing, direct exit from the corpora at the connection site is advised. Corporotomies are closed as for the malleable prosthesis.

Place the reservoir/pump or reservoir in a space created in the subdartos scrotum using the index finger or a Hegar dilator. Prior to placement irrigate the space with antibiotic solution. The tubing from each cylinder to the pump can be separated using sutured tissue as this may reduce tubing-to-tubing wear.

Placement of the suprapubic reservoir in three-piece inflatable devices requires a space created behind the rectus muscle. This is achieved via a midline vertical incision in the rectus fascia and creation of the space under direct vision behind the rectus muscle preitoneally. An alternative is to puncture the inguinal canal floor via the superficial inguinal ring and dilate the space behind the rectus muscle with the aid of a long-nose nasal speculum. It is important to create an adequate space for the reservoir or auto-inflation via entrapment can occur. This can be achieved by placing the reservoir in the space, filling it to 5 mL above its capacity via a connected syringe, and leaving the tubing open to the filling syringe. The syringe should spontaneously fill to 5 mL. If it fills by more than this, the reservoir position needs to be checked and the space expanded so that no more than 5 mL drains. The Mentor prosthesis now contains a lock-out valve which prevents reservoir auto-inflation. With the reservoir in place and filled, the tubing is shod clamped and the rectus fascia closed with 0 Vicryl. Make the appropriate connections between the three pieces of tubing. Release the shods and inflate and deflate the device several times to ensure correct function. Then leave it in the deflated state. Close the skin with 4–0 Vicryl. Follow similar post-operative measures as for the malleable prosthesis.

First inflate the device 4–6 weeks following surgery.

Outcomes and complications[3–22]

Crural perforation occurs in <1% in uncomplicated cases. Proximal perforations can be repaired via a separate perineal direct closure. The other cylinder can still be placed and the device left deflated for 6 weeks. If a distal perforation occurs on the first side of dilatation, the procedure should be abandoned and rescheduled at least 6 weeks later. If the patient already has severe distal corporeal scarring or a history of a previous distal perforation, a catheterized diverting perineal urethrostomy or suprapubic vesicostomy is created. The perforation is then repaired via a circumcision-like incision. The patient is put on broad-spectrum antibiotics for 3 weeks and a retrograde urethrogram is performed prior to definitive removal of the catheter. If the distal perforation occurs at dilatation of the second corpora, the injury should be repaired. The options are then to place the cylinder on the non-ruptured side together with a urinary diversion or abandon the procedure and irrigate both corpora via a fenestrated drain with the antibiotic solution every 4 hr for 2 days. The first option will prevent corporeal fibrosis on the side that the cylinder is placed. The antibiotic solution also decreases the subsequent fibrosis.

Penile implant surgery carries the highest success rate for treatment of erectile dysfunction: 70–76% for malleable devices and 79–92.5% for three-piece devices. Failure rates (mechanical or otherwise) between 1.3% (enhanced Mentor Alpha-1) and 9% (AMS CX) have been reported. Infections occur in 0.6–8.9%, increasing to 10% in diabetic patients and 21% after pelvic trauma with urethral injury. Salvage protocols allow these infections to be managed acutely, salvaging the prosthesis in selected cases. Erosion is reported in 5% (and is most common in patients with loss of distal penile sensation secondary to spinal cord injury/diabetes or irradiation).

Positional problems including inadequate cylinder length with SST deformity, high-riding pump/reservoir, and pump or kinked reservoir neck have been reported.

References

1 Montague DK, Jarow JP, Broderick GA et al. Chapter 1: The management of erectile dysfunction: an AUA update. J Urol 2006; **174**:230–9.

2 European Association of Urology Guidelines. Arnhem: European Association of Urology, 2006.

3 Zermann DH, Kutzenberger J, Sauerwein D et al. Penile prosthetic surgery in neurologically impaired patients: long-term followup. J Urol 2006; **175**:1041–4.

4 Mulcahy JJ. Crural perforation during penile prosthetic surgery. J Sex Med 2006; **3**:177–80.

5 Minervini A, Ralph DJ, Pryor JP. Outcome of penile prosthesis implantation for treating erectile dysfunction: experience with 504 procedures. BJU Int 2006; **97**:129–33.

6 Carson CC. Penile prosthesis implantation: surgical implants in the era of oral medication. Urol Clin North Am 2005; **32**:503–9.

7 Brinkman MJ, Henry GD, Wilson SK et al. A survey of patients with inflatable penile prostheses for satisfaction. J Urol 2005; **174**:253–7.

8 Abouassaly R, Montague DK. Penile prosthesis coating and the reduction of postoperative infection. Curr Urol Rep 2004; **5**:460–6.

9 Rahman NU, Carrion RE, Bochinski D, Lue TF. Combined penile plication surgery and insertion of penile prosthesis for severe penile curvature and erectile dysfunction. J Urol 2004; **171**:2346–9.

10 Carson CC. Diagnosis, treatment and prevention of penile prosthesis infection. Int J Impot Res 2003; **15**(Suppl 5):S139–46.

11 Montague DK, Angermeier KW. Surgical approaches for penile prosthesis implantation: penoscrotal vs infrapubic. Int J Impot Res 2003; **15**(Suppl 5):S134–5.

12 Mulhall JP, Ahmed A, Branch J et al. Serial assessment of efficacy and satisfaction profiles following penile prosthesis surgery. J Urol 2003; **169**:1429–33.

13 Montague DK, Angermeier KW, Lakin MM. Penile prosthesis infections. Int J Impot Res 2001; **13**:326–8.

14 Montague DK, Angermeier KW. Penile prosthesis implantation. Urol Clin North Am 2001; **28**:355–61.

15 Carson CC, Mulcahy JJ, Govier FE. Efficacy, safety and patient satisfaction outcomes of the AMS 700CX inflatable penile prosthesis: results of a long-term multicenter study. AMS 700CX Study Group. J Urol 2000; **164**:376–80.

16 Montorsi F, Rigatti P, Carmignani G et al. AMS three-piece inflatable implants for erectile dysfunction: a long-term multi-institutional study in 200 consecutive patients. Eur Urol 2000; **37**:50–5.

17 Mulcahy JJ. Long-term experience with salvage of infected penile implants. J Urol 2000; **163**:481–2.

18 Jhaveri FM, Rutledge R, Carson CC. Penile prosthesis implantation surgery: a statewide population based analysis of 2354 patients. Int J Impot Res 1998; **10**:251–4.

19 Garber BB, Marcus SM. Does surgical approach affect the incidence of inflatable penile prosthesis infection? Urology 1998; **52**:291–3.

20 Govier FE, Gibbons RP, Correa RJ, Pritchett TR, Kramer-Levien D. Mechanical reliability, surgical complications, and patient and partner satisfaction of the modern three-piece inflatable penile prosthesis. Urology 1998; **52**:282–6.

21 Dubocq F, Tefilli MV, Gheiler EL et al. Long-term mechanical reliability of multicomponent inflatable penile prosthesis: comparison of device survival. Urology 1998; **52**:277–81.

22 Evans C. The use of penile prostheses in the treatment of impotence. Br J Urol 1998; **81**:591–8.

Surgical treatment for Peyronie's disease

Surgery is offered to correct the penile deformity when the disease has stabilized or to insert a penile prosthesis in those with erectile dysfunction that has been resistant to oral, injection, or vacuum therapy.[1] Most patients opt for a Nesbit type procedure or a grafting technique. Dorsal deformities <45° are often manageable without surgery. Lesser degrees of ventral or lateral deformity, due to penetration difficulties, are more often corrected surgically. These patients need assessment with an IIEF questionnaire, photographic documentation of the deformity from home, or combined injection and stimulation in the outpatient department. Following injection, colour Doppler can be used to assess the collaterals between cavernosal artery and the deep dorsal vein in cases of dorsal curvature.

Nesbit's procedure

Described in 1965.[2] Aims to shorten the long side of the penis by excising an ellipse of tunica at the most prominent part of the curvature.

Indications[1]

- Simple dorsal/lateral/ventral penile curvatures <60°.
- Difficulty/inability to penetrate due to curvature ± pain on penetration.

Absolute contraindications[1]

- Pre-existing erectile dysfunction not responsive to pro-erectile agents.
- Hourglass deformity or hinge effect.

Relative contraindications[1]

- Small penis where loss of length from surgery is critical (minimum of 13 cm on concave side when erect recommended to proceed with Nesbit's procedure).

Immediate pre-operative preparation

- TED stockings.

Patient positioning

- Supine with hands by side.

Operative technique[2]

Make a circumglanular incision. Deglove the foreskin down to the base of the penis. Perform an artificial erection test as follows. Apply a rubber tourniquet to the base of the penis. Insert a large butterfly needle into one of the corpora and infuse normal saline to create the erection. Note the point of maximum curvature and release the tourniquet. Incise Buck's fascia opposite the maximal curvature point. If the corpus spongiosus or dorsal vascular pedicle is on this line it needs to be carefully elevated off the corpora. Mark out the Nesbit ellipse. Excise 1 mm of ellipse width for each 10° of deformity. Close the defect with 0 polydioxanone suture (or 2–0 Vicryl/dexon) with the knots on the inner aspect. Repeat the artificial erection to check on the straightening.

Outcomes and complications[3-6]

- In patients with normal erections satisfaction rates are high (67–100%) with successful penile straightening in 79–91%. In those with erectile problems this drops to 74–77%.
- The overall complication rate is 17%, including urethral injury (1.4%), urinary retention (1.4%), UTI (0.6%), wound infection (2.2%), haematoma (5.3%), suture granuloma (0.6%), painful sutures (0.2%), glans numbness (1.9%), and paraphimosis (1.1%). Circumcision is now recommended to avoid paraphimosis.
- Recurrent or persistent significant deformities (>30°) occur in 10.6%. Failures occur due to suture breakage, ligatures which are too tight, or problems arising from use of absorbable sutures.
- Significant penile shortening (>2 cm) is seen in 4.7%, with some shortening reported in 17.4–100%.
- Secondary operations (re-do Nesbit's procedure (1.7%) and prosthesis insertion (1.7%)) have been reported.

Alternative approaches

Numerous variations on the Nesbit's procedure have been described. These include a simple plication technique rather than excising the ellipse of corpora.[7,8,9] This technique relies on the strength of suture used, and several rows of non-absorbable sutures are probably required to achieve durable results similar to those obtained with Nesbit's procedure. Yachia[8] described making longitudinal incisions opposite the point of maximal curvature and closing them transversely with effective straightening. However, Yachia's technique requires extensive dissection of the neurovascular bundle. Donatucci and Lue[10] modified this to avoid neurovascular bundle dissection. The tunica albuginea on the opposite side to the curvature is grasped with an Allis clamp to achieve straightening and two plication sutures are placed not more then 0.5 cm apart between the bites of the Allis clamp. The artificial erection test is repeated to check the degree of correction.

Compared with the standard Nesbit procedure, plication has lower success rates of 57–91% because of the higher rates of recurrent deformity (probably due to suture failure).[1,11]

Lue procedure

Indications[1]

- Dorsal/lateral/ventral penile curvatures <60°.
- Difficulty/inability to penetrate due to curvature ± pain on penetration.
- 'Hourglass' penile deformity or hinge effect.

Absolute contraindications[1]

- Pre-existing erectile dysfunction not responsive to pro-erectile agents.

Relative contraindications[1]

- Pre-existing erectile dysfunction particularly in veno-occlusive dysfunction and arterial insufficiency.

Immediate pre-operative preparation

- TED stockings.

Patient positioning
- Supine with hands by side.

Operative technique
Incise the penile skin and deglove as in Nesbit's procedure. Mobilize Buck's fascia and isolate the dorsal neurovascular bundle. Isolate the plaque and incise an H-shape in the plaque. Harvest a long saphenous vein graft and suture endothelial side down into the H-shaped defect. Repeat the artificial erection test and use further patches or plication sutures to maximize penile straightening.

Outcomes and complications[12–14]
- Penile straightening is reported in 67–96%, and some shortening in 0–40%.
- Decreased potency is seen in 5–12%.
- The operation has greater morbidity than Nesbit's procedure because of additional dissection and the vein harvesting. Commercially available autologous grafts can reduce this morbidity but long-term results are awaited. Other autologous grafts such as dermis, fascia lata, tunica vaginalis/albuginea, temporal fascia, buccal mucosa, rectus sheath and muscular aponeurosis have been tried but do not have any obvious advantages over saphenous vein.

Penile prostheses[15–17]

This is the treatment of choice for men with Peyronie's and erectile dysfunction that has not responded to oral, injection, or vacuum therapy. The Mentor Alpha-1 and AMS CX700 prostheses have narrow cylinders which facilitates their insertion in the scarred corpora of patients with Peyronie's disease. This makes them the prosthesis of choice in these circumstances. Eighty per cent of patients will achieve penile straightening from the dilatation and prosthesis insertion. Those patients with persistent curvature can be improved by modelling. This process involves grasping the penis and bending it over inflated cylinders at the maximum curvature point. The deflection is maintained for 90 sec and repeated if necessary. Modelling success is reported in >85%. In those who fail, plaque incision may be required.

References

1 Levine LA, Lenting EL. A surgical algorithm for the treatment of Peyronie's disease. *J Urol* 1997; **158**:2149–52.
2 Nesbit RM. Congenital curvature of the phallus: report of three cases with description of corrective operation. *J Urol* 1965; **93**:230–2.
3 Savoca G, Sciera F, Pietropaolo F et al. Straightening corporoplasty for Peyronie's disease: a review of 218 patients with median follow up of 89 months. *Eur Urol* 2004; **46**:610–14.
4 Ralph DJ, al-Akraa M, Pryor JP. The Nesbit operation for Peyronie's disease: 16 year experience. *J Urol* 1995; 4:1362–3.
5 Daitch JA, Angermeier KW, Montague DK. Modified corporoplasty for penile curvature: long term results and patient satisfaction. *J Urol* 1999; **162**:2006–9.
6 Rehman J, Benet A, Minsky LS et al. Results of surgical treatment for abnormal penile curvature: Peyronie's disease and congenital deviation by modified Nesbit plication. *J Urol* 1997; **157**: 1288–91.
7 Lemberger RJ, Bishop MC, Bates CP. Nesbit's operation for Peyronie's disease. *Br J Urol* 1984; **56**:721–3.
8 Yachia D. Corporal plication for surgical correction of Peyronie's disease. *J Urol* 1993; **149**:869.
9 Gholami SS, Lue TF. Correction of penile curvature using the 16-dot plication technique: a review of 132 patients. *J Urol* 2002; **167**:2066–9.
10 Donatucci CF, Lue TF. Correction of penile deformity assisted by intracavernous injection of papaverine. *J Urol* 1992; **141**:1108–10.
11 Schultheiss D, Meschi MR, Hagemann J et al. Congenital and acquired penile deviation treated with the Essed placation method. *Eur Urol* 2000; **38**:167–71.
12 El-Sakka AI, Rashwan HM, Lue TF. Venous patch graft for Peyronie's disease. Part II: Outcome analysis. *J Urol* 1998; **160**:2050–3.
13 Kalsi J, Minhas S, Christopher N et al. The results of plaque incision and venous grafting (Lue procedure) to correct the penile deformity of Peyronie's disease. *BJU Int* 2005; **95**:1029–33.
14 Montorsi F, Salonia A, Briganti A et al. Five year follow up of plaque incision and vein grafting for Peyronie's disease. *J Urol* 2004; **171**:331.
15 Wilson SK, Delk JR, 2nd. A new treatment for Peyronie's disease: modelling the penis over an inflatable penile prosthesis. *J Urol* 1994; **152**:1121–3.
16 Carson CC. Penile prosthesis implantation in the treatment of Peyronie's disease and erectile dysfunction. *Int J Impot Res* 2000; **12**:122–6.
17 Wilson SK, Cleves MA, Delk JR, 2nd. Long-term follow up of treatment for Peyronie's disease: modelling the penis over an inflatable penile prosthesis. *J Urol* 2001; **165**:825–9.

Management of the neuropathic bladder

Innervation of the lower urinary tract

Motor innervation of the bladder

Parasympathetic motor innervation of the bladder

Pre-ganglionic parasympathetic nerve cell bodies are located in the intermediolateral column of spinal segments S2–4. These pre-ganglionic parasympathetic fibres pass out of the spinal cord through the anterior primary rami of S2, S3, and S4, and, contained within nerves called the nervi erigentes, they head towards the pelvic plexus. In the pelvic plexus (in front of the piriformis muscle) the pre-ganglionic parasympathetic fibres synapse, within ganglia, with the cell bodies of the post-ganglionic parasympathetic nerves which then run to the bladder and urethra. Half of the ganglia of the pelvic plexus lie in the adventitia of the bladder and bladder base (the connective tissue surrounding the bladder) and half are lie within the bladder wall. The post-ganglionic axons provide cholinergic excitatory input to the smooth muscle of the bladder.

Sympathetic motor innervation of the bladder

- In the male, pre-ganglionic sympathetic nerve fibres arise from the intermediolateral column of T10–12 and L1–2. These pre-ganglionic neurons synapse in the sympathetic chain, and post-ganglionic sympathetic nerve fibres travel as the hypogastric nerves to innervate the trigone, the blood vessels of the bladder, and the smooth muscle of the prostate and pre-prostatic sphincter (i.e. the bladder neck).
- In the female, there is sparse sympathetic innervation of the bladder neck, and urethra.
- In both sexes, some post-ganglionic sympathetic nerves also terminate in parasympathetic ganglia (in the adventitia surrounding the bladder and within the bladder wall) and exert an inhibitory effect on bladder smooth muscle contraction.

Afferent innervation of the bladder

- Afferent nerves from receptors throughout the bladder ascend with parasympathetic neurons back to the cord and from there up to the pontine storage and micturition centres or to the cerebral cortex. They sense bladder filling.
- Other receptors are located in the trigone, and afferent neurons from these neurons ascend with sympathetic neurons up to the thoracolumbar cord and thence to the pons and cerebral cortex.
- Other receptors are located in the urethra. The afferent neurons pass through the pudendal nerve and again ascend to the pons and cerebral cortex. All these neurons have local relays in the cord.

Somatic motor innervation of the urethral sphincter

The distal urethral sphincter mechanism

Anatomically this is located slightly distal to the apex of the prostate in the male (between the verumontanum and proximal bulbar urethra) and in the mid-urethra in the female. It has three components.

- Extrinsic skeletal muscle: this is the outermost layer, the pubo-urethral sling (part of levator ani). It is composed of striated muscle and is innervated by the pudendal nerve (spinal segments S2–4, somatic nerve fibres). It is activated under conditions of stress and augments urethral occlusion pressure.
- Smooth muscle within the wall of the urethra: cholinergic innervation, tonically active, relaxed by NO.
- Intrinsic striated muscle i.e. skeletal muscle *within* the wall of the urethra, hence known as the 'intrinsic rhabdosphincter'. It forms a U-shape around the anterior and lateral aspects of the membranous urethra and is absent posteriorly (i.e. it does not completely encircle the membranous urethra). It may produce urethral occlusion by kinking the urethra rather than by circumferential compression.

Pre-ganglionic *somatic* nerve fibres (i.e. neurons which innervate *striated* muscle) are, along with *parasympathetic* nerve fibres (which innervate the bladder), derived from spinal segments S2–4, specifically from Onuf's nucleus (also known as spinal nucleus X) which lies in the medial part of the anterior horn of the spinal cord (Onuf's nucleus is the location of the cell bodies of somatic motoneurons which provide motor input to the *striated* muscle of the pelvic floor—the external urethral and anal sphincters). These somatomotor nerves travel to the rhabdosphincter via the perineal branch of the pudendal nerve (documented by direct stimulation studies and horseradish peroxidase (HRP) tracing—HRP accumulates in Onuf's nucleus following injection into either the pudendal or the pelvic nerves). There also seems to be some innervation of the rhabdosphincter from branches of the pelvic plexus (specifically the inferior hypogastric plexus) via pelvic nerves. In dogs, complete silence of the rhabdosphincter is seen only if both the pudendal and pelvic efferents are sectioned. Thus pudendal nerve block or pudendal neurectomy does not cause incontinence.

The nerve fibres which pass distally to the distal sphincter mechanism are located in a dorsolateral position (5 and 7 o'clock). More distally, they adopt a more lateral position.

Sensory innervation of the urethra

Afferent neurons from the urethra travel in the pudendal nerve. Their cell bodies lie in the dorsal root ganglia, and they terminate in the dorsal horn of the spinal cord at S2–S4, connecting with neurons which relay sensory information to the brainstem and cerebral cortex.

The pudendal nerve, a somatic nerve derived from spinal segments S2–4, innervates striated muscle of the pelvic floor (levator ani, i.e. the pubo-urethral sling). Bilateral pudendal nerve block[1] does not lead to incontinence because of maintenance of internal (sympathetic innervation) and external sphincter function (somatic innervation: S2–4 nerve fibres travelling to the external sphincter alongside parasympathetic neurons in the nervi erigentes).

Clinical consequences of damage to the nerves innervating the LUT

Bladder neck function in the female

Approximately 75% of continent young women and 50% of peri-menopausal continent women have a closed bladder neck during the bladder filling phase. Twenty-five per cent of continent young women and 50% of peri-menopausal continent women have an open bladder neck and yet they remain continent because of their functioning distal sphincter mechanism (the external sphincter).[2,3] Presacral neurectomy (to destroy afferent pain pathways) does not lead to incontinence because of maintenance of the somatic innervation of the external sphincter.

Sympathetic motor innervation of the bladder

Division of the hypogastric plexus of nerves during a retroperitoneal lymph node dissection for metastatic testis tumours results in paralysis of the bladder neck. This is of significance during ejaculation, where normally sympathetic activity results in closure of the bladder neck so that the ejaculate is directed distally into the posterior and then anterior urethra. If the bladder neck is incompetent, the patient develops retrograde ejaculation; they remain continent of urine because the distal urethral sphincter remains functional, being innervated by somatic neurons from S2–4.

During pelvic fracture the external sphincter and/or its somatic motor innervation may be damaged, such that it is incompetent and unable to maintain continence of urine. Preservation of bladder neck function (the sympathetic innervation of the bladder neck usually remains intact) can preserve continence. However, if in later life the patient undergoes a TURP or bladder neck incision for symptomatic prostatic obstruction, they may well be rendered incontinent because their one remaining sphincter mechanism (the bladder neck) will be divided during these operations.

Further reading

1 Gosling JA, Dixon JS. Structure of the bladder and urethra. In *Textbook of Genitourinary Surgery*, ed. Whitfield HN, Hendry WF, Kirby R, Duckett J. Oxford: Blackwell Science, 1998, p 456.

References

1 Brindley GS. The pressure exerted by the external sphincter of the urethra when its motor nerve fibres are stimulated electrically. *Br J Urol* 1974; **46**:453–62.
2 Chapple CR Helm CW, Blease S, Milroy EJ, Rickards D, Osborne JL Asymptomatic bladder neck incompetence in nulliparous females. *Br J Urol* 1989; **64**:357–9.
3 Versi E *et al.* Distal urethral compensatory mechanisms in women with an incompetent bladder neck who remain continent and the effect of the menopause. *Neurourol Urodyn* 1990; **9**:579–90.

The physiology of urine storage and micturition

Urine storage

During bladder filling, bladder pressure remains low despite a substantial increase in volume. The bladder is thus highly *compliant*. Its high compliance is due partly to the elastic properties (viscoelasticity) of the connective tissues of the bladder and partly to the ability of detrusor smooth muscle cells to increase their length without any change in tension. The detrusor is able to do this as a consequence of prevention of transmission of activity from pre-ganglionic parasympathetic neurons to postganglionic efferent neurons, a so-called 'gating' mechanism within the parasympathetic ganglia. In addition, inhibitory interneuron activity in the spinal cord prevents transmission of afferent activity from sensors of bladder filling.

Micturition

A spino-bulbar–spinal reflex, coordinated in the pontine micturition centre (PMC) in the brainstem (also known as Barrington's nucleus or the M region), results in simultaneous detrusor contraction, urethral relaxation, and subsequent micturition. Receptors located in the bladder wall sense increasing *tension* as the bladder fills (rather than stretches). This information is relayed by afferent neurons to the dorsal horn of the sacral cord. Neurons project from here to the peri-aqueductal grey matter (PAG) in the pons. Thus the PAG is informed about the state of bladder filling. The PAG and other areas of the brain (limbic system, orbitofrontal cortex) input into the PMC and determine whether it is appropriate to start micturition.

At times when it is appropriate to void, micturition is initiated by relaxation of the external urethral sphincter and pelvic floor. Urine enters the posterior urethra and this, combined with pelvic floor relaxation, activates afferent neurons which result in stimulation of the PMC. Activation of the PMC switches on a detrusor contraction via a direct communication between neurons of the PMC and the cell bodies of parasympathetic pre-ganglionic motoneurons located in the sacral intermediolateral cell column of S2–4. At the same time that the detrusor contracts, the urethra (the external sphincter) relaxes. The PMC inhibits the somatic motoneurons located in Onuf's nucleus (the activation of which causes external sphincter contraction) by exciting GABA- and glycine-containing, inhibitory neurons in the intermediolateral cell column of the sacral cord, which in turn project to the motoneurons in Onuf's nucleus. In this way, the PMC relaxes the external sphincter.

Micturition is an example of a positive feedback loop; the aim is to maintain bladder contraction until the bladder is empty. As the detrusor contracts, tension in the bladder wall rises. The bladder wall tension receptors are stimulated and the detrusor contraction is driven harder. One of the problems of positive feedback loops is their instability. Several inhibitory pathways exist to stabilize the storage–micturition 'loop.'

- Tension receptors activate bladder afferents, which via the pudendal and hypogastric nerves inhibit S2–4 parasympathetic motor nerve output. An ongoing detrusor contraction cannot be overridden.
- Afferents in the anal and genital regions and in the distribution of the posterior tibial nerve stimulate inhibitory neurons in the sacral cord, and these neurons inhibit S2–4 parasympathetic motor nerve output. This pathway can override an ongoing detrusor contraction. It is hypothesized that this system prevents involuntary detrusor contraction during sexual activity and defecation, and while walking, running, and jumping.

Excitatory neurotransmission in the normal detrusor is exclusively cholinergic, and reciprocal relaxation of the urethral sphincter and bladder neck is mediated by NO released from post-ganglionic parasympathetic neurons.

Further reading

1 De Groat WC. Anatomy and physiology of the lower urinary tract. *Urol Clin North Am* 1993; **20**:383–401.

Bladder and sphincter behaviour in the patient with neurological disease

A variety of neurological conditions are associated with abnormal bladder and sphincter function, e.g. spinal cord injury (SCI), spina bifida (myelo-meningocele), and multiple sclerosis (MS). The bladder and sphincters of such patients are described as 'neuropathic.'

They may have abnormal bladder function or abnormal sphincter function, or more usually both. The bladder may be over- or underactive, as may the sphincter, and any combination of bladder and sphincter over- or underactivity may coexist. 'Activity' here means bladder and sphincter pressure.

In the normal lower urinary tract, the detrusor muscle is inactive and the sphincter pressure is high during bladder filling. Therefore bladder pressure is low and the high sphincter pressure maintains continence. During voiding, the sphincter relaxes and the detrusor contracts. This leads to a short-lived increase in bladder pressure, which is sustained until the bladder is completely empty. Thus the detrusor and sphincter function in synergy: when the sphincter is active the detrusor is relaxed (storage phase), and when the detrusor contracts the sphincter relaxes (voiding phase).

An overactive bladder intermittently contracts during bladder filling, thus developing high pressures when normally bladder pressure should be low. Between these waves of contraction, bladder pressure returns to normal or near normal levels. In a patient with an underlying neurological problem bladder overactivity is called detrusor hyper-reflexia (DH). In other patients the bladder wall is stiffer than normal, a condition known as poor compliance. Bladder pressure rises progressively during filling, as such bladders are unable to store urine at low pressures. Some patients have a combination of DH and poor compliance. The other end of the spectrum of bladder behaviour is the underactive bladder, in which pressure is low during filling and voiding. This is called detrusor areflexia.

An overactive sphincter generates high pressure during bladder filling, but it also does so during voiding, when normally it should relax. This is known as detrusor–external sphincter dyssynergia (DSD or DESD) (Fig. 13.1). During EMG recording, activity in the external sphincter increases during attempted voiding (the external sphincter should normally be 'quiet' during voiding) (Fig. 13.2). An underactive sphincter is unable to maintain enough pressure, in the face of normal bladder pressures, to prevent leakage of urine.

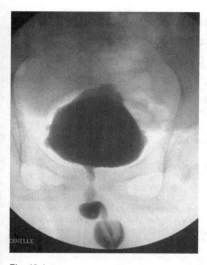

Fig. 13.1 Detrusor–external sphincter dyssynergia seen during video-cystourethrography. Reproduced from Reynard *et al.* 2006, *Oxford Handbook Urology* with permission Oxford University Press.

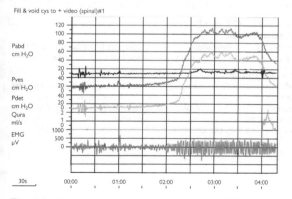

Fig. 13.2 Filling and voiding cystometry in a patient with DSD. Reproduced from Reynard *et al.* 2006, *Oxford Handbook Urology* with permission Oxford University Press.

The neuropathic lower urinary tract: clinical consequences of storage and emptying problems

Neuropathic patients experience two broad categories of problem, bladder filling and bladder emptying problems, depending on the *balance* between bladder and sphincter pressures during filling and emptying. The effects of these bladder filling and emptying problems include incontinence, retention, recurrent UTIs, and renal failure.

High-pressure sphincter

High-pressure bladder

If the bladder is overactive (detrusor hyper-reflexia) or poorly compliant, bladder pressures during filling are high. The kidneys have to function against these chronically high pressures. Hydronephrosis develops and ultimately the kidneys fail (renal failure). At times the bladder pressure overcomes the sphincter pressure and the patient leaks urine (incontinence). If the sphincter pressure is higher than the bladder pressure during voiding (DSD), bladder emptying is inefficient (retention, recurrent UTIs).

Low-pressure bladder

If the bladder is underactive (detrusor areflexia), pressure during filling is low. The bladder simply fills up—it is unable to generate enough pressure to empty (retention, recurrent UTIs). Urine leaks at times if the bladder pressure becomes higher than the sphincter pressure (incontinence), but this may occur only at very high bladder volumes or not at all.

Low-pressure sphincter

High-pressure bladder

If the detrusor is hyper-reflexic or poorly compliant, the bladder will only be able to hold small volumes of urine before leaking (incontinence).

Low-pressure bladder

If the detrusor is areflexic, such that it cannot develop high pressures, the patient may be dry for much of the time. However, they may leak urine (incontinence) when abdominal pressure rises, e.g. when coughing, rising from a seated position, or transferring to or from a wheelchair. Their low bladder pressure may compromise bladder emptying (recurrent UTIs).

Bladder management techniques

A variety of techniques and procedures are used to treat retention, incontinence, recurrent UTIs, and hydronephrosis in the patient with a neuropathic bladder. Each of the techniques described below can be used for a variety of clinical problems. Thus a patient with a high pressure, hyperreflexic bladder which is causing incontinence can be managed with ISC (with intravesical Botox injections if necessary) or a suprapubic catheter, or by sphincterotomy with condom sheath drainage, or by deafferentation combined with a sacral anterior root stimulator (SARS). Precisely which option the patient chooses will depend on their individual clinical problem, their hand function, their lifestyle, and other personal factors such as body image, sexual function, etc. Some patients will opt for a suprapubic catheter, as a simple, generally safe, and generally very convenient and effective form of bladder drainage. Others wish to be free from external appliances and devices, because of an understandable desire to look and feel normal. They might opt for deafferentation with a SARS.

Intermittent self catheterization (ISC)

📖 See p. 26, 720.

Indwelling catheters

📖 See p. 26, 720.

Intravesical botulinum toxin injections

Botulinum-A neurotoxin (Botox) is produced by *Clostridium botulinum*, a Gram-positive anaerobic spore-producing bacterium. It is synthesized as a single-chain polypeptide with a molecular weight of 150 kDa. This 'parent' chain is cleaved into an active two-chain polypeptide consisting of a heavy chain (100 kDa) and a light chain (50 kDa). It causes a temporary block of release of the neurotransmitter acetylcholine (ACh) from the presynaptic nerve terminals of parasympathetic neurons which innervate the detrusor (it has the same effect on skeletal muscle). It does so by cleaving a synaptosomal-associated protein of molecular weight 25 kDa (SNAP-25) which moves ACh-containing vesicles towards the presynaptic membrane. In so doing a flaccid muscle paralysis results and the effects of sudden uninhibited bladder contractions that are the pathophysiological basis of the overactive bladder are negated. Affected nerve terminals recover function by a process of axonal sprouting and formation of new synaptic contacts. This process takes months.

Botox has clinical effects (namely a reduction in the sensation of urgency) over and above that resulting from detrusor paralysis, i.e. it has both efferent and afferent effects. There is evidence that the afferent effects may be due to inhibition of release of neurotransmitters involved in sensory nerve pathways (including pain pathways), such as ATP and substance P.[1] These neurotransmitters are believed to be released from a suburothelial network of myofibroblasts and interstitial cells which may represent the site of the bladder stretch-receptor.

Bladder Botox injections increase bladder capacity, bladder volume at first hyperreflexic contraction, and bladder compliance in patients with neuropathic detrusor overactivity, and these urodynamic effects are believed to account, at least in part, for their clinical effect.[2,3]

Contraindications
• Peripheral motor neuropathy, e.g. amyotrophic lateral sclerosis.
• Neuromuscular junction disorders, e.g. myasthenia gravis.

Dosage
There are seven immunologically distinct forms of botulinum toxin: A, B, C, D, E, F, and G. Type A is the type used in urological disease. Two commercially available preparation of Botulinum-A neurotoxin are available: Botox®, (Allergan, Irvine, CA) and 'Dysport®' (Ipsen, Slough, UK). The minimum clinically effective dosage has not been determined, but in general terms a dose of 1000 units of Dysport or 200–300 units of Botox is used. The toxin comes in powder form and is dissolved in normal saline. The precise volume of saline is variably reported (5–20 mL). Vigorous shaking of the dissolved Botox should be avoided as this may cause dissociation of the heavy and light chains and reduce clinical efficacy.

Injection technique
Detrusor Botox injections can be administered under local, spinal, or general anaesthetic, depending on patient preference. A rigid or flexible cystoscope can be used. Two needle types are available: the Williams cystoscopic needle (Fig. 13.3a, b) and the Olympus needle (Fig. 13.4a, b). The latter must be stabilized within a flexible metal sheath (the needle does not have the rigidity to allow it to puncture the urothelium, and without the flexible metal sheath it bounces off the surface of the bladder). Both can be used in the rigid cystoscope, but only the Olympus needle is small enough to be used in the instrument channel of the flexible cystoscope.

Some surgeons avoid injecting in the region of the trigone. The rationale of this is to prevent relaxation of the ureter at the vesico-ureteric junction and thereby prevent reflux (there is no evidence base for this). Other surgeons do not bother with so-called trigonal sparing. There is no fixed number of injections. Anything between 20 and 40 injections have been reported.

Repeat injections can be performed once the beneficial effects have worn off. This may be many months or as a long a year.

It has been suggested that aminoglycoside antibiotic prophylaxis or treatment should be avoided in patients undergoing Botox injections because of its inhibitory effects on transmission at the neuromuscular junction. We routinely use gentamicin for prophylaxis and in our experience of over 1000 Botox injections, we have had three cases of generalized weakness lasting for a few months.

(a)

(b)

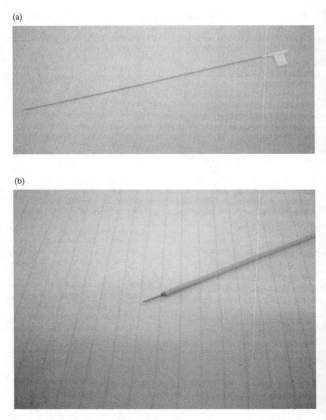

Fig. 13.3 (a) The Williams cytoscopic needle; (b) Close up of the tip of the needle.

(a)

(b)

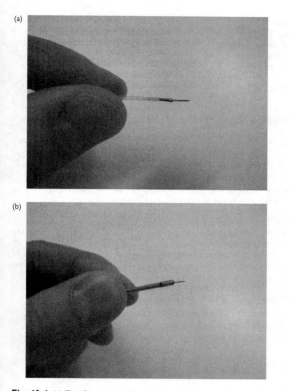

Fig. 13.4 (a) The Olympus needle; (b) The Olympus needle contained within the flexible injection sheath that stabilises the needle, thereby allowing it to puncture the bladder wall.

Side-effects
- Potential systemic side-effects include generalized weakness (upper and/or lower extremity), blurring of vision, and difficulty swallowing.[4] These may last many months.
- Allergic reaction.
- Influenza-like reaction.
- Urinary retention: this is clearly of no consequence for those patients who are already doing intermittent self-catheterization and are having Botox injections because of inter-catheter incontinence. For the non-neuropathic patient with detrusor overactivity, the risk of retention is on the order of 2 in 10. The patient should be warned that this may necessitate ISC several times daily, until the effect of the Botox wears off (which may be many months).
- Transient erectile dysfunction.
- Respiratory compromise.

Neutralizing antibodies to Botox may form and this may impact on the efficacy of bladder Botox injections ('immunoresistance').[5]

Other applications of botulinum toxin

Botulinum toxin is used to treat detrusor sphincter dyssynergia (so-called medical sphincterotomy) where this is causing hydronephrosis or recurrent urinary infections due to inefficient bladder emptying or episodes of autonomic dysreflexia.[5] We use a transurethral approach with a Williams cystoscopic needle to allow adequate penetration of toxin into the sphincter. Others have used a transperineal approach. Some surgeons use electromyographic (EMG) guidance.

References

1 Apostolidis A, Dasgupta P, Fowler CJ. Proposed mechanism for the efficacy of injected botulinum toxin in the treatment of human detrusor overactivity. *Eur Urol* 2006; **49**:644–50.
2 Reitz A, Stohrer M, Kramer G et al. European experience of 200 cases treated with botulinum-A toxin injections into the detrusor muscle for urinary incontinence due to neurogenic overactivity. *Eur Urol* 2004; **45**:510–15.
3 Schurch B, de Seze M, Denys P et al. Botulinum toxin type A is a safe and effective treatment for neurogenic urinary incontinence: results of a single treatment, randomized, placebo controlled 6-month study. *J Urol* 2005; **174**:196–200.
4 Wyndaele JJ, van Dromme SA. Muscular weakness as side-effect of botulinum toxin injection for neurogenic detrusor overactivity. *Spinal Cord* 2002; **40**:599.
5 Schurch B, Hauri D, Rodic B et al. Botulinum-A toxin as a treatment of detrusor-sphincter dyssynergia: a prospective study in 24 spinal cord injury patients. *J Urol* 1996; **155**:1023.

External sphincterotomy

This is deliberate division of the external sphincter to convert the high-pressure, poorly emptying bladder due to DSD to a low-pressure, efficiently emptying bladder.

Indications
- Detrusor-sphincter dysynergia causing urinary retention.
- Recurrent UTIs.
- Hydronephrosis.
- Vesico-ureteric reflux (VUR) secondary to high bladder pressures.
- Autonomic dysreflexia.

Techniques
Surgical

A Collings knife is used to make an anterior incision at 11, 12, or 1 o'clock, beginning at the level of the proximal part of the veru montanum and extending distally into the corpus spongiosum of the bulbar urethra. The anteromedian (as opposed to a 6 o'clock) incision is thought to reduce the risk of heavy bleeding and erectile dysfunction. The depth of incision is difficult to gauge. Some surgeons recommend that the incision is continued until the plane of the periurethral venous sinuses is reached.[1] This plane becomes self-evident when heavy bleeding is encountered. In anticipation of the potential problem of post-operative clot retention, leave a 22 Ch irrigating catheter for 24–48 hr.

An Nd:YAG laser can be used as an alternative to a Collings knife. There are no randomized controlled trials comparing blood loss in conventional and laser sphincterotomy.

Outcomes of surgical external sphincterotomy[2]

'Success' is defined according to the indication for sphincterotomy.
- Resolution of hydronephrosis or VUR: 70–80%.
- Reduction in frequency of or complete resolution of UTIs: 75%.
- Reduction in frequency or complete resolution of autonomic dysreflexia: 90%.

Failure of sphincterotomy
- Occurs in 15–40% of reported cases: may be due to inadequate sphincterotomy (balance of risks between heavy bleeding and cutting deep enough to achieve the desired effect), detrusor hypocontractility resulting in inefficient bladder emptying (can cause persistent UTIs where this was the indication for sphincterotomy), or urethral stricture.
- Management: repeat sphincterotomy or division of stricture, or alternative management (e.g. suprapubic catheter).

Consequences and side-effects
- Irreversible.
- Post-operative bleeding: 10% need blood transfusion and/or return to theatre.
- Permanent loss of erection: 7%.
- Septicaemia.
- Stricture formation: 3–13%.
- Many patients with DSD have enough continence to allow them to shower, dry themselves, and apply a condom sheath without leaking. Warn them that they may lose this control after a sphincterotomy.

Intra-sphincteric Botox (botulinum toxin)
Increasingly popular because it is minimally invasive and reversible. Precise 'targeting' of the zone of highest pressure within the membranous urethra (i.e. of the external sphincter) can be difficult, and this may account for variable outcomes.

Disadvantages
- Repeat injection required every 6–12 months.
- Careful monitoring of the kidneys for developing hydronephrosis is necessary.

Alternatives to sphincterotomy
- Oral or sublingual NO donor (e.g. nifedipine, glyceryl trinitrate). NO is a neurotransmitter which relaxes the external sphincter. Hypothesized as a treatment for DSD, and preliminary studies support this hypothesis.[3,4]
- Urethral stents (UroLume Wallstent, Memotherm): a randomized trial of the UroLume Wallstent versus sphincterotomy showed approximately equivalent outcomes in terms of reduction of maximum detrusor pressure and residual urine volume,[5] resolution of hydronephrosis and autonomic dysreflexia, and fall in haemoglobin. Encrustation over the long term and stent migration into the bladder are concerns.

References
1 Mundy AR. Incisions and exposure. In *Urodynamic and reconstructive surgery of the lower urinary tract*, ed. Mundy AR. Edinburgh: Churchill Livingstone 1996, p 36.
2 Reynard JM, Vass J ,Sullivan M, Mamas MA. Sphincterotomy and the treatment of detrusor–sphincter dyssynergia: current status, future prospects. *Spinal Cord* 2003; **41**:1–11.
3 Mamas MA, Reynard JM, Brading AF. Augmentation of external sphincter nitric oxide: a potential pharmacological treatment for detrusor-external sphincter dyssynergia in spinal cord injury. *Lancet* 2001; **357**:1964–7.
4 Reitz A, Knapp PA, Müntener M, Schurch B. Oral nitric oxide donors: a new pharmacological approach to detrusor–sphincter dyssynergia in spinal cord injured patients. *Eur Urol* 2004; **45**: 516–20.
5 Chancellor MB, Bennett C, Simoneau AR et al. Sphincteric stent versus external sphincterotomy in spinal cord injured men: prospective randomized multicenter study. *J Urol* 1999; **161**:1893–8.

Augmentation

Augmentation is the technique of increasing bladder volume to lower pressure by implanting detubularized small bowel into the bivalved bladder ('clam' ileocystoplasty) or by removing a disk of muscle from the dome of the bladder (auto-augmentation or detrusor myectomy). Indications are incontinence and hydronephrosis. There has been a substantial reduction in the use of augmentation with the advent of intravesical Botox injections.

📖 See also Augmentation cystoplasty, p. 710.

Deafferentation

Division of dorsal spinal nerve roots of S2–4, to convert the hyper-reflexic, high pressure bladder into an areflexic, low pressure one. Can be used where the hyper-reflexic bladder is the cause of incontinence or hydronephrosis. Bladder emptying can subsequently be achieved by ISC or implantation of a nerve stimulator placed on the ventral roots (efferent nerves) of S2–4 to 'drive' micturition when the patient wants to void—this is known as the Brindley sacral anterior root stimulator (SARS) (a pager-sized externally applied radiotransmitter activates micturition) (Fig. 13.5, Fig. 13.6). This is also useful for DSD/incomplete bladder emptying causing recurrent UTIs and retention.

Bladder neck closure

Bladder neck closure, with long-term bladder drainage via a suprapubic catheter, is an option for the patient with persistent leakage of urine per urethra, despite the presence of a suprapubic catheter, who does not want to have or is not fit for an ileal conduit. It may also be necessary for female patients whose bladder has been managed by a long-term urethral catheter, which by a pressure effect has led to urethral and bladder neck erosion, leading to a patulous urethra. Bladder neck closure is irreversible and access to the bladder via the suprapubic track is not always easy, particularly if access to the ureteric orifices is required for upper tract endoscopy.

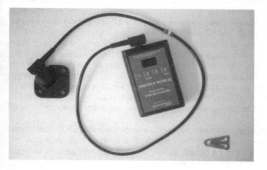

Fig. 13.5 The external nerve stimulator. Reproduced from Reynard et al. 2006, *Oxford Handbook Urology*, with permission Oxford University Press.

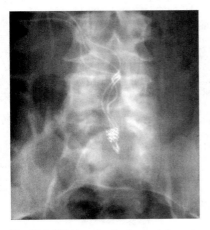

Fig. 13.6 KUB X-ray showing the sacral electrodes, positioned on the ventral roots of S2, S3, and S4. Reproduced from Reynard et al. 2006, *Oxford Handbook of Urology*, with permission Oxford University Press.

Techniques in women
Vaginal approach
Lithotomy position. Suture the labia out of the way. Place an Ovid's retractor in the vagina to allow exposure of the anterior vaginal wall. Place a traction suture through the external urethral meatus. Applying traction to this, make a circumferential incision around the urethra (Fig. 13.7). Get into the plane between the urethra and vagina and develop this to free the urethra from the vagina as far as the bladder neck. Anteriorly, divide the endopelvic fasica and work your way upwards in the retropubic space towards the bladder neck. The pubo-urethral ligament will be found within this space, and this must be divided using sharp dissection so that the urethra can be fully mobilized up to the bladder neck. If the urethra remains tethered by this ligament, it cannot be invaginated into the bladder. Excess urethra may be removed, thus shortening the length of urethra to be invaginated into the bladder. It is then inverted into the bladder using a series of sutures (or several purse-string sutures) to oversew it. The peri-urethral fascia is approximated with absorbable sutures.

Alternatively an inverted U-flap of anterior vaginal wall can be raised off the posterior aspect of the urethra. The urethra is dissected in the retropubic space as described above, divided, and invaginated into the bladder. The anterior vaginal wall flap can then be used as an additional layer to secure the closure.

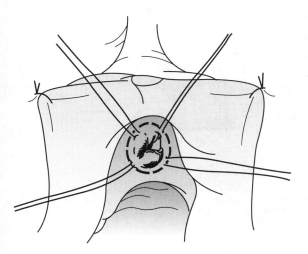

Fig. 13.7 Bladder neck closure: vaginal approach. A circumferential incision is made around the urethra.

Transvesical approach
Low midline or Pfannenstiel incision. Divide the pubo-urethral ligament. Dissect the urethra free from the underlying vagina (a finger in the vagina is helpful). Once it is free, divide the urethra and ligate its distal end with a 3–0 absorbable suture (Fig. 13.8). Open the bladder in the midline. Insert ureteric catheters to identify and protect the ureters. Make a circumferential incision around the bladder neck and excise a circular disk of bladder neck (Fig. 13.9). Invaginate the urethra into the bladder (Fig. 13.10). Excess urethra can be removed and the end oversewn. A purse-string suture can be used to close the bladder neck (Fig. 13.11) or alternatively simply close the opposing edges of the bladder in two layers.

Persistent leakage of urine is due to the development of a vesicovaginal fistula (caused by breakdown of the wound).

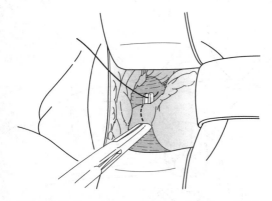

Fig. 13.8 Bladder neck closure: bladder approach. The urethra is mobilized, divided, and ligated.

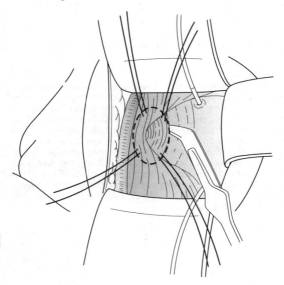

Fig. 13.9 Bladder neck closure: bladder approach. A circumferential incision is made around the bladder neck and a circular disk of bladder neck is excised.

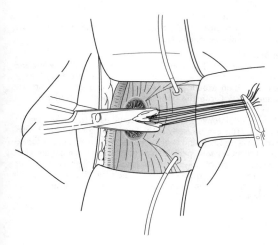

Fig. 13.10 Bladder neck closure: bladder approach. The urethra is invaginated into the bladder.

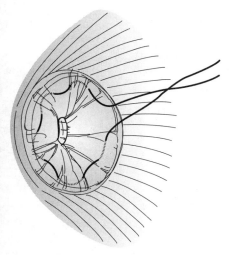

Fig. 13.11 Bladder neck closure: bladder approach. The urethra is invaginated into the bladder.

Alternative to bladder neck closure

A tension-free vaginal tape (TVT), tightened more than normally, may achieve an acceptable level of continence.

Techniques in men

Low midline or Pfannenstiel incision. Open the bladder in the midline and insert ureteric catheters to identify and protect the ureters. Make a circumferential incision around the bladder neck and excise a circular disk of bladder neck. Close the opposing edges of the bladder in two layers.

A pedicled rectus abdominis muscle flap can be used to protect against fistula formation.[1] This can be easily mobilized into the pelvis on an inferior epigastric artery pedicle and avoids the need to enter the peritoneal cavity to mobilize an omental pedicle in a patient who is almost certainly frail and disabled. Many of these patients have lower limb contractures such that it is difficult or impossible to abduct their legs to allow harvesting of a Martius graft. In this situation a rectus abdominis pedicle is much more easily harvested.

References

1 McGrath JS, MacDermott SP. Use of a pedicled rectus abdominis muscle flap to protect against fistula formation after bladder neck closure. *BJU Int* 2005; **95**:450–1.

Cystoplasty

There are two types of cystoplasty:
- Augmentation.
- Substitution.

Augmentation cystoplasty: rationale

- Designed to increase bladder capacity and thereby lower bladder pressures in patients with high bladder pressures secondary to detrusor hyper-reflexia or poor compliance. These patterns of bladder dysfunction are common in patients with neurological conditions such as spinal cord injury or spina bifida.
- Designed to ameliorate the effects of sudden uninhibited bladder contractions in patients with idiopathic bladder overactivity (formerly called detrusor instability). 'Idiopathic' in this context means that there is no overt neurological disease.

In the neuropathic patient with detrusor hyper-reflexia or poor bladder compliance, the raised bladder pressures, often combined with high external sphincter pressures, lead to incontinence and/or high pressure reflux. In the absence of treatment, the latter leads to renal failure. In the non-neuropathic patient with bladder overactivity, the uninhibited bladder contractions lead to urgency and urge incontinence.

Indications

Neuropathic bladder
- High-pressure bladder causing hydronephrosis and/or incontinence. In the case of poor compliance, the 'classic' bladder pressure above which impairment of kidney function and long-term renal damage are likely is 40 cm H_2O (the 'McGuire leak point pressure').[1]
- Where medical therapy (anticholinergic drugs) or minor surgical therapy (intravesical botulinum toxin injections) combined with ISC has failed to lower bladder pressures sufficiently to result in resolution of hydronephrosis or achievement of continence.

Non-neuropathic bladder
- Persistence of frequency, urgency, or urge incontinence after medical or minor surgical therapy (anticholinergics, intravesical botulinum toxin injections, sacral neuromodulation (Interstim implant)) for detrusor instability (bladder overactivity).
- To increase bladder capacity in conditions such as chronic interstitial cystitis, TB, and radiation cystitis, and thus to ameliorate the symptoms of marked urinary frequency that occur with such conditions.

Diagnostic work-up

Most, if not all, patients with abnormal bladder function and in whom a cystoplasty is being contemplated as a treatment option (e.g. neuropathic patients or those with idiopathic bladder overactivity) will undergo urodynamics prior to a decision being made about whether or not cystoplasty is indicated.

Substitution cystoplasty: rationale and indications

- Designed to replace the bladder with a reservoir made from bowel in (usually) patients undergoing cystectomy for bladder cancer or interstitial cystitis (see p. 257).

Alternatives to augmentation cystoplasty

Before the advent of intravesical botulinum toxin injections (and to a lesser extent the Medtronic Interstim), the patient with bladder overactivity who had failed to respond to anticholinergics had no other treatment option than an augmentation cystoplasty. The same was true for the neuropathic patient with DH-induced urinary incontinence. Intravesical botulinum toxin is increasingly being used as a minimally invasive option for such patients. Although it has not been compared with augmentation in a randomized study (and it is difficult to imagine that such a trial could ever be done, or indeed needs to be done), it seems to be effective in resolving urgency and urge incontinence in a substantial proportion of patients. Understandably, many patients prefer a minimally invasive option such as botulinum toxin injections to major surgery, even if the former is only a temporary treatment and regular repeat injections are required.

Alternative surgical options to augmentation cystoplasty are autoaugmentation, ileal conduit urinary diversion, and continent urinary diversion.

Contraindications to cystoplasty

- Renal function that is not adequate to cope with urine absorption (some say that enterocystoplasty is contraindicated if creatinine clearance is <40 mL/min).
- Inability to perform ISC. Bladder pressure will often be so effectively lowered that the patient will be unable to empty their bladder other than by ISC.

Augmentation ileocystoplasty

Pre-operative preparation

Arrange for the patient to be trained in ISC techniques. Bowel preparation is not necessary (unless you anticipate that large bowel may be used for the augmentation, e.g. an ileocaecocystoplasty). Latex allergy is common in patients with spina bifida; use non-latex products for those with known allergies.

The procedure is carried out under general anaesthesia. Give antibiotic prophylaxis and anti-thromboembolic prophylaxis which will usually be AK-TEDs with subcutaneous heparin or intermittent pneumatic compression boots.

Catheterize the patient using a reasonably large two-way Foley catheter (e.g. 16Ch). This will provide post-operative drainage of urine. A small catheter is more easily blocked with mucus produced by the small intestine. Connect the two-way catheter via a giving set to a sterile 1 L bag of water. Keep the inlet control within the sterile field so that you can control the flow of water into the bag and thus inflate and deflate the bladder at appropriate times during the operation (with the bag elevated above the bladder to inflate it and positioned below the patient to deflate it).

Operative technique

Midline transperitoneal incision (some surgeons prefer a Pfannenstiel incision, but others find that this gives poor access for bowel mobilization) (Fig. 13.12). Mobilize a piece of ileum, in theory at least 20 cm from the ileocaecal junction, but in reality whatever piece will come down easily into the pelvis without tension on the loop. Isolate a segment of ileum 20–25 cm long and re-anastomose the bowel, above the isolated loop, with your preferred method of small bowel anastomosis.

Swing the isolated loop down into the pelvis. Check that it will reach without tension. If there is tension, make small incisions in the cut edges of the mesentery to lengthen this. Wash any small bowel contents out of the segment of ileum using a 50 mL bladder syringe. Detubularize the loop. Start this by placing two stay sutures at each end of the isolated loop (Fig. 13.12). Leave a large enough gap between the stay sutures to allow you to cut between them. Detubularization is made easier by passing the sucker through the lumen of the bowel and cutting along the antimesenteric border of the bowel onto the sucker. Clean the bowel with saline in a kidney dish (avoid spilling bowel contents into the peritoneal cavity).

Now divide the bladder between two stay sutures in the midline (sagittal) or, alternatively, in a coronal plane. It does not matter which as long as an adequate length of the bladder is divided such that the two halves of the bladder cannot produce a coordinated contraction. The key to this part of the procedure is to use multiple stay sutures (e.g. 3–0 vicryl). Inflate the bladder with water via the pre-positioned urethral catheter. Control the inflow until the bladder is well distended. Place three pairs of stay sutures along the intended line of the incision: one pair at the dome, one pair anteriorly, and one pair posteriorly. For a sagittal incision start at the dome and work anteriorly to within about a centimetre of the bladder neck and posteriorly to a roughly equivalent point. Use the diathermy blade for the incision, cutting between the paired stay sutures, so that you end up with three stays on either side of the incision. These stay sutures help hold the bladder open while the bowel is anastomosed to the bladder. Consider placing infant feeding tubes into the ureters to identify their position and avoid damaging them during the bowel to bladder anastomosis.

Bring the ileal patch down into the pelvis. Make sure that its vascular pedicle is not twisted. Some surgeons prefer to configure the ileal patch into the shape of an inverted U, thus creating a cup which can be anastomosed to the bladder (Fig. 13.13). Others simply place the entire un-reconfigured ileal patch directly into the bivalved bladder. Anastomose the bowel to bladder with 3–0 vicryl starting on one side of the bladder and bowel (Fig. 13.14). Use two lengths of vicryl, one to work up the right side and one for the left side. Precisely where you start (front, middle, back) is up to you. I find it easier to start at the front and work backwards, completing a bit of the right side, then the left, then going back to the right, and so forth (the anterior part of the anastomosis is down a slightly deeper hole than the posterior part and therefore is slightly less accessible). Remove the stay sutures as you reach them. Lock

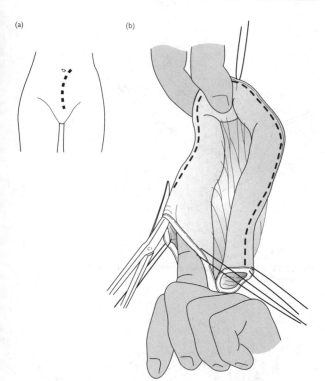

Fig. 13.12 (a) Midline incision (b) The isolated small bowel segment is detubularized.

every third stitch. Not infrequently the circumference of the bowel is greater than that of the bladder, so that you end up having to anastomose bowel to bowel to complete the closure.

Before you finish the closure place a 14Ch suprapubic catheter (silicone if latex-free procedure). Pass a clamp from inside to outside of the bladder and then through the skin. Grab the end of the Foley catheter with the clamp and pull the catheter into the bladder. Inflate the balloon (to stop it from falling out!). If possible, avoid passing the catheter through the bowel which has been anastomosed to the bladder; the bladder has a better blood supply than the bowel and therefore will heal very quickly once the suprapubic catheter is removed (there could be persistent

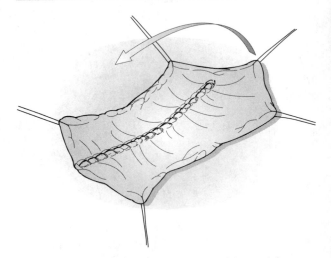

Fig. 13.13 The ileal patch has been configured into a 'U' shape ready for anastomosis onto the bladder.

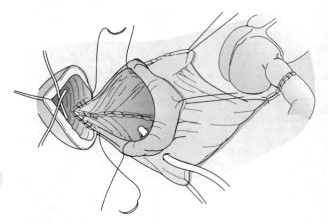

Fig. 13.14 The patch of ileum is anastomosed to the bladder.

leakage of urine through the suprapubic track if this was through bowel rather than bladder). Finish the bladder closure, taking care not to puncture the balloon with your needle.

Place a 10Ch tube drain down to the closure (avoid suction drains; the high pressure these exert will simply encourage urine to continue draining). Bring down some omentum, if possible, to cover the augmentation. Close the fascia and skin.

Post-operative care

Three daily bladder washouts (20 mL of normal saline per nursing shift change) to prevent accumulation of mucus. Ask for the urine output to be recorded every hour. This is to ensure that the catheters are flushed if the urine output falls below say 40 mL/hr. Overdistension of a recently performed cystoplasty because catheters are blocked by mucus will lead to rupture of your carefully performed suture line.

Remove the drain in 24–48 hr. Keep the patient nil by mouth, other than sips of water, for 3 days. Give clear fluids thereafter. Give food once they have passed flatus. Remove the suprapubic catheter on day 13 and the urethral catheter on day 14 (leaving the urethral catheter on drainage encourages the suprapubic puncture site to heal). Some surgeons are confident enough to remove the catheters on day 10; others prefer to wait a few extra days while others (the author included) like to get a cystogram prior to catheter removal to check for urine leaks.

Outcomes and complications

Only 50–60% of patients with idiopathic bladder overactivity undergoing ileocystoplasty report long-term symptomatic success.[2] Mortality is 0–3%; Mundy reports 0% mortality in 267 patients[2] but not all surgeons are able to mimic this outcome.

Early complications (all figures are approximate)

- Wound infection 5%.
- Pelvic abscess.
- Wound dehiscence.
- Re-operation for bleeding 0–3%.
- VP shunt infection 0–20%.
- Enterocutaneous fistula 1%.
- Pulmonary embolus 1%.

Late complications (all figures are approximate)

- *Nutritional* Diarrhoea due to an increased solute load being delivered to the colon as a consequence of decreased bile salt absorption in the ileum; vitamin A and D malabsorption; vitamin B_{12} deficiency.
- *Metabolic* hyperchloraemic metabolic acidosis and hypokalaemia are the classic metabolic abnormalities following ileocystoplasty and augmentation using colon[3] (this is the opposite problem to that encountered in augmentation using the stomach, where loss of chlorine and acid lead to hypochloraemic metabolic alkalosis). The hyperchloraemic metabolic acidosis and hypokalaemia result from active absorption of NaCl by the ileum with loss of bicarbonate and passive loss of potassium. In the presence of normal renal function compensatory mechanisms come into play.

- *Osteomalacia* Presents with lethargy and joint pains in weight-bearing joints. Likely to be multifactorial: chronic acidosis, excess calcium loss by the kidneys, vitamin D resistance (treat with active forms of vitamin D such as 1α-hydroxycholecalciferol).
- *Intestinal obstruction* due to adhesions (and less commonly volvulus or internal hernia). The lifetime incidence is said to be approximately 10%.[4] Adhesive small bowel obstruction requiring operation 3–6%.
- *UTI* is the most common problem over the long term.
- *Bladder rupture* due to trauma to the distended augmented bladder or can occur spontaneously. It is more likely to occur with ileocystoplasty when compared with other bowel segments used for cystoplasty. It has been described in 5–10% of patients, and can occur months or even years later.[5] Regular ISC (with a catheter interval of no longer than 4 hr) probably reduces the risk, presumably by limiting episodes of overdistension. Mucus obstruction may also be a causative factor. The presentation may include abdominal pain (with abdominal tenderness), poor urine output, abdominal distension, fever, and sepsis. In the neuropathic patient with diminished abdominal and pelvic sensation, pain may be absent and this may lead to delayed diagnosis. Thus any patient who has undergone an augmentation cystoplasty and who presents with fever, sepsis, or abdominal pain should undergo a cystogram to determine whether they have a bladder rupture. Exploration and repair is usually required.
- *Cancer* within the augmented bladder. While there is most definitely an increased risk of cancer in an intestine that is chronically in contact with urine *and* faeces (e.g. ureterosigmoidostomy),[6] the precise risk of cancer development in intestinal segments in contact with urine, but *not* faeces, is less clear. A variety of different histological tumour types have been reported in intestinal segments in urinary diversions and augmentations including, most commonly, adenocarcinomas (suggesting origin from the intestine rather than the bladder), but also squamous carcinomas, sarcomas, and transitional cell carcinomas.[7] Whether such tumours occur with an increased incidence is not known. Some say that there is no increased incidence of cancer in ileocystoplasties (over and above that of the normal incidence of tumours in the ileum),[8] whereas others suggest that there is an increased incidence. Even less certain is whether surveillance cystoscopy is warranted in this group of patients. Because the incidence of such cancers is low, it remains uncertain whether a cystoscopy surveillance policy enhances survival or simply diagnoses cancers at a stage when they cannot actually be cured.

Pregnancy and augmentation cystoplasty

There is an increased risk of urinary infection, but fetal and maternal outcomes are usually excellent. Vaginal delivery is safe and is preferred to Caesarian section because of the risk of injury to the clam cystoplasty during surgery. If a Caesarian section is needed, a classical approach rather than lower-segment Caesarean section is usually needed to avoid injury to the bowel mesentery, and ideally a urologist familiar with the patient's anatomy should be available.

Detrusor myectomy

This is an alternative to ileocystoplasty, with the advantage that it does not use bowel. As a consequence there is no potential for morbidity from the bowel anastomosis and the procedure can be carried out entirely extra-peritoneally. The avoidance of bowel also avoids the potential for metabolic complications.

Operative technique

Cystoscope the patient to exclude other pathology. Insert a 20 or 22Ch three-way catheter (in case of haematuria so that you can wash out the bladder and irrigate if necessary). Connect this to a 1 L bag of saline containing methylene blue, with the giving set sterile so that you can control it. Place the legs down.

Use a Pfannenstiel incision for access. Identify the junction between the bladder and the peritoneum. By a combination of sharp and blunt dissection separate the peritoneum from the dome of the bladder. During this dissection you will see the urachus. When enough length of this has been exposed clamp it, divide the urachus, and tie the umbilical end. Keep a clip on the bladder end for traction. Using the coagulating diathermy current at a low setting, circumscribe an inverted U-shape on the antero-superior bladder wall. Now, using Addson's scissors, divide the muscle fibres carefully until an area of underlying urothelium 'pouts' up (dilute methylene blue instilled into the bladder via the catheter helps to identify this), thus identifying the depth of the urothelium. Dissect the muscle off the urothelium very carefully, changing sides as necessary, using Addson's scissors to identify the plane between the muscle and the urothelium (Fig. 13.15). Remove the muscle posteriorly, behind the urachus, and continue down the lateral surfaces of the bladder and as far down anteriorly as you can. The flaps of tissue so created can be cut off with the diathermy probe and the cut edge oversewn with 3–0 vicryl.

Peri-operative perforations of the mucosa are very common, occurring in 50% of patients, whether neurogenic or non-neurogenic.[9,10] Close any holes in the mucosa with very fine (e.g. 6–0) absorbable suture material, using a small buttress of excised detrusor muscle to prevent the stitch cutting through the mucosa. Leakage stops with bladder drainage. If, at the end of the operation, the bladder does not leak when slowly distended, bladder cycling can start that evening (gentle expansion of the bladder with 100–150 mL of saline). If there is a leak, delay cycling for a couple of days. Peri-operative perforations do not seem to lead to an adverse symptomatic outcome.[9]

Once the diverticulum has been created, deflate the bladder. It will start to ooze a lot of blood. Control any obvious bleeders and apply Surgicel as necessary. Place a tube drain (e.g. 15Ch Easyview or 20Ch Robinson) through the belly of one rectus muscle, taking care to avoid the inferior epigastric vessels. Close the space between the two recti. Close the Pfannenstiel incision using PDS. Empty the bladder, do a gentle bladder washout, and connect the catheter to an hourly urobag.

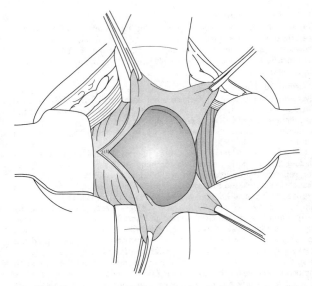

Fig. 13.15 Detrusor myectomy. The muscle of the bladder is dissected off the underlying urothelium.

Post-operative care

Check urine output hourly (so that the staff check that the bladder is not becoming overdistended), 48 hr IV antibiotics, gentle washouts with 60 mL saline every 8 hr. If the catheter blocks, gently wash out the bladder. If it remains blocked, change the catheter. Do not allow the bladder to become overdistended because of the risk of rupture.

If there have been no perforations during the operation, leave the catheter for 24–48 hr, removing it when the patient is mobile and able to get to the toilet. If the mucosa was breached and has been repaired, arrange a cystogram on day 7 and remove the catheter if there is no extravasation. Take the drain out a day later.

Outcomes and complications of detrusor myectomy

The outcomes are related to the indication for auto-augmentation: patients with idiopathic refractory detrusor overactivity have a greater chance of symptomatic improvement than patients with neurogenic voiding dysfunction.[9]

Eighty per cent of patients with idiopathic refractory detrusor overactivity report symptom improvement,[9] compared with just 33% of patients with neurogenic voiding dysfunction.

In patients with spinal cord injury:[10]

• In the early post-operative period hyper-reflexic contractions often require anticholinergics.

- Those with at least 6 month follow-up urodynamics show increase in maximal cystometric capacity from an average of 121 to 406 mL, increase in compliance from 6 to 30 mL/cmH$_2$O, decrease in maximum voiding capacity from 86 to 51 cmH$_2$O, and increase in post-void residual urine volume from 20 to 76 mL.
- 60% need post-operative ISC.
- Bladder rupture in 2% (probably secondary to the obstructive effect of an artificial urinary sphincter if inserted at the same time as or subsequent to the myectomy).
- Symptomatic outcome: some series report improvement in 90% of patients; others less. Symptomatic improvement may not occur for a year.

Ileocaecocystoplasty

The procedure is essentially the same as for ileocystoplasty, but the caecum is removed in continuity with the terminal ileum. Detubularize the whole length of the bowel, fold the ileum into the caecum, and suture it with with 3–0 vicryl, thereby creating a wide-necked cup of bowel (leave the appendix *in situ* if there is a possibility of later having to create a Mitrofanoff stoma). Check that the cup of bowel will come down to the bladder without tension. Divide the bladder in the sagittal plane from just proximal to the bladder neck to just proximal to the inter-ureteric bar, using bilateral ureteric catheters to identify and protect the ureters. Suture the cup of bowel onto the bladder using 3–0 vicryl, from within the bladder on the posterior and lateral walls and from outside anteriorly. Before closing the bladder place a 12Ch suprapubic catheter through the bladder wall, rather than the bowel (the bladder will heal very quickly when the catheter is removed; the bowel may not). Insert a 14Ch urethral catheter and wash out the bladder with saline. Inflate the augmented bladder to 200–300 mL to check for leaks and leave a 20Ch pelvic drain.

Further reading

1 Tomezsko JE, Sands PK. Pregnancy and intercurrent diseases of the urogenital tract. *Clin Perinatol* 1997; **24**:343–68.
2 McRae P, Murray KH, Nurse DE et al. Clam enterocystoplasty in the neuropathic bladder. *Br J Urol* 1987; **60**:523.

References

1 McGuire EJ, Woodside JR, Borden TA et al. Prognostic value of urodynamic testing in myelo-dysplastic patients. *J Urol* 1981; **126**:205.
2 Greenwell TJ, Venn SN, Mundy AR Augmentation cystoplasty. *BJU Int* 2001; **88**:511–25.
3 Nurse DE, Mundy AR. Metabolic complications of cystoplasty. *Br J Urol* 1989; **63**:165.
4 Aboseif SR, Carroll PR. Augmentation cystoplasty. In *Traumatic and reconstructive urology*, ed. McAninch JW. Philadelphia, PA: WB Saunders, 1996, pp 295–309.
5 DeFoor W, Tackett L, Minevich E et al. Risk factors for spontaneous bladder perforation after augmentation cystoplasty. *Urology* 2003; **62**:737–41.
6 Stewart M, MaCrae FA, Williams CB. Neoplasia and ureterosigmoidostomy: a colonoscopic survey. *Br J Surg* 1982; **69**:414.
7 Filmer RB, Spencer JR. Malignancies in bladder augmentations and intestinal conduits. *J Urol* 1990; **143**:671.
8 Nurse DE, Mundy AR. Assessment of the malignant potential of cystoplasty. *Br J Urol* 1989; **64**:489.
9 Kumar SPV, Abrams PH. Detrusor myectomy: long-term results with a minimum follow-up of 2 years. *BJU* 2005; **96**:341–4.
10 Stohrer M, Kramer G, Goepel M et al. Bladder autoaugmentation in adult patients with neurogenic voiding dysfunction. *Spinal Cord* 1997; **35**:456–62.

Catheters and condoms and the neuropathic patient

Many patients manage their bladders by intermittent catheterization (IC) done by themselves (intermittent self-catheterization (ISC)) or by a carer if their hand function is inadequate, as is the case with most tetraplegics. Many others manage their bladders with an indwelling catheter (urethral or suprapubic). Both methods can be effective for managing incontinence, recurrent UTIs, and bladder outlet obstruction causing hydronephrosis.

Some patients prefer the convenience of a long-term catheter. Others regard it as a last resort when other methods of bladder drainage have failed. The suprapubic route (suprapubic catheter (SPC)) is preferred over the urethral route because of pressure necrosis of the ventral surface of the distal penile urethra in men (acquired hypospadias—'kippering' of the penis) and pressure necrosis of the bladder neck in women, which increases in width until urine leaks around the catheter ('patulous' urethra) or frequent expulsion of the catheter occurs with the balloon inflated.

Catheter-related problems take up a substantial amount of district nursing time.[1] Many of the problems experienced by patients with neuropathic bladders who are managed by long-term catheterization are similar to those experienced by patients with long-term catheters but no neurological disease.

Recurrent urinary tract infection and manifestations of UTI

There is no strict definition of catheter-associated urinary tract infection (CAUTI). It has been variably defined as a patient with a urine culture with 10^5–10^8 CFU/mL with (one definition) or without (another definition) symptoms of infection (offensive cloudy urine, suprapubic pain, urgency, urethral burning on voiding, malaise, fever, headache, leucocytosis) in association. The problem for the neuropathic patient, particularly those with spinal cord injury, is that the symptoms which might ordinarily been taken as 'classic' symptoms of infection can be manifestations of wide-ranging conditions such as constipation and pressure sores. Thus, the classic symptoms of infection can occur in the presence of sterile urine, and conversely a patient with urine full of bacteria may remain perfectly well over the long term.

Thus there is no universally accepted definition of CAUTI. The presence of bacteriuria may simply represent colonization of the catheter with bacteria. The incidence of CAUTI varies widely depending on definition, and thus statements that CAUTI is the most common cause of nosocomial or hospital-acquired infection, accounting for over a million cases in US hospitals and nursing homes every year, must be interpreted with caution. What evidence there is suggests that CAUTIs are rarely symptomatic.[2]

Antimicrobial catheters have been developed with the aim of reducing the incidence of CAUTI. Some have a coating of an antibacterial, nitrofurazone. Others are coated with a silver alloy. In the short term (<30 days) they prevent or reduce the likelihood of bacteriuria in hospitalized patients. However, whether this translates into a reduction in symptoms or in the long-term complications of catheters (blockages, stones, other infective complications) remains doubtful.[3]

Recommendations
- Treat with antibiotics only when symptomatic (although as stated above establishing UTI as the cause of the symptoms can be difficult). Antibiotics may achieve clearance of bacteria from the urine over the short term, but long-term re-colonization is inevitable.
- Anecdotally, low-dose (prophylactic) antibiotics may help symptoms which are assumed to be due to CAUTI. Promotion of antibiotic-resistant strains is a concern.
- If you and the patient believe that their symptoms are due to recurrent UTI, consider changing the method of bladder management, if feasible.

Other manifestations of UTI
These include bladder stones, pyelonephritis, epididymitis, peri-urethral abscess, and septicaemia.[4,5]

Catheter blockages and the development of bladder stones are manifestations of CAUTI. CAUTI with urease-producing bacteria leads to a chronically elevated urinary pH. This provides the chemical environment in which calcium salts become insoluble. The combination of a biofilm build-up of bacteria with calcium salt deposition within the biofilm leads to catheter encrustation and ultimately catheter blockage.

Catheter blockages
Blockages caused by encrustation of the lumen of the catheter with bacterial biofilms are common.[6,7] *Proteus mirabilis*, *Morganella* spp and *Providencia* spp secrete a polysaccharide matrix. Within this matrix, urease-producing bacteria generate ammonia from nitrogen in urine, raising urine pH and precipitating magnesium phosphate and calcium phosphate crystals. The matrix–crystal complex blocks the catheter. Catheter blockage causes bypassing, which soils the patient's clothes. Bladder distension can cause autonomic dysreflexia, leading to extreme rises in blood pressure which can cause stroke and death! Regular bladder washouts and increased catheter size sometimes help. There is a suggestion, based on *in vitro* experiments on catheters in the laboratory, that intermittent catheter drainage (by using a valve inserted between the catheter and the drainage bag) can reduce the likelihood of catheter blockages. Whether this holds true in patients remains to be established.

Bladder stones
Stones necessitating surgical removal (cystolithotomy) develop in one in four patients over 5 years.[8]

Catheter bypassing either around the suprapubic site or per urethra
Management is empirical. Try as small a balloon size as possible. If the leakage is due to bladder spasms, a smaller balloon may reduce their intensity and frequency. Anticholinergics may help, as may intravesical Botox injections.

Cancer

There is conflicting evidence regarding the incidence of bladder cancer in spinal-cord-injured patients, with some studies suggesting an increased risk and others suggesting that the risk is the same as in the non-spinal-injured population.[9] Screening cystoscopy studies have either failed to result in a downstaging of bladder cancer when compared with non-screened patients or have simply not detected any cases of bladder cancer. Screening cystoscopy remains a subject of debate.[10]

Intermittent catheterization

This technique was popularized by Lapides.[11] It requires adequate hand function. The technique is 'clean' (simple handwashing prior to catheterization) rather than 'sterile'. Gel-coated catheters become slippery when in contact with water, thus providing lubrication. Usually done every 3–4 hr.

Problems

- Recurrent UTIs: review catheter technique to ensure that adequate drainage of the last few millilitres of urine is being achieved. Increase catheter frequency and consider catheterization once or twice in the middle of the night. Aim to keep each catheter volume <400 mLs to reduce frequency of UTIs.[12]
- Recurrent incontinence: check technique (adequate drainage of last few drops of urine). Suggest increasing frequency of ISC to minimize volume of urine in the bladder (reduces bacterial colonization and minimizes bladder pressure). If incontinence persists, consider intravesical botulinum toxin.

Condom sheaths

These are an externally worn urine collection device consisting of a tubular sheath applied over the glans and shaft of the penis (just like a contraceptive condom, only without the lubrication to prevent it slipping off!). Usually made of silicone rubber with a tube attached to the distal end to allow urine drainage into a leg bag. They are used as a convenient way of preventing leakage of urine, but are obviously only suitable for men. Detachment of the sheath from the penis is prevented by using adhesive gels and tapes. They are used for patients with reflex voiding (where the hyper-reflexic bladder spontaneously empties, and where bladder pressure between voids never reaches a high enough level to compromise kidney function). They are also used as a urine collection device for patients after external sphincterotomy (for combined detrusor hyper-reflexia and sphincter dyssynergia where incomplete bladder emptying leads to recurrent UTIs and/or hydronephrosis).

- Penoplasty for receding phallus to prevent dislodging of external urinary collecting device:
  - Catheterize.
  - Two circumferential incisions at 3 mm and 2.5 cm proximal to coronal sulcus, through skin.
  - Invert edges of this continuous isolated skin band and suture them together using fine absorbable suture. The ring can be secured to Buck's fascia with a few sutures.
  - Cover with the proximal penile skin.

Problems

The principle problem experienced by some patients is sheath detachment. In some cases a complete change of bladder management is required. Skin reactions sometimes occur.

References

1 Getliffe KA. The characteristics and management of patients with recurrent blockage of long-term urinary catheters. *J Adv Nurs.* 1994; **20**:140–9.

2 Tambyah PA, Maki DG. Catheter-associated urinary tract infection is rarely symptomatic. *Arch Intern Med* 2000; **160**:678–2.

3 Johnson JR, Kuskowski MA, Wilt TJ. Systematic review: antimicrobial urinary catheters to prevent catheter-associated urinary tract infection in hospitalized patients. *Ann Intern Med* 2006; **144**:116–26.

4 Warren JW, Muncie HL, Hebel JR, Hall-Craggs M. Long-term urethral catheterisation increases risk of chronic pyelonephritis and renal inflammation. *J Am Geriatr Soc* 1994; **42**:1286–90.

5 Stickler DJ, Zimakoff J. Complications of urinary tract infections associated with devices for long-term bladder management. *J Hosp Infect* 1994; **28**:177–94.

6 Stickler DJ, Jones GL, Russell AD. Control of encrustation and blockage of Foley catheters. *Lancet* 2003; **361**:1435–7.

7 Sabbuba NA, Stickler DJ, Long M et al. Does the valve-regulated release of urine from the bladder reduce the encrustation and blockage of indwelling catheters by crystalline *Proteus mirabilis* biofilms? *J Urol* 2005; **173**:26–6.

8 Ord J, Lunn D, Reynard J. Bladder management and risk of bladder stone formation in spinal cord injured patients. *J Urol* 2003; **170**:1734–7.

9 Subramonian K, Cartwright RA, Harnden P, Harrison SCW. Bladder cancer in patients with spinal cord injuries. *BJU Int* 2004; **93**:739–43.

10 Hamid R, Bycroft J, Arya M, Shah PJ. Screening cystoscopy and biopsy in patients with neuropathic bladder and chronic suprapubic indwelling catheters: is it valid? *J Urol* 2003; **170**:425–7.

11 Lapides J, Diokno AC, Silber SJ, Lowe BS. Clean intermittent self-catheterization in the treatment of urinary tract disease. *Trans Am Assoc Genitourin Surg* 1971; **63**:92–6.

12 Bakke A, Digranes A, Høisaeter. Physical predictors of infection in patients treated with clean intermittent catheterization: a prospective 7-year study. *BJU Int* 1997; **79**:85–90.

The artificial urinary sphincter

History

The artificial urinary sphincter (AUS) was introduced in 1973 by Brantley and Scott. The first generation (AS721) consisted of a cuff for implantation around the bulbar urethra in adult males or around the bladder neck in either sex, an inflation and a deflation bulb, and a zero-pressure reservoir designed to prevent urethral leakage which offset the effect of rises in abdominal pressure. A series of valves controlled pressure within the system. Various modifications followed, incorporating a pressure-regulating balloon to transfer a set pressure to the urethral cuff. The AS800, which is in current use, is the fifth model. It has been modified over the past 20 years (sutureless connectors, kink-resistant tubing, narrow back cuff), but the essential design has remained the same.

Indications

Incontinence:

- Following prostatectomy (after TURP or radical prostatectomy).
- In the neuropathic patient (spinal cord injury, spina bifida) because of intrinsic sphincter deficiency.
- Following trauma to the pelvis or perineum.

The precise management of sphincter weakness incontinence in the neuropathic patient depends on the 'balance' between bladder and sphincter behaviour, as assessed by urodynamics. In patients with a combination of detrusor hyper-reflexia and detrusor sphincter dyssynergia, the high-pressure sphincter is often able to achieve continence if bladder pressure can be lowered by anticholinergics (rarely), increased frequency of ISC (sometimes), intravesical botulinum toxin injections (often), bladder augmentation (usually), or sacral deafferentation (usually).

Where the patient has a combination of sphincter weakness and high-pressure bladder, as a general principle attempts to lower bladder pressure should be the first-line treatment. For those who remain wet despite these manoeuvres, a urethral bulking agent might occasionally help. In women a tension-free vaginal tape (TVT) may help. Where the patient does not wish to resort to a long-term suprapubic catheter, an artificial urinary sphincter is the next option.

The patient who is wet after radical prostatectomy or TURP may be so because of uninhibited bladder contractions, which may become manifest only once the prostatic obstruction has been relieved. Empirical treatment with anticholinergics might help, but if it does not a video-urodynamic assessment will establish whether or not the sphincter is weak.

Relative contraindications

- Poor bladder compliance: in some neuropathic patients with detrusor hyper-reflexia or poor bladder compliance, normal kidney function is maintained because of sphincter weakness which leads to incontinence (i.e. leak point pressure is low). Increased urethral resistance following AUS implantation can lead to a dangerous and silent elevation of bladder pressure, with the development of hydronephrosis. New transient hydronephrosis developed in 7% of 120 patients with neuropathic bladders (75% spina bifida, 16% spinal injury) who underwent AUS insertion, and new progressive hydronephrosis developed in 3%.[1]

- Untreated involuntary bladder contractions: the AUS is usually unable to achieve continence in this situation. As a general rule where a patient has bladder overactivity treat the bladder first (anticholinergics, Botox injections). Continence will be achieved in a proportion. If it is not, insert an AUS. For the neuropathic patient who is still wet, the next step is clam cystoplasty.
- Urethral stricture: if treatment of a stricture becomes necessary at some stage following AUS implantation, the cuff of the AUS could be damaged, e.g. the AUS cuff could have been incised by the knife of the optical urethrotome.
- Poor cognitive function such that the patient is unable to appreciate the need to deflate the cuff of the AUS several times a day, when the need to void arises.

Preparation prior to insertion

- Video-urodynamics (to assess bladder compliance and presence/absence of uninhibited contractions, and confirm presence of sphincter weakness incontinence). Usually not necessary in 'simple' post-radical prostatectomy patients without symptoms of urgency and urge-associated leakage. The cause of the incontinence is usually obvious from the characteristic history: 'I leak urine when I cough or get up from a seated position.'
- Flexible cystoscopy to exclude urethral stricture. Worth doing in all patients, but particularly those who have had a radical prostatectomy where there may be stricturing at the vesico-urethral anastomosis.
- Urine culture: ensure that the patient's urine is sterile by culturing the urine 3 weeks before to give time to treat any infection with an appropriate antibiotic.

Immediate pre-operative preparation

This is directed towards preventing the feared complication of device infection.

- If positive urine culture, commence an appropriate oral antibiotic about a week before hand to sterilize the urine (and thereby reduce the risk of device infection).
- Enema.
- Hibiscrub bath or shower twice (the night before and morning of operation).
- Antibiotic prophylaxis: this will be partly be determined by local hospital flora. Provide cover for Gram-negative bacteria and against staphylococcus infection. We use IV gentamicin 240 mg once daily plus Augmentin 1.2 g three times daily, commencing 24 hr before the operation, and load the patient with IV vancomycin 1 g, starting 1 hr before the call to theatre (infused over 1 hr). These IV antibiotics are continued for 48 hr post-operatively (total of four doses of vancomycin).

Operative technique

Focus on prevention of device infection:
- Shave in theatre.
- 10 min scrub with Hibiscrub followed by formal surgical prep.
- All staff hooded and masked.
- Limit theatre traffic.
- Consider double gloving and change outer gloves whenever you touch areas of potential bacterial contamination (e.g. urethral catheter).
- Catheterize the patient (we use a 16Ch catheter which assists with dissection around the bulbar urethra).
- An assistant liberally applies 5–10 mL aliquots of a gentamicin and vancomycin flush to the operative site throughout the procedure (gentamicin 240 mg plus vancomycin 1 g in 1 L of normal saline).

Evidence in the form of randomized trials to support this advice is lacking, but we adopt these methods on the basis of parallels from other fields of surgery (e.g. orthopaedic implant surgery) and because it seems intuitive to do everything reasonably possible to avoid the devastating complications of device infection.

A bulbar cuff is usually placed for post-radical prostatectomy incontinence and history of previous operations around the bladder neck or of pelvic fracture incontinence (both are associated with the potential for marked fibrosis around bladder neck, which increases the risk of rectal perforation).

A bladder neck cuff is placed for women (obviously), children (bulbar urethra is too small for the available cuffs), men who wish to maintain fertility by preserving antegrade ejaculation, and neuropathic patients where ISC is or may be required. ISC can safely be performed with an AUS provided that the cuff is placed around the more robust bladder neck and not the bulbar urethra which is thinner and more liable to perforation. Bladder neck placement is contraindicated with previous surgery around the bladder neck or previous pelvic trauma.

For the neuropathic bladder where you plan to do an augmentation cystoplasty and insert a sphincter the chance of infection may be higher than for insertion of a sphincter in the absence of an augmentation. Therefore in cases where it is anticipated that an AUS may be required in addition to an augmentation, and where for fear of device infection the surgeon decides not to place an AUS at the time of augmentation, consider placing an omental pedicle around the bladder neck, to limit the develop of fibrosis. If the patient is still incontinent despite the augmentation, subsequent dissection around the bladder neck may be easier in the presence of this omental 'wrap.'

Ask the patient whether they are right- or left-handed (which side of the scrotum or labia do they want the pump to be). Use the modified lithotomy position.

Choosing a balloon

A 61–70 cmH$_2$O pressure regulating balloon is usually adequate for bulbar urethral cuff placement. Flush all air bubbles out of the balloon and pump. A 71–80 cmH$_2$O balloon is usual for bladder neck cuff placement.

A higher-pressure balloon or a smaller cuff (or both) should be used for re-operation for urethral atrophy otherwise leakage through the urethra will occur (obviously higher-pressure balloons and tighter cuffs run the risk of subsequent re-atrophy). An alternative choice is to use the same pressure cuff but to go down 0.5 cm in size (i.e. from 4.5 to 4 cm). Use a lower-pressure balloon if there is considerable pelvic devascularization secondary to radiation or previous surgery. Clearly, the risk of persistent incontinence is higher.

Filling the components

The AMS 800 sphincter (Fig. 13.16) is made of semipermeable silicone elastomer (not latex) and therefore the filling fluid must be isotonic. Normal saline or a radiographic contrast medium can be used, but since isotonic contrast medium is not commercially available standard contrast solutions must be diluted with water (the sphincter comes with recommendations on the proportion of contrast solution to water). A 15 gauge needle is used for filling and a smaller 22 gauge needle for flushing the ends of the tubing so that debris (blood, fat) is not introduced into the system.

The capacity of the system (balloon + cuff) for a 4.5 cm cuff (the most common bulbar cuff size) is 22 mL. The cuff usually contains ~2 mL and the balloon ~20 mL. Some surgeons pressurize the cuff by initially filling the balloon with 22 mL of solution, connecting the balloon directly to the implanted cuff which has had all air removed) and allowing a minute or two for pressure equilibration. Other surgeons (Barrett) do not bother with pressurization for bulbar cuffs, but simply fill the balloon with 22 mL of solution and connect all the components.

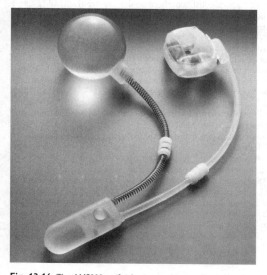

Fig. 13.16 The AMS800 artificial urinary sphincter. Reproduced courtesy of American Medical Systems UK Ltd.

For bladder neck cuffs, which are larger than the usual 4.5 cm bulbar cuff size, pressurization is required in order to fill the cuff with the correct volume of fluid. Fill the balloon with 22 mL of solution, connect it to the cuff, allow equilibration, and then disconnect the balloon. Empty it completely and refill with 20 mL of solution. For implantation of a Tandem cuff fill the balloon with 25 mL to allow for the extra volume of the extra cuff and tubing.

All the components should have the air removed from them. A syringe is required to do this for the balloon and cuff. Rubber-shod haemostats are used to clamp the tubing whenever disconnections are made to prevent air being sucked into the components. Close them by one ratchet only to avoid damage to the tubing. The cuff is positioned empty. Some surgeons position the balloon empty; others position it already filled.

Dissecting around the bulbar urethra, measuring for the cuff size, and placing the cuff

Pass a 12–16Ch catheter or sound to help identify the urethra. This can be left throughout the procedure (remove it temporarily for cuff pressurization if this is your preference).

Using a knife divide the skin with a midline perineal incision (Fig. 13.17). Pick up the subcutaneous fat with DeBakey forceps, tent it towards yourself, and using scissors cut down onto the urethra, dividing the bulbocavernosus muscles in the midline and dissecting them off the bulbous spongiosum until you are just superficial to the urethra (Fig. 13.18). Leave a layer of bulbocavernosus muscle overlying the urethra if you wish. Insert a ring retractor to help with exposure during this dissection (Fig. 13.19). Enter the plane behind the urethra, using a right-angled clamp to get around the urethra, and pass a tape around it to act as a retractor during subsequent mobilization. The best place to put the cuff is just proximal to the corpora cavernosa which can be seen as two bulging structures on either side of the urethra. The AMS 800 cuff is 2 cm long, so this length of urethra should be exposed. There is a natural tendency to expose a more distal section of urethra so try to make the periurethral dissection very posterior (Webster makes his dissection very posterior, proximal to the point where the corporal bodies bifurcate). Measure the circumference of the urethra with the cuff sizer; remove the catheter or sound first (Fig. 13.20). In most cases a 4.5 cm cuff is most appropriate. It is better for it to be too loose than too tight, as the latter will lead to tissue atrophy. At 4.5 cm the cuff will appear to be too loose, but unless this looseness is considerable a 4.5 cm cuff should be used. However, in a revision for atrophy a 4 cm cuff is more appropriate. Position the cuff (deflated) around the urethra so that the tubing is on the patient's right side (if they are right-handed). Once the cuff is in place, trim the tab. Cover the cuff with an antibiotic soaked swab.

Making the pre-vesical space pocket

Change your gloves so as not to contaminate the abdominal wound with bacteria from the perineum. Now make a pre-vesical space for the balloon through a transverse incision through the rectus fascia and through the belly of the right rectus itself. Insert a tube passer onto the end of the tubing from the cuff. Pass the tubing from the cuff from the perineal incision through to the pre-vesical pocket, making sure the cuff passer passes anterior to the pubic bone. Place a rubber-shod haemostat on the tubing to prevent air getting into the system.

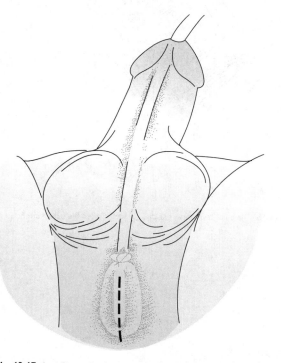

Fig. 13.17 A midline perineal incision is made to expose the bulbar urethra.

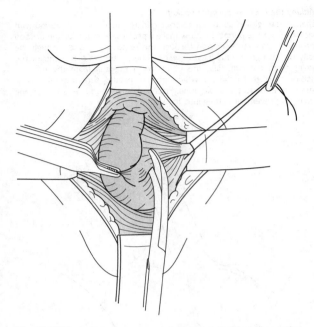

Fig. 13.18 The bulbocavernosus muscle is dissected off of the bulbar urethra.

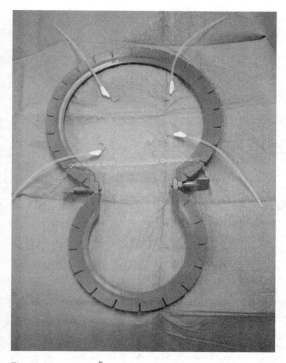

Fig. 13.19 A LoneStar® ring retractor is very helpful for exposing the bulbar urethra.

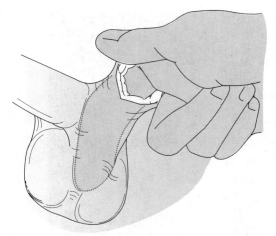

Fig. 13.20 The circumference of the bulbar urethra is measured with a cuff sizer.

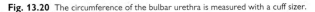

Positioning the balloon

Position the balloon in the prevesical pocket. Route the balloon tubing through the rectus muscle using a clamp or tubing passer. Close this pocket. Be particularly careful not to damage the balloon with the needle. Place the pump in a dartos pouch created in the scrotum or labia on the same side as the balloon. Avoid scissors in making this pouch; a finger or Hegar dilator is safer (Fig. 13.21). Orientate the pump so that the deactivation button is facing forwards. Hold the pump in the scrotum with Babcock forceps applied to the skin overlying the pump.

Connecting all the components

The *clear* tubing of the pump connects to the tubing from the *cuff*. The *black* tubing from the pump will connect to the *black* tubing from the *balloon*. Trim excess tubing with straight scissors which are used only for this purpose to avoid contaminating the tubing with blood. Then connect the pump to the balloon (black tubing, straight connector) and the pump to the cuff (clear tubing, right-angled connector). A connector ring (several small connector rings are found on a blue rod in the components tray) is slipped onto the ends of the tube to be connected. Flush the ends with fluid. The ends of the tubing are pushed into the connector (the

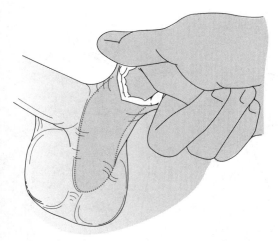

Fig. 13.21 A dartos pouch is created in the scrotum to accommodate the control pump.

ends of the tubing should be cut at right angles rather than bevelled to provide a really good fit). The connector rings are squeezed into the connector with the special clamp. The quick connect assembly tool will need to be used twice for right-angled connectors, once on each end of the connector. Close all the wounds in layers using absorbable sutures (Fig. 13.22).

Cycle the pump to check that fluid is flowing through the device. Now deactivate the device. Having squeezed the pump, let it refill by about half its full volume and then push the deactivation button. The pump will not fill any more if properly deactivated. If you deactivate the AUS without any fluid contained within it, it can be very difficult to reactivate it by 'blowing out' the deactivation valve when the time comes for activation.

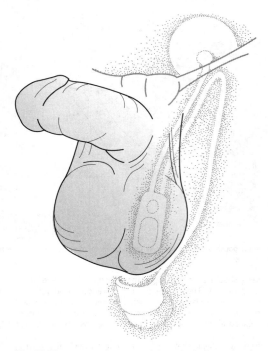

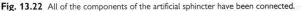

Fig. 13.22 All of the components of the artificial sphincter have been connected.

Leave a 12–16Ch catheter at the end of the procedure and remove it after 48 hr. Continue IV antibiotics post-operatively: three further doses of vancomycin, cefuroxime and gentamicin for 48 hr, and send home on 7 days of antibiotics. Draw a picture of the position of the components in your operation note. Obtain an X-ray a day after the operation to confirm that the cuff is empty, i.e. that deactivation has really been achieved. Occasionally you may think that the device is deactivated when it is activated. The device should be deactivated for at least 6 weeks. The patient should be instructed to gently retract the pump into his scrotum on a daily basis. Daily showers should be taken from day 5. Avoid soaking in a bath for 4 weeks from the day of surgery.

Alternative technique for implantation of bulbar urethral cuff: the transverse scrotal approach

Recently a novel technique of implantation of the AUS around the bulbar urethra in patients post-prostatectomy has been described using a single upper scrotal incision.[2] The scrotal incision allows good access to the proximal bulbar urethra and retropubic and subdartos spaces. All the components can be implanted via this single incision. Operating time is less because exposure of the urethra is easier and a second incision for placement of the pressure regulating balloon is not necessary.

The patient is positioned supine on the operating table. In this position the urethra is more mobile than in the lithotomy position where it tends to be under a degree of stretch. As for the conventional perineal approach, pass a urethral catheter to facilitate urethral dissection. Make a transverse scrotal incision just below the peno-scrotal junction. Move the incision onto the penis and secure it there using the blunt stay hooks of the LoneStar retractor at 1, 3, 5, 7, 9 and 11 o'clock. As the incision is deepened, reposition these stay hooks in a deeper position. Lift the skin edges and using a combination of blunt dissection with your index fingers and sharp dissection with McIndoe scissors, divide the subcutaneous tissues in order to expose the corpora cavernosa and the urethra. Coagulate the many small subcutaneous scrotal vessels before they are torn.

The key to correct exposure of the bulbar urethra is to expose the corpora cavernosa proximally. This is made easier by inserting infant Deaver or Langenbeck retractors in the 5 and 7 o'clock positions, with your assistant pulling caudally to expose the proximal ends of the corpora cavernosa. The scrotal septum, which connects the skin to the urethra, is then divided. Now the proximal corpus spongiosum has been exposed, divide Buck's fascia between the corpora cavernosa and the corpus spongiosum, thus circumferentially mobilizing the urethra. Posteriorly the urethra is densely attached to the corpora cavernosa and sharp dissection is required to fully mobilize the urethra. A slightly smaller cuff size (generally 4 cm) is more usual than with the perineal approach.

Move the incision over the region of the external inguinal ring. Divide the transversalis fascia just above the pubic tubercle (displace the spermatic cord downwards) and gently develop a space deep to this incision within which the pressure regulating balloon is placed. Ensure that the bladder is empty (with the urethral catheter) in order to avoid inadvertently perforating the bladder.

The control pump can be easily placed in a subdartos pouch in the scrotum and is easily secured in this position with a few sutures. Close the incision in layers.

Bladder neck implantation

Make a Pfannenstiel incision. Divide the endopelvic fascia (Fig. 13.23). Expose the bladder neck and urethra. Use right-angled forceps to get around the bladder neck; the position of the bladder neck is identified by the balloon of the catheter. Use your middle finger and thumb to identify the plane between the trigone anteriorly (feel the catheter) and the vas deferens posteriorly. Dissect a way through this plane by gently opening and closing curved scissors (Figs. 13.24 and 13.25). If you are having difficulty in identifying the correct plane it is safer to open the bladder (a little distant from the bladder neck so that the closure suture line is not under the cuff) and introduce a finger into the bladder neck while you do this dissection. In this situation leave a catheter for 7–10 days. A 61–70 cmH$_2$O or more usually a 71–80 cmH$_2$O balloon should be used. Cuff size is determined with the cuff sizer.

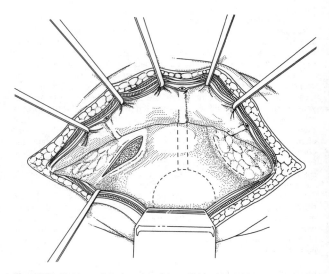

Fig. 13.23 Bladder neck implantation of the artificial urinary sphincter. The endopelvic fascia is divided. Reproduced from Whitfield, *Rob and Smith's Operative Surgery*, 1993, Butterworth-Heinemann. Permission sought.

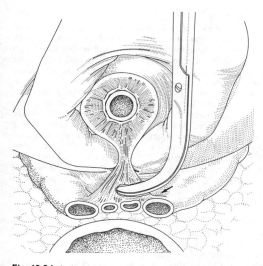

Fig. 13.24 A plane is dissected between the trigone and the vas deferens. Reproduced from Whitfield, *Rob and Smith's Operative Surgery*, 1993, Butterworth-Heinemann. Permission sought.

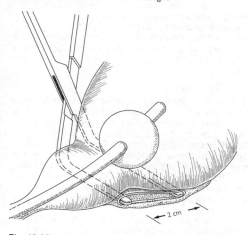

Fig. 13.25 This plane is widened to accommodate the 2 cm width of the cuff. Reproduced from Whitfield, *Rob and Smith's Operative Surgery*, 1993, Butterworth-Heinemann. Permission sought.

Operating the device

Squeezing the pump deflates the cuff, thus allowing voiding, and provides the force to pump fluid from the cuff to the balloon in the opposite direction to the normal direction of flow (the normal pressure head) from reservoir to cuff. The cuff and pump then slowly refill over 30 sec as the fluid squeezed out of the cuff and pump into the reservoir slowly moves back from reservoir into the cuff and pump. When the pump is full, the cuff is also inflated. To catheterize a patient with an AUS, squeeze the pump to force fluid out of the cuff, let the pump fill a little, and then deactivate the pump. If catheterization is necessary this should ideally be for <48 hr. Advise the patient to avoid rising suddenly from a sitting position as this can sometimes inadvertently activate the device, so causing leakage. Sometimes leakage can occur as a result of cuff compression by sitting on a hard surface. Sitting on a doughnut ring when driving long distances can be helpful. Two or three cycles may be required for complete bladder emptying. Some surgeons advise their patients to deactivate the device at night if they are dry when recumbent in an attempt to reduce the risk of tissue atrophy.

Advice to patients prior to AMS 800 insertion

- Continence will never be quite the same as it was prior to the onset of incontinence, but in most cases incontinence is markedly reduced. Overall patient satisfaction rate is about 90%.
- The device is subject to mechanical wear and tear and will eventually fail, requiring revision surgery.
- There have been reports in the literature of adverse events, including allergic-like and autoimmune-like symptoms, in patients with implantable silicone devices. However, no causal relationship has been established between these events and solid silicone elastomer.
- Mechanical malfunction (e.g. device leak) can occur at any time.
- Catheterization should only be done when the device has been deactivated, and the device should remain deactivated as long as the catheter remains in place.

Outcomes and complications[3]

- *Continence rates* depend on the patient population and the definition of 'satisfactory' continence. If the latter is defined as the need to use two or fewer pads per day (and the majority of patients prior to AUS insertion will be using more), 90% of post-radical prostatectomy patients and 70% of patients with spinal cord injury report improved continence.[4] Consider implanting an additional cuff in tandem with the original (so-called double cuff) in those with persistent incontinence.
- *Infection*: the most feared complication as removal of the entire device is almost always required. In non-neuropaths infection occurs in approximately 2–5% of cases; 24% of spinal injury patients required device removal for infection.[4]
- *Mechanical failure* (leaks in the tubing, cuff, or balloon; failure of the pump; blockages due to tube kinking): 8% prior to introduction of kink-resistant tubing and sutureless connections. Revision AUS is required.

- *Cuff erosion*: another feared complication. Approximately 5% incidence. More common in those who have had previous radiotherapy or previous cuff erosions. Usually leads to infection, necessitating removal of the cuff and often all the other components. Erosions in the first year after device implantation almost always occur because of injury to the bulbous urethra during mobilization. Thought to be less likely with introduction of narrow-back cuff design, which results in a more even spread of pressure on the urethra.
- *Atrophy of the urethra beneath the cuff*: pressure (ischaemia) induced atrophy of the peri-urethral tissues beneath the cuff results in reduced pressure transmission to the urethra and recurrent incontinence. Occurs in approximately 10% of cases 1–5 years after implantation.
- *Pump malposition*: the pump sometimes rides up from the scrotum towards the inguinal canal, in which position it may be impossible to use. Repositioning within the scrotum is required.
- *Overall re-operation rate*: depends on the length of follow-up report and case mix (post-prostatectomy versus neuropathic incontinence). Re-operation rate is higher with longer follow-up and in neuropaths. Five-year revision rates are between 40% and 50%,[5,6] and 80% with minimum of 10-year follow-up;[7] revision for erosion was required in 31% of patients in the latter series. The narrow-back cuff design reduces the need for cuff revision.

Management of recurrent incontinence in a patient with a previously implanted AUS

- Cycle the pump to ascertain whether or not it is working.
- KUB X-ray: look for leaks in the system (the balloon may have lost its spherical shape).
- Flexible cystoscopy to look for urethral erosions. For bladder neck erosion take particular care to obtain a reverse view of the bladder neck, as an erosion may only be apparent by looking back onto the bladder neck.
- In selected cases, video-urodynamics to identify bladder overactivity (where LUTS suggest this possibility) and in neuropaths where you suspect bladder behaviour may have changed (to measure bladder compliance).

If the pump cycles normally, the X-ray shows a spherical balloon (i.e. no leakage of fluid from the balloon), and there is no erosion, the cause of the recurrent incontinence is, by exclusion, tissue atrophy and you will need to replace the sphincter, either in a different urethral location or with a 4 cm as opposed to a 4.5 cm cuff, or use a higher pressure balloon.

Alternatives to the AUS

- The male urethral sling. There are 3 types—bulbourethral (suprapubic to suburethral); bone anchored perineal (InVance™); transobturator (AdVance™). They are said to improve continence by bulbar urethral repositioning (rather than compression). Good (short term) outcomes for less severe incontinence (5 or fewer pads per day) have been reported; poorer outcome are reported if 6 or more pads per day[8]. Long term outcomes and those for transobturator slings remain undetermined.
- Extraurethral retropubic adjustable compression devices. Under local or regional anaesthesia 2 small silicone balloons are introduced percutaneously via a perineal approach and positioned on each side of the urethra close to the bladder neck. Subcutaneous ports allow volume adjustment postoperatively to increase (for persistent leakage) or decrease urethral resistance (for voiding difficulty). Questions remain over its safety (e.g. 10% urethral or bladder perforation, balloon migration, fluid leakage) and continence outcomes.

References

1 Scott FB, Fishman IJ, Shabsigh R. The impact of the artificial urinary sphincter in the neurogenic bladder on the upper tracts. *J Urol* 1986; **136**:636.
2 Wilson SK, Delk JR, Henry GD, Siegel AL. New surgical technique for sphincter urinary control system using upper transverse scrotal incision. *J Urol* 2003; **169**:261–4.
3 Leo ME, DM Barrett. Success of the narrow-backed cuff design of the AMS800 artificial urinary sphincter: analysis of 144 patients. *J Urol* 1993; **150**:1412–14.
4 Light JK, Scott FB. Use of artificial urinary sphincter in spinal cord injury patients. *J Urol* 1983; **130**:1127.
5 Clemens JQ, Schuster TG, Konnak JW, McGuire EJ, Faerber GJ. Revision rate after artificial urinary sphincter implantation for incontinence after radical prostatectomy: actuarial analysis. *J Urol* 2001; **166**:1372.
6 Venn SN, Greenwell TJ, Mundy AR. The long-term outcome of artificial urinary sphincters. *J Urol* 2000; **164**:702.
7 Fulford SCV, Sutton C, Bales G, Hickling M, Stephenson TP. The fate of the 'modern' artificial urinary sphincter with a follow-up of more than 10 years. *Br J Urol* 1997; **79**:713–16.
8 Castle EP, Andrews PE, Itano N. The male sling for post-prostatectomy incontinence: mean follow-up of 18 months. *J Urol* 2005;**173**:1657.

Additional reading

Parulkar BG, Barrett DM. Combined implantation of artificial sphincter and penile prosthesis. *J Urol* 1989; **130**:1127.

Management of incontinence

Causes
- High-pressure bladder (DH, reduced bladder compliance).
- Sphincter weakness.
- UTI.
- Bladder stones.
- Rarely, bladder cancer (enquire about UTI symptoms and haematuria).
- Hyper-reflexic peripheral reflexes suggest that bladder may be hyper-reflexic (increased ankle jerk reflexes, S1–2, and a positive bulbocavernosus reflex indicating an intact sacral reflex arc i.e. S2–4 intact).
- Absent peripheral reflexes suggest that the bladder and sphincter may be areflexic, i.e. sphincter unable to generate pressures adequate for maintaining continence.

Initial investigations
- Urine culture (for infection).
- KUB X-ray for bladder stones.
- Bladder and renal ultrasound for residual urine volume and to detect hydronephrosis.
- Cytology and cystoscopy if bladder cancer suspected.

Empirical treatment
Start with simple treatments. If the bladder residual volume is large, regular ISC may lower bladder pressure and achieve continence. Try an anticholinergic drug (e.g. oxybutynin, tolterodine). Many SCI patients are already doing ISC and simply increasing ISC frequency to every 3–4 hr may achieve continence. ISC more frequently than every 3 hr is usually impractical, particularly for paraplegic women who usually have to transfer from their wheelchair to a toilet and then back to their wheelchair.

Management of failed empirical treatment
Voiding cystourethrogram to determine bladder and sphincter behaviour.

Detrusor hyper-reflexia or poor compliance
- High pressure sphincter (i.e. DSD): treating the high-pressure bladder is usually enough to achieve continence.
  - Bladder treatments: intravesical botulinum toxin, detrusor myectomy (auto-augmentation), bladder augmentation (ileocystoplasty). All will usually require ISC for bladder emptying.
  - Long-term suprapubic catheter.
  - Sacral deafferentation plus ISC or Brindley implant (SARS).
- Low-pressure sphincter: first treat the bladder as above. If bladder treatment alone fails, consider a urethral bulking agent, TVT or bladder neck closure in women, or an artificial urinary sphincter in either sex.

Detrusor areflexia plus low-pressure sphincter
- Urethral bulking agents.
- TVT.
- Bladder neck closure in women.
- Artificial urinary sphincter.

Table 13.1 Management of incontinence

	High bladder pressure	**Low bladder pressure**
High sphincter pressure	Lower bladder pressure by: ISC + anticholinergics or Botox or Augmentation	ISC*
Low sphincter pressure	Lower bladder pressure (by ISC + anticholinergics or Botox or augmentation) plus: Urethral bulking agent TVT or Bladder neck closure or Artificial urinary sphincter	Urethral bulking agent TVT Bladder neck closure Artificial urinary sphincter

* High sphincter pressure is usually enough to keep the patient dry.

Management of recurrent urinary tract infections

Causes of recurrent UTIs in the neuropathic patient

- Incomplete bladder emptying.
- Kidney stones.
- Bladder stones.
- Presence of an indwelling catheter (urethral or suprapubic).

History

What the patient interprets as a UTI may be different from your definition of UTI. The neuropathic bladders is frequently colonized with bacteria and frequently contains pus cells (pyuria). From time to time it becomes cloudy due to precipitation of calcium, magnesium, and phosphate salts in the absence of active infection. The presence of bacteria, pus cells, or cloudy urine in the presence of non-specific symptoms (abdominal pain, tiredness, headaches, feeling 'under the weather') is frequently interpreted as a UTI. Warn your patient that the constellation of symptoms thought to represent active infection may not resolve following the various treatments or management options outlined in Table 13.2. This is frustrating for both you and the patient.

Indications for treatment of 'urinary tract infection' in the neuropathic patient

It is impossible to eradicate bacteria or pus cells from the urine in the presence of a foreign body, e.g. a catheter. In the absence of fever and cloudy smelly urine, we do not prescribe antibiotics, the indiscriminate use of which encourages growth of antibiotic-resistant organisms. We prescribe antibiotics to the chronically catheterized patient where there is a combination of fever and cloudy smelly urine and where the patient feels unwell. Culture urine and immediately start empirical antibiotic therapy with nitrofurantoin, ciprofloxacin, or trimethoprim (the antibiotic sensitivities of our local 'bacterial flora'), changing to a more specific if the organism is resistant to the prescribed antibiotic.

Investigations

For recurrent UTIs (frequent episodes of fever, cloudy smelly urine, and feeling unwell), organize the following:

- KUB X-ray looking for kidney and bladder stones.
- Renal and bladder ultrasound to determine the presence/absence of hydronephrosis and to measure pre-void bladder volume and post-void residual urine volume.

Treatment

In the presence of fever and cloudy smelly urine, culture the urine and start antibiotics empirically (e.g. trimethoprim, nitrofurantoin, amoxicillin, ciprofloxacin), changing the antibiotic if the culture result suggests resistance to your empirical choice. 'Response' to treatment is suggested by the patient feeling better and their urine clearing and becoming non-offensive to smell. Persistent fever, with constitutional symptoms (malaise, rigors) despite treatment with a specific oral antibiotic in an adequate dose is an indication for admission for treatment with IV antibiotics.

Management of recurrent UTIs (Table 13.2)

If there is residual urine present, optimize bladder emptying by intermittent catheterization (males, females) or external sphincterotomy for DSD (males). Intermittent catheterization can be done by the patient (ISC) if hand function is good (paraplegic), or by a carer if tetraplegic. An indwelling catheter is an option, but the presence of a foreign body in the bladder may itself cause recurrent UTIs (although in some it seems to reduce UTI frequency). Aim to keep ISC volumes <400 mLs.

Antimicrobial catheters have been developed with the aim of reducing the incidence of CAUTI. Some are coated with an antibacterial (nitrofurazone) and others with a silver alloy. In the short term (<30 days) they prevent or reduce the likelihood of bacteriuria in hospitalized patients. However, whether this translates into a reduction in symptoms or in the long-term complications of catheters (blockages, stones, other infective complications) remains doubtful.[1]

Summary of treatment for recurrent UTIs

- Remove stones if present: cystolitholapaxy for bladder stones; PCNL for staghorn stones.
- A new potential option for DSD is augmentation of external sphincter NO, a neurotransmitter which relaxes the external sphincter, thereby encouraging antegrade flow of urine and potentially lowering residual urine volume. NO donors such as nifedipine or glyceryl trinitrate can be used. There is theoretical and some experimental evidence to support this.[2,3]

Table 13.2 Management of recurrent UTIs

Low bladder pressure	High bladder pressure + DSD
ISC	ISC
IDC	IDC
	External sphincterotomy: surgical, Botox, stent
	Deafferentation/SARS

References

1 Johnson JR, Kuskowski MA, Wilt TJ. Systematic review: antimicrobial urinary catheters to prevent catheter-associated urinary tract infection in hospitalized patients. *Ann Intern Med* 2006; **144**:116–26.
2 Mamas MA, Reynard JM, Brading AF. Augmentation of external sphincter nitric oxide: a potential pharmacological treatment for detrusor-external sphincter dyssynergia in spinal cord injury. *Lancet* 2001; **357**:1964–7.
3 Reitz A, Knapp PA, Müntener M, Schurch B. Oral nitric oxide donors: a new pharmacological approach to detrusor–sphincter dyssynergia in spinal cord injured patients. *Eur Urol* 2004; **45**:516–20.

Management of hydronephrosis

An overactive bladder (detrusor hyperreflexia) or poorly compliant bladder is frequently combined with a high-pressure sphincter (detrusor–sphincter dyssynergia). Bladder pressures during both filling and voiding are high. At times the bladder pressure may overcome the sphincter pressure and the patient leaks small quantities of urine. However, for much of the time the sphincter pressures are higher than the bladder pressures, and the kidneys are chronically exposed to these high pressures. They are hydronephrotic on ultrasound and renal function deteriorates slowly but inexorably.

Treatment options

- Bypass the external sphincter:
  - Indwelling catheter.
  - Intermittent self catheterization plus anticholinergics.
- Treat the external sphincter:
  - Sphincterotomy: surgical incision via a cystoscope inserted down the urethra (electrically heated knife or laser), Botox injections into sphincter, urethral stent.
  - Deafferentation plus ISC or SARS.
- Treat the bladder:
  - Intravesical Botox plus ISC.
  - Augmentation plus ISC.
  - Deafferentation plus ISC or SARS.

Deafferentation converts the high-pressure sphincter into a low-pressure sphincter and the high-pressure bladder into a low-pressure bladder.

Neuromodulation in lower urinary tract dysfunction

This is the electrical activation of *afferent* nerve fibres to modulate their function. Electrical stimulation applied anywhere in the body preferentially depolarizes nerves (higher current amplitudes are required to directly depolarize muscle). In patients with LUT dysfunction, the relevant spinal segments are S2–4.

Indications
- Urgency.
- Frequency.
- Urge incontinence.
- Chronic urinary retention where behavioural and drug therapy has failed.

Stimulation sites
The electrical stimulus is applied directly to nerves, or as close as possible. Several stimulation sites are available:
- Sacral nerve stimulation (SNS).
- Pudendal nerve: direct pelvic floor electrical stimulation (of bladder, vagina, anus, pelvic floor muscles) or via stimulation of the dorsal penile or clitoral nerve.
- Posterior tibial nerve stimulation (PTNS).

Posterior tibial nerve stimulation[1]
The posterior tibial nerve (PTN) shares common nerve roots (L4,5 and S1–3) with those innervating the bladder. Stimulation of the PTN can be applied transcutaneously (adhesive surface electrodes) or percutaneously (needle electrodes). Percutaneous needle systems include the SANS (Stoller) and the UrgentPC system. Stimulation is applied via an acupuncture needle inserted just above the medial malleolus with a reference (or return) electrode, initially for 30 min per week over a period of 12 weeks. Thereafter, 30 min of treatment every 2–3 weeks can be used to maintain the treatment effect in those who respond. PTNS has not been compared with placebo ('sham' stimulation) and therefore reported efficacy may represent a placebo response.

Sacral nerve stimulation
A sacral nerve stimulator (Medtronic InterStim®) delivers continuous electrical pulses to sacral nerve root 3 via an electrode inserted through the sacral foramina and connected to an electrical pulse generator which is implanted subcutaneously. The effects of SNS are believed to occur at a spinal and supraspinal level and involve inhibition of spinal neurons involved in the micturition reflex and post-ganglionic neurons. Its effects on urinary retention may be due to changes in pelvic floor function or may be mediated at a brainstem level on the pontine storage/micturition centres.

A test stimulation lasting at least 3 days (peripheral nerve evaluation (PNE)) is performed under local anaesthetic by placing a percutaneous test electrode in the S3 foramina (secured to the skin with tape) to confirm an appropriate clinical response (a reduction in urgency, frequency, or incontinence episodes). A permanent implant is offered if there is a 50% reduction in frequency and urgency episodes. The implantable pulse generator is placed in a subcutaneous pocket over the buttocks and is connected to the sacral electrode. It can be switched on and off and the amplitude varied within set limits.

Approximately 50% of patients have a successful PNE and undergo subsequent permanent implantation. Of these, 50% report resolution of their urge incontinence, and 80% report a >50% reduction in incontinence episodes, persisting for at least 3–5 years. The Medtronic Interstim is supported by NICE for patients with urge incontinence who have failed lifestyle modification and behaviour and drug therapy.[2]

Failure to respond to the PNE is often due to lead migration during the test period. The introduction of tined leads (designed to be self-anchoring within musculofascial tissues), which are used for the PNE and, if successful, are then retained *in situ* as the permanent electrode, has reduced migration rates to as low as 2% and has reduced PNE failure.[3] However, anterior migration can still occur even with tined leads.

References

1 Andrews B, Reynard J. Transcutaneous posterior tibial nerve stimulation for treatment of detrusor hyperreflexia in spinal cord injury. *J Urol* 2003; **170**:926.

2 NICE. *Interventional Procedure Guidance 64*, June 2004. Available online at: www.nice.org.uk/ip082systematic review.

3 Deng DY, Gulati M, Rutman M et al. Failure of sacral nerve stimulation due to migration of tined lead. *J Urol* 2006; **175**:2182–5.

Chapter 14

Paediatric urology

Paediatric urology: general comments

Paediatric urology is a subspeciality derived from urology and paediatric surgery. It is generally an elective surgical specialty with few acute conditions. Development of a good team incorporating a paediatric nephrologist, a radiologist, and a pathologist assists in the clinical diagnosis, management options, and follow-up. A paediatric anaesthetist and skilled experienced and compassionate nursing staff to manage the children. A continence nurse with expertise in clean intermittent catheterisation (CIC) assists with teaching CIC and trouble shooting catheter related issues. In some paediatric urological conditions there are issues where an experienced psychologist is helpful for coping with growing up with a disability affecting the genitourinary tract.

More surgery is being undertaken laparoscopically. However, the benefits of minimally invasive surgery are less in children and the risks are greater. The trend towards laparoscopy is likely to continue. From a radiological perspective, MRI will probably become the single diagnostic modality of choice for congenital urological conditions as it shows both structural and functional anomalies, despite needing a general anaesthetic. This single study can replace other more invasive studies and involves no ionizing radiation. The surgical management of common conditions such as reflux and upper tract obstruction is still debated. There is need for further natural history and outcomes research to clarify the most appropriate treatment and indications for these successful surgeries.

Undescended testis

Introduction

An undescended testis (UDT) cannot be brought down into the scrotum during physical examination. UDT represents a collection of disorders related to the abnormal position of the testis. Groin surgery to correct this condition is one of the most common paediatric urological operations. Despite this, the long-term functional outcome of orchidopexy in terms of fertility remains unknown as the current practice of surgery at about 1–2 years of age has only been recommended for a limited number of years.

Classification

In practical terms it is best to classify UDT as either palpable or impalpable, and unilateral or bilateral. Palpable undescended testes can either be ectopic (outside the line of normal descent, e.g. perineal, femoral, pre-penile), or more commonly along the normal descent pathway, being palpable somewhere between the internal inguinal and external inguinal rings (incompletely descended). Retractile testes (generally palpated in the inguinal region) are not undescended, but need follow-up. If a retractile testis becomes undescended (ascended), orchidopexy is required. The best management for palpable testes is a standard orchidopexy.

Prevalence

The incidence of UDT is slowly increasing, possibly because of an increase in oestrogens in the environment.[1] Prematurity is associated with an increased risk of UDT. Approximately 3–4% of term boys have an UDT (85% unilateral, 15% bilateral), and 50% of these will descend within the first 6 months of life. Eighty per cent of UDTs are palpable and 20% are impalpable. Clinical examination is easier in this age group as the cremasteric reflex has yet to develop (6–12 months). Boys with previously descended but retractile testes may 'ascend,' accounting for a small number of orchidopexies. The right testis is affected twice as commonly as the left.

Impalpable testes need to have their presence (they may be atrophic or absent) and location clarified: 75% are present but impalpable; in 25% of cases where no testis is palpable, it proves to be absent at surgical exploration. Bilateral impalpable testes are a special situation with ambiguous genitalia a possibility. Thus a boy with bilateral impalpable testes may have ambiguous genitalia and need karyotype and endocrine testing, and radiological studies. This is done in conjunction with a multidisciplinary team. If the XY male karyotype is present, an hCG stimulation test is undertaken to determine the presence of functioning testes.[2] If the test is negative, no further investigations are necessary and supportive hormone therapy is required. Usually the test is positive and management is to determine the location of impalpable testes. The surgical management is similar for unilateral impalpable testes. Radiological studies to locate the testis are costly and inaccurate, and thus rarely undertaken. Diagnostic and therapeutic laparoscopy as a day patient is appropriate.

Patient assessment
- A history of whether the testis has previously been descended is useful, along with that of any previous groin surgery.
- Examination begins with careful observation to see if a testis is present and to look at the scrotal size. A small scrotum may indicate UDT. Palpate gently and begin by laterally sweeping the contents of the inguinal canal medially. Then with gentle pressure draw the hand deep and laterally. A palpable testis is commonly seen high in the scrotum. Assessment of size and position is important.

Surgical management
The aim of surgery is to place the testis in the scrotum without tension to allow normal development in a cooler environment and testicular self-examination (the chance of developing testicular cancer is approximately 1 in 100 in males with UDT, roughly 25–30 times that of males without UDT).

Approximately 20% of undescended testes are impalpable. A repeat examination under anaesthetic is mandatory, and if the testis is palpable a standard orchidopexy is performed. If the testis remains impalpable, trans-umbilical laparoscopy will show: an absent testis (defined by absent gonadal vessels) (~25% of cases), or vas and vessels entering the deep ring (possible atrophic testis) (~40%), or an intra-abdominal testis (~40%).

If the testis is absent, surgical fixation of the contralateral testis may be performed. If the testis is in the groin, a standard groin exploration is performed and a small atrophic nubbin of testis may be removed, if present. This probably represents a remnant of *in utero* testis torsion. If the testis is intra-abdominal there are a number of options:
- A one-stage orchidopexy is usually possible if the testis is close to the deep ring.
- A two-stage Fowler–Stevens operation (a clip is placed separate from the testis on the testicular vessels).
- Rarely, if the testis is small or the child >10 years old with a normally descended contralateral testis, proceed with orchidectomy.[3]

Standard inguinal orchidopexy
This is usually undertaken at around 1–2 years of age as a day case procedure. Repeat examination is undertaken prior to surgery. The principles include isolation and mobilization of the testis, preservation of the structures of the spermatic cord, high ligation of the patent processus, and fixation of the testis in the scrotum.

An ilio-inguinal nerve block is useful for analgesia. Insert a small gauge needle 1 cm medial and inferior to the anterior superior iliac spine at a right angle to the skin. As the needle passes through the aponeurosis of external oblique, a slight 'give' is felt. The nerve lies immediately deep to this layer. Infiltrate with local anaesthetic. Then infiltrate the skin with local anaesthetic, partly for analgesia, but also to better define the tissue planes.

Make a transverse groin incision from just above the pubic tubercle laterally to the mid-inguinal point. Ask an assistant to insert some cat's paws retractors to elevate the tissues and so demonstrate Scarpa's fascia which should be picked up with toothed forceps and then divided with scissors. Having divided Scarpa's fascia, insert the scissors and spread their ends to free the tissues over external oblique.

Now insert your finger towards the scrotum. As it is pulled back out the gubernaculum, an attached testis is delivered. The testis is carefully dissected free from the fibres of the gubernaculum distally. Slide your scissors beneath the external oblique to push the superficial lying ilio-inguinal nerve out of the way. Then split the external oblique towards the deep ring. Free the cord of cremasteric fibres to gain extra length.

To dissect off the patent processus, the testis and cord are reflected laterally and the vas and vessels are preserved under direct vision. Watch out for a small cremasteric vessel near the deep ring. This is easily divided and can cause troublesome bleeding. The patent processus is mobilized to the deep ring and ligated with an absorbable suture. A dartos pouch is created by carefully dissecting onto a finger placed within the scrotum, and a space twice the size of the mobilized testis is created. The tunica is opened and an appendix testis removed if present. The testis is drawn tension free into this space and the neck of the pouch closed with a suture. Care is taken not to suture fixate the testis; this is only done in rare circumstances (for fear of inducing an autoantibody response). Wounds are closed with subcuticular suture such as a 4–0 monocryl suture.

If there is inadequate spermatic cord length for tension-free testis fixation, additional length can be gained by dividing bands lateral to the vessels in the retroperitoneum, and mobilizing the cord and testis medial to the inferior epigastric vessels (Prentiss manoeuvre).[4] Once dissection of the vas and vessels has been done, a Fowler–Stevens orchidopexy is not possible.

Re-operative orchidopexy is a difficult operation and there are some important principles: early testicular isolation with careful dissection, wide mobilization of the spermatic cord with a strip of external oblique retained, and mobilization of the peritoneum lateral to the deep ring along with suture fixation to the scrotum.

Complications of standard orchidopexy are uncommon and <5% of patients should have testicular atrophy or subsequent testicular ascent.

Long-term outcome
- Unilateral orchidopexy: 90% paternity (the same as with normally descended testes).
- Bilateral orchidopexy: 60% paternity.
- No proven reduction in malignancy risk but improved ability to perform testis examination.

Fowler–Stevens operation

The Fowler–Stevens operation relies on the testis having three blood supplies: testicular, cremasteric, and via the artery of the vas. The testicular artery can be safely divided remote from the testis and the testis consistently remains viable. This operation is usually done in two stages approximately 6 months apart to allow the secondary blood supply to become more robust. The second stage is undertaken by an open approach with careful dissection of the testis and the surrounding peritoneum. In some centres this is being undertaken laparoscopically as a one-stage procedure with good success in experienced hands.

Re-operative orchidopexy is a difficult operation and there are some important principles. Early testicular isolation with careful dissection, wide mobilisation of the spermatic cord with a strip of external oblique retained and mobilisation of the peritoneum lateral to the deep ring along with suture fixation of the testis to the scrotum.

Overall, complications are uncommon and less than 5% of patients should have testicular atrophy or subsequent testicular ascent. Long term outcome of unilateral orchidopexy—90% paternity (the same as that with normally descended testes), bilateral orchidopexy 40–60% paternity. There is no proven reduction in malignancy risk by orchidopexy proven, but there is improved ability to perform testis examination.

Further reading

1 Schneck FX and Bellinger MF. Abnormalities of the testes and scrotum and their surgical management. In *Campbell's Urology* 8th edn, ed Walsh PC, Retik AB, Vaughan ED, Wein AJ. Philadelphia, PA: WB Saunders, 2002, p 2353.

References

1 Toppari J, Skakkebaek NE. Sexual differentiation and environmental endocrine disrupters. *Ballières Clin Endocrinol Metab* 1998; **12**:143.
2 Sultan C, Paris F, Jeandel C, Lumbroso S, Galifer RB Ambiguous genitalia in the newborn. *Semin Reprod Med* 2002; **20**:181.
3 Patil KK, Green JS, Duffy PG. Laparoscopy for impalpable testes. *BJU Int* 2005; **95**:704.
4 Prentiss RJ, Teickgenant CJ, Moses JJ, Frazier DB. Undescended testes: surgical anatomy of the spermatic vessels, spermatic surgical triangles, and lateral spermatic ligament. *J Urol* 1960; **83**:686.

Urinary tract infection and voiding dysfunction

Introduction

UTI is common in childhood and may indicate an underlying structural urinary tract problem. All children with a proven UTI should be investigated in order to rule out these anatomic anomalies. A wide spectrum of severity of presentation is seen, ranging from a severe acute illness to troublesome recurrent infections, leading to social problems. Increasingly bowel elimination disorder is recognized as a cause of these infections.

Prevalence

Around 5% of girls and a smaller number of boys suffer a UTI during childhood. Girls have more UTIs than boys at all ages except under 12 months where the incidence in boys is greater. Neonatal circumcision reduces this risk 10-fold.[1] *Escherichia coli* is the most common bacterium involved, followed by *Klebsiella* and *Proteus*.[2]

Voiding dysfunction commonly presents with daytime wetting, and is increasingly recognized as being associated with UTI in children. Up to 10% of children aged between 4 and 6 years have voiding dysfunction; this reduces to 5% at age 10 years. This symptom complex, when severe, was previously known as Hinman syndrome. It varies in severity but is associated with UTI, daytime wetting, and bowel elimination delay. It is rare to obtain a clear history of bowel symptoms and the pathogenesis is poorly understood. Rarely, these children have associated renal dilatation and, if so, should be managed similarly to children with a neuropathic bladder.

Further investigations are designed to establish whether significant reflux and/or obstruction is present in children diagnosed with UTI. Children with these conditions need additional management to prevent further UTI and renal damage.

Diagnosis

Clinical symptoms may be vague in childhood and so urine analysis is vital. UTI requires pure growth of bacteria and pyuria. The urine specimen can be collected as bag urine, clean catch, catheter urine, or by suprapubic aspiration. Invasive urine sampling (via a catheter) is reserved for younger children and those who are unwell. There is diagnostic controversy where there is bacteriuria but no pyuria. Many urologists will regard the presence of bacteriuria UTI without pyuria as diagnostic of urinary infection and treat and investigate accordingly. Contaminated specimens are common and should be repeated.

Clinical features

In the neonatal and infant age groups symptoms of urinary infection are vague, usually a fever, vomiting, diarrhoea, and rarely failure to thrive. Haematuria is seen in severe cases and, in males, epididymo-orchitis is occasionally seen.

Children over the age of 2 years usually have localizing symptoms such as dysuria, frequency, wetting, and lower abdominal pain. If pyelonephritis is present, a fever, vomiting, and vague abdominal pain are common. The classic adult symptom of loin pain is rare. It is usually difficult to differentiate upper tract from lower tract infections on symptoms alone. Constipation is rarely found on history, and occasionally faecal soiling may be reported.

Clinical examination is rarely helpful but should focus on the lower abdomen, genitals, and peripheral neurology.

Investigations

All children with proven UTI need investigation regardless of age or sex. However, there is controversy about which test at which age. There may be a lower risk to the kidneys with increasing age. The younger the child with a UTI, the more potential there is for renal damage with infection. Since invasive investigations are distressing for both parent and child, there is a tendency to limit invasive investigations to the older child. We currently restrict the use of routine micturating cysto-urethrography (MCU) to UTI under 2 years, recurrent UTI, or febrile UTI.

Ultrasound of the renal tracts should be performed in all children. Modern directed renal ultrasound is an excellent non-invasive structural investigation. However, it may miss small renal scars, reflux, and other minor renal anomalies. All children with ultrasound abnormalities need further tests. As younger children are more prone to renal damage with pyelonephritis, investigations and treatment are more aggressive in this age group (see Table 14.1).

A plain KUB X-ray is very useful to diagnose constipation, but there are no agreed radiological criteria for bowel elimination disorder. Ultrasound can also visualize the rectum, and if it is dilated with stool, constipation is also likely.

Table 14.1 Investigation of UTI in children

UTI <2 years	Renal US scan + MCU
Simple UTI >years(not systemically unwell, common organism)	Renal US scan + DMSA renal scan
Complex UTI >2 years(systemically unwell, unusual organism	DMSA renal scan + MCU
Abnormal renal US scan or DMSA renal scan >2 years	MCU

Micturating urethro-cystogram

This invasive test should be undertaken in children <2 years old with a UTI, those with an abnormal DMSA scan (i.e. scars), and those with febrile UTIs. It is also recommended for those children with recurrent UTIs but, as it is invasive, it should be undertaken with careful consideration. MCU may be undertaken with sedation to make it more tolerable. Indirect MAG3 cystography can be used without the need for catheterization in older children.

Radio-isotope scanning

• A DMSA scan will detect renal parenchymal scarring and establish differential renal function. It is most useful in the management of reflux.
• MAG3 renography is used to determine obstruction and can also determine differential renal function.

Other radiology

• IVU is rarely undertaken nowadays.
• MR urography is a promising modality that can determine both structural and functional renal abnormalities. It is free of radiation, but is more expensive, requires IV gadolinium contrast, and requires general anaesthetic in younger children to prevent excessive movement artefact.

Management

Antibiotics are the mainstay of treatment to clear infection, and IV gentamicin remains the medication of choice in severe infections. The vast majority of infections can be treated with oral medications, such as co-trimoxazole, trimethoprim, and amoxicillin. Treatment should be continued for 5–7 days and a clear urine analysis should be obtained post-treatment to ensure the infection has been adequately treated.

• Antibiotic prophylaxis should be maintained in all infants while organizing investigations and in children with recurrent UTIs.
• Aggressive bowel treatment is required for older children with recurrent UTIs and daytime wetting. Natural laxatives initially together with acidophyllis yoghurt (probiotic) and cranberry are also helpful. If this regimen is unsuccessful, a prescription laxative, such as lactulose, in increasing dose may be required for prolonged times.
• Oxybutinin may also be beneficial in children with urgency once urine analysis is clear. This medication is well tolerated in children.
• Behavioural modification therapy is recommended for some children with recalcitrant voiding dysfunction. However, reassurance is also required as the majority of children improve with time.

Further reading

1 Kunin CM. Urinary tract infections in children. In *Pediatric urology*, 3rd edn, ed. O'Donnell B, Koff SA. Oxford: Butterworth-Heinemann, 1977, pp 171–96.

References

1 Wiswell TE, Roscelli JD. Corroborative evidence for the decreased incidence of urinary tract infections in circumcised male infants. *Pediatrics* 1986; **78**:96.
2 Riccabona M. Urinary tract infection in children. *Curr Opin Urol* 2003; **13**:59–62.

Surgery for vesico-ureteric reflux

Vesico-ureteric reflux (VUR) is the retrograde flow of urine from the bladder into the upper urinary tract through an incompetent vesico-ureteric junction. Reflux of infected urine can lead to pyelonephritis and subsequently renal scarring, hypertension, and renal failure.

VUR may be diagnosed pre-natally (fetal renal dilatation on pregnancy ultrasound) following investigation for urinary infection (usually pyelone-phritis) or as an associated abnormality during investigation of another genitourinary abnormality. About 20–50% of children with UTI have VUR, and so UTI is a marker for reflux.

Primary VUR is due to incompetence of the vesico-ureteric junction, whereas secondary VUR is due to another cause such as neuropathy (spinal cord injury, spina bifida) or obstruction (posterior urethral valves, ectopic ureteroceles). Secondary VUR is treated by correcting the under-lying abnormality (surgical correction of the VUR itself is rarely required).

Grading of VUR

VUR is diagnosed and graded on the basis of voiding cystourethrography (VCUG):

- Grade 1   Contrast in the ureter only
- Grade 2   Contrast in the ureter and renal pelvis with no pelvic dilatation or calyceal blunting
- Grade 3   Mild calyceal dilatation
- Grade 4   Moderate calyceal dilatation
- Grade 5   Severe calyceal dilatation with tortuosity of the ureter

The aim of management is to preserve renal function and prevent UTI. There has been a recent move away from aggressive management of VUR, with greater attention directed towards UTI prevention by focusing on bowel and bladder management. The indications for surgical correction of VUR remain controversial.

Indications for surgery

- Absolute: UTI while on antibiotic prophylaxis; development of new renal scarring.
- Relative: parental request; persistent high-grade VUR; bladder anatomical abnormalities with VUR.

Operative techniques

- Open surgery with the Cohen technique is the most popular operation.
- Endoscopic injection has become less popular because of particle migration and low success rates, but Deflux® is regaining some popularity. This is a copolymer of dextranomer and hyaluronic acid which is injected into the wall of the bladder beneath the opening of the relevant ureter. The lower morbidity of endoscopic injection allows it to be done as a day-case procedure, but this must be counterbalanced against its lower efficacy for high-grade VUR (resolution of reflux: grade 2, 95%; grade 3, 70%; grade 4, 40%).[1] As a consequence follow-up VCUG tests and repeat injections may be required if endoscopic injection therapy is used as the method of management. Complications include ureteric obstruction (rare) and UTI.
- Laparoscopic correction of VUR has been reported but is not as popular as open correction.[2]

Pre-operative work-up

Surgery is contraindicated with a current UTI and should be postponed for 4–6 weeks after successful treatment of infection. Ensure that the patient's X-rays are present in the operating theatre. Give antibiotic prophylaxis.

Operative technique

The patient is placed supine in a warm environment with a small towel under the lower back to rotate the pelvis. Point diathermy is helpful for bloodless dissection. A Pfannenstiel incision is used with wide dissection up and down the midline to help pelvic access. The retropubic space is entered and the peritoneum is swept up off the bladder, which is higher in children. A Dennis-Browne retractor is positioned to expose the bladder. Two stay sutures are placed in the bladder, which is then incised between the stays with diathermy, thereby allowing visualization of the posterior surface. Carefully aspirate the urine with a sucker, avoiding suction on the mucosa (the consequent oedema could obscure visualization of the ureter) and place two to four moist swabs in the dome of the bladder. Then place the third retractor blade cranially to elevate the posterior bladder wall and bring the trigone into view. A stay suture is placed caudally in the midline bladder incision and hooked round the retractor. Infant feeding tubes are placed up the ureters. Look carefully for duplex openings.

A stay suture is placed just distal to the ureteric orifice, and dissection is carried out circumferentially through the mucosa, using diathermy. Dissection with sharp scissors laterally to the ureteric orifice allows a ureteric plane to be identified outside the bladder. Diathermy dissection of the bladder muscle off the distal ureter is carried out circumferentially using a small right-angle to separate the ureter and bladder. The ureter is stripped of adventitial attachments and drawn out into the bladder until it reaches, without tension, the skin level. In bilateral cases this is repeated on the other side. Use a couple of sutures to close the small bladder defect loosely. Use sharp dissection to create a long submucosal tunnel, avoiding ureteric angulation. The length of this tunnel should be three to four times the ureteric width. In bilateral cases the tunnels should not cross. The ureteric catheters are now removed, and the ureters are passed down the tunnels with stay sutures and carefully sutured to the mucosa without tension. The first suture should be deep to anchor the ureter and is best placed laterally on the bladder wall. In unilateral re-implant a Y–Vplasty distal to the non-refluxing ureter prevents development of contralateral reflux. Mucosal defects are closed, the swabs are removed and counted, and the bladder is closed in a standard two-layer closure. In boys it is usual to leave an SPC to avoid urethral trauma. Girls may have bladder drainage with a urethral catheter. A drain may be left in the retropubic space, and then fascia and skin are closed with a subcuticular stitch. Drains and the SPC should be well sutured and taped to the patient's skin to ensure they do not fall out.

If tapering of the ureter is required, the ureter wall should be loosely rolled in on itself over an 8FR catheter. The sutures are best interrupted, especially distally, and should be re-implanted with a longer submucosal channel. A J stent is placed to prevent obstruction and is removed 6 weeks post-operatively.

Post-operative management

An epidural for 48 hr provides excellent analgesia. Antibiotic prophylaxis continues for 4 weeks. A renal ultrasound is undertaken at 6 weeks to rule out obstruction. A repeat VCUG is not required unless UTI occurs. A repeat renal ultrasound is usually undertaken at 6 and 12 months to check interval renal growth. Long-term follow-up is determined by the degree of renal scarring. In children with significant renal scars, prophylactic ACE inhibitors may reduce the risk of development of reflux nephropathy.

Complications

Recurrent reflux is rare and should occur in <1% of cases unless tapering is undertaken. Where there has been a tapered re-implant, especially into a small bladder, recurrent reflux and/or obstruction is more frequent. In the setting of persistent reflux, antibiotic prophylaxis continues but can usually stop 1–2 years later. Obstruction is heralded by increasing dilatation on post-operative ultrasound and usually requires renal drainage by nephrostomy as antegrade stenting is very difficult after re-implant. A JJ stent is best passed antegrade through an obstructed re-implant and usually resolves in time following resolution of post-operative oedema. Very rarely re-do surgery is required because of reflux and this is more easily undertaken by dissecting the ureter outside the bladder.

References

1 Capozza N, Caione P. Dextranomer/hyaluronic acid copolymer implantation for vesico-ureteral reflux: a randomized comparison with antibiotic prophylaxis. *J Pediatr* 2002; **140**:230–4.
2 Greenbaum LA, Mesrobian HG. Vesicoureteric reflux. *Paediatr Clin North Am.* 2006; **53**:413–47.
3 Heidenreich A, Ozgur E, Becker T, Haupt G. Surgical management of vesicoureteral reflux in paediatric patients. *World J Urol.* 2004; **22**:96–106.

Hypospadias

Introduction

Hypospadias is characterized by three penile anatomical abnormalities: a ventrally sited urethral meatus, ventral penile curvature (chordee), and a ventrally deficient hooded foreskin.

Classification

Hypospadias is classified by the position of the urethral meatus. A glanular or subcoronal meatus is seen in 50% of cases, a mid-shaft meatus in 30%, and a proximal scrotal meatus in 20%.[1] The ventral skin may be very thin in some cases and the meatus may be falsely assumed to be distal. Chordee may be present without hypospadias.

Prevalence

Hypospadias is seen in 1 in 100 boys, and is more common in siblings with a family history. The incidence is increasing. It has been suggested that hypospadias may be due to increased environmental oestrogens.[2] If UDT is present (10% of boys with hypospadias; 25% of boys with peno-scrotal and more severe forms of hypospadias), consider the possibility of intersex. However, if the hypospadias is isolated no further urological investigations are required.

Surgical repair

The aim of surgery is to correct penile chordee (straighten the penis), create a neo-urethra in the glans (glanular urethral meatus), and replace absent ventral penile skin with dorsal 'excess' foreskin, thus improving cosmetic appearance. Penile surgery is best completed between 6 and 12 months of age as the penis is simply too small in younger boys and the risks of surgery and anaesthesia are less in the older child.

General principles

Optical magnification (commonly 2.5×) is used by the majority of surgeons. A variety of techniques are employed to reduce bleeding, both operative and post-operative. For haemostasis during the operation use either a tourniquet or subcutaneous injection of a vasoconstrictor. A sterile rubber band, tightened round the penile base with artery forceps, can be used as a tourniquet. The safe tourniquet time is unknown, but the shorter the better. The author's preference is subcutaneous adrenaline which is easily available by diluting local anaesthetic with adrenaline 1:100 000, (50:50 with normal saline). This vasoconstrictor is placed in a labelled syringe and can be injected safely if *placed superficially*, just under the skin. This is the most commonly used tool to reduce bleeding intra-operatively. Historically there was concern with regard to injecting vasoconstricting agents into the penis and other extremities because of possible ischaemic injury. It is safe if the injection is kept subcutaneous. If inadvertent injection of adrenaline into the corporal body occurs, flush the corporal body with saline and also with papaverine as a vasodilator. Bipolar diathermy is used by some but has an irritating tendency to stick to tissue. Monopolar diathermy is safe if used sparingly at low power without the penis on stretch. High-power monopolar diathermy with a small penis under stretch can cause vascular damage and has caused penile loss. If monopolar diathermy is used appropriately, it is safe. There is no evidence that use of monopolar diathermy in hypospadias repair leads to erectile dysfunction. Use fine (6–0 or 7–0) absorbable sutures such as PDS or Monocryl. Post-operatively use a compression dressing with a sandwich of non-stick dressing, gauze, and a bio-occlusive dressing (Tegaderm). Post-operative urinary drainage with a 6Ch 'dripping' stent, sutured in for 3–7 days is usual, although not mandatory.

Surgical options
- Tubularized incised plate (TIP).[3]
- MAGPI (meatal advancement and glanuloplasty procedure).
- Onlay island flap repair.
- Staged repairs for severe hypospadias.

Many procedures for hypospadias repair have been described, of which the TIP[3] is the most popular. It can be used in the majority of repairs from the distal to the very proximal meatal position. It has excellent cosmetic and functional outcomes. However, long-term results are still awaited.[4]

A stay suture placed in the glans makes surgery easier. The author's preference is a 6–0 nylon suture. Initially the penile skin is dropped back (degloved) and a saline artificial erection is undertaken to determine if chordee is corrected. A 25 gauge needle is placed directly into the corpora and, with digital pressure at the penile base, saline is injected until the penis is erect and firm. By observing laterally, the chordee can be assessed. If this skin mobilization does not correct the chordee, fibrous corpus spongiosum is excised by dissection of the thick tissue lateral to the hypospadiac urethra. Rarely, dorsal plication of the corpus cavernosa is required. A midline suture (5–0 or 6–0 nylon) is placed dorsally opposite the maximum bend and artificial erection undertaken. More than one suture may be required to correct severe chordee.

The TIP urethral repair is performed by deeply incising the urethral plate in the midline and rolling it over an 8Ch catheter (Duplay procedure). Care is taken not to incise too distally so as to avoid meatal stenosis. To reduce the fistula rate, a second fascial layer covers the urethral repair, either reflected from the ventral penile surface or from the subcutaneous foreskin rotated dorsally. Glansplasty requires deep mobilization of the glans flaps laterally and a two-layer repair is fashioned over the distal urethra. Penile skin is rotated ventrally from the excess foreskin.

A compression dressing with an inner non-stick pad (Telfa) reduces post-operative ooze. The stent is removed 3–5 days post-operatively. Long-term follow-up of this repair is required to detect urethral narrowing and to check that uroflow is not obstructed.

Glanular hypospadias can be managed with a simple meatoplasty and hemi-circumcision or a modified MAGPI procedure. This operation, popularized by Duckett, may retract the urethral meatus and can lead to unsightly meatal regression.[5]

Rarely, more proximal repairs require a one-stage vascularized preputial onlay flap augmenting the urethral plate.

Staged repairs for severe hypospadias

Two-stage repairs are still occasionally undertaken and give consistent results with good cosmesis. They are usually reserved for very proximal cases or where the urethral plate is very thin.[6] In the first stage, the penis is straightened and well-vascularized excess dorsal preputial skin is transferred to the ventral aspect of the penis. In the second stage, the new urethra and the glans is reconstructed.

Complications of hypospadias repairs

Complications occur in approximately 10% of cases.

- Urethrocutaneous fistula is the most common complication. Principles of fistula repair are to rule out distal obstruction, excise fistula tract, and perform multi-layer repair with a fascial layer interposed to prevent overlapping suture lines. Absorbable sutures with compression dressing and usually a catheter are placed. Ten per cent fistula recurrence is expected after a fistula repair.
- Excess penile skin occasionally needs excision for adequate cosmesis. It is removed at least 6 months post-operatively to let the wounds fully recover. Under general anaesthetic a stay suture is placed in the glans and a penile block with plain local anaesthetic injected. A marker pen is used to identify excess skin. Sharp dissection is used to excise the skin with a full-thickness incision down to the corpora. Interrupted Monocryl is used for skin apposition and a compression dressing.
- Persistent chordee is rare, but if present repair may be delayed until after adolescence, by which time the penis has stopped growing.
- Stricture of the neourethra or delayed BXO may develop, and surgical correction is with a two-stage buccal mucosal repair.
- Urethral diverticulum: ballooning of the urethra due to too large a urethroplasty or distal obstruction.

Further reading

1 Retik A. Borer JG. Hypospadias. In *Campbell's Urology* 8th edn, ed Walsh PC, Retik AB, Vaughan ED, Wein AJ. Philadelphia, PA: WB Saunders, 2002, pp 2305–24.

References

1 Caldamone AA. Diamond DA Contemporary hyspadiology. *Contemp Urol* 1999; **11**:61–77.
2 Sharpe RM, Skakkebaek NE. Are oestrogens involved in falling sperm counts and disorders of the male reproductive tract? *Lancet* 1993; **341**:1392–5.
3 Snodgrass W. Tubularised incised plate hypospadias repair. *J Urol* 1994; **151**:464–5.
4 Wilcox D, Snodgrass W Long-term outcome following hypospadias repair. *World J Urol* 2006; **24**:240–3.
5 Duckett JW Snyder HM Meatal advancement and glanuloplasty repair after 1000 cases: avoidance of meatal stenosis and regression. *J Urol* 1992; **147**:665–9.
6 Bracka A. A versatile two stage hypospadias repair. *Br J Plastic Surg* 1995; **48**:345–52.

Ureteric duplication, ureteroceles, and ectopic ureter

Duplication of the ureter

Duplication of the ureter is common. It is seen in 1% of the population but in up to 5% of patients investigated for UTI. Forty per cent are bilateral and the great majority are incomplete. Many are now diagnosed antenatally as a consequence of finding hydronephrosis on the maternal ultrasound scan. UTI and incontinence are other common presentations.

Embryology

Early division of the ureteric bud leads to a duplication. The more complete the division, the more complete the duplication. The lower ureteric bud attaches to the lower pole of the kidney and inserts superolaterally on the trigone. It has an abnormally short intramural course so that it has a tendency to reflux. The upper ureteric bud attaches to the upper pole of the kidney and inserts in a distal location in the lower urinary tract such that it may even lie below the sphincter mechanism in girls. Ectopic ureters in boys always lie above the sphincter, and so boys never present with incontinence. As a consequence, incontinence or obstruction (particularly if the ureter inserts *into* the sphincter mechanism) may occur. Thus the lower pole ureter is shorter and inserts into the bladder in a proximal location, whereas the upper pole ureter is longer and inserts distally—the so-called Meyer–Weigart law. A ureteric bud rising further from the normal position will make contact with the developing kidney more peripherally, resulting in poor function (dysplasia) in that moiety.

Clinically, patients may present with a duplex system, ureterocele from a single or duplex system, a single system or duplex ectopic, and rarely bilateral ectopic ureter. Duplicated ureters may be incomplete or complete, and both empty into the bladder.

Surgical management

As stated above (Meyer–Weigart law) reflux into the lower pole is commonly seen and is initially managed as for single-system reflux. As reflux does not resolve in duplex systems at the same rate as in a single system, surgery to correct reflux is more commonly required with duplex ureters. A common sheath Cohen type re-implantation is undertaken, as the ureteric adventitia and blood supply is common between both ureters.

If the renal function of the lower pole is very poor (dysplastic moiety) a lower pole hemi-nephrectomy is performed, taking care not to damage the upper pole ureter.

Ectopic ureter in a single system

If the kidney is small and non-functioning a nephro-ureterectomy is performed (open or laparoscopically). If the kidney is functioning, the ureter is re-implanted.

Ureterocele

A ureterocele is a cystic dilatation of the terminal intravesical segment of the ureter. It occurs in 0.2% of the population and is four to seven times more common in females. They are bilateral in 10%, and 80% are associated with a duplex system, usually being associated with the upper pole. Sixty per cent are located in an ectopic location.

Ureteroceles are classified as intravesical or ectopic. They usually present antenatally (on maternal ultrasound scan) with fetal hydronephrosis or clinically are associated with a UTI or, rarely, urethral obstruction. Renal ultrasound shows a cystic mass on the posterior aspect of the bladder with a dilated ureter behind. The kidney has an echo-dense or dysplastic upper pole with an associated dilated ureter. The lower pole is usually normal. A VCUG is mandatory as up to 50% have reflux into the ipsilateral lower pole and 25% into the contralateral kidney. A DMSA renal scan will determine differential parenchymal function of each kidney and the respective poles. A MAG3 scan is occasionally used to determine obstruction. At cystoscopy the ureterocele has a variable appearance and is best seen with the bladder empty and the irrigant fluid bag low (to minimize pressure). Sometimes pressure on the flank fills the cystic mass. The upper pole ureteric orifice is low and medial in position, while the upper pole ureter is wide and lateral.

Treatment is required only where obstruction or significant reflux is present. Initial treatment is designed to relieve obstruction, and is usually endoscopic. An endoscopic incision is made low and medially on the ureterocele with a cold knife, cautery, or (more recently) a holmium laser. The aim is to relieve obstruction and avoid reflux. However, most do reflux post-operatively and antibiotic prophylaxis is usually required.

A DMSA renal scan which determines differential function of the affected pole is the cornerstone to determine definitive management. If function is adequate (>10%) reconstruct the distal ureters with a double-barrel re-implant and occasionally bladder wall repair.

The procedure is essentially the same as a Cohen re-implant, but the ureterocele is fully excised and both ureters are cannulated with infant feeding tubes. Both ureters are mobilized to their common sheath with a mixture of sharp and blunt dissection. The ureters are mobilized into the bladder and the wide ureter tapered by loose plication over an 8Fr catheter. If tapering is undertaken, a JJ stent is usually left. The stent is removed at 6 weeks and a follow-up cystogram is usually obtained. If the renal function is poor, hemi-nephrectomy is performed. This is increasingly being undertaken laparoscopically but the principle is the same as for open surgery. Usually a retroperitoneal approach is used. The abnormally wide ureter is located, taking care to preserve as much adventitia round it. It is divided and carefully passed anteriorly to the vessels. Traction upwards exposes the upper pole vessels medially which can be divided. A demarcation plane is found easily between the poles and cautery is used to divide the upper pole off. Haemostasis is secured and a drain is usually left. The ureter is left tied off in the pelvis unless it is ectopic. Antibiotics are stopped post-operatively. Follow-up is with occasional ultrasound scans at 3 and 12 months.

Ectopic ureter

An ectopic ureter is usually found in a position caudal to the normal ureteric orifice, along the pathway of normal development. In boys this may mean that the ureter opens at the bladder neck, prostate, or epididymis. In girls it may open at the bladder neck, urethra, or vagina, and possibly lead to incontinence. The further the ureter opens from the normal site, the worse the renal function.

Ectopic ureter occurs six times more commonly in girls than in boys, and 70% are associated with a complete duplication. Boys are more likely to have a single system. If an ectopic ureter is present with duplication, 80% will be bilateral. Boys and girls may present antenatally or with a UTI. In boys epididymo-orchitis may be present, and in girls continuous incontinence with a normal voiding pattern. Renal ultrasound may show a dilated ureter behind the bladder with a duplex kidney and a variable amount of cortex. CT and MRI are more accurate if the diagnosis needs to be ruled out. Also, a DMSA scan not only checks for differential but can be used to rule out an ectopically located kidney in difficult cases. An IVU is rarely used nowadays. A cystoscopy is not required but is a useful adjunct.

Management depends on the function of the ectopic system. Function is rarely good, so a hemi-nephrectomy is performed in the majority. If the ureter is ectopic, the distal ureteric stump is excised, sometimes via a separate incision to reduce the risk of post-operative UTI and discharge.

Further reading

1 Cooper S. Duplicated ureters and ureteroceles. In *Pediatric Urology*, ed Gearhart JP. Totowa, NJ: Humana Press, 2003, pp 85–210.
2 Frank JD, Rickwood AMK. Duplication anomalies, ureteroceles and ectopic ureters. In *Essentials of paediatric urology*, ed. Thomas D, Duffy PG, Rickwood AMK. London: Martin Dunitz, 2002, pp 75–86.

Pelvi-ureteric junction obstruction

PUJ obstruction is a narrowing at the PUJ with restriction to flow of urine which, if left untreated, will lead to a reduction in renal function. It is the most common congenital urinary tract obstruction and presents following detection of antenatal renal dilatation at routine screening ultrasound scan, following a UTI in a young child, or with loin pain in the older child. Renal ultrasound can accurately predict the level of obstruction. PUJ level obstruction is suggested if the ureter is not visible behind the bladder. IVU is rarely done nowadays. MAG3 scan is a functional study that can show differential renal function and washout of contrast, which is delayed in obstruction. The need to treat renal dilatation that may be a PUJ obstruction in the asymptomatic child is an area of controversy. Where interval ultrasound shows increasing dilatation, or a MAG3 scan shows reduced function and delayed washout, obstruction is present and surgery is indicated. Where renal dilatation is being observed it is usual to perform renal ultrasound every 3 to 6 months, especially in the first 2 years, and repeat MAG3 scan if significant dilatation persists. CT scans looking for abnormal lower pole vessels are not performed as this does not affect treatment decisions.

Indications for surgical correction of PUJO in children

All symptomatic patients require surgery. In asymptomatic patients serial ultrasound is useful and surgery is required where significant increasing dilatation is seen. Where renal dilatation extends into the calyces, dilatation is significant. Otherwise there may just be renal pelvic dilatation alone, where obstruction is rare. A MAG3 scan is helpful where renal dilatation is significant, and indications for surgery include reduced function on the affected side and delayed washout. Where renal function is preserved and washout is delayed, careful observation with serial ultrasound will predict when surgery is required. The majority of these cases resolve and do not need surgery.[1] Controversy exists where washout is delayed and normal function exists. Management of cases with bilateral renal dilatation provides a particularly difficult problem. In this situation serial ultrasound scans are helpful, with progressive dilatation providing evidence to support surgical intervention.

Techniques of surgical correction of PUJO

Open dismembered pyeloplasty remains the gold standard. This is commonly done via the anterior or lateral approach. Occasionally the lumbotomy incision is preferred, but this may restrict access to a low PUJ. Laparoscopic pyeloplasty is becoming more popular, but is technically challenging in children because of reduced perinephric space and laparoscopic suturing of a narrow ureter to the renal pelvis.[2] Laparoscopy can reduce hospital stay in adults, but because of the short hospital stay with open surgery in children, it gives little benefit in paediatric cases.

Pre-operative work-up

Antibiotic prophylaxis is given. We use gentamicin 3–5 mg/kg as a single intravenous dose. Make sure that the appropriate X-rays are in the operating theatre!

Operative technique

The patient is placed in the supine position with a rolled towel under the appropriate loin. A transverse anterior 12th rib incision is made, keeping extra-peritoneal with careful use of the diathermy point. In children the muscle layers of the abdominal wall are well defined. The transverse layer is split, beginning laterally at the rib tip. The dissection is deepened laterally, taking care to stay retroperitoneal until lumbar fat is seen. Once the fat is seen further finger-tip blunt dissection is used to sweep the peritoneum medially and gain access to the kidney. Gerota's fascia is sharply incised laterally and opened with careful dissection anteromedially to expose the PUJ region. If the peritoneum is opened accidentally, it should be closed and careful dissection continued. A Dennis-Browne retractor helps with exposure. Using blunt dissection with non-tooth forceps, remove the fascia overlying the PUJ. Place a stay suture in the renal pelvis. This suture is used to elevate and stabilize the operative site. Further blunt dissection exposes the ureter. Take care not to damage any lower pole vessels. Despite these being uncommon in children, as in adults they should be preserved. The PUJ region is divided at the point of narrowing, the ureter is spatulated where convenient, and the renal pelvis opened. The renal pelvis does not need to be reduced in size.

A careful anastamosis is fashioned tension free with at least three interrupted sutures at the apex and on each side as this is the narrowest aspect of the repair. We use absorbable sutures (4–0 and 5–0 Vicryl). The completion of the anastamosis with continuous or interrupted sutures is undertaken with the posterior wall first. A JJ stent can be placed with guidewire assistance. Confirm passage of the stent into the bladder by feeling for a slight degree of tightness at the VUJ as it passes through and by visual confirmation of urine flow out of the bladder out of the side-holes of the stent once the guidewire is withdrawn. Once the stent is in position, the repair is completed. The repair should be tension free, dependent, and not rotated or kinked. A suction drain is placed. The muscle layers are closed, the skin is closed with a subcuticular suture, and a drain is sutured in. A urethral catheter is placed.

Post-operative managemant

An epidural provides excellent analgesia. Antibiotic prophylaxis, such as co-trimoxazole or trimethoprim, is used until stent removal. Remove the drain at 24 hr unless the drain fluid is urine, in which case take off the suction and leave the drain until dry. Take the catheter out at 48 hr. Most children can be discharged on day 2. Remove the stent under general anaesthetic at 4–6 weeks. Get a renal ultrasound at 3 months, and then 6 and 12 months later if dilatation is reducing.

Complications

- Early complications:
    - UTI.
    - Wound infection.
    - Urine leaks: usually seal spontaneously if the drain is taken off suction and the catheter left in place. In this setting the drain should be left in for 24 hr after the leak stops and the catheter should be left for a further 24 hr.
- Late complications:
    - Recurrent obstruction is rare and occurs in less than 1–2%.

Outcomes

Follow-up of laparoscopic cases is too short to give long-term results. However, in the short term results are similar to open surgery.

Further reading

1 Gough DCS. Upper urinary tract obstruction: pathophysiology and diagnosis. In *Essentials of paediatric urology*, ed. Thomas D, Duffy PG, Rickwood AMK. London: Martin Dunitz, 2002, pp 57–62.
2 Gough DCS and Thomas DFM. Upper urinary tract obstruction. In *Essentials of paediatric urology*, ed. Thomas D, Duffy PG, Rickwood AMK. London: Martin Dunitz, 2002, pp 63–71.

References

1 Thorup J, Jokela R, Cortes D, Nielsen OH. The results of 15 years of consistent strategy in treating antenatally suspected pelvi-ureteric obstruction. *BJU Int* 2003; **91**:850–2.
2 El-Ghoneimi A, Farhat W, Bolduc S et al. Laparoscopic dismembered pyeloplasty by a retroperitoneal approach in children. *BJU Int* 2003; **92**:104–8.

Ambiguous genitalia (intersex)

Ambiguous genitalia or intersex is a rare, complex, and potentially life-threatening condition. Because of confusing and controversial historic nomenclature, a recent consensus statement has proposed the term 'disorders of sexual development' (DSD) to indicate congenital conditions with atypical development of chromosomal, gonadal, or anatomic sex.[1] This new classification system allows up-to-date investigation with accurate diagnosis and also meets the need for psychologically sensitive yet descriptive terminology (Table 14.2).

Psychosexual development is influenced by a many factors including X and Y genes, brain structure, social and cultural circumstances, and the *in utero* environment. A number of 'standards of care' have been proposed for the management of these children:

• Avoiding gender assignment before expert evaluation of the newborn.
• Open communication with family.
• Experienced multidisciplinary team evaluation and management.
• Family and patient involvement in decision-making.
• Strict confidentiality.

The multidisciplinary team should include paediatric endocrinologists, surgeons (urologist and gynaecologist), psychologists/psychiatrists, geneticists, neonatologists, social workers, nurses, and medical ethicists. Consensus regarding diagnosis, gender assignment, and management options must be reached, and one member should primarily interact with the family. The surgeon's role involves outlining and undertaking surgical procedures with a focus on functional genital anatomy.

Evaluation of a neonate with genital ambiguity requires accurate objective assessment of genitalia. Investigations include karyotyping, measurement of 17-hydroxyprogesterone, testosterone, gonadotropins, anti-Müllerian hormone, and electrolytes. Pelvic ultrasound and laparoscopy are used to clarify pelvic anatomy. Some children may present late with unrecognized gender ambiguity, such as virilized female at puberty and primary amenorrhea. Sex determination may occasionally be difficult and should be delayed until an accurate diagnosis is made (usually available within 48 hr). Factors influencing the sex assignment include diagnosis, genital appearance, treatment options, fertility potential, social and cultural issues, and parental request. Parents should be advised not to register the sex of their child until all investigations are complete. Appearance-altering surgery is not urgent.

Table 14.2 New classification system for disorders of sexual development (DSD)

Previous	Proposed
Intersex	DSD
Male pseudohermaphrodite, undervirilization of an XY male, and undermasculinization of an XY male	46,XY DSD
Female pseudohermaphrodite, overvirilization of an XX female, and masculinization of an XX female	46,XX DSD
True hermaphrodite	Ovotesticular DSD
XX male or XX sex reversal	46,XX testicular DSD
XY sex reversal	46,XX complete gonadal dysgenesis

Reproduced from Lee PA, Houk CP, Faisal Ahmed S *et al*. Consensus statement on management of intersex disorders. *Pediatrics* 2006; **118**:488–500.

Normal sex differentiation

Sex is determined by a gene on the short arm of the Y chromosome— the 'sex-determining region on Y' (SRY). In fetal development phenotypic sex is undifferentiated until the sixth week. Without the SRY gene, female development is a passive process. In male development, genetic and endocrine factors actively develop the male phenotype. Müllerian inhibitory substance (MIS) is produced by the Sertoli cells, and induces resorption of the Müllerian ducts and stimulates the Leydig cells. Testosterone is produced by the Leydig cells and reaches a peak at 15–18 weeks of gestation. Intra-cellular testosterone is converted to dihydro-testosterone (DHT), and maintains the mesonephric ducts and causes virilization of the urogenital sinus and external genitalia. Masculinization requires both the local and systemic effect of testosterone. Genetic and hormonal factors alter the structure and function of the brain contributing to male behaviour.

Surgical principles

The timing and extent of genital surgery in DSD is controversial. Early surgery has some benefits including the effect of oestrogen on tissues, satisfactory outcomes, and minimizing family concern of atypical genital appearance. Adverse outcomes have led to delay in unnecessary genital surgery. Vaginal reconstruction should be undertaken at puberty and dilatation should not be performed in childhood. If reconstructive surgery is performed early, it is common to perform an examination under anaesthesia and dilatation at or around puberty. Intra-abdominal testes should be removed because of the high risk of malignancy. The goals are to maximize anatomy and enhance sexual function. Long-term follow-up of these children continues to alter both the type and timing of surgery, with the aim of giving the best functional outcome for both physical and psychological development.

Congenital adrenal hyperplasia (CAH)

This is the most common cause of DSD with XX sex chromosomes, making up >80% of the cases. All are genetic females. Because of an enzyme defect in the adrenal gland, there is excess production of a precursor steroid. This is converted to male sex steroids and thus there is virilization of a genetic female. 21-Hydroxylase deficiency is the most common enzyme defect and is an autosomal recessive condition. 11b-Hydroxylase deficiency and 3b-hydroxysteroid deficiency are the other rarer enzyme defects. Other rarer causes include maternal exogenous steroid consumption in pregnancy and steroid-producing tumours.

The presentation is variable and includes severe electrolyte imbalance (salt retention and potassium loss) requiring emergency treatment. Diagnosis may be made pre-natally, especially with a positive family history confirmed by fetal tissue sampling. Pre-natal treatment using maternal steroid supplementation has been reported to be successful. Elevation of blood 17a-hydroxyprogesterone is diagnostic of 21-hydroxylase deficiency in a karyotypic female (XX).

Management consists of steroid replacement, female gender assignment, and genitoplasty.[2] The steps to genitoplasty are initial clitoral reduction, retaining sensation to the glans, leaving the dorsally sited neurovascular structures and glans fully intact. Vaginal reconstruction requires separation of the vagina and urethra to create two perineal openings. Where the vagina opens up high into the urethra, vaginoplasty may be technically challenging. Urinary continence is not usually affected. Excess perineal 'scrotal' skin is used for labial reconstruction. Vaginal dilatation may be required post-operatively to prevent the orifice narrowing and thus vaginal reconstruction is commonly delayed until puberty. Occasionally, an examination under anaesthetic and Y–Vplasty may be required for introital stenosis. Normal fertility is usual in CAH.

Androgen insensitivity syndrome (AIS)

This condition is a group of disorders with varying degrees of feminization of a genetic male and may be partial or complete. In the most severe (complete) form, the external genitalia are female in appearance. This condition may be diagnosed late because of primary amenorrhoea. Partial androgen insensitivity may present with varying degrees of masculinization. Gender assignment is determined by penile size and response to hCG stimulation. In cases of severe micropenis, gender conversion to female is undertaken and a feminizing genitoplasty is performed. More recently, genetic males with a micropenis have not been surgically altered and initial results are that they may also have good long-term results living as males. Severe hypospadias is repaired if present, and occasionally de-scrotalization of the penis may be required. Care should be taken to avoid unrealistic expectations of genital surgery in this group.

Mixed gonadal dysgenesis

This genetic abnormality leads to an abnormality of gonadal development and a non-functioning 'streak' gonad. There are varying degrees of phenotypic abnormality associated with a mosaic or mixed chromosomal anomaly. A streak gonad carries a malignant risk and should be removed. Growth of external genitalia in males can be stimulated by testosterone.

References

1 Lee PA, Houk CP, Faisal Ahmed S *et al.* Consensus statement on management of intersex disorders. *Pediatrics* 2006; **118**:488–500.
2 Rink RC and Kaefer M. Surgical management of intersexuality, cloacal malformation and other abnormalities of the genitalia in girls. In *Campbell's Urology* 8th edn, ed Walsh PC, Retik AB, Vaughan ED, Wein AJ. Philadelphia, PA: WB Saunders, 2002, Chapter 69.

Cystic renal disease

Introduction

Cystic renal disease in childhood is less common than in adults, with autosomal recessive polycystic disease rarely seen. Multicystic dysplastic kidney (MCDK) is more common and management is still controversial.

Polycystic renal disease

This inherited renal disease is autosomal dominant when seen in adults and commonly leads to renal failure, with little impact in childhood. Autosomal recessive polycystic renal disease is a rare childhood condition. The kidneys retain a normal shape but are large because of the presence of many small (1–2 mm) cysts which replace the renal cortex. The liver and biliary tree may be involved. This condition often presents antenatally and termination is a management option.

Clinically, the presentation depends on the level of renal function. If renal function is poor in pregnancy, pulmonary hypoplasia and Potter syndrome are present because of the volume amniotic fluid volume. Early perinatal death may occur. Occasionally autosomal recessive polycystic renal disease does not present until later, with hypertension and secondary effects of hepatic fibrosis. Diagnosis is by renal ultrasound.

Treatment depends on the degree of renal impairment. Renal failure at birth carries a poor prognosis. Initial dialysis and subsequent transplantation are reported and are the only option for survival with renal failure. Native nephrectomy for control of hypertension or to make space for transplantation may be undertaken. Medical management is to preserve renal function with treatment of hypertension and ACE inhibitors for improved renal blood flow.

Multicystic dysplastic kidney

This unilateral cystic condition is associated with renal dysplasia caused by ureteral obstruction *in utero* and invariably no renal function on the affected side. The prevalence is unknown as it may remain asymptomatic. However, routine screening ultrasound during pregnancy has led to an increased detection rate of MCDK. Clinically, MCDK may present with a renal mass, predicted with pre-natal ultrasound or by incidental ultrasound finding post-natally. MCDK is a diagnosis made on the basis of ultrasound scanning and is identified as a collection of variable-sized cysts with echogenic material between them.[1] A DMSA renal scan shows no function. MCU is usually undertaken to see if contralateral reflux is present as this may need treatment in its own right. Contralateral reflux is present in 15–20% of cases.

The natural history of MCDK is variable, but a number involute and completely disappear on ultrasound. Up to 50% may resolve spontaneously and need follow-up only. Very rarely MCDK may be misdiagnosed as a cystic Wilms' tumour. Hypertension is a rare but well-documented complication and is cured by nephrectomy.

The management of MCDK is controversial, with prophylactic nephrectomy recommended by some and surveillance by others.[2] With the advent of minimally invasive laparoscopic nephrectomy, surgery remains the most common management. Laparoscopic nephrectomy is retroperitoneal and may be difficult in children because of the small perinephric space.

If surveillance rather than surgery is chosen, regular ultrasound every 6 months and then annually is undertaken, with nephrectomy only if the kidney does not involute. Management of the contralateral kidney, if refluxing, is directed towards preservation of renal function in the context of what is essentially a solitary functioning kidney. Therefore surgical management of persistent reflux may be favoured over conservative management.

Multilocular renal cyst

This is a rare renal lesion. It presents with haematuria, loin pain, and occasionally an abdominal mass. Ultrasound is usually sufficient for a definitive diagnosis, but CT or MRI gives clearer anatomical definition. Rarely, a multilocular renal cyst is misdiagnosed as a cystic Wilms' tumour. It is not a pre-malignant condition. Surveillance or partial or total nephrectomy are management options, depending on the size of the cyst and renal function.

Simple renal cyst is rare in childhood. Be aware that a dilated upper pole of a duplex renal tract may be reported by the ultrasonographer as a simple renal cyst.

References

1 Sanders RC, Hartman DS. The sonographic distinction between neonatal multicystic kidney and hydronephrosis. *Radiology* 1984; **151**:621–5.
2 Welch TR, Wacksman J. The changing approach to multicystic dysplastic kidney in children. *J Paediatr* 2005; **146**:759–63.

Haematuria

Haematuria, either macroscopic or microscopic, rarely requires surgical intervention in the paediatric age group.

Haematuria usually represents a benign self-limiting condition. Evaluation requires a urine microscopy (haematuria is defined as >5 RBCs per high power field). Because of the transient nature of haematuria, consider repeat analysis. Further diagnostic investigations should be reserved for select children at higher risk for harbouring an underlying urological condition. A renal tract ultrasound is the most useful test.

Important aspects of history include symptoms of UTI, recent upper respiratory tract infection, trauma, and medication. A family history of haematuria is common in cases of benign haematuria. During examination check blood pressure and examine the abdomen and genitalia. Look for a skin rash which could indicate Henoch–Schönlein purpura.

Urinalysis (WBCs, RBCs, casts, protein, and dysmorphic RBCs) is the cornerstone test for bacterial infection and renal causes for haematuria. The urine calcium-to-creatinine ratio is undertaken as this is an indicator of hypercalcuria and may predispose to stone disease. Serum creatinine, anti-streptolysin-O (ASO) and anti-DNAase antibody titres look for post-streptococcal causes such as acute glomerulonephritis secondary to a recent upper respiratory infection. The exact aetiology is unknown, but appears to be an inflammatory reaction to the glomerular basement membrane. This may commonly cause of haematuria or brownish discoloration of the urine. Refer children with significant proteinuria and casts to a paediatric nephrologist.

The common medical causes of haematuria include glomerulonephritis (e.g. IgA nephropathy), basement membrane disorders (benign familial haematuria), and UTI. African Caribbean children should be tested for sickle cell disease.

A renal ultrasound will assess renal size and cortical and medullary echogenicity, which are altered in acute inflammation and will determine whether there is dilatation and stone disease. If these investigations are normal, reassurance is required. Cystoscopy should be reserved for children with irritative lower urinary symptoms, macroscopic haematuria, and bladder abnormality on ultrasound.

Further reading
1 Mathias R. Haematuria. In *Handbook of pediatric urology*, 2nd edn, eds Baskin LS, Kogan BA. Baltimore, MD: Lippincott–Williams & Wilkins, 2005, pp 203–16.

Bladder extrophy

Introduction

Bladder extrophy is a rare devastating condition affecting the urinary tract, genital tract, musculoskeletal system, and sometimes the intestinal tract. The incidence is about one in 50 000–100 000 with a male-to-female ratio of 3:1. Bladder extrophy is the most common in a spectrum of conditions ranging from the less severe epispadias through to the most severe cloacal extrophy. Pre-natal ultrasound may identify a fetus with extrophy and delivery at a specialist centre can be organized.

Embryogenesis

Persistence of the cloacal membrane prevents medial migration of meso-derm. When the cloacal membrane disappears, there is no anterior bladder wall and the posterior wall of the bladder is exposed. Failure of the urethra to fold on its dorsal surface leads to epispadias. In cloacal extrophy, the most severe form of the condition, the cloacal membrane perforates before division of the cloaca by the urorectal septum into an anterior bladder and a posterior rectum.

Possible abnormalities

- Exposure of the bladder which develops squamous metaplasia and fibrosis and is colonized with bacteria. The bladder on the lower abdominal wall which rapidly develops squamous may be a small vestige or measure 6–7 cm in diameter.
- Vesico-ureteric reflux (once the bladder has been closed).
- Separation of the pubic bones.
- In boys, a short dorsally curved penis (chordee), with separated corporal bodies which diverge to attach to the inferior pubic rami.
- In girls, the clitoris is divided on either side of the urethral plate.
- The vagina is tilted anteriorly and may be stenosed.
- Uterine duplication may occur.
- Inguinal hernias are common.
- Upper tract abnormalities occur in 60–70% of those with cloacal extrophy.
- Rectal prolapse in 10–20%.
- Fertility may be normal.

Surgical correction

Surgical correction is very demanding, and urgent referral to a specialist centre with experience gives the best results. Careful sensitive communi-cation to the parents is important. Initial management is supportive, together with a clear plastic wrap over the exposed bladder. This protects the fragile bladder mucosa and minimizes heat loss through the exposed organ. Abdominal ultrasound is important as a baseline to identify associated renal abnormalities.

The aim of surgery is to repair the bladder, bladder outlet, and urethra in order to provide a capacious low-pressure reservoir with a competent functioning bladder outlet and unobstructed urethra. Long-term surgical results can be poor and further multiple surgeries may be required to gain continence and an adequate phallus. There has been a move away from staged reconstruction (with bladder closure first, then a continence procedure, and lastly a penile repair) towards a single complete repair, although long-term outcomes with this approach are awaited. Where it is not possible to achieve a continent bladder outlet or where clean inter-mittent catheterization (CIC) is difficult because of maintenance of urethral sensation, a continent catheterizable diversion with a Mitrofanoff channel gives good results. This is used for salvage of an incontinent patient.

Operative technique for single-stage procedure

Surgery is performed in a centre with experience in neonatal surgery with appropriate anaesthetic and other support services. Pelvic bones are flexible in the newborn period, and iliac osteotomies to bring the pubic bones together are not required. Bladder repair is initially undertaken and bilateral ureteric re-implantation is carried out. The bladder is closed down to the bladder neck where additional wrap or tightening is under-taken using either bladder neck mucosa or local fascia.

Next the epispadias repair is performed by complete mobilization of the urethra off the corporal bodies. The corporal bodies are separated so that the penile corporal body and urethra are mobile with two sepa-rate glans segments. The urethra is dropped between the corporal bodies ventrally, and the penis and urethra are reconstructed. A urethral catheter is placed and skin closure achieved.

Long-term continence ranges from a low level up to 80% in some series. In males, continence tends to improve as the prostate grows around the time of adolescence. Incontinence may be due to inadequate bladder capacity, poor compliance, bladder neck incompetence, or urethral obstruction. Assessment involves cystoscopy, video-urodynamics, and discussion of options taking into account the patient and family expectations. Renal function may deteriorate if bladder pressure is high or emptying is poor. Regular renal ultrasound is important to monitor kidney growth and manage any dilatation. Where urinary incontinence persists despite further surgical management, consider a continent catheterizable urinary diversion. Since urethral sensation is preserved, a catheterizable channel may be required.

In female patients with extrophy repairs who subsequently become pregnant, obstetric complications such as uterine prolapse occur because of weak pelvic floor muscles. Patients with previous bladder neck recon-struction or urinary diversion are best managed by Caesarian section with urological input. Vaginal delivery is associated with a higher risk of maternal incontinence.

Further reading

1 Gearhart J. Extrophy, epispadias, and other bladder anomalies In *Campbell's Urology* 8th edn, ed Walsh PC, Retik AB, Vaughan ED, Wein AJ. Philadelphia, PA: WB Saunders, 2002, Chapter 61.
2 Gearhart J, Matthews R. Combined bladder closure in epispadias and reconstruction of bladder extrophy. *J Urol*. 1998; **160**:1182.
3 Lotteman H, Melon Y, Lombrail P, Cendron J Reconstruction of bladder extrophy: retrospective study of 57 patients with evaluation of factors in favour of acquisition of continence. *Ann Urol*; **32**:233–9.
4 Mitchell M, Bagley. Complete penile disassembly for epispadias repair: The Mitchell technique. *J Urol* 1996; **155**:300.
5 Ransley P, Duffy P *et al.* Bladder extrophy closure and epispadias repair. In *Operative surgery: paediatric surgery*.

Posterior urethral valves

Posterior urethral valves (PUVs) are a thin obstructing membrane running from the veru montanum and spreading round the urethra anteriorly to attach more distally. They occur only in boys, with an incidence of one in 5000 live births. They may present as a neonatal emergency with severe urosepsis and renal failure, but nowadays they more usually present ante-natally as renal dilatation and/or oligohydramnios (most amniotic fluid volume is composed of fetal urine from week 16 onwards). PUVs are the most common congenital cause of urethral obstruction with a spectrum of anomalies affecting the renal tracts proximally. The diagnosis is made with a VCUG. Management depends on severity, but a multidisciplinary approach with medical and surgical input is usually required. PUVs remain the most common cause of paediatric renal failure and need for subsequent transplantation. In these patients, the bladder commonly requires reconstructive surgery to make it safe to drain a successful transplant.

Presentation

Antenatally, PUV presents with an ultrasound appearance of a full thick walled bladder, renal dilatation, and a dilated visible posterior urethra (keyhole sign). In severe cases associated renal dysplasia and obstruction leads to reduced fetal urine output, oligohydramnios, and pulmonary hypoplasia (Potter syndrome). The timing and degree of oligohydramnios is an important predictor of post-natal outcome. Pre-natal intervention with vesico-amniotic shunts or premature delivery have not improved renal function or survival.[1] Antenatal dilatation with suspicion of PUV has allowed early investigation, diagnosis, and prevention of early urosepsis with improved outlook.

Post-natal investigations in asymptomatic neonates include baseline renal function plus early renal ultrasound and MCUG. MCUG characteristically shows a dilated trabeculated bladder and an elongated dilated posterior urethra with a dramatic calibre change distal to the valves. Reflux is present in up to 50% of cases, and occasionally rupture of a calyceal fornix or diverticulum leads to urinary ascites. Ultrasound usually shows renal dilatation and cortical thinning with a bladder that is thick walled and not emptying. A DMSA renal scan is useful to determine differential renal function. Antibiotic prophylaxis is begun immediately. A nadir creatinine at day 5–7 gives good indication of long-term renal function. Symptomatic neonates may present with respiratory distress, sepsis, renal failure, abdominal distension. and a poor urinary stream. Late presentation is rare, but is sometimes seen with incontinence, UTI, and poor urinary flow.

Management

Initial management in acute presentation is to resuscitate, treat sepsis, and drain the urinary tract with a small infant feeding catheter (rather than a Foley balloon catheter which can cause bladder spasm and obstruction of the ureteric orifices). MCUG is the gold standard for diagnosis, and endoscopic valve resection is performed when the boy is medically fit. Valve resection is undertaken with a paediatric resectoscope; meatal dilatation is usually required. The valves are visualized and cauterized just lateral to the veru montanum on both sides. If the child is premature, or appropriate equipment or an experienced surgeon is unavailable, a cutaneous vesicostomy can be undertaken. This is performed with a transverse incision midway between the umbilicus and pubic bone, and the linea alba is split. The dome of the bladder is mobilized, opened, and sutured to the fascia and skin with absorbable sutures (3–0 or 4–0 absorbable) to prevent prolapse.

The aim of subsequent management is to preserve renal function, prevent UTI, and perform continence-preserving surgery for specific indications. Surveillance follows with multidisciplinary care with medical and surgical input. Antibiotic prophylaxis continues in children with reflux. Follow-up MCUG is required to show relief of obstruction with valve ablation. A redo cystoscopy is occasionally required.

Regular creatinine and renal ultrasound is undertaken to determine renal function, growth and dilatation. If renal function deteriorates, UTIs occur, or kidney dilatation develops during observation, upper tract diversion can be considered. This is controversial and rarely improves renal function. Temporary drainage via nephrostomy may be an alternative.

Management of reflux in boys with valves is controversial as it is secondary reflux due to obstruction. Surgery to correct reflux has poorer outcomes because of persistent abnormal bladder function. Circumcision is recommended in boys with reflux and valves, especially with a breakthrough UTI.

Bladder dysfunction, or 'valve bladder' is seen in up to 30% of boys and may lead to secondary renal deterioration due to high pressure and poor bladder emptying. Poor renal concentrating ability may lead to polyuria which compounds this problem, especially overnight.[2] Management is by lowering bladder pressure, and increasing capacity and emptying efficiency. Clinically, these boys may have incontinence and dilating upper tracts, with progressive reduction in renal function Urodynamics confirms this bladder behaviour, and anticholinergics, low-dose alpha-blockers, and occasionally CIC are required. CIC is difficult as these boys have a sensate urethra and a Mitrofanoff channel is usually required. Nocturnal urine drainage can assist in renal preservation.

In children with renal failure, transplantation offers the best quality of life. Bladder dysfunction needs to be treated prior to transplantation, and surgery to produce a high-volume low-pressure reservoir is required. Augmentation of the bladder can be accomplished using a dilated ureter draining a non-functioning kidney, or more commonly, ileum. A Mitrofanoff channel is important for emptying. Transplantation may be undertaken approximately 6 weeks later with similar outcome to transplantation into a normal bladder.[3]

Further reading

1 Frank JD, Rickwood AMK. Posterior urethral valves and other urethral anomalies. In *Essentials of paediatric urology*, ed. Thomas D, Duffy PG, Rickwood AMK. London: Martin Dunitz, 2002.
2 Gonzales E. Posterior urethral valves and other urethral anomalies. In *Campbell's Urology*, 8th edn, ed Walsh PC, Retik AB, Vaughan ED, Wein AJ. Philadelphia, PA: WB Saunders, 2002, Chapter 63.

References

1 Salam MA. Posterior urethral valve: outcome of antenatal intervention. *Int J Urol* 2006: **13**:1317–22.
2 Koff SA, Mutabagani KH, Jayanthi VR. The valve bladder syndrome: pathophysiology and treatment with nocturnal bladder emptying. *J Urol* 2002; **167**:291–7.
3 Ali-El-Dein B, Abol-Enein H, El-Husseini A, Osman Y, Shehab El-Din AB, Ghoneim MA. Renal transplantation in children with abnormal lower urinary tract. *Transplant Proc* 2004; **36**:2968–73.

Neuropathic bladder

The most common cause of neuropathic bladder in children is spina bifida (myelomeningocoele) and sacral agenesis, the latter often being associated with imperforate anus. Acquired neuropathic bladder is rare (spinal cord injury from trauma, spinal cord tumours, or transverse myelitis). The incidence of spina bifida is decreasing because of prevention by folate supplementation during pregnancy and therapeutic abortion.

Historically, renal failure was the main cause of death in such children and urinary diversion was the mainstay of treatment. Modern urological management of the neuropathic bladder is aimed at preserving renal function and promoting urinary and faecal continence. Long-term conduit management does not always protect the kidneys. With improved understanding of 'safe' bladder storage and CIC, the majority of children with a neuropathic bladder can be dry and free from urinary infections, and have well-preserved renal function with an improved quality of life.

Prevalence

Up to one in 1000 live births have a neural tube defect. There is increasing interest in fetal surgery with closure of the open neural defect and bladder drainage. Early results suggest that it is feasible but benefits are yet to be proven in improved urinary tract function.

Classification

The normal urinary tract 'stores' urine at low pressure and high volume, requiring a highly compliant bladder and a competent outlet. At a socially appropriate moment the bladder empties. This requires coordinated outlet relaxation and bladder contraction. Complete bladder emptying at low pressure protects the kidneys and prevents UTIs.

From a clinical perspective, the most useful classification of the neuropathic lower urinary tract is a functional system since this allows management to be based around specific clinical problems. Classification in children is the same as that in adults (📖 see Chapter 13).

Patient assessment

Neonatal management is a team approach with careful consideration of the huge emotional trauma associated with the birth of a child with this anomaly. Renal ultrasound to determine kidney size, dilatation, and bladder emptying is undertaken early (within the first few days). Back closure can alter bladder function, so consider arranging a repeat ultrasound.

Renal tract surveillance is the mainstay of management combined with intervention to protect the kidneys, prevent UTI, and achieve and maintain continence. Urinary infection may be difficult to diagnose and should be based on a combination of symptoms and abnormal urinalysis. Commonly urinalysis will show bacterial contamination or colonization (mixed organisms).

Urodynamics has improved our understanding of the neuropathic bladder, and a 'safe' bladder is defined as one with a low storage pressure (below 30–40 cmH$_2$O).[1] Some advocate early urodynamics and management based on these findings alone; others recommend a more expectant management with serial renal ultrasound.

Patient management

The goal of management is to prevent renal damage and promote continence. Because of individual patient and caregiver factors, management options are individualized. Only rarely are patients able to spontaneously void to completion at low pressures, and therefore for the majority surveillance alone is not adequate to achieve these goals of management.

The high-pressure bladder is managed by CIC and anticholinergic medication or bladder augmentation. CIC is safe and effective in children, and it can be instigated in the neonatal period. If this is not possible a vesicostomy can be performed and left for a prolonged time. Anticholinergic medication (oxybutinin) is well tolerated by children and effectively lowers bladder pressure. New long-acting formulations and other anticholinergics appear equally effective and have fewer side-effects.

Intravesical Botox injection has recently been advocated as a treatment option. However, the effect of this is temporary and its place in long-term care is yet to be fully established.

Bladder augmentation can be undertaken a number of ways: auto-augmentation, ureteric augmentation, and enterocystoplasty. Enterocystoplasty, which provides a consistent low-pressure high-volume bladder, remains the most common surgical procedure for bladder augmentation.[2] Bowel segments used are ileum, sigmoid, and rarely stomach (see p. 710 for operative details and complications). Auto-augmentation, where the bladder muscle dome is stripped from the mucosa and a thin-walled diverticulum left, rarely gives a consistent high capacity and appears to contract in the long term. Ureteral augmentation can only be performed where there is a redundant capacious ureter, and again consistent safe bladder storage is rarely seen. However, there are theoretical benefits of not incorporating bowel into the urinary tract.

An incompetent bladder outlet is more difficult to treat consistently and many surgical techniques are described, an indication that no single procedure guarantees success. In nearly all cases an augmentation is undertaken with an outlet procedure. Outlet resistance may be static, such as with a sling, bladder neck reconstruction, and injectable substance, or dynamic (open to void), such as an artificial sphincter (AUS). In static procedures all patients need to do CIC; in theory, a dynamic outlet procedure may allow voiding. This is rarely the case and CIC is usually undertaken in all cases of surgical bladder reconstruction.

Where CIC of the native urethra is difficult because of hand function or body position, a Mitrofanoff continent catheterizable channel can be constructed. As the appendix is usually used for bowel management, this can be constructed out of the small bowel (Monti).[3] In severe cases, such as poor dexterity, low intellect or poor caregiver support, ileal conduit drainage may still be employed.

Latex allergy is a special situation in children with spina bifida. This may be due to early multiple exposures to latex products (catheters and other medical devices). Precautions now are to remove all latex products from the operating theatre and other management areas. A high index of suspicion is required, especially where children give a history of atopy.

Bowel management

Faecal incontinence is a common finding in spina bifida and this severely limits quality of life. A variety of methods are used to treat this: voluntary bowel movement, manual evacuation, stool softeners, and retrograde enemas. Bowel management should be addressed at the time of correction of urinary incontinence. If previously used bowel management has failed, an antegrade colonic enema (ACE procedure) can prove highly effective in allowing better bowel management.

ACE procedure

A trial of conservative measures should be performed first. An ACE procedure can be undertaken laparoscopically or by open surgery.[4]

- *Laparoscopic ACE* Patients do not need bowel preparation. An initial peri-umbilical direct transperitoneal port should be inserted, the peritoneal cavity inspected, and the appendix visualized. Usually mobilization is not required and a right iliac fossa port can be placed and the appendix drawn out tip first without buttressing the junction with the caecum. The appendix is mobilized to the skin, spatulated, and catheterized. Interrupted absorbable sutures are placed between appendix and skin, and a 10Fr catheter is inserted for flushing.

- *Open surgery* The ACE procedure can be undertaken separately or in conjunction with bladder reconstruction. If the operation is undertaken separately, a muscle splitting incision over the right iliac fossa is used. The appendix can be left *in situ* or, as originally described, mobilized and divided at the appendico-caecal junction. The appendix tip is opened and catheterized, and then anastomosed into the caecum with interrupted 4–0 Vicryl sutures. The taenia coli is separated down to the mucosa and the appendix buried within the wall with interrupted serosal sutures. The large bowel end is bought out to the skin in a straight short direction and approximated with interrupted Vicryl sutures. The appendix is catheterized with a 10Fr catheter and flushed, with the catheter left *in situ* for 1–2 weeks post-operatively.

Bowel evacuation is undertaken by flushing with 500–1000 mL of irrigant fluid daily or every second day. Patients compliant with clinic visits, young patients (<8 years), and non-obese patients have a better outcome with improved quality of life.

Summary

The aim of urological care of children with neuropathic bladder is to preserve renal function, establish urinary and faecal continence, and prevent UTIs, with a commitment to minimize early surgery. A combination of surveillance, intervention, and education helps to provide a successful outcome.

Further reading

1 Rickwood AMK, Malone PS. Neuropathic bladder In *Essentials of paediatric urology*, ed. Thomas D, Duffy PG, Rickwood AMK. London: Martin Dunitz, 2002, pp 135–48.

References

1 McGuire EJ, Woodside JR, Borden TA et al. Prognostic value of urodynamics testing in myelo-dysplastic patients. *J Urol* 1981; **126**:205–9.
2 Goldwasser B, Webster GD. Augmentation and substitution enterocystoplasty. *J Urol* 1986; **135**:215–24.
3 Tekant G, Emir H Esenturk N et al. Catheterisable continent urinary diversion (Mitrofanoff principle): clinical experience and psychological aspects. *Eur J Pediatr Surg* 2001; **11**:263–7.
4 Malone PS, Ransley PG, Kiely EM. Preliminary report: the antegrade continence enema. *Lancet* 1990; **336**:1217–18.

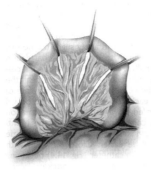

Fig. 14.1 Separate a 4–5 cm length of ileum with its blood supply from the length of ileum that will be used for the augmentation. Reproduced from Ghoniem and Ali-El-Dein, *B J Urol*, 2005, **95**: 455–70, Blackwell. Permission sought.

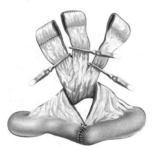

Fig. 14.2 Use coagulation diathermy to incise the bowel longitudinally. Reproduced from Ghoniem and Ali-El-Dein, *B J Urol*, 2005, **95**: 455–70, Blackwell. Permission sought.

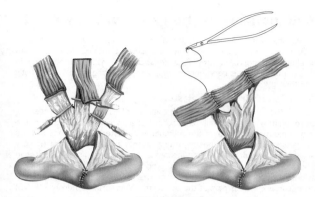

Fig. 14.3 Suture the three bowel segments into a long plate of ileum. (a) Each ring of intestine is incised to create a 'plate' of intestine; (b) The plates are anastomosis to form a long plate of ileum. Reproduced from Ghoniem and Ali-El-Dein, *B J Urol*, 2005, **95**: 455–70, Blackwell. Permission sought.

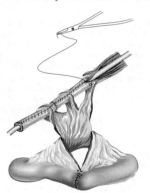

Fig. 14.4 Close the tube with interrupted 3–0 or 4–0 Vicryl over the 12Ch catheter. Reproduced from Ghoniem and Ali-El-Dein, *B J Urol*, 2005, **95**: 455–70, Blackwell. Permission sought.

Further reading

1 Adams MC, Joseph DB. Urinary tract reconstruction in children. In *Campbell's Urology* 8th edn, ed Walsh PC, Retik AB, Vaughan ED, Wein AJ. Philadelphia, PA: WB Saunders, 2002, Chapter 71.

References

1 Mitrofanoff P. Cystotomie continente trans-appendiculare dans le traitement des vessies neurologiques. *Chir Pediatr* 1980; **21**:297–305.
2 Monti, PR, Lara RC, Dutra MD *et al*: New techniques for construction of efferent conduits based on the Mitrofanoff principle. *Urology* 1997; **49**:112–15.

Malignancies of the genitourinary tract

These rare malignancies of childhood, including Wilms' tumour, rhabdomyosarcoma, neuroblastomas, and testicular tumours, now have an excellent prognosis. Treatment is collaborative with chemotherapy in combination with surgery (increasingly organ sparing) and occasionally radiotherapy.

Wilms' tumour (nephroblastoma)

This is the most common renal tumour of childhood, representing approximately 6–7% of all paediatric malignancies. It arises from the embryonic mesenchyme of the metanephric blastema. Incidence in boys and girls is equal, with the majority presenting before 6 years (it very rarely affects adults). A higher incidence is noted in African Caribbean children. Children with 'overgrowth' syndromes also have a much higher incidence. Such syndromes are characterized by hemi-hypertrophy which can occur alone or as part of the Beckwith–Wiedemann syndrome (BWS) (macroglossia, nephromegaly, hepatomegaly, and hemi-hypertrophy). Wilms' tumours occur in ~5% of children with BWS and ~10% of children with hemi-hypertrophy. Therefore renal surveillance ultrasonography every 3–4 months is recommended in such groups.

Presentation

A painless abdominal mass is the usual presentation. Rarely, pain and haematuria may be seen. Hypertension is said to occur in as many as 25% of cases (attributed to elevated plasma renin levels). Look for associated abnormalities (e.g. hemi-hypertrophy, genitourinary anomalies).

Ultrasound confirms the mass and staging radiology is performed with CT or MRI together with a bone scan. The contralateral kidney is carefully studied to rule out bilateral disease; if this is present, differential renal function is assessed with a DMSA scan and a careful review of tumour location is undertaken. Approximately 5% of children have inferior vena caval tumour extension which can be identified on ultrasound (or MRI if ultrasound is indeterminate).

There are two main histological types: favourable (triphasic cell population) and unfavourable (anaplastic, rhabdoid and clear cell).

Evaluation is cooperative and multidisciplinary with overall results improved due to collaborative multicentre research into multimodal therapy. Treatment depends on whether disease is completely resectable; if so, a transperitoneal nephrectomy is performed along with palpation of the contralateral kidney. If the tumour is not resectable, a renal biopsy and pre-operative chemotherapy are undertaken. Dose and type of chemotherapy depends on the stage and histology of the tumour. Radiotherapy is reserved for residual or metastatic disease.

Remember that ~7% of children with synchronous bilateral Wilms' tumour have normal preoperative CT or MR imaging.[1] The contralateral kidney may have disease which is of small volume, and therefore exploration for the larger contralateral tumour will be required at the time of nephrectomy. However, as the accuracy of CT or MRI staging improves, the requirement for exploration of the contralateral kidney will no longer be routine.

Surgical approach to nephrectomy for Wilms' tumour

The approach to nephrectomy for Wilms' tumour in children differs somewhat to that in adults undergoing nephrectomy for renal cell carcinoma. Accurate staging is crucial to subsequent management, as radiotherapy and chemotherapy may be required post-operatively. The surgeon is the final arbiter of staging, and should be mindful that pre-operative imaging may understage the extent of disease. Regional nodes, the IVC, and the contralateral kidney may be involved. Therefore the abdominal cavity should be explored to determine the presence or absence of local tumour extension, metastases to liver and regional nodes, and peritoneal seeding. The contralateral kidney is formally explored prior to nephrectomy. Open Gerota's fascia and palpate and visually inspect the kidney on all its surfaces, looking for evidence of a synchronous bilateral tumour. Palpate the renal vein and inferior vena cava to determine intravascular tumour extension. Suspicious nodes should be sampled.

Wilms' tumours are often very large. Pre-operative imaging may suggest invasion of adjacent organs, such as the liver, and at operation they frequently compress and adhere to structures, but without actual invasion. The extent of resection of adjacent organs will be determined by the experience of the surgeon and the balance of the potential benefit of extensive surgery versus the potential for complications. It is important to manipulate the tumour gently during nephrectomy to avoid tumour spillage (which leads to a substantially increased risk of local abdominal relapse). Resection of adjacent structures may help to prevent tumour spillage and violation of the tumour capsule. Where resection is incomplete, post-operative chemotherapy will be necessary.

For patients with bilateral nephroblastoma confirmed before surgical exploration, the preferred approach is initial biopsy of the tumour in both kidneys (to determine precisely what it is) followed by pre-operative chemotherapy. The aim is to preserve as much functioning renal tissue as possible and thereby lower the chance that renal replacement therapy will be required. An attempt to resect residual disease is made at a second operation after completion of chemotherapy (about 2–3 months after commencement).

Wilms' tumours are usually too large for partial nephrectomy (without prior chemotherapy). Nephron-sparing surgery is principally indicated to preserve renal tissue where there is bilateral disease, a solitary kidney, or renal insufficiency.

Prognosis is excellent with >90% long-term survival in the good prognosis group. Patients with unfavourable disease do not enjoy such a good outcome. Bad prognostic variables include positive lymph nodes, tumour spillage, and unfavourable histology. Recurrence after primary treatment can also be stratified for prognosis dependent on the initial stage, site of relapse, time from initial diagnosis to relapse, and prior therapy. There appears to be a higher incidence of secondary tumours in survivors and future research will be directed towards maintaining good outcomes and reducing treatment-related morbidity.

Rhabdomyosarcoma (RMS)

This rare connective tissue tumour accounts for 10–15% of childhood tumours, with a third arising in the urinary tract. The most common sites are the prostate, bladder, vagina, and para-testicular. There are three histological subtypes (embryonal, alveolar, and pleomorphic), with a poor prognosis in the anaplastic group.

Patients present with urinary symptoms such as frequency, abdominal pain, strangury, or retention. In boys, a scrotal mass may be para-testicular and solid. In girls, a protruding vaginal mass is rarely a RMS but more commonly a benign condition such as urethral prolapse or protruding ureterocele. Haematuria is rare. Diagnostic and staging studies include ultrasound, CT, and MRI plus a bone scan. A percutaneous biopsy may be possible if the tumour is outside the bladder, but the majority of biopsies are undertaken cystoscopically.

Management has improved over time, with emphasis on organ preservation. Relief of urinary tract obstruction is required before initial chemotherapy. Surgery follows to fully excise residual disease and preserve the organ of origin if possible. Radiation is only used for incomplete excision.

The role of surgery varies by site. In recent years, surgical treatment of RMS has become more conservative. Anterior pelvic exenteration is no longer considered to be the initial therapy in pelvic RMS.[2] Partial resection of the bladder wall for primary tumours affecting the dome or sides of the bladder distant from the trigone is recommended either as initial therapy or as a delayed procedure after chemotherapy. Although conservative surgical therapy for bladder tumours has not been as successful as for vaginal primaries, the bladder salvage rate has increased.[3,4] With the intensification of treatment for pelvic RMS in IRS-III (Intergroup Rhabdomyosarcoma Study), 60% of patients retained a functional bladder at 4 years after diagnosis and the overall survival rate exceeded 85%.[5]

There are some concerns about this approach, particularly the number of cases with residual disease after partial cystectomy. Among 22 patients undergoing conservative surgery as primary surgery, there were five cases of local relapse and one of distant relapse.[5] The estimated 3-year survival rate of 79% was similar to that noted for all patients with primary bladder tumours. However, others have noted that a very select group of patients should be expected to have a better prognosis than those with involvement of the bladder base and prostate.[6] In the most recent report from the IRS, partial cystectomy had been employed in 40 patients, in 33 before any other therapy.[4] Seventy-three per cent of the long-term survivors in IRS-I and IRS-II had no bladder-related symptoms.[2] Bladder augmentation or substitution has achieved good functional results in some of these patients.[7]

Most of these tumors arise from the trigonal area or prostate and are not amenable to local or partial resection. Prostatic involvement has been reported to be a significant predictor of a poor outcome.[8] Local recurrence is highly likely if there is incomplete resection or if radiotherapy is omitted. If chemotherapy does not result in adequate shrinkage to allow partial resection, radical cystectomy may be necessary. Pelvic exenteration is also employed for relapsed tumours.[4] Prostatectomy without cystectomy has been performed in selected patients with persistent disease or local relapse.[4,9–11] However, local relapses have occurred in 40% of these patients. The completeness of surgical resection may be difficult to determine by frozen section, and there may be an increased likelihood of local recurrence. On the other hand, if the tumour is shrinking during chemotherapy and repeat biopsy after completing radiotherapy shows maturing rhabdomyoblasts without frank tumour cells, total cystectomy may be postponed or avoided altogether.[12] Serial cystoscopic biopsies are particularly useful in assessing tumour status in patients with intra-vesicular RMS.[13]

Up to 80% survival is seen, with over two-thirds retaining the organ of origin. However, significant long-term symptoms exist in some cases.

Neuroblastomas

Neuroblastomas are the most common solid tumours of childhood and arise in the adrenal medulla or sympathetic ganglia. Interestingly, they may spontaneously regress in children less than 1 year old. These tumours can be classified histologically as favourable or unfavourable. Unfavourable histology is 'stroma poor,' or lacking stroma with a high mitotic rate, and less cellular maturity.

Presentation is most commonly an abdominal mass which may cross the midline. There is sometimes pain, and vaso-active agents secreted from the tumour can produce symptoms (ataxia or behavioural problems, diarrhoea, weight loss). Urinary metabolites, vanillymandillic acid, and homovanillic acid are elevated in 90% of patients. These substances can be monitored for tumour surveillance. n-myc is a tumour oncogene which is commonly present in poor prognosis tumours.

Staging is important to determine treatment and prognosis. Ultrasound, CT, and MRI are used plus bone scan. Meta-iodobenzylguanidine (MIBG) scintography scanning can also show bone marrow outlining primary and metastatic involvement and is useful in staging. MRI has the advantage of showing intraspinal disease.

Treatment is based on completeness of surgical excision which is usually open. However, laparoscopic is being increasingly utilized. Chemotherapy and radiation are reserved for those with residual disease or used prior to surgery where it is unresectable.

There is excellent outcome for lower-risk groups (i.e. children <1 year old, low-stage disease, and no n-myc amplification) with >90% survival.

Testicular tumours

These are very rare tumours in childhood, and they metastasize even more rarely. They present as a painless scrotal mass. A hydrocoele can be differentiated from a tumour by transillumination with a normally palpable testis within. If concern exists, a scrotal ultrasound scan is diagnostic. They are more commonly yolk sac tumours and AFP is positive. Teratomas may occur and orchidectomy is curative for these. Approximately 10% of yolk sac tumours have metastases with an elevated AFP after orchidectomy. Close follow-up is recommended.

Further reading

1 Cook A, Farhat W, Khoury A. Update on Wilms' tumour in children. *J Med Liban* 2005: **53**:85–90.
2 Ferrer FA, Isakoff M, Koyle MA. Bladder/prostate rhabdomyosarcoma: past, present and future. *J Urol* 2006; **176**:1283–91.
3 Grundy P, Perlman E, Rosen NS et al. Current issues in Wilms' tumour management. *Curr Probl Cancer* 2005; **29**:221–60.
4 Kaefer M, Rink RC. Genitourinary rhabdomyosarcoma: treatment options. *Urol Clin North Am* 2000; **27**:471–87.
5 Kim S, Chung DH. Paediatric solid malignancies: neuroblastoma and Wilms' tumour. *Surg Clin North Am* 2006; **86**:469–87.
6 Ritchey ML, Coppes M, Raney RB et al. Paediatric urologic oncology. *Campbell's Urology* 8th edn, ed Walsh PC, Retik AB, Vaughan ED, Wein AJ. Philadelphia, PA: WB Saunders, 2002, pp 2069–507.
7 Rodeberg D, Paidas C. Childhood rhabdomyosarcoma. *Semin Paediatr Surg* 2006; **15**:57–62.
8 Weinstein JL, Katzenstein HM, Cohn SL. Advances in the diagnosis and treatment of neuroblastoma. *Oncologist* 2003; **8**:278–92.

References

1 Ritchey ML, Green DM, Breslow NE, Norkool P. Accuracy of current imaging modalities in the diagnosis of synchronous bilateral Wilms' tumor. *Cancer* 1995; **75**:600–4.
2 Raney RB, Jr, Heyn D, Hays DM et al. Sequelae of treatment in 109 patients followed for 5 to 15 years after diagnosis of sarcoma of the bladder and prostate. *Cancer* 1993; **71**:2387–94.
3 Hays DM. New approaches to the surgical management of rhabdomyosarcoma in childhood. *Chir Paediatr* 1990; **31**:197.
4 Hays DM. Bladder/prostate rhabdomyosarcoma: results of the multi-institutional trials of the Intergroup Rhabdomyosarcoma Study. *Semin Surg Oncol* 1993; **9**:520–3.
5 Hays DM, Raney RB, Wharam MD et al: Children with vesical rhabdomyosarcoma (RMS) treated by partial cystectomy with neoadjuvant chemotherapy, with or without radiotherapy: a report from the Intergroup Rhabdomyosarcoma Study (IRS) Committee. *J Pediatr Hematol Oncol* 1995; **17**:46–52.
6 Fisch M, Burger R, Barthels U, Gutahr P, Hohenfellner R. Surgery in Rhabomyosarcoma of the bladder, prostate and vagina. *World J Urol* 1995; **13**: 213
7 Hicks BA, Hensle TW, Burbige KA, Altman RP. Bladder management in children with genitourinary sarcoma. *J Paed Surg* 1993; **28**: 1019.
8 Crist WM, Garnsey L, Beltangady MS, Gehon E, Ruymann F, Webber B, Haus DB, Wharam M, Maurer HM. Prognosis in children with rhabdomyosarcoma: a report of the intergroup rhabdomyosarcoma studies 1 and 2. Intergroup Rhabdomyosarcoma Committee. *J Clin Oncol* 1990; **4**:443.
9 McLorie GA, Abana OE, Churchill BB, Greenberg M , Mancer K. Rhabdomyosarcoma of the prostate in childhood: current challenges. *J Paed Surg* 1989; **24**:977.
10 Lobe TE, Weiner E, Andrassy RJ, Bagwell CE, Hays D, Crist WM, Webber B, Breneman JC, Reed HM, Teft MC, Heyn R. The argument for conservative, delayed surgery in the management of prostate rhabdomyosarcoma. *J Paed Surg* 1966; **21**: 1084.
11 Merguerian PA. Paediatric genitourinary tumours. *Curr Opin Oncol* 2003; **15**:222–6.
12 Ortega JA, Rowland J, Montforte H, Malogolosski M, Triche T. Presence of well differentiated rhabdomyoblasts at the end of therapy for pelvic rhabdomyosarcoma: implications for the outcome. *J Paed Haematol Oncol* 2000; **22**: 106.
13 Heyn R, Newton WA, Raney RB, Hamond A, Bagwell C, Vietti T, Wharan M ,Gehan E, Maurer HM, Preservation of the bladder in patients with rhabdomyosarcoma. *J Clin Oncol* 1997; **15**:69.

The urachus

This structure lies between the dome of the bladder and the umbilicus, adjacent to the umbilical arteries. It usually closes, resulting in urination via the urethra, and becomes a fibrous cord.

A congenitally patent urachus is rare. It results in a urinary fistula through the umbilicus and may be associated with failure of the bladder to descend. A urachal cyst is also rare, but is seen more commonly and may present in childhood or as an adult. In a urachal cyst there is isolated epithelium between the bladder dome and umbilicus which may become infected or, rarely, malignant. Presentation of an inflammatory mass is with local symptoms, with the diagnosis confirmed by ultrasound or CT.

A urachal diverticulum is a blind internal bladder sinus which usually does not require treatment.

Surgical treatment usually requires complete urachal removal with the bladder dome but umbilical preservation. The incision is usually midline, but peri-umbilical incision is also reported. The incision is opened to the peritoneum and the triangle of tissue excised, bounded by the umbilical arteries laterally. The dome of the bladder is closed in two layers over a catheter with absorbable sutures. A cystogram may be done prior to removal to avoid a urine leak.

Further reading

1 Park JM. Normal and abnormal development of the urogenital system. *Campbell's Urology*, 8th edn, ed Walsh PC, Retik AB, Vaughan ED, Wein AJ. Philadelphia, PA: WB Saunders, 2002 Chapter 49.

Chapter 15

Medicolegal aspects of urology

Why do people sue surgeons?

Much clinical litigation is due to medical error, although in reality the majority of cases of medical error do not end in a lawsuit. The incidence of medical error (an event due to medical management resulting in disability or prolonged hospitalization) is roughly similar across developed countries, occurring in approximately 5–10% of hospital admissions.[1]

Although the incidence of medical errors seems to be roughly similar across developed countries, the likelihood that such errors will lead to litigation is variable. US urologists may be expected to be sued for malpractice at least twice during their career.[2] The 'lifetime risk' of a malpractice suit for UK urologists has not been quantified.

Since the majority of clinical errors do not end in a lawsuit. So why do some patients sue surgeons while others do not? The single most important factor is communication with patients and relatives, or rather the lack of it. Other reasons include:[3]

- So that it would not happen to anyone else (90%).
- I wanted an explanation (90%).
- I wanted the doctors to realize what they had done.
- To get an admission of negligence (80%).
- So that the doctors would know how I feel (70%).
- My feelings were ignored (67%).
- I wanted financial compensation (65%).
- Because I was angry.
- So that the doctor did not get away with it (50%).
- So that the doctor would be disciplined.
- Because it was the only way I could cope with my feelings (45%).
- Because of the attitude of the staff afterwards (42%).
- To get back at the doctor involved (23%).

References

1 Vincent C, Neale G, Woloshynowych M. Adverse events in British hospitals: preliminary retrospective record review. *BMJ* 2001; **322**:517–9.
2 Kaplan GW. Malpractice risks for urologists. *Urology* 1998; **51**:183.
3 Vincent C, Young M, Philips A. Why do people sue doctors? A study of patients and relatives taking legal action. *Lancet* 1994; **343**:1609–13.

What actually precipitates litigation?

Litigation after any operation often arises because something unexpected has happened—a known complication of the operation that the surgeon may not find surprising, or simply a poor outcome. The salient point is that it is entirely unanticipated by the patient. The patient or the relatives believe that something has gone wrong which ought not to have gone wrong. They interpret this as having been due to an error by the surgeon, and make the assumption that such an error on his/her part must have involved negligence. Litigation may follow.

Clinical negligence is defined by the courts as making an error (by act or omission) of which no ordinary doctor, professing the relevant skill, would have been guilty, if acting with reasonable care. To be held negligent in English law an error must be demonstrated to fall below the standards of skill and care which are reasonably to be expected of one carrying out the task or procedure in question. Junior doctors or general practitioners will not be judged by the higher and different standards which are expected of experienced and specialized colleagues, but the junior and the generalist must recognize the limits of their abilities and experience, and seek help from a senior or a specialist in areas where they are unqualified.

It is a defence to a civil action in negligence if it can be shown that, in relation to a particular act or omission, a body of doctors of similar experience and skill would have done (or not done) the same, even if there are others who disagree. This is the *Bolam* defence, more recently qualified in that there must be a logical basis for the act or omission (the *Bolitho* modification of the *Bolam* defence).

Poor communication is a precipitating factor leading to many claims, whether justified or not. Good communication is essential in the pre-operative and post-operative period even if nothing untoward has happened. Explanation from nurses or junior doctors may not carry the same weight as from a more senior doctor, and sometimes is not completely accurate. If complications do occur, if something goes wrong during the operation, or if something unexpected occurs, good communication becomes even more vital. A clear and accurate explanation that is understood by the patient and the relatives needs to be provided, by as senior a member of the surgical team as possible, preferably the consultant in charge. This clear explanation will go a very long way towards preventing suspicions from growing into subsequent litigation. Remember that an apology is not an admission of liability, and in many situations it is only human to say 'I'm sorry for what has happened.'

What can be done to prevent possible litigation?

- The referral letter:
    - Read it from beginning to end—the most relevant piece of information may be buried in the last line of the letter. Act appropriately on the information contained.
- The clinic appointment:
    - Make sure that a doctor of appropriate skill and seniority sees the patient.
- Patient identification:
    - Use 'active' rather than 'passive' identification. To 'actively' identify a patient after calling their name, ask them to confirm their date of birth and address.
    - Check that the blood, urine, or pathology results or X-rays correspond to the patient sitting in front of you. Occasionally the results of blood and urine tests are filed in the wrong set of notes.
- Modesty and humility:
    - Treat people in the way you would like to be treated. Be patient and courteous. Listen to what they have to say. Do not be arrogant.
- History taking, examination, and note writing:
    - Remember that history and examination remain the mainstays of diagnosis.
    - Consider the need for a physical examination, even if this might not seem necessary at the time, and record what you find. It may well be a negative examination, but occasionally something unexpected turns up which needs investigation. The accusation that 'the doctor did not even examine me' is not uncommon in complaints. You can only prove that an abnormality was not present when you met the patient by examining them and *recording* your findings in the notes.
- Chaperones during intimate physical examination:
    - Always ask for a chaperone when examining a patient and document who it was.
    - The definition of 'intimate' is defined by the patient. It is not necessarily confined to examination of the breast, genitalia, pelvis, or perineum.
- Other aspects of communication:
    - Avoid vivid descriptions and colourful language, either when speaking to patients or in your written records. Be prepared for anything you say to be quoted in a court of law.
    - Avoid cracking jokes or laughing during a consultation, unless you really know the patient very well.
    - Avoid euphemisms. If you mean 'cancer', use the term 'cancer' rather than 'warts' (the two have completely different connotations).
- Talking to the angry patient:
    - Never, ever, become angry with a patient who is angry with you. This will not only make *you* more stressed, but it is also very unlikely to calm the patient down. People often become angry because they have been kept waiting, or because tests or treatment

have taken a long time to complete, or because things have genuinely not gone according to plan. Try to put yourself in the position of the patient. Try to understand why they are angry.

- In the operating theatre:
  - Patient identification and wrong side/wrong site surgery. Wrong patient and wrong side errors are rare but, not surprisingly, usually end in litigation. In the UK the National Patient Safety Agency has developed nationally applicable guidelines designed to reduce the risk of wrong site surgery.[1]

The Medical Defence Union has issued the following suggestions to reduce the risk of such errors:

- Avoid the use of abbreviations in referring to site, side, or anatomical location in written notes, consent forms, and on operating lists.
- Use multiple sources of written information to confirm that you are doing the correct operation on the correct side and in the correct patient. These sources can include the patient's original referral letter, consent form, and X-rays.
- The appropriate site and side of the operation should be marked by a member of the surgical team who is going to be present at the operation.
- The process of marking should involve more than one member of clinical staff.
- When marking the patient, you should ask them to identify themselves actively by stating their name, their date of birth, and their address. You should ask them what procedure they think they are about to undergo and the anatomical site/side. (Clearly, in the case of nephrectomy, the patient will usually not have symptoms referable to the diseased side and they will only know which kidney is to be removed because you have told them which side. Therefore if you make a mistake at the beginning of the 'patient pathway,' the patient's confirmation of the side of surgery may not be a safe source for confirming the correct side).
- The operating surgeon should see the patient before administration of anaesthesia and ensure that all clinical documentation is available (referral letter, source of referral, a signed consent form, supporting radiological images).
- Marking should be done with a clear unambiguous indelible method.
- The operating surgeon must be satisfied about the intended site and side of the operation before the patient is draped.
- Marks should be clearly visible to the operating surgeon after the drapes have been positioned.
- A 'time-out' should be called before the procedure starts, so that the patient details and the site and side of the operation can be confirmed against the clinical records.

References

1 Green S. NPSA guidelines on 'wrong site' surgery. *MDU J* 2005; **21**:6. Available online at: www.npsa.nhs.uk.

Record keeping

Remember, no records of the events that took place in a clinic consultation, during an admission, or during an operation may equal no defence, and poor records may equal a poor defence.[1,2]

Keep clear, accurate, legible, and contemporaneous records which report the clinical findings, the decisions made, the information given to patients and any drugs or treatment prescribed.[3] The Royal College of Surgeons of England recommends that the patient's name, date of birth, and record number should be clearly written on every sheet of notepaper on which you write.[4] For each entry write the date, including the year, the time you made the note, and who you are, including your grade (e.g. consultant, registrar, house officer). Cases often come to court many years after the events which led to the litigation, so it can sometimes be difficult to establish in which year the notes were made if they are not dated carefully.

One of the fundamentals of good note-keeping is good handwriting. If it is impossible to read what you have written, vital information that could be used to justify your actions is lost. If you know that your handwriting is difficult to read, write in capital letters. Avoid the use of abbreviations, or if you do so try to remember to explain the abbreviation the first time that you use it. Use clear diagrams of your physical findings. Record why you have chosen a particular course of action, particularly in the context of operative notes. There may be a perfectly reasonable explanation for a particular decision, but only by recording this reason will you be able to recall, months or years later, why you did what you did.

Never make critical comments at the expense of the patient in the records, no matter how irritating he/she may have been. Not only may your rude remarks be exposed in a court of law, but patients also have access to their records on request.

Some patients can be regarded as medicolegally high risk. While it is not always easy to anticipate who these patients are going to be, there are certain clues which can be used to identify them. These include patients and relatives who find fault with their carers, patients who refuse treatment or discharge themselves from hospital, patients where adverse events have occurred, and patients who require re-admission because their symptoms fail to resolve. In these cases in particular you should be especially careful to maintain notes of a high standard.

Operative records

Write a clear and comprehensive note of the operation performed, including any unexpected problems and complication encountered, as well as the steps taken to neutralize any problems arising. If you leave this to a junior, it is your responsibility to make sure that the account is reasonable and accurate. It is acceptable to dictate an operative note for your secretary to include in the notes, especially if your handwriting is illegible, but make sure that it really is contemporaneous and comprehensive. Ensure that it is inserted into the patient's note folder without unreasonable delay.

You cannot write too much on an operative note. Accompany your text with diagrams. Document precautions you took to avoid complications. Note antibiotic and venous thromboembolic prophylaxis used. Specify drains and catheters and draw a clear diagram to demonstrate to the nursing staff and your surgical team what all the tubes are draining and when they should be removed. Note your intended post-operative plan, including length of antibiotic and DVT prophylaxis.

References

1 Goodwin H. Litigation and surgical practice in the UK. *Br J Surg* 2000; **87**:977–9.
2 Gorney M. Accurate medical records: your primary line of defence. *Health Care Risk Report* 1998; **May**: 10–11.
3 General Medical Council. *Good medical practice*, 2001. Available online at: www.gmc-uk.org
4 Royal College of Surgeons of England. *Guidelines for clinicians on medical records and notes.* London: RCSE, 1994. Available online at: www.rcseng.ac.uk.

Consent

It is part of a doctor's duty of care to inform a patient of the options for treatment, the nature of that treatment, and its potential outcomes and complications. A doctor who fails to consent a patient adequately about a treatment will be in breach of his duty of care to that patient and, if the patient suffers ill consequences from that treatment, he/she may be judged to have been negligent in carrying out his/her duty. Consent for operation is a *process* to be gone through carefully with the patient, rather than an event of signing a consent form. This process is designed to ensure that the patient gives valid consent. Valid consent means consent which makes lawful what the surgeon is proposing to do to the body of the patient, which is only possible if that patient, at the time of consenting, has a real understanding of what it is that will be done. An operation done without the true consent of the patient is in law technically an assault.

In the absence of valid consent, the patient will have the opportunity, in the event of a bad outcome, and even if that bad outcome is not your fault, to argue that if fully informed before signing the form he/she would have refused the procedure, or opted for a second opinion, and so escaped the unfortunate consequences of the operation at your hands. In certain circumstances, and provided that the judge accepts that the patient would indeed have avoided your operation if properly informed about it, you may be held liable in damages for the consequences in fact suffered. Therefore be sure to document carefully your consent process in the clinical records. If a problem does arise subsequently, the evidence of a full and thorough discussion with the patient, clearly recorded as a contemporaneous note in the medical records, is a much more powerful defence than a signed consent form.

Much of consent is about good communication—communication of alternative management options, communication of the nature of the procedure and the post-operative course, communication of likely outcomes, and communication of risks. It is a sensible idea, particularly for major surgery where there is a real risk of serious complications or poor outcomes, to consent your patients with a relative of the patient present. The patient may not think or remember to ask important questions. Their relative may do this on their behalf. Obtaining consent well in advance of the intended procedure has significant advantages for the patients and the relatives. It provides a time for reflection, an opportunity to change their mind, and an opportunity to ask for more information.

In the UK the General Medical Council sets out 12 items of information which the patient will need:
- Details of the diagnosis and prognosis, including what will happen if the condition is left untreated.
- Any uncertainties about diagnosis, including what options there are for further investigation before treatment.
- Options for the treatment or management of the condition, including the option of not treating.
- The purpose of any proposed investigation or treatment: details of the procedures involved, including any additional treatment, such as pain relief, how the patient should prepare, and what they can expect during or after the procedure, including common or severe side-effects.
- The likely benefits and probabilities for success for each option: what the likely risks are and what changes may they have to make to their lifestyle.
- Whether the treatment is experimental.
- How the patient's progress will be monitored.
- Who has overall responsibility for the treatment and who are the other senior members of the team.
- To what extent students or trainees will be involved.
- A reminder that patients can change their mind at any time.
- A reminder that they can request a second opinion.
- Details of any charges there may be for the treatment, if applicable.

Avoid writing 'options and complications discussed.' It is relatively easy for a prosecuting lawyer to argue that on this one occasion you forgot to mention the particular complication that arose. If you do not write down what you said, there is a risk that the court will find that you did not say it. 'I didn't have time' is not a basis for a defence.

Available online at: www.gmc-uk.org/standards/consent.htm

Further reading

1 Reference guide to consent for examination and treatment. Available online at: www.dh.gov.uk.
2 Good practice guide. Available online at: www.dh.gov.uk.
3 www.gmc-uk.org/standards/consent.htm.
4 General Medical Council Seeking patient's consent: the ethical considerations. London: GMC, 1998.
5 Bolam v. Friern Hospital Management Committee, 1957, 1 WLR 58.
6 Sidaway v. Board of Governors of the Bethlem Royal and the Maudsley Hospital, 1985, 1 All ER 643.
7 Rogers v. Whittaker, 1992, 67 ALJR 47.
8 Pearce v. United Bristol Healthcare NHS Trust, 1996, EWCA Civ 702.
9 Chester v. Afshar, 2002, EWCA Civ 724.

Consent: frequently asked questions

For what sort of procedures or treatments do I need to seek consent from patients?

You must obtain consent from a patient prior to any examination or treatment, whether this is taking blood from the patient's arm or carrying out a cystectomy. However, during the process of taking blood, the fact that the patient voluntarily offers you their arm is an indication that they have consented for you to take blood from them. This is enough to allow you to take blood and you need not get them to complete a formal consent form.

When should consent be sought?

Consent is a process rather than an event. Ideally, the process of consent should start well in advance of the planned procedure. This allows the patient to ask appropriate questions without feeling under pressure and it allows you, the doctor, to provide adequate information about the planned treatment, alternative treatment options, potential outcomes, and risks. The time immediately before an operation is a stressful for the patient and they are particularly vulnerable at this time. Therefore it is sensible to avoid trying to obtain consent immediately prior to surgery.

Do I need to get the patient to sign a consent form in order for consent to be valid?

No. A patient may give verbal consent to a procedure, and this is a perfectly adequate 'form' of consent. However, absence of documentation to support the fact that you went to certain lengths to explain the procedure to the patient may make it difficult for you to defend yourself against allegations that you did not inform the patient fully about a certain risk or outcome. The use of a specific consent form prior to a surgical procedure is regarded as good practice. Its role is to provide a record of the patient's decision. There is no substitute for carefully written notes made in the patient's medical records outlining the procedure you went through to explain the nature of a treatment, alternatives to that treatment, and its possible outcomes and risks.

Does the process of signing the consent form need to be witnessed?

No. Having said this, going through the outcomes and complications of a procedure with a close relative, particularly prior to major surgery, is a sensible idea. If you have done this, record the fact that a relative (named) was present during the consultation.

Who should obtain consent?

The consultant responsible for the patient's care is ultimately responsible for ensuring that a patient has been provided with enough information about a treatment or procedure for them to decide whether or not they wish to undergo that treatment or procedure. Consent may be obtained by a junior doctor (or another health professional) as long as that doctor (or health professional) is suitably qualified and trained in performing that procedure.

That means that they may obtain consent as long as they are capable of explaining alternative options, the nature of the procedure, and its potential outcomes and risks. Where the health professional has inadequate knowledge of the procedure, such that they cannot provide full information for the patient about the proposed treatment, the consent may not be valid.

How much should I tell the patient about the operation?

You must inform the patient of any risks that they might regard as 'material' or 'significant'. This will vary from patient to patient. The General Medical Council states that doctors should find out about the patient's individual needs and priorities when providing information about treatment options. Err on the side of giving more information rather than less. Remember that some patients will attach great significance to a one in 1000 chance of a particular side-effect occurring whereas others will not be concerned about such a risk. Absolute percentages are meaningless when it comes to obtaining consent. The fact that a patient may be upset by hearing certain information or might refuse treatment as a consequence of hearing that information is not sufficient cause to withhold that information. Remember, any misrepresentation of possible benefits and risks of a procedure will invalidate consent.

In summary, the type of information that you should consider discussing with the patients includes:
- The treatment options.
- The benefits of each option.
- The risks of each option.
- The success rates of each option: nationally, for your unit, for you as an individual surgeon.
- Why is an operation necessary?
- What are the risks of not having the operation?
- How will the patient feel after the operation?

This is not an exhaustive list and there may well be other things that should be discussed with the patient depending on their circumstances and the procedure in question.

Can another person provide consent for a patient?

No-one can give consent on behalf of an incompetent adult. Incompetent adults include unconscious adults. If you believe that a treatment or operation is in the patient's best interests, then you may go ahead with that treatment or procedure in the absence of consent from the patient. Thus, for example, you do not need to ask permission from anyone to stop life-threatening haemorrhage in an unconscious patient, because you will, in almost every case, be acting in their best interests (most Jehovah's Witnesses excluded). If a patient has never been competent, then it is sensible to ask relatives, carers, and friends about the needs and preferences of the patient, but these people cannot give consent for that incompetent adult. If an incompetent patient has in the past, at a stage when they were competent, indicated that they would refuse treatment in certain circumstances (a so-called 'advance refusal') you must abide by that refusal.

Can children consent for themselves?

People aged 16 and 17 have the competence to give consent for themselves. Younger children who understand fully what is involved in a proposed procedure can also give consent, although their parents will usually be involved in the process. If a competent child consents to treatment, a parent cannot over-ride that consent. However, a child cannot refuse consent. A parent can consent for a child if that child refuses consent (such situations are likely to be rare).

Can I consent a patient if they have been given pre-operative medication?

The simple answer is no. If the patient has been given sedation prior to an operation, but has not consented for that operation, you will need to wait until the patient has fully recovered from the sedation, even if this means postponing the operation until a later date.

How long is consent valid for?

Indefinitely, unless consent is withdrawn by the patient, or if the circumstances of the case change in some relevant way (e.g. a new treatment option becomes available or the patient's problem changes in some way such that there is a change in the risks or likely benefits of a procedure). If circumstances do change, the process of consent must be repeated.

What should I do if a patient withdraws consent during a procedure?

This can occur if the patient is undergoing a procedure under local or spinal anaesthesia. Stop the procedure. Find out why the patient is concerned. Explain the consequences of not completing the procedure. Clearly, if not continuing the procedure would endanger the patient in some way (e.g. if there is continued bleeding) you should continue the operation until the patient is no longer at risk. Document carefully the conversation you had with the patient, ask attending staff to witness what you say to the patient, and ask them to countersign your version of events to corroborate what has occurred.

Index